ACRONYMS AND ABBREVIATIONS

JUN	protein synthesized by the onco-gene c-jun	pCO$_2$	partial pressure of carbon dioxide
LGS	lateral head of the gastrocnemius plus soleus muscle	PET	positron emission tomography
LTM	low-threshold mechanoreceptor	PG	prostaglandin
LTR	local twitch response	PGE$_2$	prostaglandin E$_2$
LTs	leukotrienes	pH	hydrogen ion concentration
μM	micromolar (see Glossary)	PO	*per os* (Latin): by mouth
MEPP	miniature endplate potential	pO$_2$	partial pressure of oxygen
Mg	magnesium	qhs	every bedtime
MG	medial head of the gastrocnemius muscle	qid	*quater in die* (Latin): four times a day
MMPI	Minnesota Multiphasic Personality Inventory	qod	every other day
MPS	myofascial pain syndrome	RA	rheumatoid arthritis
MRI	magnetic resonance imaging	RF	receptive field
mRNA	messenger ribonucleic acid	SEA	spontaneous electrical activity
ms	millisecond	SLE	systemic lupus erythematosus
m/s	meters per second	SOM	somatostatin
NGF	nerve growth factor	SP	substance P
NK-1	neurokinin-1	tid	*ter in die* (Latin): three times a day
NMDA	*N*-methyl-D-aspartate	TP	tender point (of fibromyalgia syndrome)
NO	nitric oxide	TPI	tender point index (see Glossary)
NRM	nucleus raphe magnus	TrP	trigger point (of myofascial pain syndrome)
NSAID	nonsteroidal anti-inflammatory drug	TRP	tryptophan
O$_2$	oxygen	T-TH	tension-type headache
OTC	over the counter	TTX	tetrodotoxin
p	pond (1 p is the force a mass of 1 g exerts under the influence of earth's gravity)	VAS	visual analog scale
		VRS	verbal rating scale
PAG	periaqueductal gray matter	Z band	connection between sarcomeres (see Glossary)

Muscle Pain

Understanding Its Nature, Diagnosis, and Treatment

Muscle Pain
Understanding Its Nature, Diagnosis, and Treatment

SIEGFRIED MENSE, Prof Dr med
Institut für Anatomie und Zellbiologie
Ruprecht-Karls-Universität Heidelberg
Heidelberg, FRG

DAVID G. SIMONS, MD, FAAPM&R, MS, DSC(Hon)
Clinical Professor, Rehabilitation Medicine
Emory University School of Medicine
Atlanta, Georgia

I. JON RUSSELL, MD, PhD
Associate Professor of Medicine
Director, The University Clinical Research Center
Department of Medicine
The University of Texas
Health Science Center at San Antonio
San Antonio, Texas

LIPPINCOTT WILLIAMS & WILKINS
A **Wolters Kluwer** Company
Philadelphia • Baltimore • New York • London
Buenos Aires • Hong Kong • Sydney • Tokyo

Acquisitions Editor: Peter J. Darcy
Managing Editor: Linda S. Napora
Marketing Manager: Anne E. P. Smith
Production Editor: Bill Cady

351 West Camden Street
Baltimore, Maryland 21201-2436 USA

530 Walnut Street
Philadelphia, Pennsylvania 19106-3621 USA

Printed in the United States of America

Library of Congress Cataloging-in-Publication Data

Mense, Siegfried.
  Muscle pain : understanding its nature, diagnosis, and treatment / Siegfried Mense, David G. Simons, I. Jon Russell.
    p. ; cm.
  Includes bibliographical references and index.
  ISBN 0-683-05928-9
  1. Myalgia. I. Simons, David G. II. Russell, I. Jon. III. Title.
  [DNLM: 1. Muscular Diseases—diagnosis. 2. Fibromyalgia. 3. Muscular Diseases—therapy. 4. Pain—diagnosis. 5. Pain—therapy. WE 550 M549m 2000]
  RC935.M77 M46 2000
  616.7′4—dc21
                                                              00-041262

To purchase additional copies of this book call our customer service department at **(800) 638-3030** or fax orders to **(301) 824-7390**. International customers should call **(301) 714-2324**.

Lippincott Williams & Wilkins customer service representatives are available from 8:30 am to 6:00 pm, EST, Monday through Friday, for telephone access. **Or *visit Lippincott Williams & Wilkins on the Internet:* http://www.lww.com.**

00 01 02 03
1 2 3 4 5 6 7 8 9 10

Foreword

The subject of this book is a huge practical challenge and, at the same time, probes our intellectual understanding. Any population survey reveals large numbers of people in steady pain labeled as being of musculoskeletal origin. The incidence increases with age, up to the level where there are few senior citizens of my age who are not candidates for the diagnosis.

There is a groan that unites men and women, rich and poor, in any nation. These pains are "explained" in every culture, but the universal fact of this persistence must mean that no adequate therapy exists. The impressive multiplicity of therapies with varying degrees of rationality and effectiveness is part of the problem because it implies a failure of understanding. It represents a particular threat to the rich, who invite more and more vigorous therapeutic intrusion in their search for relief and thereby add the risk of iatrogenic deterioration.

For 200 years, since the Age of Reason, diagnosis and therapy have been pathology driven. The cause of each disease was to be confidently identified by the presence of some objectively identified disturbance of anatomy, physiology, or chemistry. Pity those who suffered a disease unaccompanied by an identified pathology. It is these patients who are the subject of much of this book.

In the 18th century, Heberden described precisely the signs and symptoms of angina pectoris. He carried out postmortem examinations and failed to locate a cause. In the subsequent 150 years, every structure in the region—muscles, heart, joints, nerve, pleura, lung, arteries, and veins—was proposed as the site of the disorder. Finally, in this century, the condition was attributed by Lewis and White to cardiac ischemia.

This, in turn, led to the present high-tech therapies that improve the vascularization of the heart. In spite of this undoubted diagnostic and therapeutic success, there remain some patients with intractable angina in whom the most elaborate probes fail to show any signs of ischemic heart muscle. Evidently, we still do not fully understand the cause of angina, and so it is with many of the pains discussed in this book.

It is reasonable and excellent tactics to start with the simplest hypothesis. In the case of muscle pain, that hypothesis would be specifically that nociceptors are excited at the site of the pain. Much remains to be discovered, even in situations in which the simple idea is almost certainly correct. For example, in the case of the ubiquitous night cramps, the explanation of the massive and synchronous discharge of motor neurons is not understood, nor is the precise chemical link between muscle contraction and the excitation of afferents, nor the origin of muscle tenderness that persists for hours and days after the contraction has ceased.

To return to the example of angina, it teaches us that the cause of the pain is not necessarily at the site of the pain. This goes beyond a localization error, since the site of the pain is tender, meaning that gentle stimulation of normal tissue exaggerates the pain of distant origin and that anesthesia of the painful area decreases the anginal pain. This means that even the clearest localization of pain in one area may, in fact, be originating from a distant area, as Travell and Simons have shown in their seminal work on trigger points. The reference of pain implies the existence of convergence of inputs within the spinal cord. This leads to the necessary involvement of central neural circuits in the simplest of peripheral disorders. It also leads to the possibility that the basic disorder is entirely central where disordered hyperexcitable cells are driven to excessive activity by afferent impulses from normal peripheral tissue over normal sensory afferents. A growing number of neuroscientists consider this a likely explanation for the pains in trigeminal neuralgia and migraine, two obviously painful disorders in which no primary peripheral pathology has been identified. Similarly, in the extreme case of brachial plexus avulsion, the intense pain cannot originate in peripheral afferents, since they do not exist.

This book is welcome because close collaboration between neuroscientists and clinicians is long overdue. Hopefully, we are emerging from an era of fantasy explanations for real phenomena. The authors certainly have to face a community of therapists who are obsessionally committed to explanations for disease and for therapy unsupported by a scrap of evidence except for their claimed therapeutic success. Part of the problem is to define precisely what are the fractions of elaborate therapeutic maneuvers that change the patient's pathology in the periphery and in the central nervous system, and their attitude toward their undoubted misery.

Professor Patrick D. Wall, FRS, DM, FRCP
London, United Kingdom

Preface

Background

The history of this book reaches back to the year 1978, when the authors met for the first time in Montreal on the occasion of the Second World Congress on Pain, organized by the International Association for the Study of Pain (IASP). Contact between the authors was maintained and intensified in ensuing years. The contacts were used for long and vivid discussions of all aspects of muscle pain.

In 1978, the mechanisms of muscle pain were largely unknown. One of the authors (S. M.) had just started to perform animal experiments on this topic in the Department of Physiology at Kiel University in Germany, which at that time was chaired by Prof. Robert F. Schmidt. The other author (D. G. S.) was already an experienced clinician who had been trained by Prof. Janet G. Travell and who had acquired a working knowledge in the field of clinical muscle pain, particularly pain caused by trigger points.

Very often, the discussions started with an effort to account for a clinical observation and ended with the frustrating conclusion that it could not be solved because too little was known about the neurobiology and pathophysiology of muscle pain. In the late 1970s, pain research in general was a relatively new discipline, and the bulk of the available knowledge was obtained in experiments on cutaneous pain. Even though many mechanisms controlling cutaneous pain could be assumed to be functioning also in muscle pain, it became increasingly clear that muscle pain differed from cutaneous pain in many aspects.

Over the years, many clinical and basic science groups of researchers have collected so much data on muscle pain that it appeared justified to publish this book. The authors do not think that all questions regarding muscle pain have been solved (the contrary is true), but the scientific basis now appears broad enough to offer the reader a relatively coherent picture of muscle pain. Aside from attempting to communicate this knowledge to a broader readership, the authors wanted to bridge the unnecessarily wide gap between clinical and basic research.

It became clear while writing the first draft of this book that solid information on drug therapy would be essential. The authors (and readers) are most fortunate that Dr. I. Jon Russell contributed the sections on drug therapy, and he also critically reviewed the entire text from his unique point of view as an experienced clinician and editor of the *Journal of Musculoskeletal Pain*. Most important, Dr. Russell, a leading world authority on the field of fibromyalgia syndrome, has contributed Chapter 9: Fibromyalgia Syndrome.

Purpose

In recent years, knowledge of muscle pain in the field of neurobiology has increased considerably. Data continues to accumulate on the components of pain pathways and mechanisms (e.g., neuropeptides, integration and modulation of information processing, neuroplasticity). Many of the concepts that for many years have been considered valid now need to be modified. For example, the pain-spasm-pain concept does not appear to exist in the assumed simple form (see Chapter 6).

The primary aim of this book is to present an overview of the clinical diseases and syndromes associated with muscle pain and to combine the clinical view with new concepts based on neuroanatomic and electrophysiologic research. In many instances, existing basic and clinical models of thinking will be challenged, and sometimes a new concept to replace the old one cannot be offered. The authors are convinced, however, that the reader will profit from this sometimes difficult approach, since a better understanding of the basic mechanisms of muscle pain will lead to more effective management of difficult cases and will make clinical practice more satisfying.

In those chapters that have sections on drug therapy, the therapy is divided in two subsections: (1) a general overview of the therapeutic principles and drugs that are appropriate for the painful conditions mentioned in the chapter, and (2) a list of the drugs that can be used for treatment, including dosage, mode of action, and side effects. The information here is for general guidance and may not be complete in all respects. The reader is reminded to consult a pharmacologic textbook or package insert for full details. The authors cannot take any responsibility for errors that may have occurred in the production of this book.

While preparing the chapters and glossary, the authors encountered a number of commonly used terms with two or more meanings that are incompatible with each other. It became obvious that we needed to clearly define and consistently identify exactly what we mean when we use a given term. In each case, we have included the rationale by which we selected the meaning best suited to this book. The reader is strongly encouraged to become acquainted with the various meanings commonly used for the same term. Rarely are such terms as muscle tone, stiffness, or spasm defined by an author, and all too often the writer and the reader ascribe different meanings to a term. Simply understanding the usage can help the reader more quickly recognize the meaning intended by the author.

Another aim of this book is to replace older, rather mechanistic views with modern concepts. Older textbooks convey the impression that all reflex pathways consist of simple chains of neurons that produce a particular reflex effect every time receptors are activated to a sufficient degree. We now know that motor reflexes (even the monosynaptic stretch reflex) are strongly dependent on the activity in descending motor pathways. When descending facilitating influences are missing—for example, during spinal shock—the monosynaptic stretch reflex cannot be elicited in spite of maximal activation of muscle spindle afferents. The flexibility of the reflex connections in the central nervous system is illustrated by the case of voluntary movement, in which inhibition of the transmission in a reflex pathway can change into facilitation (see Chapter 6). Therefore, the term "reflex" (from the Latin *reflexus,* meaning reflected), in most cases, is a misnomer. Under physiologic circumstances, a given input does not always evoke a stereotyped output (unlike a mirror that always reflects a light beam in the same way). The term "reflex" is developing a new meaning.

The versatility of reflex-controlled movements is demonstrated in situations in which an identical input leads to different motor reactions in humans. For instance, during tactile exploration of the environment, the hand makes contact with objects and maintains pressure on the explored surface by slight activation of muscles that increase the pressure. When a person in a dark room is trying to find the light switch and touches an object of unexpected tone and texture, however, the tactile input from the skin of the hand will evoke a brisk activation of muscles that withdraw the hand.

Most reflexes are the result of a complicated spinal and supraspinal integration of input from a large variety of receptors in the skin, joints, muscles, and cognitive judgments of the brain. An example of such complicated integration (even in a decerebrate animal) is the wiping reflex a decerebrate frog performs with its hindlimb when a filter paper soaked with an acid solution is placed on the skin of the forelimb. The hindlimb makes a target-oriented movement to the forelimb and removes the noxious stimulus. This movement is controlled by motor interneurons in the spinal cord; the spinal cord even appears to have a certain body image of the frog's topography, since the wiping reflex is always aimed at the body region where the stimulus is located.

Thus, the output of a reflex arc is highly dependent on the physiologic situation. In neurophysiologic terms, output will depend not only on segmental input but also on descending motor activity, intrinsic activity of spinal neurons, and afferent activity in other than the activated pathway.

Repeated usage of nociceptive pathways has been shown to change the properties of the involved neurons in a manner similar to learning. Therefore, the neurons in the spinal cord and in higher centers are likely to process nociceptive information differently in a patient suffering from chronic muscle pain than in one who is generally pain-free. To understand how nervous sys-

tem function relates to pain, one must abandon linear thinking and view the central nervous system as a versatile and highly adaptable network of neurons. The concepts presented in *Muscle Pain: Understanding Its Nature, Diagnosis, and Treatment* will give readers an understanding of the basic mechanisms of muscle pain and will ultimately benefit those who seek professional help for relief of muscle pain.

Acknowledgments

The authors would like to express gratitude to their coworkers, who contributed large pieces to the overall picture. They owe a very special debt of gratitude to their wives, Inge Mense and Lois Statham Simons, who provided the continuous support, encouragement, and understanding that have made this work possible.

Contents

CHAPTER 1
Background and Basic Principles

SUMMARY: Musculoskeletal disturbances are the leading causes of disability in people in their working years. Three important, common disturbances are **myofascial pain** caused by trigger points (TrPs), **fibromyalgia** recognized by the presence of tender points (TPs), and **articular dysfunction**. When muscles are being examined for painful conditions, the greater sensitivity of women to painful stimuli has to be taken into account. This **gender difference** is not based on a propensity of women to complain more; research indicates that it is due to a higher sensitivity of the pain system in females.

Many terms commonly used in the description of painful disturbances have frequently not been used according to the definitions published by the International Association for the Study of Pain (IASP). For the sake of uniformity, the **definitions of the most important terms** are given in this chapter. A major problem for communication between the practitioner and the patient is that pain, in essence, is a subjective sensation and can be described only in the patient's words with meanings that may or may not correspond to those of the clinician. This is particularly true for **chronic pain**, which must be considered a complex personal experience of **suffering** rather than a **sensation**. In patients with chronic pain, the subjective suffering is in the foreground; for describing the character of their pain to another person, many of the common pain terms are not suitable because they belong to the sensory-discriminative category. A quantitative estimate of the severity of a patient's pain can be obtained with the visual analog scale (VAS) or the verbal rating scale (VRS).

Pain from muscle, viscera, and skin are subjectively and objectively distinct. For instance, **muscle pain** is described as aching and cramping, while **cutaneous pain** is characterized by its sharp and pricking nature. In contrast to muscle pain, which is difficult to localize, pain from the skin is localized with great accuracy. **Visceral pain** is similar to muscle pain in many respects; one of the main differences is that visceral pain is often referred to the skin, whereas muscle pain is mostly referred to other deep somatic structures, such as tendons, fascia, joints, or other muscles. In recent years, the neurophysiologic research of many laboratories has indicated that objective differences also exist between pain from muscle and pain from other organs. These differences start with the processing of the nociceptive information at the spinal level and continue at the brainstem level, where nociceptive impulses from the skin and muscle terminate in different regions.

A. IMPORTANCE AND PREVALENCE OF MUSCLE PAIN

1. Common Sources of Muscle Pain

"The leading causes of disability in people in their working years are **musculoskeletal conditions**."[43] The clinical disorders can be classified into two main categories, articular and nonarticular. Articular disorders include articular diseases and involve varying degrees of inflammation and progressive injury to diarthrodial (synovial) joints. Typical examples include rheumatoid arthritis and osteoarthritis. They also include articular dysfunctions that are characterized by pain-limited active joint range of motion and by limited passive joint mobility, both of which respond to manual mobilization techniques. Nonarticular disorders primarily affect soft tissues such as muscles, tendons, ligaments, bursae, and nerves. Common examples include mechanical low back pain resulting from one or more dysfunctional aspects of truncal anatomy, myofascial pain syndrome caused by trigger points (TrPs), and fibromyalgia syndrome characterized by tender points (TPs).

Quantitative studies reporting the prevalence of **articular disease** as a source of musculoskeletal pain indicate that rheumatoid arthritis occurs in approximately 1% of the general population.[25] Osteoarthritis is uncommon in the young but increases in prevalence with age, approaching 70% among those who are older than 70 years.[5, 26] In the case of rheumatoid arthritis, the general body inflammation and the inactivity associated with chronic articular pain can contribute to progressive muscle wasting, which is at least partially responsive to exercise.[14] Obesity and pain-induced skeletal muscle dysfunction contribute to the development of disability among people with osteoarthritis.[30, 32] Studies documenting the prevalence of specific articular dysfunctions requiring manual mobilization are hard to find. Clinicians skilled in identifying this condition note that it is not uncommon and is frequently associated with increased tension of functionally related muscles.[28, 29]

Back pain is the most common of these nonarticular conditions, accounting for 1.3 billion person-days lost annually. Headache accounted for 0.6 billion person-days lost.[18] Even children can be affected. Nearly one third (32.3%) of 1,637 nonhypermobile Finnish third- and fifth-grade schoolchildren were found to have musculoskeletal pain at least once a week.[37] In this age group it is not surprising to find that muscular sources of pain are more likely than skeletal sources of pain.

Myofascial pain, detectable by the presence of TrPs, can go unrecognized if the physician is not prepared to identify them and does not actively look for them. The patient gives a history of acute, sustained, or repeated overload. Examination of the afflicted muscle reveals painfully restricted full range of motion and localized tenderness of a nodule in a palpable taut band. Pressure on such a tender spot that is an active TrP evokes pain that patients recognize as familiar. The prevalence of myofascial pain syndrome in the community is not known, but a recent study[49] indicates that it is a relatively common cause of regional musculoskeletal pain, occurring in up to 30% of general medical clinic patients. Whether it affects primarily the muscles of mastication or the girdle muscles, it can exhibit a clinical severity comparable with other painful conditions that cause the patient to seek medical assistance.[6, 8, 10, 41] See also Chapter 8.

Fibromyalgia occurs in 2% of the general public.[59] It accounts for approximately 15% of the patients seen in rheumatology clinics and for 6 to 10% of all patients in general internal medicine clinics.[3] Widespread chronic pain and soft-tissue tender points are diagnostic of this condition.[60] Several other organ systems, however, are usually involved. See Chapter 9.

2. Gender Differences

The female neurophysiologist, Berkley,[1, 2] reviewed differences in the physiology of pain and responses to analgesic treatment between men and women. Gender differences in the neurochemical mediation of analgesia suggest an important role for hormonal mediation of neuronal mechanisms of analgesia. These differences have important clinical and research implications.[42] Both authors point out how important it can be to collect data specific to women and not to assume that what applies to a study of males can be applied directly to females.

Numerous studies indicate that women have greater sensitivity to deep-tissue (muscle) pain than do men. Fischer[7] found the average pressure pain threshold for a group of nine normal men to be 50% higher than that of a matching group of nine women. Average thresholds were greater in men in all 10 muscles tested, significantly so in all but the gluteus maximus muscle. The upper trapezius muscle was the most sensitive in both genders. A more detailed study of the pressure sensitivity of head and neck muscles by Lee et al.[27] categorized males and females by age from the second through sixth decades of life. With only one exception (upper trapezius muscle), females from 10 to 40 years of age were more tender than males in the same age group. Beyond the age of 40 years the difference between genders became less marked. A few muscles became more tender in males than in females for subjects in their 50s, but for most muscles, those in females were still measurably more tender than those in males.

This greater sensitivity of women to painful stimuli may help to explain why there are approximately seven times as many women as men with fibromyalgia. After all, the disorder is characterized by an increased pain sensitivity that is probably mediated by abnormalities in nociception within the central nervous system (CNS).

This difference applies not only to the fibromyalgia population but also to the general population. Only 20 to 30% of males reported symptoms of facial pain, whereas 70 to 80% of females reported such symptoms in the preceding 6 months.[42] This is not due to a propensity for women to complain more, as some clinicians have suspected. In a study of muscle tenderness among male and female patients with migraine headache, episodic headache, and chronic tension-type headache (compared with headache-free controls), the women consistently had a higher total tenderness score to manual palpation and lower pressure pain thresholds by algometry.[20] It comes as a surprise to many male practitioners that women frequently experience more pain than do men in response to the same noxious stimulus. Not only are women more sensitive to pain, but a study of 121 Swedish patients showed that the benefits of cognitive behaviorally based treatments for neck, shoulder, and back pain were confined to women.[21]

B. COMMON TERMS AND CONFUSIONS (DEFINITIONS AND USAGE)
1. Established Pain Terms[36]

Established terms for pain fall into two categories: general terms and terms that describe increased or decreased sensitivity.

General Terms

Pain: An unpleasant sensory and emotional experience associated with actual or potential tissue damage, or described in terms of such damage.

Causalgia: A syndrome of sustained burning pain, allodynia, and hyperpathia after a traumatic nerve lesion, often combined with vasomotor and sudomotor dysfunction and later trophic changes.

Central pain: Pain initiated or caused by a primary lesion or dysfunction in the CNS.

Increased Sensitivity

Allodynia: Pain caused by a stimulus that does not normally provoke pain (decreased pain threshold: the stimulus and response are of different sensory modalities [categories]); for instance, tactile stimuli evoke pain.

Dysesthesia: An unpleasant abnormal sensation, whether spontaneous or evoked.

Hyperesthesia: Increased sensitivity to stimulation, excluding the special senses (the increased sensation is in the same category as the applied stimulus).

Hyperpathia: A painful syndrome characterized by an abnormally painful reaction to a stimulus, especially a repetitive stimulus, and an increased threshold (increased threshold and increased response: stimulus and response are the same kind of sensation).

Hyperalgesia: An increased pain response to a stimulus that is normally painful (stimulus and response are in the same mode). Many cases of hyperalgesia also have features of allodynia.

Decreased Sensitivity

Analgesia: Absence of pain in response to stimulation that would normally be painful.

Hypoalgesia: Diminished pain in response to a normally painful stimulus (increased threshold and decreased response: stimulus and response are the same kind of sensation).

2. Diagnostic Terms

Fibromyalgia. The criteria for diagnosing fibromyalgia were presented in 1990[60] by a group of rheumatology investigators and officially endorsed by the American College of Rheumatology. The patient must have widespread pain of at least 3 months duration, and 11 of 18 tender point sites must be painful on digital palpation with approximately 4 kg of pressure. These criteria are described in more detail in Chapter 9. Many laboratory abnormalities have been found in fibromyalgia that are potentially explained by the serotonin deficiency hypothesis.[44] This means that fibromyalgia probably results from a CNS dysfunction that causes a pathologic increase in pain sensitivity (lowered pain threshold, allodynia) throughout the body.

Fibrositis. Use of the term "fibrositis" is now outmoded as a diagnostic entity for at least two reasons. First, it has undergone

a transition of meanings through the years since its original description by Gowers,[12] who seemed to view it as we would now think of mechanical low back pain. Later, in the early part of this century, it was described in terms that were most compatible with myofascial TrPs but did not exclude fibromyalgia. Because of frustration with the lack of consistent histologic findings, it was increasingly identified with pain of a psychogenic and not organic origin. Briefly, in the late 1970s, Smythe and Moldofsky[50] described fibrositis in terms that are now more closely associated with fibromyalgia. Second, the term "fibrositis" was considered unsuitable as a label for that syndrome because the suffix "itis" implied an inflammatory pathogenic process for which there was no supportive evidence.

Myofascial Pain. Unfortunately, two applications of the term "myofascial pain syndrome" have evolved.[47] Originally, it was applied specifically to the symptoms caused by myofascial TrPs.[55] That concept has continued unchanged[47a, 56, 57] and continues to relate specifically to myofascial TrPs throughout this book. In recent years, many authors have adopted a general definition that usually includes a regional pain syndrome of any soft-tissue origin. Therefore, it is critically important that authors clearly identify whether their use of the term "myofascial pain" applies specifically to TrPs or is being used in the more general sense.

Myogelosis and "Muscle Indurations" (Myogelosen, Muskelhärten) (Old Terminology: Fibrositis). This muscular pain condition is characterized by a localized tender spot in the palpable ropiness of the muscle and is likely to be caused by myofascial TrPs.

Nonarticular Rheumatism (Weichteilrheumatismus). Nonarticular rheumatism is a more general term comparable with the outmoded term "fibrositis."

Tendomyopathy (Tendomyopathie or Tendomyose). The term "tendomyopathy" usually includes a distinction between generalized and localized tendomyopathy. Generalized tendomyopathy is often considered synonymous with fibromyalgia.

3. Descriptive Terms Commonly Used

Spread of Pain. The term "spread of pain" is used for describing the expansion of a region in which pain is felt. In contrast to referral of pain (see below), the expansion is continuous with the origin of the site of pain. The mechanisms underlying spread of pain are probably identical with those controlling referral of pain (see Chapter 4).

Projected Pain. Projected pain describes pain that is caused by a lesion of nerve fibers along their course in a peripheral nerve or dorsal root. At the site of the lesion, action potentials are generated that reach the central nervous neurons via the same afferent fibers that normally signal the presence of a stimulus at the receptive ending. The central neurons cannot recognize the origin of the action potentials and interpret any activity in a nerve fiber as coming from the receptive ending. Therefore, projected pain is felt in the innervation territory of lesioned nerve fibers.

Referred Pain. Referred pain is characterized by the fact that it is felt not at the site of its origin but remote from it. Typically, the area of referred pain is discontinuous with the site of the lesion. Referred pain can occur together with local pain (at the lesion site) or in isolation. Since pain originating in a given muscle tends to exhibit a relatively constant pattern of referral, it is often possible to identify the muscle from which the pain originates if the pattern is known. If the pain is referred from one site to several remote locations, it is often described as "radiating."

Muscle Tone. The tone of a muscle is usually defined as its resting tension, clinically determined as resistance to passive movement. Muscle tone has two components: (1) The contractile component is caused by a low-frequency activation of a small number of motor units. Its presence can be detected in the electromyogram (EMG). (2) The viscoelastic component is independent of nervous activity and reflects the passive physical properties of the elastic tension of muscle fiber elements and the osmotic pressure of cells. Note that a completely relaxed muscle has only viscoelastic tone; i.e., it is "silent" with respect to EMG activity. See also Chapter 5.

Muscle Spasm. Spasm is a contraction of striated muscle that cannot be released voluntarily (in this book, spasm of smooth muscle is not addressed). If the contraction is painful, it is often called "cramp." Spasm and cramp in the sense of this definition are associated with EMG activity. If chronic involuntary shortening of a muscle occurs without EMG activity, the term "contracture" is more appropriate. See also Chapter 5.

Muscle Stiffness. Muscle stiffness is not usually included in medical dictionaries as a medical term, but it is commonly used to describe discomfort with movement of a joint. It is also used in the engineering sense: with increased stiffness, greater force is required to produce the same movement or the same force produces smaller movement. In this sense, spastic muscles have increased stiffness. See also Chapter 5.

Subjective Quality of Pain Terms. A major communication problem in this field of pain is the totally subjective nature of pain. There is no objective standard against which to test the extent to which the sensation that one individual describes as a burning pain is physiologically the same as what another individual thinks of when he or she hears that term. This becomes more difficult with terms such as tearing pain, since few of us have had the experience of feeling a muscle being torn.

These problems—the subjective quality of pain perception and the descriptive terminology regarding it—are more than semantic. Recent studies to identify the area of the brain activated by a given noxious stimulus show that individuals with pain arising for the same reason in the same part of the body may activate quite different parts of the brain. Pain can be a physiologically individual experience, particularly if it is chronic. These differences have been interpreted as reflecting personal reactions influenced by past life experiences.

Chronic pain takes on a suffering dimension not characteristic of acute pain. This has been demonstrated by positron emission tomography.[17] In that study, acute pain activated primarily the sensory cortex, whereas chronic neuropathic pain activated Brodmann area 24 in the anterior cingulate gyrus, which is associated with an affective-motivational dimension. This finding suggests that patients attempting to describe chronic neuropathic "pain" are actually trying to describe suffering caused by the persistence of pain. The examining practitioner is unlikely to have had a comparable experience and therefore is likely to have difficulty understanding what the patient is trying to communicate.

For these reasons, the health care provider should assume that patients are trying to communicate as clearly as they can their personal pain experience. They are using the words and metaphors that seem appropriate to them, and the provider must accept their "pain" at face value. If the descriptions seem exaggerated, it may be in response to the patient's impression that the examiner is discounting what they are saying, which too often is the case. The suffering that evolves from chronic pain is more difficult to express adequately in words than was the initial pain.

The visual analog scale (VAS) has become a popular tool for measuring the severity of a patient's pain.[39] It does not require any interpretation by the investigator because the patients assess the severity of their pain in terms of their own personal standards. The patient is asked to make a mark on a line, usually 10 cm long, that has 0 designated at one end and 10 at the other. Zero represents no pain and ten represents the most severe pain that the patient can imagine. A centimeter ruler is used to measure the number of millimeters (or centimeters) the patient's mark lies from the zero end of the scale. This number is the VAS pain scale number. In clinical practice, a simplified version, the verbal rating scale (VRS), is easier to administer and showed a high correlation with the VAS.[39] These scales are useful in both clinical practice and research studies of pain but must then be localized to body location by additional questioning.

An expansion of this phenomenon can be obtained with a quantitative body drawing, as described by Wigers and associ-ates.[58] In this application, patients were instructed to shade all areas that had been painful during the past 3 days on two small (35 mm high) printed figures representing the ventral and dorsal sides of the body, respectively. No shading meant no pain. The distribution then was calculated by the Wallace's "rule of nine,"[33] which counts the head as 9%, one arm as 9%, one leg as 18%, one side of the trunk as 18%, and the genitalia as 1%. The sum of the total was the pain distribution. Combined with the VAS, this methodology provides a screening or a serial means to document the location and severity of nonarticular pain.

C. DISTINCTIVE CHARACTERISTICS OF MUSCLE PAIN
1. Subjective

Typically, the pains associated with muscle lesions are described as aching and cramping, while cutaneous pain is described as sharp, pricking, and stabbing. In contrast to cutaneous pain, which is localized with great accuracy, muscle pain is difficult to localize. However, pain from other deep structures, the fascia and periosteum, is often described as originating in a single spot.[24, 51] Electrical stimulation of muscle nerve fascicles with a needle electrode has been shown to elicit localized muscle pain at low intensities of stimulation; as the stimulation strength was increased, the area of pain expanded first, and then there was pain referred to regions not innervated by the stimulated nerve.[53] High-intensity stimulation of a cutaneous nerve fascicle did not result in pain referral to the territory of a neighboring nerve.[31]

Visceral pain, like muscle pain, is difficult to localize and is hard to distinguish from muscle pain. The main difference between these two forms of pain is that visceral pain is mainly referred to the skin, whereas muscle pain is generally referred to deep somatic structures (subcutaneous tissues excluding viscera). The skin rarely refers pain to other regions.

Tissue-threatening (noxious) stimulation of any muscle and of skin always elicits pain, if strong enough (see Chapter 2). However, noxious stimulation of viscera does not always produce pain, and not all viscera are pain-sensitive.[11] Both muscle and visceral pains are associated with autonomic symptoms such as a drop in blood pressure, sweating, and nausea. Cutaneous pain does not incite this kind of reaction.

2. Objective

The relative innervation density of skin and muscle is difficult to estimate because the skin is approximately two-dimensional and muscle is three-dimensional. It is generally assumed that innervation density decreases in this order: skin, muscle, and viscera. In the cat gastrocnemius-soleus muscle nerve, approximately half of all fibers are afferent; i.e., they conduct impulses from receptive nerve endings to the spinal cord.[38]

Receptive fields of dorsal horn cells processing information from muscle nociceptors are relatively small (i.e., the neuron can be excited only from a small region in a muscle) and show a decrease in size toward the distal part of a limb, similar to cells processing cutaneous input.

Dorsal horn cells processing information from cutaneous nociceptors show little convergence; i.e., they cannot be driven by input from different types of tissue (e.g., skin, muscle, viscera). Many appear to receive input exclusively from nociceptors in the skin. This statement is hard to prove, however, since in most studies on cutaneous nociception the deep input is not checked. Dorsal horn cells driven by muscle nociceptors show marked convergence of input from skin and viscera.[61] Conversely, most dorsal horn neurons with visceral input show additional convergent input from the skin and/or deep somatic structures.[4, 9]

In the CNS, the information from muscle and cutaneous nociceptors is processed differently. One example is that the nociceptive information from deep tissues and the skin, respectively, terminates in different regions of the mesencephalon. Neurons responding to stimulation of muscle nociceptors are located in the ventral periaqueductal gray matter (PAG), whereas cells responding to cutaneous nociceptors are located in the lateral PAG.[23] Another example of a differential processing of nociception from muscle and skin is that the input

to dorsal horn neurons from muscle nociceptors is subject to a stronger descending inhibition than is the input from cutaneous nociceptors.[62]

3. General

From a teleologic point of view, there is no need for good localization of muscle pain. In contrast, many forms of cutaneous pain show the high spatial resolution necessary for removing external noxious stimuli by well-directed motor reflexes; muscle pain is not avoided or abolished by such reflexes.

D. HYPOTHESES AS TO HOW ACUTE PAIN BECOMES CHRONIC PAIN

Muscle pain is well known for its tendency to become chronic. Chronic pain has been defined as pain that persists past the normal time of healing; in clinical practice, a period of 3 months is recognized as a convenient dividing line between acute and chronic nonmalignant pain, but for research purposes 6 months is often preferred.[36]

Acute pain functions as a warning signal that prevents damage to the tissue and, if a lesion has occurred, promotes healing processes (e.g., by activating reflexes and behavior that promote immobilization of the injured part). In patients with chronic painful conditions, the pain has lost the warning system function. The reflexes associated with chronic muscle and joint pain (e.g., muscle spasms) often do not alleviate but instead aggravate the painful condition and may become the main reason for the patient's suffering. In this way, chronic pain becomes more than a symptom of disease: It becomes a change of state that affects the entire organism.

The factors controlling the transition from acute to chronic muscle pain are largely unknown. In the paragraphs below, several mechanisms are presented that may be involved in the transition, although confirmatory evidence for some of the assumptions is still lacking.

1. Chronic Sensitization of Nociceptors

The mechanisms leading to sensitization of nociceptors are described in Chapter 2, Section A. The sensitization probably lasts

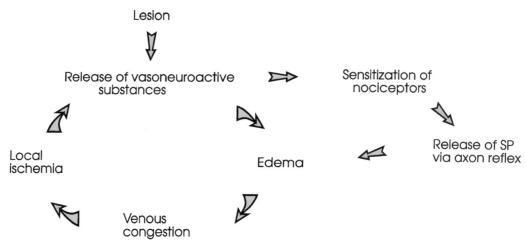

Figure 1-1. Hypothetical mechanism explaining the long-lasting tenderness of myofascial trigger points (TrPs). The basic assumption is that a muscle lesion releases so-called vasoneuroactive substances that sensitize muscle nociceptors and, by their vasodilating and permeability-increasing action, induce a local edema. The edema may impair the blood supply by compressing venules (venous congestion), causing local ischemia. Ischemia enhances the release of vasoneuroactive substances. The events of the upper half of the vicious cycle are well established. The causal relation between the local edema and ischemia, however, is largely speculative. For details, see the text. This figure is complementary to the vicious cycle model described in Chapter 8 (Fig. 8-20) as an explanation for the formation of TrPs. The local ischemia shown in this figure is an important factor for the development of an energy crisis associated with dysfunctional neuromuscular endplates. *SP*, substance P; *axon reflex*, propagation of action potentials in nonexcited side branches of a receptive nerve ending.

as long as the sensitizing substances are present in the vicinity of the nerve ending. If the release of the substances continues over a longer period of time, the sensitization is likely to persist. A possible mechanism explaining a chronic sensitization of this kind is shown in Figure 1-1. The sensitizing process is assumed to start with a tissue lesion, e.g., trauma or overuse. The lesion is followed by the release of so-called neurovasoactive (or vasoneuroactive) substances,[46] which include bradykinin (BK, cleaved from plasma proteins), prostaglandins (synthesized from endothelial and other tissue cells), and histamine (released from mast cells). By their vascular action these substances cause vasodilation and increased vascular permeability. The result is a local edema.

Simultaneously, the substances sensitize nociceptors in the vicinity of the lesion by their neural effects. The increased activity of the sensitized nociceptors is associated with the release of substances stored in the nerve endings (for instance, the neuropeptides substance P [SP] and calcitonin gene-related peptide [CGRP]). This release also can be brought about by action potentials that originate in one branch of the ending and invade antidromically (against the normal direction of impulse conduction) other branches of the same ending. This release mechanism is called **axon reflex**. The substances set free by the axon reflex (particularly SP) have a powerful vascular action and enhance the local edema.

In most patients, the formation of the edema is the end of the chain of events: the lesion is repaired and the pain and tenderness go away. Under unfavorable circumstances, however, the edematous region may increase in size and compress venous vessels. The resulting venous congestion impairs the blood supply of the damaged tissue and leads to local ischemia. Ischemia is one of the most potent factors releasing BK. Thus, a vicious cycle is formed that maintains the edema and the sensitization of the nociceptive nerve endings. If this cycle is not interrupted by proper treatment, it can continue for long periods of time.

As shown in Chapter 2, Section B, ischemia is particularly troublesome in skeletal muscle because it means a lack of energy. The energy is normally provided by oxidative metabolism but can also be obtained from glycolytic processes (which need energy to replace the glycogen). Both processes supply energy in the form of adenosine triphosphate. In muscle tissue are several mechanisms that are vulnerable to a lack of energy, such as the calcium pump. The pump terminates voluntary contractions by transporting the calcium ions from the cytoplasm of the muscle cell back into the sarcoplasmic reticulum (a network of cisternae that hold the intracellular stores of calcium. For details, see Chapter 2, Section A). If the function of the pump is impaired, the cytoplasmatic calcium concentration remains elevated and the actin and myosin filaments stay continuously activated. It is conceivable, albeit not proven, that under these conditions a local muscle contracture may ensue, which is presently being discussed as one of the central factors for the formation and maintenance of myofascial TrPs. See Chapter 8.

2. Changes in Innervation Density

The subjective sensations originating in a tissue are dependent on the type and quantity of nerve endings in that tissue. If the innervation density changes in the course of a pathologic alteration, this may lead to a chronic change in the sensations. Interestingly, recent evidence from experiments on rats indicates that a muscle inflammation of relatively short duration (12 days) is associated with marked increase in the innervation density of thin fibers that contain neuropeptides.[40] The effect was particularly large in fibers that can be visualized with antibodies to SP (Fig. 1-2); the innervation density of these SP-immunoreactive fibers increased by approximately twofold (Fig. 1-3). Because some of the SP-immunoreactive fibers are likely to be nociceptors, the increase in innervation density is probably associated

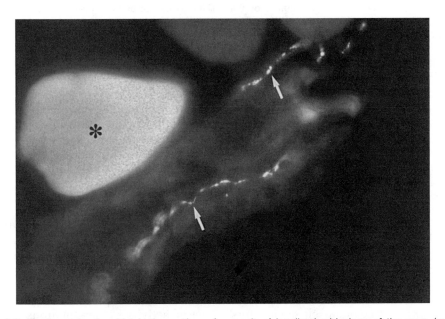

Figure 1-2. Photograph of a histologic section of the rat gastrocnemius muscle showing two nerve fibers (*arrows*) that are immunoreactive for substance P (SP). The fibers were visualized by using SP antibodies coupled to a fluorescent marker. The uneven width of the fibers is the result of localized widenings of the axon (so-called varicosities) that contain vesicles filled with SP-immunoreactive material. From these varicosities, SP (and other neuropeptides) is released when the nerve fibers are electrically active. Asterisk indicates the cross section of a muscle fiber.

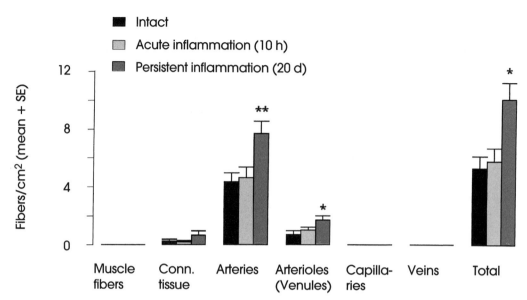

Figure 1-3. Influence of an experimental muscle inflammation on the innervation density by SP-immunoreactive fibers in various tissue components of rat gastrocnemius muscle. Only free nerve endings and preterminal axons (exhibiting varicosities) were counted. The numbers largely reflect the density of receptive free nerve endings. On the *ordinate*, the numerical area density (fibers per cm² section) is given. The *abscissa* shows the distribution of the fibers in six components of muscle tissue. *Black-filled bars*, intact (noninflamed) muscle; *light red bars*, acute inflammation of 10 hours duration, induced by infiltration of the muscle with carrageenan; *dark red bars*, persistent (subacute) inflammation of 12 days duration, induced by a single injection of Freund's complete adjuvant into the muscle. Notice the significant increase in innervation density after 12 days of myositis. *, significant at the 5% level; **, significant at the 1% level (U test). Also note that these nerve fibers of muscle are closely associated with arteries but not with veins or muscle fibers. Because some of the SP-immunoreactive endings are likely to be nociceptive, their increase in numerical density is probably associated with an increase in pain sensitivity. (Modified from Reinert A, Mense S: Inflammatory influence on the density of CGRP- and SP-immunoreactive nerve endings in rat skeletal muscle. *Neuropeptides* 24:204–205, 1993.)

with changes in pain sensations. In a muscle with increased innervation density, a given noxious stimulus will excite more nociceptive endings and thus cause more pain. Therefore, the increase in innervation density may be one peripheral mechanism explaining chronic hyperalgesia of the affected muscle.

3. Vicious Cycles Including the CNS

A widely held but questionable concept is that positive feedback mechanisms (vicious cycles) involving the CNS perpetuate the pain. Figure 1-4 shows an example of a reflex arc originating in muscle nociceptors and terminating in the neuromuscular endplates of the same muscle. There can be no doubt that the synaptic connections as presented in the figure exist. Because the synaptic transmission in the spinal cord is subjected to strong inhibitory influences, however, the mere existence of a neuronal reflex arc does not mean that every time the muscle nociceptors are excited, the muscle contracts. Nevertheless, this reflex arc has been used to explain chronic muscle spasms, based on the following (largely unproved) assumptions. The circuit is thought to be triggered by a painful lesion of the muscle, such as occurs from overuse of that muscle. The painful lesion activates muscle nociceptors, which have synaptic connections with α- and γ-motor neurons. The increased activity in these neurons induces a contraction of the muscle, either directly via α-motor neurons or indirectly via the γ-loop. The γ-loop is a neuronal circuit that leads from γ-motor neurons via muscle spindles to α-motor neurons. The γ-motor neurons activate the muscle spindles, which in turn can excite α-motor neurons monosynaptically.

If the force generated by the contracting muscle is strong enough, it may compress blood vessels and thus lead to ischemia. Ischemic contractions are painful and excite nociceptors. Thus, a vicious cycle could be formed that induces and maintains chronic muscle spasms. According to the available experimental data, a relatively high percentage of maximal muscle force is required for the occlusion of muscular arteries (a minimum of 30%[45, 48]). Fifty percent may be required. Spasm of this magnitude is exceptional, making this cycle unlikely.

It is thought that chronic muscle spasms can also be triggered by nociceptive signals emanating from a joint. In this case, a painful dysfunction of the joint is considered to be the primary lesion; it leads to muscle contractions that may reflexly stabilize the joint. However, this mechanism cannot be generalized. In many cases of painful joint lesions the neighboring muscles are reflexly inhibited (see Chapter 6).

A similar vicious cycle can be constructed for the activation of sympathetic efferent fibers by muscle nociceptors, which in turn are sensitized by the catecholamines released by the sympathetic fibers. Such a mechanism may help to perpetuate reflex sympathetic dystrophies (see Chapter 3), even though the initiating

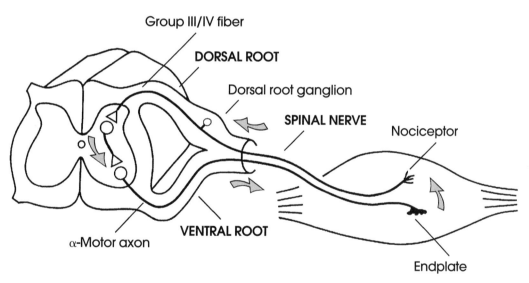

Group III/IV fiber

DORSAL ROOT

Dorsal root ganglion

SPINAL NERVE

Nociceptor

α-Motor axon

VENTRAL ROOT

Endplate

Figure 1-4. Hypothetical spinal reflex pathway that has been presumed to connect muscle nociceptors with neuromuscular endplates of the same muscle. This reflex arc has been used in many publications to construct a vicious cycle that leads to persistent muscle spasms via activation of α-motor neurons (the so-called pain-spasm-pain cycle). The cycle is assumed to start with a muscle lesion that excites nociceptors. The small-diameter (slowly conducting) group III and IV muscle afferent fibers from the muscle nociceptors excite interneurons in the dorsal horn, which in turn activate α-motor neurons. Via their efferent fibers (α-motor axons), these motor neurons activate the neuromuscular endplate and cause spasm of the muscle. A longer-lasting spasm is painful and further activates muscle nociceptors.

The excitation of dorsal horn neurons by muscle nociceptors is well established. Activation of homonymous α-motor neurons, however, is by no means proven. An acute noxious stimulus to a muscle is likely to *inhibit* rather than excite homonymous motor neurons if the muscle is an extensor. Flexor motor neurons typically show only a short-lasting excitation, if any. Painful muscles frequently show no resting electrical activity. Resting electrical activity is rarely correlated with pain level. Therefore, the postulated reflex is not functional in every muscle and cannot explain long-lasting spasms (see Chapter 6 for details).

causes of these dysfunctions are still un-known.[19]

Another possible mechanism for trigger-ing a vicious cycle is the activation of descending motor pathways by supraspinal centers. Such an activation may occur as part of a stress response to painful disor-ders of various origins. A variety of vicious cycle phenomena are dealt with in detail in Chapter 6.

As stated above, many aspects regard-ing the concept of these vicious cycles are still unproved. Therefore, the concept of

vicious cycles should be considered a working hypothesis, not a complete and satisfying explanation for chronic pain phenomena.

4. Neuroplasticity

Neuroplastic transformations in the be-havior of nerve cells are generally assumed to start as transient functional changes that eventually become fixed in the form of morphologic alterations. Plastic functional changes can be considered as long-lasting deviations from the normal synaptic func-

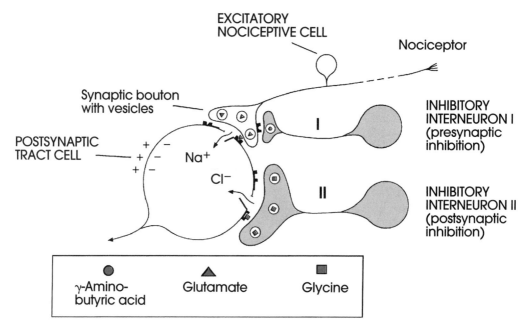

Figure 1-5. Basic synaptic events during activation and inhibition of a sensory neuron of the CNS. The excitatory input from a nociceptor arrives at the post-synaptic tract cell in the dorsal horn of the spinal cord via a nociceptive afferent axon that releases gluta-mate as a transmitter (*dark red triangles*). Gluta-mate is packed in vesicles in the presynaptic bouton and is released into the synaptic cleft when an action potential arrives at the bouton. In this sim-plified scheme, glutamate is assumed to bind to a single type of receptor molecule in the postsynap-tic membrane that controls the opening of a sodium channel. (Actually, there are several types of glutamate receptors, and other ions may also use this channel; see text for details.) The positive ions entering the cell cause a short-lasting depolar-ization of the postsynaptic membrane potential (EPSP).

Two inhibitory interneurons provide input to the same cell. Their action reduces the depolarizing effect of the excitatory input. One interneuron (I) uses γ-aminobutyric acid as a transmitter (*dark red circles*) and influences the synaptic bouton of the excitatory nociceptive cell so that it releases less glutamate. This effect is called presynaptic inhibition. Remark-ably, this inhibition does not directly influence the postsynaptic cell.

In contrast, inhibitory interneuron II forms a synapse with the postsynaptic tract cell. By releasing glycine (*dark red squares*), this neuron hyperpolarizes the postsynaptic cell and thus moves its membrane potential away from the firing threshold (postsynaptic inhibition). Possibly, this hyperpolarization occurs because glycine causes the influx of Cl^- ions into the tract cell, which increase the negative charges on the inside of the cell membrane.

tion, which are triggered by a short-lasting input.[52] Examples of synaptic processes that underlie normal signal transmission in the spinal cord are shown in Figure 1-5. Basically, two synaptic processes influence a postsynaptic neuron.

One synaptic process is release of an excitatory transmitter substance (for nociceptive transmission, mainly glutamate and aspartate[15]) from the presynaptic bouton. The transmitter binds to receptor molecules in the postsynaptic membrane that control ion channels or, in the case of metabotropic receptors, activate G proteins and other membrane-bound molecules. The formation of a glutamate-receptor complex is associated with the opening of ion channels that permit small positively charged molecules to enter the cell. This results in a short-lasting depolarization of the postsynaptic membrane, referred to as an excitatory postsynaptic potential (EPSP). If the EPSP is large enough, the postsynaptic cell is depolarized to threshold and fires an action potential; if not large enough, the result is a subthreshold EPSP that only increases the probability that the cell will fire an action potential. Alternatively, it can increase the firing frequency of an active neuron. Subthreshold EPSPs appear to be important for the adaptation of central nervous neurons to altered demands, because under special circumstances they may become suprathreshold and thus change the response properties of the cells. Normally, several simultaneous EPSPs have to combine to make a cell fire; i.e., the normal EPSP elicited by a single afferent terminal is subthreshold.

The second synaptic process is release of an inhibitory transmitter (mainly glycine for postsynaptic and GABA for presynaptic inhibition), which likewise binds to postsynaptic receptor molecules and, at least in the case of glycine, causes the opening of channels for small negatively charged ions. The influx of negative charges increases the negative membrane potential of the postsynaptic cell. The resultant shift of the membrane potential away from threshold is referred to as an inhibitory postsynaptic potential (IPSP). This reduces the excitability of the cell.

Individual central nervous neurons are known to have several thousand excitatory and inhibitory synapses on their surface.[22] Many of these synapses are simultaneously active, so the discharge frequency of the cell depends on the balance between excitatory and inhibitory inputs. This balance is an important central nervous factor determining pain in patients. The goal of most pain therapies is to reduce the excitatory input to nociceptive neurons and/or increase the inhibitory influences.

In recent years, neuroplastic processes in the CNS have attracted much interest because they offer an alternative explanation for the transition from acute to chronic pain. The basic assumption is that a nociceptive input to the spinal cord or brainstem induces long-term changes in synaptic processes in dorsal horn neurons similar to a learning process. Following such an input, the neurons are thought to increase their excitability and exhibit enhanced responses to both pathologic and normal afferent inflow. This central sensitization would then perpetuate the activity of nociceptive neurons even after the peripheral lesion has been "cured" and the nociceptive input from it is no longer present. Neuroplastic processes are dealt with in detail in Chapter 7, Section A.

5. Disturbance of the Antinociceptive System

Painful clinical syndromes have traditionally been interpreted as resulting from increased activity in afferent nociceptive fibers, with the assumption that the processing of the nociceptive information at the spinal level is normal. Recent experimental data indicate that the impulse activity in spinal sensory neurons, which process input from deep nociceptors, is subjected to a strong inhibitory influence that originates in supraspinal centers (Fig. 1-6) (probably, there are also descending pain-facilitating tracts; for details, see Chapter 7, Section A). Therefore, the magnitude of deep pain is largely dependent on the activity in this system. It is conceivable that a malfunction of the descending antinociceptive system, which might occur

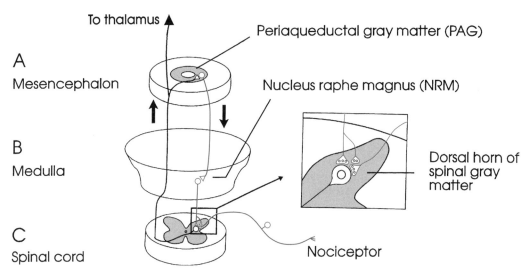

Figure 1-6. Basic organization of the descending antinociceptive system. At level C, nociceptive information (*red pathway* entering the spinal cord) is synaptically transmitted to a neuron whose axon ascends in the contralateral white matter (e.g., the spinothalamic tract). The ascending activity is relayed to a neuron at level A in the periaqueductal gray matter (PAG) of the mesencephalon at the origin of a descending pathway that ends in the medulla oblongata in the nucleus raphe magnus (NRM) at level B. Here are located inhibitory neurons whose descending axons contact the neuron at the origin of the ascending tract at level C. The inhibition exerted by the descending neuron can be either presynaptic or postsynaptic (see enlarged **inset** of dorsal horn gray matter). By the action of the descending antinociceptive system, the nociceptive activity is blocked *before* it is processed in the spinal cord. This type of antinociception is more effective and economical than an inhibition at supraspinal sites because the nociceptive information has not yet been distributed over large neuron populations. In this scheme, the descending antinociceptive system can be activated by nociceptive information entering the spinal cord, and thus operates like a negative feedback loop. More recent concepts put more emphasis on the activation of the antinociceptive system by descending input from the limbic system and hypothalamus.

spontaneously or following a central or peripheral lesion, leads to chronic pain sensations from deep tissues, even in the absence of a peripheral lesion. Such a malfunction of the antinociceptive system is presently being discussed as one of the possible causes of the pain of fibromyalgia.

6. Psychosomatic Interactions

Much controversy surrounds the issues of psychologic modulation of abnormal pain perception. Because affective status can influence pain perception, the questions at the heart of the controversy are by what mechanisms and by what magnitude do psychologic influences cause somatic dysfunctions. Why should one patient with an acute lesion recover normal function and another patient with what appears to be the same lesion develop chronic pain? A simplistic answer is that in one patient the lesion resolved, relieving the pain, whereas in the other patient the lesion did not resolve and the pain persisted. Because the lesions appeared to be the same initially, other factors must be involved. Commonly, these factors can be referred to as aggravating or perpetuating factors that were present in one patient and not in the other. Frequently, these factors were present before the occurrence of the new lesion but, alone, were not sufficiently bothersome to represent a source of distress. These factors are commonly overlooked because they are so varied and it takes so much training, experience, and attention to identify and resolve them. The persistent pain in the second type of patient is not psychogenic; it is aggravated and perpetuated by somatic problems and dysfunctions. Psychologic stress can be a potent aggravating factor.

It certainly seems to increase the electrical activity of an active TrP locus (see Chapter 8).

In this connection, as we learn more about the pathophysiology concerning the origin of muscle pain, the less psychogenic and the more somatic it becomes. The proposed pathogenesis of fibromyalgia, a disturbance of the largely serotonergic antinociceptive pathways, has replaced what was at one time classified as psychogenic rheumatism.[44]

Myofascial pain caused by TrPs provides a clear example whereby one stress or situation initially activates the TrP, but an entirely different perpetuating or aggravating factor keeps it activated. Graff-Radford et al.[13] demonstrated that attention to these factors made a definitive difference in the treatment of chronic myofascial TrP pain of the head and neck.

7. Aggravating and Perpetuating Factors

A common situation leading to chronicity is the interaction of two or more diagnostic problems. A patient who has both fibromyalgia and TrPs has more severe symptoms and a chronic pain problem that is more difficult to treat than a patient who has only one or the other.[16] Another example is the presence of both an articular dysfunction and TrPs of the muscles that are functionally related to that joint. These conditions can play Ping-Pong and persist because one tends to reactivate the other if they are treated alternately, one at a time. Both problems must be identified and appropriately treated immediately.

The resolution of factors that perpetuate the clinical activity of TrPs is often critically important in preventing an acute TrP pain situation from evolving into a chronic pain problem. The two kinds of factors, mechanical and systemic, have been extensively covered in previous publications.[47a, 56, 57] Management of the two kinds of factors demands different skills that take time and effort to learn.

Mechanical perpetuating factors involve posture, body asymmetries or disproportions, and disturbed muscle function. Poor posture (e.g., head-forward and round-shouldered) leaves some muscles in the shortened position for prolonged periods and others under chronic tension (see Chapter 6). Leg length inequality can cause compensatory muscle contraction and overload from the pelvis to the head. Relatively short upper arms overload the shoulder elevators. The recognition of muscle weakness caused by TrP inhibition is often a critical step in the restoration of normal function. Other muscles suffer from compensatory overload. Simply trying to strengthen the inhibited muscle with an exercise program often reinforces the abnormal compensatory pattern, making it more difficult for the patient to recover normal function. The cause of the muscle imbalance must be identified and addressed (see Chapter 6).

Systemic perpetuating factors encompass many conditions that compromise muscle energy metabolism. These conditions include anemia, low serum ferritin, inadequate thyroid function, vitamin B_1 (the energy vitamin) inadequacy, folic acid inadequacy, and/or vitamin B_{12} inadequacy.[57] Frequently, several of these are present at once, and the laboratory reports low-normal values. Because of the energy crisis nature of TrPs, they are especially vulnerable to impairment of the energy supply. The minimum need is highly variable from patient to patient, and it would be expected that patients with a greater need (and therefore a relatively greater inadequacy) are more vulnerable than usual to these perpetuating factors. The confusing thing about these factors is that they usually give no hint of a problem until the patient activates TrPs. For instance, the entire lower quartile of normal can be a vulnerable range for these patients. The TrP causes the pain, but the perpetuating factor facilitates chronicity. Resolution of most, sometimes all, of the perpetuating factors may be required to prevent or treat chronicity.

E. PATIENT HISTORY

In addition to a conventional thorough history of past traumas, operations, and serious illnesses, a specific muscle history is needed. The muscle history establishes the details of the situation at the onset of the pain, the relation of the pain to muscular activity and/or position, a detailed pain pattern, and the severity and constancy of the pain.

The exact time, posture, and movement or forceful activity at the time of onset are used as a guide to indicate which muscle or muscles were most likely overloaded. Characteristic of mildly active TrPs is increased pain with muscle exertion and reduced pain with rest. Severely active TrPs cause referred pain all the time, but latent TrPs cause no spontaneous pain.[54] TrPs are aggravated when the muscle is left in the shortened position and especially when the muscle is contracted in the shortened position. Stretch range of motion is limited by onset of pain. What specific activities, if any, are limited by muscle weakness? The detailed referred pain pattern serves as a guide to which muscle or muscles are most likely involved. Severe TrP pain of recent onset demands urgent attention to avoid chronicity. TrP pain of long duration and moderate to marked severity with serious disruption of the patient's previous lifestyle suggests a complex and challenging problem that will require considerable time, effort, and resourcefulness to correct.

F. APPROACH TO EXAMINING PATIENTS WITH MUSCULOSKELETAL PAIN

One reason the cause of a patient's musculoskeletal pain is so enigmatic is that an adequate examination to cover most common causes requires skills characteristic of as many as five disciplines. The clinician may be required to examine for functional muscle imbalance in the kinesiologic sense, neurologic function, myofascial TrPs, fibromyalgia, and articular dysfunction. Such a complete examination is indicated for the patient with chronic musculoskeletal pain who has seen many specialists without finding a satisfactory answer to the cause of his or her pain.

The examination for functional muscle balance is part of a physical therapist's training. The examination detects weak muscles, inhibited muscles, compensatory movement patterns, antalgic movement patterns, and muscles recruited in abnormal sequence. These dysfunctions help to identify which muscle or muscles are in

trouble and what may be causing the problem.

The neurologic examination as performed by a trained neurologist is fundamental to an adequate differential diagnosis. Projected pain or hypoesthesia along the course of a sensory nerve must be distinguished from the referred pain/anesthesia pattern of a TrP. The weakness of muscles in the distribution of a motor nerve must be distinguished from the dysfunctional patterns of weakness induced by TrPs that are related to functional muscle groups, regardless of innervation. The examination for identifying a myofascial TrP has been fully described,[47a] and appropriate diagnostic criteria included in Chapter 8 of this book. An effective examination requires the development of adequate palpation skills, the details of which vary from muscle to muscle, and, to date, are not routinely taught by most medical training programs. Frequently, physical therapists, some physiatrists, osteopathic physicians, and chiropractors, and a few practitioners of other clinical specialties have subsequently learned the necessary skills.

The physical examination for diagnosing fibromyalgia is easily learned and requires only a few minutes to perform. The examiner must determine how many of 18 TP sites are painful when pressed with 4 kg of pressure. A TP, in this setting, is one of 18 anatomically defined body sites that was found to help discriminate the fibromyalgia syndrome from other painful conditions, such as articular diseases and other nonarticular conditions.[60] Three specific distinctions from active TrPs are the absence of a palpable taut band, the inconsistent referral by TPs to another body site, and the widespread, symmetric nature of TPs in fibromyalgia. Four kg of pressure can be approximated by the amount of pressure from the broad surface of the examining thumb required to blanche the blood flow from its distal nail bed. This examination should be conducted on all patients with any complaint of musculoskeletal pain, even when the patient's presenting symptoms are unilateral or regional in nature. It is not uncommon for a patient to present with a clinical pattern of pain that mimics migraine headache, myocardial angina, low back pain, or sciatica when the actual cause is fibromyalgia. Often, the majority of the designated bilateral TPs will be remarkably tender in a person who was not aware of the contribution of widespread pain to his or her symptoms (for more details, see Chapter 9). Patients commonly have both fibromyalgia and TrPs.

An adequate examination for articular dysfunction, like that for TrPs, requires the acquisition of a special skill. Rheumatologists are the medical subspecialists for rheumatologic diseases. Osteopathic physicians, chiropractors, physical therapists, and manual medicine practitioners are most likely to have received the necessary training and to have developed the skills needed to identify and treat joint dysfunctions requiring manual mobilization.

Because the musculoskeletal conditions under consideration are common in general medical practice, practitioners need to develop a working knowledge in all of these disciplines. In addition, it is essential that the practitioner learn to recognize when the patient needs to be seen by a clinician with additional expertise in working with these conditions.

G. DISTINGUISHING BETWEEN LOCAL, PROJECTED, REFERRED, AND CENTRAL PAIN AND TENDERNESS
1. Local Pain and Tenderness

It is important to distinguish local from referred pain and tenderness because the cause of referred pain is rarely where the patient complains of pain, yet the examiner often finds tenderness in the zone of referred pain. Because muscle pain and tenderness can be referred from TrPs, articular dysfunctions, and enthesitis, the examiner must examine these sites for evidence of a condition that would cause referred muscle pain and tenderness. Local pain and/or tenderness in muscle is commonly caused by myofascial TrPs reliably associated with a palpable taut band, which the examiner must know how to identify by palpation; by an inflammatory process such as bursitis, which is not associated with a palpable taut band and which usually has tenderness that is less circumscribed than a

TrP; and by painful muscle spasm, which causes a uniformly tense muscle that has associated measurable EMG activity.

2. Projected Pain and Tenderness

Projected pain and, less commonly, tenderness must be distinguished from referred pain and tenderness. Projected pain is caused by peripheral nerve irritation that initiates sensory action potentials at the site of irritation. This afferent input is interpreted by the brain as originating at the receptive endings of the irritated (excited) nerve fibers. Projected pain follows closely the distribution of the nerve. A good example is the lightning-like shock felt down the ulnar side of the forearm and hand when one impacts the ulnar nerve at the elbow. This pain is distinctly different from the more diffuse ache characteristic of pain referred from TrPs. TrP pain and tenderness have distinctive referral patterns that are not restricted to a nerve distribution. Characteristic patterns have been described and illustrated for each of the major muscles.[47a, 56, 57]

3. Referred Pain and Tenderness

Distinguishing referred pain from central pain can be difficult. Referred pain from muscle can be identified as such whenever the pain can be reproduced by pressure on the peripheral source of the pain, as noted above. Referred pain from muscle generally has a diffuse aching quality. Reproduction of the sharper projected pain from a nerve lesion is also possible and is known as Tinel's sign when elicited by mechanical stimulation at the lesion. It has a nerve-like distribution. Referred pain and tenderness from visceral lesions can look confusingly like referred pain and tenderness of muscular origin. An example is appendicitis, which can be mimicked by active TrPs in the muscles of the lower right quadrant of the abdomen.[47a, 57]

4. Central Pain and Tenderness

Identification of central pain that the patient perceives as muscular depends on a combination of the lack of an identifiable peripheral source (which can easily be overlooked because there are so many potential sources) and a history of a lesion that can be expected to generate central pain. Common sources of central pain include spinal cord injury, CNS ablative surgery, and a severely painful peripheral lesion with subsequent interruption of its connection to the CNS. This type of central pain is eloquently demonstrated by amputees who were suffering severe pain in a limb immediately before amputation and then have a painful phantom limb that retains the preamputation pain.[34, 35] This same phenomenon is sometimes seen at the site of a painful lesion that has completely healed but has developed a comparable central source of the pain experience.

Apparently, a peripheral pain experience can produce a central imprint that can serve as a central source of pain and also modifies peripheral referral patterns. The peripheral evidence of this is the tendency for any source of referred pain in that general region of the body to refer pain to the target site, which evidences no local lesion that would account for it as an current source of pain.

REFERENCES

1. Berkley KJ: Vive la difference! *Trends Neurosci* 15:331–332, 1992.
2. Berkley KJ: Sex and chronobiology: opportunities for a focus on the positive. *IASP Newsletter* 1–5, January/February, 1993.
3. Campbell SM, Clark S, Tindall EA, *et al.*: Clinical characteristics of fibrositis. I. A "blinded," controlled study of symptoms and tender points. *Arthritis Rheum* 26:817–824, 1983.
4. Cervero F: Somatic and visceral inputs to the thoracic spinal cord of the cat: effects of noxious stimulation of the biliary system. *J Physiol* 337:51–67, 1983.
5. Cicuttini FM, Spector TD: Osteoarthritis in the aged. Epidemiological issues and optimal management. *Drugs Aging* 6:409–420, 1995.
6. Dejung B, Angerer B, Orasch J: Chronische Kopfschmerzen. *Physiotherapeut* 28(12):20–27, 1992.
7. Fischer AA: Pressure algometry over normal muscles. Standard values, validity and reproducibility of pressure threshold. *Pain* 30:115–126, 1987.
8. Fishbain DA, Goldberg M, Meagher BR, *et al.*: Male and female chronic pain patients categorized by DSM-III psychiatric diagnostic criteria. *Pain* 26: 181–197, 1986.
9. Foreman RD, Blair RW, Weber RN: Viscerosomatic convergence onto T2-T4 spinoreticular, spinoreticular-spinothalamic, and spinothalamic tract neurons in the cat. *Exp Neurol* 85:597–619, 1984.
10. Fricton JR, Kroening R, Haley D, *et al.*: Myofascial pain syndrome of the head and neck: a review of clinical characteristics of 164 patients. *Oral Surg* 60:615–623, 1985.
11. Giamberardino MA: Recent and forgotten aspects of visceral pain. *Eur J Pain* 3:77–92, 1999.
12. Gowers WR: A lecture on lumbago: its lessons and analogues. *Br Med J* 1:117-121, 1994.
13. Graff-Radford SB, Reeves JL, Jaeger B: Management of chronic headache and neck pain: the effectiveness of altering factors perpetuating myofascial pain. *Headache* 27:186–190, 1987.
14. Hakkinen A, Hannonen P, Hakkinen K: Muscle strength in healthy people and in patients suffering from recent-onset inflammatory arthritis. *Br J Rheum* 34:355–360, 1995.
15. Headley PM, Grillner S: Excitatory amino acids and synaptic transmission: the evidence for a physiological function. *Trends Pharmacol Sci (TIPS)* 11:205–211, 1990.
16. Hong C-Z, Hsueh T-C: Difference in pain relief after trigger point injections in myofascial pain patients with and without fibromyalgia. *Arch Phys Med Rehabil* 77(11):1161–1166, 1996.
17. Hsieh JC, Belfrage M, Stone-Elander S, *et al.*: Central representation of chronic ongoing neuropathic pain studies by positron emission tomography. *Pain* 63:225–236, 1995.
18. Institute of Medicine: *Pain and Disability: Clinical Behavioral and Public Policy Perspectives.* National Academy Press, Washington, DC, May 1987.
19. Jänig W: Experimental approach to reflex sympathetic dystrophy and related syndromes. *Pain* 46:241–245, 1991.
20. Jensen R, Rasmussen BK, Pedersen B, *et al.*: Muscle tenderness and pressure pain thresholds in headache. A population study. *Pain* 52:193–199, 1993.
21. Jensen I, Nygren A, Gamberale F, *et al.*: Coping with long-term musculoskeletal pain and its consequences: is gender a factor? *Pain* 57:167–172, 1994.
22. Kandel ER, Schwartz JH, Jessell TM: Elementary interactions between neurons: synaptic transmission, Chapter III. *Principles of Neural Science.* Ed. 3. Edited by Kandel ER, Schwartz JH, Jessell TM. Elsevier, New York, 1991 (p. 121).
23. Keay KA, Bandler R: Deep and superficial noxious stimulation increases Fos-like immunoreactivity in different regions of the midbrain periaqueductal grey of the rat. *Neurosci Lett* 154:23–26, 1993.
24. Kellgren JH: Observations on referred pain arising from muscle. *Clin Sci* 3:175–190, 1938.
25. Lawrence JS: Prevalence of rheumatoid arthritis. *Ann Rheum Dis* 20:11–17, 1961.
26. Lawrence JS, Bremner JM, Bier F: Osteoarthritis prevalence in the population and relationship between symptoms and X-ray changes. *Ann Rheum Dis* 25:1–7, 1966.
27. Lee K-H, Lee M-H, Kim H-S, *et al.*: Pressure pain thresholds [PPT] of head and neck muscles in a normal population. *J Musculoskeletal Pain* 2(4):67–81, 1994.
28. Lewit K: *Manipulative Therapy in Rehabilitation of the Motor System.* Butterworths, London, 1985.
29. Lewit K: Changes in locomotor function, complementary medicine and the general practitioner. *J R Soc Med* 87:36–39, 1994.

30. Madsen OR, Bliddal H, Egsmose C, *et al.*: Isometric and isokinetic quadriceps strength in gonarthrosis; inter-relations between quadriceps strength, walking ability, radiology, subchondral bone density and pain. *Clin Rheumatol* 14:308–314, 1995.

31. Marchettini P, Cline M, Ochoa JL: Innervation territories for touch and pain afferents of single fascicles of the human ulnar nerve. Mapping through intraneural microrecording and microstimulation. *Brain* 113:1491–1500, 1990.

32. Marks R, Percy JS, Semple J, *et al.*: Comparison between the surface electromyogram of the quadriceps surrounding the knees of healthy women and the knees of women with osteoarthritis. *Clin Exp Rheumatol* 12:11–15, 1994.

33. Masterton JP: Burns. *Hamilton Bailey's Emergency Surgery.* Ed. 11. Edited by Dudley HAF. John Wright & Sons, Bristol, UK, 1986 (pp. 68–76).

34. Melzack R: The gate control theory 25 years later: new perspectives on phantom limb pain, Chapter 2. *Proceedings of the VIth World Congress on Pain.* Edited by Bond MR, Charlton JE, Woolf CJ. Elsevier Science Publishers, Amsterdam, 1991.

35. Melzack R: Phantom limbs. *Sci Am* 120–126, April 1992.

36. Merskey H, Bogduk N: *Classification of Chronic Pain: Descriptions of Chronic Pain Syndromes and Definitions of Pain Terms.* Ed. 2. IASP Press, Seattle, 1994.

37. Mikklesson M, Salminen JJ, Kautiainen H: Joint hypermobility is not a contributing factor to musculoskeletal pain in pre-adolescents. *Arch Phys Med Rehabil* 77:958–959, 1996 (Abstract).

38. Mitchell JH, Schmidt RF: Cardiovascular reflex control by fibers from skeletal muscle. *Handbook of Physiology, Section 2: The Cardiovascular System, Volume III: Peripheral Circulation and Organ Blood Flow, Part 2.* Edited by Shepherd JT, Abboud FM. American Physiological Society, Bethesda, MD, 1983 (pp. 623–658).

39. Reading AE: Testing pain mechanisms in persons in pain, Ch. 17. *Textbook of Pain.* Edited by Wall PD, Melzack R. Churchill Livingstone, Edinburgh, 1989 (pp. 269–280).

40. Reinert A, Mense S: Inflammatory influence on the density of CGRP- and SP-immunoreactive nerve endings in rat skeletal muscle. *Neuropeptides* 24:204–205, 1993.

41. Rosomoff HL, Fishbain DA, Goldberg M, *et al.*: Physical findings in patients with chronic intractable benign pain of the neck and/or back. *Pain* 37:279–287, 1989.

42. Ruda MA: Gender and pain. *Pain* 53:1–2, 1993.

43. Russell IJ: A new journal. *J Musculoskeletal Pain* 1(1):1–7, 1993.

44. Russell IJ: Neurochemical pathogenesis of fibromyalgia syndrome. *J Musculoskeletal Pain* 4(1/2):61–92, 1996.

45. Sadamoto T, Bonde-Petersen F, Suzuki Y: Skeletal muscle tension, flow, pressure, and EMG during sustained isometric contractions in humans. *Eur J Appl Physiol* 51:395–408, 1983.

46. Sicuteri F: Neurovasoactive substances and their implication in vascular pain. *Resident Clinical Studies Headache, 1.* Edited by Friedman AP. Karger, Basel, 1967 (pp. 6–45).

47. Simons DG: Myofascial pain syndrome: one term but two concepts. A new understanding. [Editorial] *J Musculoskeletal Pain* 3(1):7–13, 1995.

47a. Simons DG, Travell JG, Simons LS: *Travell & Simons' Myofascial Pain and Dysfunction: The Trigger Point Manual, Volume 1. Upper Half of Body.* Ed. 2. Williams & Wilkins, Baltimore, 1999.

48. Sjogaard G: Muscle energy metabolism and electrolyte shifts during low-level prolonged static contraction in man. *Acta Physiol Scand* 134:181–187, 1988.

49. Skootsky SA, Jaeger B, Oye RK: Prevalence of myofascial pain in general internal medicine practice. *West J Med* 151:157–160, 1989.

50. Smythe HA, Moldofsky H: Two contributions to understanding of the "fibrositis" syndrome. *Bull Rheum Dis* 28:928–931, 1977.

51. Staff PH: Clinical consideration in referred muscle pain and tenderness—connective tissue reactions. *Eur J Appl Physiol* 57:369–372, 1988.

52. Sutula T, He X-X, Cavazos J, *et al.*: Synaptic reorganization in the hippocampus induced by abnormal functional activity. *Science* 239:1147–1150, 1988.

53. Torebjörk HE, Ochoa JL, Schady W: Referred pain from intraneural stimulation of muscle fascicles in the median nerve. *Pain* 18:145–156, 1984.

54. Travell JG: Chronic myofascial pain syndromes. Mysteries of the history, Chapter 6. *Myofascial Pain and Fibromyalgia, Advances in Pain Research and Therapy,* Volume 17. Edited by Fricton JR, Awad EA. Raven Press, New York, 1990 (pp. 129–137).

55. Travell JG, Rinzler SH: The myofascial genesis of pain. *Postgrad Med* 11:425–434, 1952.

56. Travell JG, Simons DG: *Myofascial Pain and Dysfunction. The Trigger Point Manual, Volume 2. The Lower Extremities.* Williams & Wilkins, Baltimore, 1992.

57. Travell JG, Simons DG: *Myofascial Pain and Dysfunction: The Trigger Point Manual, Volume 1.* Williams & Wilkins, Baltimore, 1983.

58. Wigers SH, Skrondal A, Finset A, *et al.*: Measuring change in fibromyalgic pain: the relevance of pain distribution. *J Musculoskeletal Pain* 5(2):29–41, 1997.

59. Wolfe F, Ross K, Anderson J, *et al.*: The prevalence and characteristics of fibromyalgia in the general population. *Arthritis Rheum* 38:19–28, 1995.

60. Wolfe F, Smythe HA, Yunus MB, *et al.*: American College of Rheumatology 1990 criteria for the classification of fibromyalgia: report of the Multicenter Criteria Committee. *Arthritis Rheum* 33:160–172, 1990.

61. Yu X-M, Mense S: Response properties and descending control of rat dorsal horn neurons with deep receptive fields. *Neuroscience* 39:823–831, 1990.

62. Yu X-M, Hua M, Mense S: The effects of intracerebroventricular injection of naloxone, phentolamine and methysergide on the transmission of nociceptive signals in rat dorsal horn neurons with convergent cutaneous-deep input. *Neuroscience* 44:715–723, 1991.

CHAPTER 2
Local Pain in Muscle

SUMMARY: This chapter gives an overview of known **structures and mechanisms** that lead to local muscle pain and describes diseases that exhibit this type of pain. **Local muscle pain** is defined as pain caused by excitation of muscle nociceptors. This is in contrast to other forms of muscle pain that, for example, are due to lesions of the muscle nerve or alterations of central neurons mediating muscle pain.

Muscle nociceptors most likely are free nerve endings, but not all free nerve endings are nociceptive. Muscle nociceptors are sensitive to strong mechanical stimuli and endogenous chemical stimulants (pain-producing substances) that are released from muscle tissue in the course of pathologic alterations. Extremely effective in this regard is **bradykinin (BK)**; other substances (e.g., **prostaglandin E$_2$, serotonin**) likely act mainly as sensitizing agents that increase the sensitivity of nociceptors to mechanical and chemical stimuli. This **sensitization of muscle nociceptors** is assumed to be the peripheral mechanism of the tenderness of lesioned muscle (central nervous mechanisms also cause tenderness). Nonsteroidal anti-inflammatory drugs decrease the magnitude of the sensitization of nociceptors and thus reduce the tenderness.

Clinical examples of local muscle pain include **trauma, inflammation, and intermittent claudication**. Trauma can activate muscle nociceptors directly or can induce a lesion in the muscle, from which endogenous pain-producing substances are released. Inflammation is known to release BK and prostaglandins (PGs) from the inflamed tissue. Since the amounts of these agents released during inflammation are relatively small, the main action is probably sensitization of the nociceptors, not excitation. Therefore, muscle inflammation does not cause strong spontaneous pain but instead causes **dysesthesia** and **sensations of weakness**, the latter of which is probably caused by central reflexes. The exact cause of the pain of intermittent claudication is still unknown. Some evidence, however, indicates that ischemia releases BK from its precursor molecule, kallidin. BK then sensitizes or activates muscle nociceptors. Ischemic muscle pain in experimental animals is largely caused by activity in nociceptors with unmyelinated afferent fibers (as opposed to nociceptors with thin myelinated fibers) and, therefore, can be considered an example of so-called C-fiber pain.

Non-nociceptive free nerve endings in muscle likely have an important function in the adjustment of respiration and circulation during muscular exercise. These receptors typically show marked activations during contractions of the muscle; they are unable, however, to respond differentially to physiologic and nonphysiologic (painful, ischemic) contractions and, therefore, cannot fulfill the function of nociceptors.

A. STRUCTURES AND MECHANISMS UNDERLYING LOCAL MUSCLE PAIN

1. Structure of Skeletal Muscle

Skeletal muscles are ensheathed by connective tissue, the epimysium, which in some muscles has the form of a dense fascia (Fig. 2-1, Panel A). Inside the tube-like room formed by the fascia, the muscle can contract with minimal distortion of the subcutaneous tissue or other adjacent structures. A large muscle is composed of many fascicles (bundles of muscle fibers), each of which is again surrounded by connective tissue, the perimysium. The individual muscle fibers (or muscle cells) of a fascicle are separated from each other by loose connective tissue, the endomysium (Fig. 2-1, Panel B). Each muscle fiber contains many myofibrils—the contractile elements of a muscle cell that consist of a chain of sarcomeres (Fig. 2-1, Panel C). The sarcomeres have two main constituents, molecular filaments of actin and myosin, which interdigitate and advance against each other during muscle shortening (Fig. 2-1, Panels D and E).

The myofibrils of a muscle fiber are structured so that the myosin and actin filaments of adjacent fibrils are in alignment. Thus, the aligned myosin filaments of many myofibrils form the dark band (the anisotropic or A band) of the striations in skeletal muscle fibers that can be seen with a light microscope. (Because of their small size, the filaments and sarcomeres of a single myofibril are not visible at the light microscopic level.)

The smallest functional unit of a muscle cell (or fiber) is the sarcomere, which extends from one Z band (or Z line) to the next. A sarcomere is approximately 2.5 μm (micrometers or microns) long in resting muscle and consists of the relatively thin actin filaments, which are attached to the Z band, and the thick myosin filaments, which lie in the middle of a sarcomere and interdigitate with the actin filaments. The A band has a darker outer zone (closer to the Z band) that is characterized by an overlap between myosin and actin filaments and a paler inner zone, the H (Hensen) band, that marks that region of the A band where only myosin filaments are present. Areas outside the region of the myosin filaments close to the Z band contain actin filaments only; they look pale in the light microscope and form the isotropic (I) band.

he signal for the filaments to shorten the sarcomere by sliding against each other is an increase in intracellular Ca^{++} concentration. In a resting sarcomere the calcium concentration is approximately 10^{-8} M (.00000001 molar); additional calcium is stored in intracellular stores called sarcoplasmic reticulum (sarcoplasm is the cytoplasm of a muscle cell). The reticulum consists of a network of branching and anastomosing tubules that fill the space between the myofibrils. The reticulum of each sarcomere has terminal expansions (the terminal cisternae) that are situated transversely at the level of the A-I band junction (Fig. 2-2). Between two of these cisternae is a tubular invagination (transverse tubule) of the cell membrane. Together these two cisternae and the tubule form the "triad."

When an action potential arrives at the neuromuscular junction, it releases many quantal packets of acetylcholine (ACh) from the terminal branches of the α-motor axon (Fig. 2-3). The ACh diffuses across the synaptic cleft to the muscle cell membrane and binds to specific receptor molecules on the surface of the membrane. The formation of the ACh receptor complex opens ion channels that allow positive ions (mainly sodium) to enter the muscle cell. The positive charges decrease the negative membrane potential and initiate a large number of short-lasting postsynaptic action potentials (endplate potentials, EPPs; Fig. 2-4). Normally, the great number of ACh molecules that are released simultaneously

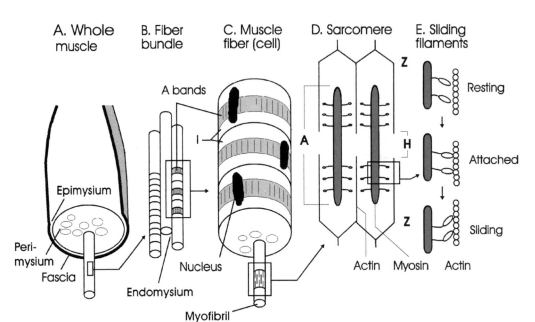

Figure 2-1. Composition of skeletal muscle tissue. **Panel A.** Whole muscle showing cross sections of muscle fiber bundles. The bundles are separated from each other by loose connective tissue (perimysium). The loose connective tissue on the surface of the muscle forms the epimysium, which can move freely against the fascia (dense connective tissue). A single muscle fiber bundle protrudes from the muscle. The bundle is composed of muscle fibers, each of which is enveloped by a fine layer of loose connective tissue (endomysium). **Panel B.** Muscle fiber bundle containing three muscle fibers (or muscle cells). **Panel C.** Single muscle fiber cell showing the typical striations and several nuclei. The round profiles at the lower end of the cell indicate cross sections of myofibrils that contain the contractile filaments. One of the fibrils protruding from the cell consists of a chain of sarcomeres. In the *box*, one of the sarcomeres is shown in more detail. **Panel D.** Composition of a sarcomere, the smallest functional unit of a striated muscle. The sarcomere extends from one Z line to the next. Thick myosin molecules *(red)* with spiny heads lie in the center of the sarcomere. They interdigitate with thin actin molecules that are anchored to the Z line. The isotropic (I) band on both sides of the Z line contains actin filaments only (see **Panel C**). The anisotropic (A) band contains both actin and myosin filaments with the exception of its middle portion (the lighter H zone), which is free from actin. During contraction, the filaments slide against each other; thus, the I band and H zone become narrower, whereas the A band maintains a constant width. **Panel E.** "Sliding filament" mechanism during contraction. In the resting state, the binding sites for the myosin heads on the globular molecules of the actin chain are not accessible. The contraction starts with the release of calcium ions from the sarcoplasmic reticulum within the muscle cell. Under the influence of a raised calcium concentration, the molecules that cover the binding sites (tropomyosin, not shown) move aside, and the myosin heads attach to the actin molecules. Subsequently, the heads make a bending movement and thus pull the myosin filament toward the Z line. Since the formed actomyosin complex has the action of an ATPase (an enzyme that splits adenosine triphosphate, ATP), energy-rich ATP molecules in the vicinity of the complex are cleaved. The released energy is used for separating the myosin heads from the actin. By repeating this sequence of attaching, bending, and separating, the myosin heads make a rowing movement that leads to movement of the filaments, which shortens the sarcomere.

drives the muscle membrane well beyond threshold and elicits an action potential in the muscle cell. This is in sharp contrast to the postsynaptic potentials in central nervous system neurons, which are typically subthreshold.

In the absence of α-motor neuron activity, a few vesicles of the presynaptic terminal occasionally merge with the axonal membrane and release their content of ACh into the synaptic cleft. These small amounts of transmitter cause minute, individual subthreshold depolarizations of the postsynaptic membrane (the miniature endplate potentials [MEPPs]). Recent studies indicate that the frequency of MEPPs can be markedly increased under abnormal conditions (see Chapter 8).

The normal suprathreshold EPP elicits a pair of action potentials that start at the endplate and traverse the length of the muscle cell in opposite directions. The action potentials also invade the body of the cell by following transverse tubules. The invasive action potentials release Ca^{++} from the cisternae of the sarcoplasmic reticulum. The intracellular Ca^{++} concentration rises approximately 100-fold (to approximately 10^{-6} M); this change causes the tropomyosin chain, which is wrapped

around the actin, to change its position relative to the actin molecule. In resting muscle, tropomyosin masks the binding sites on the surface of the actin molecule for myosin. After the binding sites have been unmasked, the myosin heads bind to actin, continuing to make flexing ("rowing") movements as long as the additional calcium is present. These movements pull the actin filament and Z band toward the middle of the sarcomere and shorten it.

The myosin heads contain ATPase, an enzyme that splits adenosine triphosphate (ATP) into adenosine diphosphate (ADP) and phosphate (P) plus energy. Actin activates the enzyme in the presence of Mg^{++} ions; i.e., as soon as the myosin heads make contact with the actin filaments, ATP is

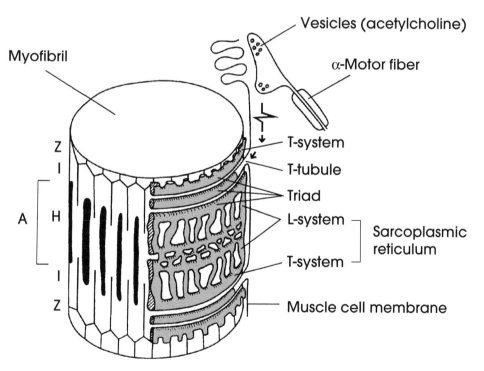

Figure 2-2. Sarcoplasmic reticulum. The reticulum of one myofibril is partly cut away to show the arrangement of its components relative to the contractile filaments. The sarcoplasmic reticulum has the function of a calcium store; it consists of two systems of tubules, the longitudinally oriented L-system and the transversely oriented T-system. The T-system forms the terminal cisternae where all tubuli of the L-system join. Neighboring cisternae are not in contact with each other; they are separated by an

invagination of the cell membrane, the so-called T-tubule. Together with the two adjacent cisternae this tubule forms the triad that is always located close to the transition between the I and A band.

During activity of the α-motor fiber, action potentials are initiated in the membrane of the muscle cell close to the neuromuscular endplate. The action potentials propagate along the muscle cell and invade the T-tubules. Here, the action potentials release calcium from the adjacent T-system of the reticulum.

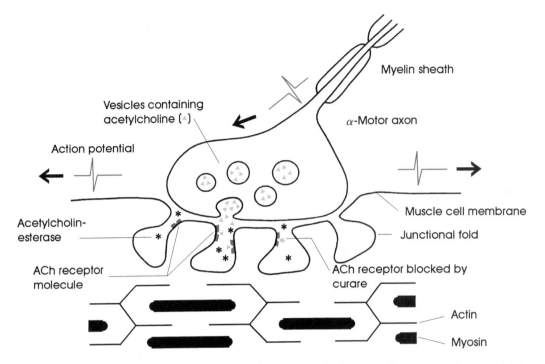

Figure 2-3. Scheme of a neuromuscular endplate. A branch of the α-motor axon terminates as a presynaptic expansion in which vesicles containing acetylcholine (ACh, *light red triangles*) are located. ACh is the transmitter substance of the neuromuscular junction. When an action potential of the motor axon arrives at the endplate, it causes fusion of many vesicles with the presynaptic membrane and release of ACh into the synaptic cleft. The ACh molecules diffuse to the postsynaptic membrane and bind to ACh receptor molecules *(dark red)*. This induces opening of membrane channels and influx of positively charged ions into the muscle cell. Release of a single packet of ACh produces a subthreshold depolarization of the postsynaptic membrane (a miniature endplate potential [MEPP]). Simultaneous release of many packets of ACh by a single nerve action potential normally causes a larger endplate potential (EPP), which depolarizes the muscle cell beyond threshold. This depolarization initiates an action potential in the membrane of the muscle cell adjacent to the endplate. The action potential is propagated throughout the entire muscle cell and releases calcium ions from the sarcoplasmic reticulum. The resulting increase in intracellular calcium concentration is the signal for the myosin filaments to pull against the actin filaments by rowing movements of the myosin heads and thus shorten the sarcomere (see Fig. 2-1). The ACh molecules in the synaptic cleft are cleaved by acetylcholinesterase *(black asterisks)*. If the number of accessible postsynaptic ACh receptors is reduced by curare *(light red diamond)*, the EPP does not reach threshold, and the muscle cell does not contract.

cleaved. The released energy is used to separate the myosin heads from the actin. If the intracellular Ca^{++} concentration is still high, the myosin heads will attach again to the actin filament. Many successive cycles of this attaching-flexing-separating process produce movement of the actin filament along the myosin.

The rowing movements of the myosin heads stop when the intracellular calcium concentration drops to the original value. This drop is brought about by the calcium pump, which transports the Ca^{++} back into the sarcoplasmic reticulum and thus terminates the effect of the muscle action potential. When the intracellular ATP concentration is very low, as occurs, for example, after death, the myosin heads cannot separate from the actin and rigor mortis ensues. This condition is characterized by the attachment of *all* myosin heads to actin, a situation that normally never occurs during life because attachment of the head is immediately followed by detachment.

A   ENDPLATE POTENTIALS

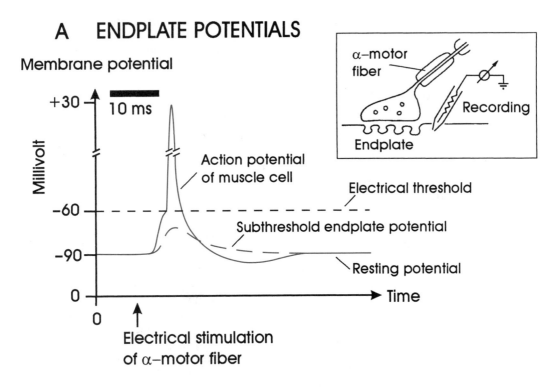

B   MINIATURE ENDPLATE POTENTIALS

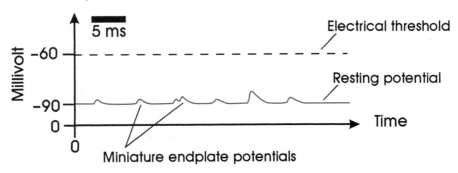

Figure 2-4. Endplate potentials (EPPs). The setup used for recording the potentials is shown in the **insert**. A microelectrode is placed intracellularly, close to the neuromuscular endplate. **Panel A.** *Solid red line,* the resting membrane potential of the muscle cell is nearly −90 mV, inside negative. Binding of acetylcholine (ACh) to the postsynaptic receptors causes a depolarization of the muscle cell, the EPP. Normally, the EPP reaches the electrical threshold of the cell *(dashed black line)* and triggers a muscle action potential. In the presence of curare, many ACh receptors are blocked, and, therefore, the EPP is subthreshold *(dashed red line).* Accordingly, the muscle cell does not generate an action potential. **Panel B.** Even under resting conditions (in the absence of impulse activity in the α-motor neuron), occasionally an ACh vesicle fuses with the pre-synaptic membrane and releases ACh into the synaptic cleft. Each "package" of ACh causes a small and transient depolarization of the muscle cell membrane, a miniature EPP (MEPP). Individual MEPPs are always subthreshold. In **A** and **B**, the time scale is 10 and 5 ms, respectively *(thick horizontal bars).*

Under the microscope, a contracted muscle fiber can be recognized by the unchanged width of the A band and a narrower I and H band. Recent data show that in the resting muscle a small proportion of the myosin heads are attached to the actin filaments.[43] An increase in this proportion ordinarily would increase the viscoelastic component of muscle tone (see Chapter 5).

Basically, a skeletal muscle can perform four types of contraction. An understanding of these different forms of muscular activity is essential for effective therapeutic exercise.

1. Shortening (concentric) contraction, defined as length reduction produced by a generation of muscle force. An example of this kind of contraction is the quadriceps femoris muscle extending the knee during stair climbing.
2. Lengthening (eccentric) contraction, defined as a muscular force resisting lengthening of the muscle by external forces. Under these circumstances the force developed by the muscle is smaller than that causing the lengthening. The muscle contracts to slow the lengthening. An example of such an action is the contraction of the quadriceps muscle during downhill walking. This type of contraction is particularly important for the development of soreness (see Postexercise Muscle Soreness in Section B1 of this chapter).
3. Isometric contraction, defined as increase in force without length change. A good example of such a contraction is activation of the masseter muscle when the maxillary and mandibular teeth are in contact. As the teeth are not compressible, the contraction is largely isometric. Under these conditions, the myosin heads perform their cyclic movements, but the developed force is used not for shortening of the muscle but for putting tension on the elastic parts of the muscle and on the insertion points. This means that the contractile elements expend energy to shorten, but the muscle as a whole does not.
4. Isotonic contraction, defined as length change without change in the force exerted. Isotonic contractions can be performed on a muscle testing and exercise machine designed to provide constant resistance through the range of movement.

Human muscles contain two main types of muscle fibers: white and red fibers. White fibers have a pale appearance because they contain less myoglobin. They are rich in phosphorylases and glycogen and obtain energy mainly by degrading glucose (glycolytic metabolism). The white fibers respond with a fast twitch (25 ms duration) when activated, and they fatigue quickly. They are used predominantly for spurts of fast movements.

The red fibers contain more myoglobin and oxidative enzymes than do the white fibers, but they are less rich in phosphorylases. They respond with slow twitches (75 ms duration) when activated and are more resistant to fatigue. They can continue contractions for a long period based on oxygen consumption (oxidative metabolism that makes use of mitochondria). Red muscle fibers are numerous in postural muscles. The white fibers correspond to type II fibers, and the red fibers correspond to type I fibers. (For a more detailed description of the various subtypes of fibers, the reader is referred to the special literature—see, for example, Ref. 28.)

In adult muscle fibers, so-called satellite cells are present underneath the cell membrane and are thought to be myoblasts, i.e., cells that develop into muscle cells (fibers) during development. With the help of these cells, small lesions of skeletal muscles can regenerate to form muscle tissue that is indistinguishable from the original skeletal muscle. Larger regions of damaged muscle cannot regenerate; they are replaced with connective (scar) tissue.

2. Morphology and Location of Muscle Receptors Relevant to Pain

The available clinical and experimental evidence indicates that small-diameter afferent (sensory) fibers have to be activated to elicit local pain from a muscle.[128] These fibers are either thin myelinated (Aδ or group III) fibers that have conduction velocities between 2.5 and 30 m/s in the cat[10, 36] or unmyelinated (C or group IV) fibers that conduct at velocities below 2.5 m/s.[98] In this book, the afferent fiber types are named groups I to IV according to the nomenclature of Lloyd,[75] which was developed specifically for muscle afferent fibers. Sensory nerve fibers in a peripheral nerve are called primary afferent fibers; they are connected to secondary afferent neurons in the central nervous system. An afferent fiber, together with its receptive ending, forms an afferent unit.

Investigations using electron microscopy have shown that the main type of receptive ending of small-diameter afferent fibers is a free nerve ending. Under the light microscope this type of ending lacks a corpuscular receptive structure. Group IV fibers are thought to terminate exclusively in free nerve endings, while group III fibers supply both free nerve endings and other types of muscle receptors (e.g., paciniform corpuscles; Fig. 2-5). Free nerve endings in skeletal muscle (which include all nociceptors) typically end in the adventitia surrounding arterioles; i.e., the capillaries proper are not supplied with these endings

(see Fig. 1-3).[119] The marked sensitivity of the free nerve endings to chemical stimuli, particularly to those accompanying disturbances of the microcirculation, may be related to their location on or in the walls of the blood vessels. The finding that the muscle fibers proper are not supplied with neuropeptide-containing free nerve endings (see Fig. 1-3)[106, 106a] may relate to the clinical experience that muscle cell death—even on a large scale, such as may occur during muscular dystrophy, polymyositis, or dermatomyositis—usually is not painful.

More recent data demonstrate that free nerve endings are not free in the strict sense, since they are almost completely ensheathed by Schwann cells. Only small areas of the axonal membrane remain uncovered by Schwann cell processes and are in direct contact with the interstitial fluid around the vessels and muscle fibers.[2] The exposed nerve membrane areas are supplied with mitochondria and vesicles and show other structural specializations characteristic of receptive areas; they are probably the site where external stimuli

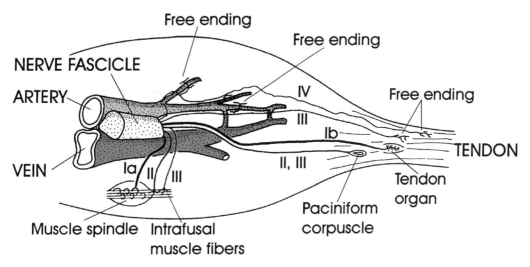

Figure 2-5. Overview of muscle receptors and afferent fibers. To the left is a nerve fascicle in the muscle, together with a larger muscle artery and vein. The afferent fibers are labeled with roman numerals according to the nomenclature of Lloyd.[75] *Group I,* thick myelinated fibers supplying muscle spindle primary endings (Ia) and tendon (Golgi) organs (Ib). *Group II,* medium-sized myelinated fibers supplying muscle spindle secondary endings and paciniform corpuscles. *Group III,* thin myelinated fibers supplying free nerve endings and paciniform corpuscles. *Group IV,* unmyelinated fibers supplying exclusively free nerve endings. The efferent sympathetic fibers as well as the α- and γ-fibers have been omitted from the figure for reasons of clarity.

act. A reconstruction of free endings in the calcaneal tendon of the cat revealed the existence of different morphologic types of endings connected to group III and group IV afferent fibers (Fig. 2-6).[2] Similar endings have also been found in skeletal muscle.[26]

Those receptive membrane areas of a single nerve fiber that are located closely together in a small volume of tissue form an ending in the strict sense. An ending can extend over relatively long distances and can have several receptive terminals that, again, have several receptive sites, as shown in light red in Figure 2-6. Whether a single ending may possess functionally different receptive terminals is a matter of discussion. The physiologic term "receptor" refers to an entire morphologic ending.

At present, it is not possible to correlate these morphologic types with the functional types found in electrophysiologic experiments (see below). Although muscle nociceptors are most probably free nerve endings, their exact ultrastructure is unknown. The existence of more than one morphologic type of free nerve ending supports the notion that this population of receptors does not form a homogeneous group but instead consists of functionally different (presumably nociceptive and non-nociceptive) types.

In quantitative evaluations of the innervation density by neuropeptide-containing

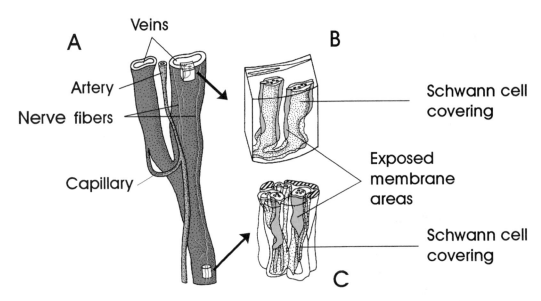

Figure 2-6. Different morphologic types of free nerve endings. Reconstructions from electron microscopic sections of two free nerve endings in the Achilles tendon of the cat. **Panel A.** A bundle of arterial and venous vessels is accompanied by two thin myelinated nerve fibers *(thin red lines)*. The *arrows* mark the regions from which the sections for the reconstructions in **Panels B** and **C** were taken. **Panel B.** A free nerve ending with two lanceolate terminals in the loose connective tissue around the venous vessel. *Dark stippling*, Schwann cell covering large portions of the axon. Exposed axon membrane areas *(light red)* are in direct contact with the interstitial fluid. Here, the axoplasm contains mitochondria and vesicles, i.e., structures that are considered typical of receptive membrane sites. **Panel C.** Receptive ending of the other axon. The axoplasm of the exposed and expanded portions *(light red)* of the axon show the same specializations as the ending in **Panel B.** Collagen fiber bundles *(hatched area)* insert close to the receptive membrane areas. The collagen fibers are capable of transmitting mechanical forces to the axonal membrane and thus suggest a mechanoreceptive function of the free nerve ending. (Redrawn from Andres KH, von Düring M, Schmidt RF: Sensory innervation of the Achilles tendon by group III and IV afferent fibers. *Anat Embryol* 172:145–156, 1985.)

Although these data were obtained from tendon tissue, preliminary results from skeletal muscle suggest that the basic features of free nerve endings, namely, exposed membrane areas and axonal expansions with mitochondria and vesicles, are also present in muscle tissue.[26]

Table 2-1   *Fiber Composition of the Nerve to the Lateral Gastrocnemius-Soleus Muscle in the Cat[a]*

Myelinated 1200								Unmyelinated 2000	
Motor		720	60%	Sensory		480	40%	Motor	Sensory
Aα	Skeleto-motor	382	53%	I	Spindle primary sensory endings (Ia)	144	30%		
					Tendon organs (Ib)	72	15%		
Aβ	Skeleto and fusimotor	14	2%	II	Spindle secondary sensory endings	144	30%		
Aγ	Fusimotor	324	45%		Spray (Ruffini) endings	5	<1%		
					Lamellated (paciniform) endings	5	<1%		
				III	Free nerve endings	110	23%	C vasomotor	IV sensory
					(nociceptive)	36	33%	1000 50%	1000 50% (nociceptive 430 43%)

[a]Notice that for muscle afferent (sensory) fibers, the nomenclature by Lloyd[75] (group I–IV) has been used. This system is based on the diameter of the fibers. The other common nomenclature, which uses Latin and Greek letters, is based on the conduction velocity of the fibers and is normally applied to efferent (motor) fibers.

The two systems are similar in the following aspects: group I and II are thick myelinated and correspond largely to Aα- and Aβ-fibers. Aγ- and Aδ-fibers are thin myelinated and correspond largely to group III. The unmyelinated C fibers are identical to the group IV afferents. (Source: Mitchell and Schmidt.[91])

fibers (substance P [SP] and calcitonin gene-related peptide [CGRP]), no difference was found between the proximal and distal portions of the rat gastrocnemius-soleus (GS) muscle. Therefore, a higher innervation density at an end of the muscle by nociceptive fibers does not seem to be an adequate explanation for the pain and tenderness of enthesopathy or enthesitis. The nerve fiber density in the peritendineum (the connective tissue around a tendon) of the rat calcaneal tendon, however, was approximately five times higher than that in the GS muscle.[106] The tendon tissue proper was almost free of immunoreactive free nerve endings. The high fiber density in the peritendineum may explain the spontaneous tenderness or pain many people have in the tissue around the tendon. Conversely, the lack of nerve endings in the center of the tendon may relate to the fact that incomplete ruptures of the tendon may occur without pain.

3. Fiber Composition of a Muscle Nerve

The nerve to a locomotor muscle in the cat (the lateral GS) is composed of approximately one-third myelinated and two-thirds unmyelinated fibers (Table 2-1).[91, 119] Nearly one quarter of the myelinated fibers had nociceptive properties in neurophysiologic experiments.[87] Of the unmyelinated fibers, 50% are sensory, and 43% of these were found to be nociceptive. In the sternomastoid nerve of the rat, the (afferent) group IV fibers likewise constitute approximately half of all the unmyelinated fibers and thus account for the great majority of afferent units in that nerve.[39, 115]

Data obtained from one muscle nerve cannot be transferred directly to other muscle nerves, as considerable differences reportedly exist between different muscles. For instance, the neck muscle nerves of the cat are known to contain unusually high numbers of sensory and γ-motor fibers,[108] and the receptive properties of group III receptors in hindlimb muscles differ from those in neck muscles. One possible explanation for these differences is that the muscles have different functions and environmental conditions. In contrast to the neck muscles, which must register the orientation of the head in relation to the body in fine detail, the locomotor hindlimb muscles often have to contract with maximal strength and under ischemic conditions.[1]

4. Neuropeptide Content of Muscle Afferent Units

The various neuropeptides are known to have different neuronal and vascular effects in different tissues. Therefore, no function for the neuropeptides in general can be given. For example, in the central nervous system, SP is assumed to modulate the transmission of sensory information; in the peripheral nervous system, the neuropeptide is known to be involved in inflammatory processes by increasing vascular permeability and releasing histamine from mast cells. CGRP has vascular and metabolic actions; it has been shown to control the synthesis of a subunit of the ACh receptor molecule in the neuromuscular endplate.[96]

The significance of neuropeptides for painful pathologic processes throughout the body is probably high because they are ubiquitously present in sensory units of small diameter and influence basic tissue functions, such as neuronal excitability, microcirculation, and metabolism. Under pathologic conditions the neuropeptides can be released from the receptive endings of these afferent fibers and influence the pathologic process.

To date, no neuropeptide has been found that is specific for afferent fibers from muscle. Dorsal root ganglion cells projecting in a muscle nerve have been shown to contain SP, CGRP, and somatostatin (SOM) and thus present a peptide pattern similar to that of cutaneous nerves.[92]

Some of the events that take place in and around a free nerve ending in muscle during its activation by a noxious mechanical stimulus are shown in Figure 2-7. The stimulus deforms the ending and thus opens ion channels that are present in its membrane; the resulting ion flux across the membrane leads to a membrane depolarization (the receptor potential). The difference in membrane potential between the stimulated (depolarized) ending and the afferent fiber drives a current that depolarizes the afferent fiber to its threshold and elicits a propagated action potential in that fiber, if the current is strong enough. Small currents lead only to a transient depolarization of the afferent fiber without generating action potentials; this is the typical nonpropagated effect of a subthreshold stimulus.

The neuropeptides present in group IV muscle afferents (e.g., SP, CGRP, SOM) are stored in small vesicles that are localized in expanded portions of the ending (the so-called varicosities). The peptides are released on activation of the ending and influence structures in its vicinity. As SP and CGRP have strong vascular and other cellular actions, the peptides influence the biochemical environment of the receptors from which they are released. Actually, it has been shown that the bulk of SP, after its production in dorsal root ganglion cells, is not transported to the spinal cord but to the peripheral endings.[9] The release of this neuropeptide from nociceptive endings triggers a cascade of events that result in neurogenic inflammation, i.e., a sterile inflammation that is caused by antidromic neuronal activity in sensory nerve fibers via the release of endogenous substances with vascular and cellular actions.[35, 72] Antidromic activity means that the action potentials propagate against the normal (afferent) direction; i.e., in sensory neurons the action potentials course in the periphery and release the above substances from the receptive ending. This means that a nociceptor not only is a passive sensor of noxious stimuli but also is capable of changing the chemical composition of the environment as part of its reaction to a tissue-threatening stimulus.

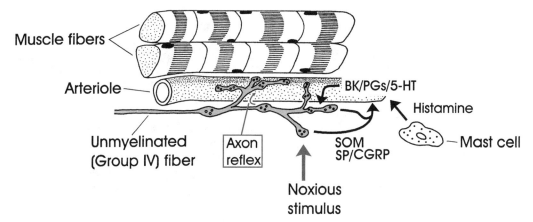

Figure 2-7. Events occurring in and around a nociceptor during noxious stimulation. An unmyelinated nerve fiber is shown terminating as a free nerve ending in the wall of an arteriole. In the expansions (varicosities) of the terminal fiber are mitochondria and vesicles containing neuropeptides: substance P *(SP)*, somatostatin *(SOM)*, and calcitonin gene-related peptide *(CGRP)*. A noxious stimulus may be a mechanical one that leads to a membrane depolarization by deforming the ending or may be a chemical one that leads to a depolarization by binding to receptor molecules on the ending and thus causing ion fluxes across the membrane or metabolic changes in the cytoplasm. The mechanical stimulus can also act indirectly on the ending by releasing endogenous algesic substances from the blood (e.g., bradykinin *(BK)*, prostaglandins *(PGs)*, or serotonin (5-hydroxytryptamine *[5-HT]*). If the depolarization is strong enough, action potentials are elicited in the afferent axon.

Activation of the nociceptor is associated with the release of the substances stored in the varicosities of the ending. SP causes vasodilation and an increase in vascular permeability. SP also degranulates mast cells; the released histamine likewise is a vasodilator. Action potentials elicited at one terminal of the ending can invade nonactivated branches of the same ending (axon reflex) and liberate substances from those branches.

CGRP and SP are particularly effective in inducing vasodilation and increasing the permeability of the microvasculature, with SP exerting its vascular effects partly via the liberation of histamine from mast cells (Fig. 2-7). All these substances diffuse to neighboring free nerve endings, leading to an expansion of the area affected by a localized stimulus.

The action potentials elicited by the noxious stimulus travel via the afferent fiber not only to the spinal cord but also into nonactivated branches of the same ending. This process is called an axon reflex (Fig. 2-7); it releases substances from the branch invaded by the action potential and thus likewise contributes to the expansion of the affected tissue volume.

The noxious stimulus influences not only afferent nerve endings but also blood vessels in the adventitia of larger vessels, where the afferent fibers are located. The blood vessels may be damaged directly by the stimulus, or their permeability may be increased by the release of SP. In both cases, fluid and proteins shift from the intravascular into the interstitial space. This process releases vasoneuroactive substances: bradykinin (BK) from protein (kallidin) in the blood plasma, serotonin (5-hydroxytryptamine [5-HT]) from platelets, and PGs (particularly PGE_2) from endothelial and other tissue cells. All these substances increase the sensitivity of nociceptors. Thus, the main tissue alteration induced by a nondestructive noxious mechanical stimulus is a localized region of edema that contains sensitized nociceptors.

Whether a particular neuropeptide or combination of neuropeptides is associated with a particular type of muscle receptor is still unknown. Data from experiments in which individual dorsal root ganglion cells were first identified functionally and then injected with a dye indicate that many cell bodies whose peripheral processes terminate in muscle nociceptors exhibit CGRP-like immunoreactivity (Fig. 2-8). It has to be emphasized, though, that such a reaction was found not only in nociceptive units but also in other types of muscle afferent units, such as those originating in low-threshold mechanosensitive (LTM) receptors. The only condition for the presence of CGRP-like immunoreactivity seemed to be that the afferent unit had a small cell body and/or a low conduction velocity. This finding suggests that CGRP may be present in many thin myelinated or unmyelinated muscle afferent units irrespective of their sensory function.[47b]

Of the above-mentioned neuropeptides, SP is of particular interest because apparently it can modulate pain sensations.[11, 25] In primary afferent fibers it coexists with CGRP[59]; both peptides are presumably released together when the fiber is active. In the spinal cord, CGRP has been reported to prolong the action of SP by inhibiting its degradation[71] and to facilitate synaptic transmission in general by enhancing the calcium influx into afferent fibers.[111] In cutaneous afferent fibers, a close correlation between the presence of SP and a nociceptive function appears to exist: In a recent study, all cutaneous afferents showing SP immunoreactivity were found to be nociceptive.[69a]

The role of SP and CGRP in the mediation of muscle pain is a matter of discussion. In comparison with skin nerves,

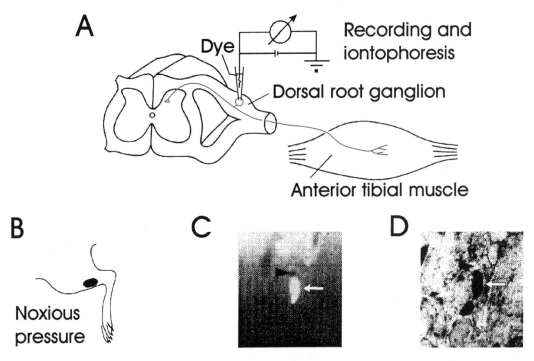

Figure 2-8. Identification of the neuropeptide, calcitonin gene-related peptide (CGRP), in a nociceptive muscle afferent unit. **Panel A.** Impulse activity of a single dorsal root ganglion (DRG) cell is recorded intracellularly by using a micropipette filled with a fluorescent dye (tip diameter of the pipette less than 1 μm). The ending in the anterior tibial muscle is tested with a variety of innocuous and noxious stimuli for determining the receptive properties of the unit. After functional identification the cell body is injected with the dye by passing an iontophoretic current through the pipette. **Panel B.** Location of the receptive field of the unit in the anterior tibial muscle. The cell required noxious local pressure for activation. Pinching of the skin alone had no effect. **Panel C.** Photomicrograph of the fluorescent cell body in a section of the DRG. The cell body is marked with a *white arrow*. **Panel D.** Same section as in **Panel C** after incubation with antibodies to CGRP coupled to horseradish peroxidase as a marker. The dark color of the injected and neighboring cells indicates the presence of CGRP.

muscle nerves appear to contain much less SP and CGRP.[79] This finding has been teleologically explained by assuming that the vasodilation and plasma extravasation caused by the release of the peptides from afferent fibers in skeletal muscle could be deleterious for muscle tissue because it is surrounded by a fascia. Because of the fascia, muscle edema, which increases interstitial pressure, can cause ischemia and muscle necrosis,[80] as seen in a compartment syndrome. Red muscles are possibly more endangered because they contain more SP than do white muscles.[129]

5. Physiologic Properties of Muscle Nociceptors

A nociceptor is a receptive ending activated by noxious (tissue-threatening, subjectively painful) stimulation and, by its response behavior, is capable of distinguishing between innocuous and noxious stimuli. As an additional feature, the nociceptor may have a high stimulation threshold; this feature is useful for the recognition of nociceptors in experiments employing mechanical or thermal stimuli.[12, 99, 100] For a review of nociceptive mechanisms, see Besson and Chaouch.[6]

The stimulus intensity required for activating a muscle nociceptor is usually lower than that for causing persistent tissue damage. In an animal experiment, a muscle nociceptor can be activated repeatedly, e.g., by squeezing the muscle, without producing a hematoma. This aspect is important for understanding the role of nociceptors as a warning system. The receptors are not supposed to signal the presence of tissue damage but instead are supposed to prevent damage by informing the central nervous system that the tissue in which they are situated is approaching its structural or functional limits.

Viscera can be strongly lesioned by knife cuts or burning, without causing subjective pain, if the stimulated area is kept small. One possible explanation for this finding is that cuts and burns will surely excite visceral receptors, but as the innervation density of viscera is low, the afferent activity generated by the few activated receptors is not sufficient to elicit subjective sensations.

It is a common clinical experience that in skeletal muscle, too, not every lesion elicits pain. Examples are movements of an electromyographic (EMG) needle inside a muscle or dissecting procedures during open muscle biopsies, many of which the patient does not perceive as painful. This phenomenon may be due to the fact that the innervation density of that part of the muscle is so low that small lesions can occur without affecting sensory receptors. In contrast to the viscera, however, where pain is elicited only if a certain degree of afferent activity is reached in a larger population of receptors, the EMG needle moving in muscle will eventually hit a nociceptor (or a nerve fiber bundle containing nociceptive afferents) and thus elicit pain.

Recordings of the electrical activity of single muscle afferent units in various species have shown that skeletal muscle nociceptors (in the sense of the above definition) are present. Figure 2-9 shows schematically this method of recording. If tested with a variety of different natural stimuli (mechanical and chemical), these receptors do not respond to everyday stimuli, such as weak local pressure, contractions, and stretches within the physiologic range, but instead require high intensities of stimulation to become activated (Fig. 2-10).[87, 97] (For details of the presentation of electrophysiologic data used in this book, see Figure 2-11.) Judging from their conduction velocity, most of the nociceptive afferent units have unmyelinated fibers and, therefore, can be expected to terminate in free nerve endings.

The discharges of muscle nociceptors elicited by noxious mechanical stimulation often outlast the duration of the stimulus; i.e., the receptors exhibit afterdischarges (Fig. 2-10, noxious pressure). The afterdischarges have a duration of a few seconds to several minutes, depending on the intensity of stimulation; these discharges might be the reason for the subjective aftersensations following strong noxious stimulation. The mechanism underlying the generation of afterdischarges is unknown; possible explanations are mechanical damage to the axon membrane of the receptive ending or release of endogenous excitatory sub-

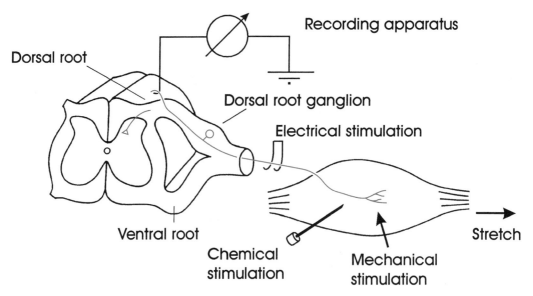

Figure 2-9. Experimental setup used for recording the impulse activity of single muscle nociceptors in anesthetized cats and rats. Small filaments of the dorsal root (or muscle nerve) were dissected by hand under the microscope and put over wire electrodes for recording unitary action potentials. The afferent unit under study was characterized by electrical stimulation of the muscle nerve for determining the fiber's conduction velocity and by natural (mechanical, chemical) stimulation of the receptive ending in the muscle for determining the physiologic function of the unit. Chemical noxious stimulation included intra-arterial (into the muscle artery) and intramuscular injections of bradykinin into the region where the nerve ending was located.

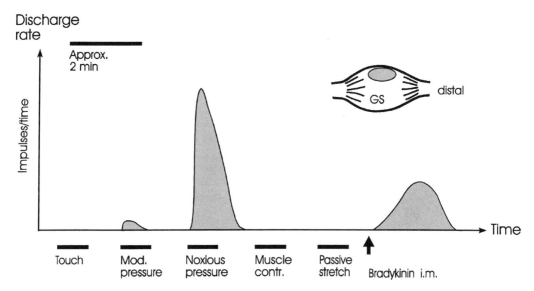

Figure 2-10. Typical discharges of a nociceptor in the gastrocnemius-soleus *(GS)* muscle in the cat. The data were obtained using the technique shown schematically in Figure 2-9. On the *ordinate*, the discharge rate of the ending is plotted against time on the *abscissa*. The *filled bars* underneath the *abscissa* mark the time and duration of the stimuli applied to the receptive field (*light red area* in **insert**) or to the muscle as a whole. *Touch*, touching the receptive field repeatedly with an artist's brush; *Mod. pressure*, innocuous local pressure exerted on the receptive field with forceps with broadened tips; *Noxious pressure*, squeezing the receptive field with the forceps at an intensity perceived as painful when applied to the thenar muscle of the experimenter; *Muscle contr.*, contractions induced by electrically stimulating the GS muscle nerve (every second a tetanic contraction of 50 Hz and a duration of 0.5 second was elicited); *Passive stretch*, innocuous stretch (6 mm); *Bradykinin i.m.*, injection of bradykinin 17.2 µg in 0.2 mL saline into the receptive field of the unit at the time marked by the *arrow*. The receptive field of an afferent unit is that body region from which the unit can be activated by external stimuli. It probably coincides mostly with the terminal branches of the receptive ending. Note that the receptor gave clear responses to painful stimuli only.

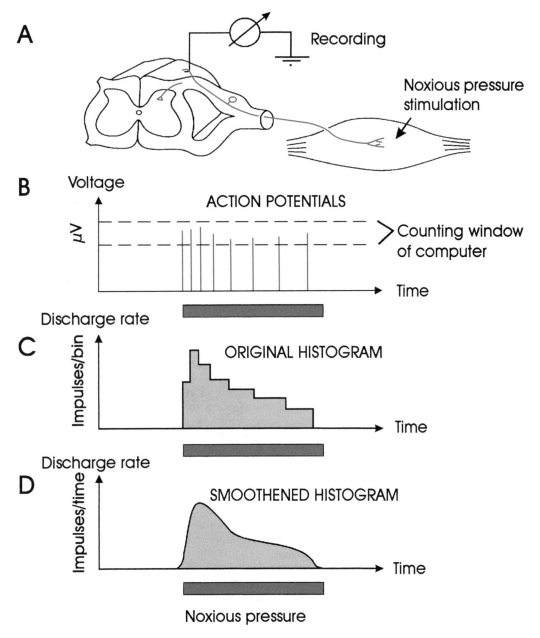

Figure 2-11. Technique used for recording the impulses of single nociceptors, as shown in Figure 2-10, and for constructing the smoothened histograms of the receptor activity, which are used throughout the book for depicting neuronal activity. **Panel A.** Experimental setup. The impulse activity of the receptive ending was recorded from its central branch in the dorsal root. A thin filament of the root containing the branch was put over a hook electrode that was connected to an amplifier. **Panel B.** Schematic reproduction of an original recording during noxious pressure stimulation of the receptive ending, maintained for the duration indicated by the *bar* underneath the *abscissa*. Each *vertical line* represents an action potential. The counting window accepts only those electrical events whose peaks lie within the window. **Panel C.** Schematic reproduction of the original histogram of the receptor's activity. The histogram was constructed by a computer that sampled the impulses for a given time (the bin width) and displayed the sum of the impulses per bin on the *ordinate*. **Panel D.** Smoothened histogram as shown in Figure 2-10 and others. The histogram was constructed by smoothening the step-like borderlines of the original histogram.

stances from tissue cells or the nerve ending by the stimulus (see below).

Particularly effective stimulants for free nerve endings are endogenous pain-producing or algesic substances[41] such as BK, 5-HT, and high concentrations of potassium ions.[31, 33, 62, 65, 68] The nonapeptide BK is cleaved from its precursor molecule kallidin if pathologic deviations from the normal environmental conditions occur (e.g., lowering in pH, ischemia, blood clotting). As kallidin is part of the plasma proteins, BK is ubiquitously present in the organism. 5-HT is released from platelets following vascular damage, and large amounts of potassium are present in the sarcoplasm of muscle cells. BK and 5-HT also have strong actions on blood vessels. These agents, therefore, have been called "vasoneuroactive substances."[117]

The effects of BK and other chemical stimulants on nerve endings are mediated by specific molecular receptors that are located on the surface of the nerve membrane. Binding of the stimulant to the receptor molecule results either in the opening of an ion channel or in changes in the state of activation of intracellular second messenger systems such as cyclic adenosine monophosphate (cAMP) and protein kinases. One possible sequel of the activation of these messengers is the activation (phosphorylation) of ion channel molecules. Collectively, these events may lead to direct excitation of the ending or to a modulation of the reaction of the nerve ending to external stimuli.

The discharges evoked in nerve endings by BK are mainly caused by the activation of the BK receptor molecule B_2, whereas under pathologic conditions the receptor B_1 is of greater importance. Likewise, different receptor molecules have been identified for PGs. For example, the sensitization of nerve endings by PGE_2 to BK has been shown to be due to activation of the EP_3 receptor molecule, one of the receptors for this type of PG (for a review of receptor molecules mediating the effects of pain-producing substances, see Kumazawa[67]). It is often overlooked that the above substances, particularly BK, excite not only nociceptors but also non-nociceptive endings with group III and IV afferent fibers.[81] BK, there-fore, cannot be considered a specific excitant of nociceptors. Nociceptors with nonmyelinated fibers, however, appear to be activated by lower concentrations of BK than are non-nociceptive receptors.[122] Muscle receptors with group I and II afferents (e.g., muscle spindles and tendon organs) are not excited by doses of BK sufficient to activate group III and IV receptors.

The doses of pain-producing substances required for the activation of muscle nociceptors in animal experiments are similar to those eliciting pain in humans on intra-arterial or intracutaneous and subcutaneous injection.[16, 74] The same applies to the time course of activation (latency and duration), which resembles closely the time course of painful sensations in humans. These findings support the assumption that chemically induced pain in humans is caused by activation of that subset of free nerve endings that were classified as nociceptors in animal experiments.

The typical muscle nociceptor responds to both noxious local pressure and close arterial or intramuscular injections of BK (see Fig. 2-10), but in animal experiments, receptors that are activated by only one type of noxious stimulation (mechanical or chemical) can also be found. This finding may indicate that different types of nociceptors are present in skeletal muscle, similar to the skin wherein mechano-, mechano-heat, and polymodal nociceptors have been reported to exist.[6, 12]

An unexpected experimental finding was that some nociceptive units in cat and rat muscle had two receptive fields; i.e., they could be activated from two separate areas in the muscle. In the deep tissues of the cat tail, afferent units were found that had one receptive field in deep tissues (muscle or joint) and another one in the skin distal to the deep receptive field.[89] The anatomic basis of this feature probably is branching of the afferent fiber close to the area of termination. Anatomic and neurophysiologic studies[20, 104] have shown that afferent units with dividing peripheral axons are relatively rare but may be functionally relevant, in that they likely reduce the spatial resolution of the nociceptive system and thus could contribute to the diffuse nature of muscle pain.

In tissues other than muscle (joint, skin, viscera), so-called silent, unresponsive or "sleeping" nociceptors have been described.[40, 42, 44] In these experiments, the receptor activity was recorded from dorsal root fibers or filaments of the peripheral nerve. The investigators found that these receptors cannot be activated by mechanical stimuli under normal conditions, but that if the tissue is inflamed, the endings respond readily to local stimuli, such as pressure stimulation, joint movement, or urinary bladder distension. The afferent input from the newly recruited receptors may have an enhancing effect on pain sensations because it leads to spatial summation in dorsal horn neurons. Whether such receptors are present in skeletal muscle is unexplored.

6. Interactions Between Stimulants at the Receptive Nerve Ending

Strong interactions exist between endogenous algesic substances with respect to their stimulating effects on nerve endings. Thus, PGE_2 and 5-HT have been shown to enhance the excitatory action of BK on slowly conducting muscle afferent units (Fig. 2-12).[82] The pain elicited in volunteers by intramuscular injection of a combination of BK and 5-HT is likewise stronger than that caused by each stimulant alone.[55] Conversely, BK is known to increase the synthesis and release of PGE_2 from various types of tissue.[58] By this mechanism, BK is capable of potentiating its own action[30]; i.e., in the presence of PGE_2 the action of BK is enhanced in a more than additive way. These interactions are probably clinically important because in damaged tissue the substances are released together. Therefore, the potentiation of the BK effects has to be considered the rule and not the exception.

Data from animal experiments show that the concentration of PGE_2 and 5-HT required for potentiating the BK action on muscle receptors is lower than that for exciting the receptive ending. In the beginning of a pathologic tissue alteration, when the concentrations of sensitizing agents are increasing, the receptive endings will probably be sensitized first and then excited. This assumption is consistent with the clinical observation that in the course of a pathologic alteration the patient first experiences tenderness (the result of nociceptor

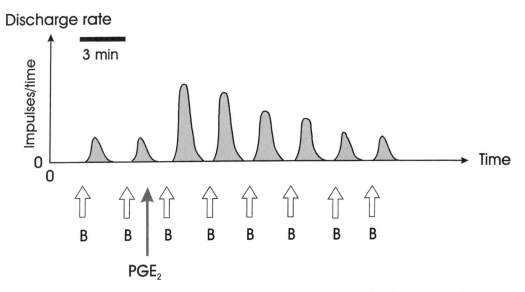

Figure 2-12. Potentiation by prostaglandin E_2 (PGE$_2$) of the responses of a free nerve ending to bradykinin (B). Intra-arterial injections of a painful dose of bradykinin (26 μg in 0.3 mL saline) were given every 3 minutes, and the responses of the muscle receptor were recorded. After the second response an intervening injection of PGE$_2$ (30 μg) was given. The PGE$_2$ in the dose applied did not excite the receptor but sensitized it to following injections of bradykinin.

sensitization [see Section A7]) and then spontaneous pain (the result of nociceptor excitation).

Because the half-time of PGs in living tissue is short, the "release" of PGE_2 by BK probably reflects an increase in the *de novo* synthesis of PGs by BK.[17, 60] From the above data it must be concluded that there is a PG component in the BK-induced activations of muscle nociceptors. Consequently, it should be possible to decrease the BK-induced excitations by blocking the PG synthesis with nonsteroidal anti-inflammatory drugs such as acetylsalicylic acid (ASA).[29, 126] Single fiber recordings in anesthetized cats have shown that this is the case: Systemic administration of ASA strongly reduces the stimulating effects of BK on muscle receptors with unmyelinated afferent fibers (Fig. 2-13).[83] These experiments demonstrate unequivocally a peripheral site of action of ASA.

7. Sensitization of Nociceptors as the Peripheral Neurophysiologic Basis of Tenderness

Besides the above-mentioned interactions between chemical stimulants, which lead to an increased sensitivity of the ending to chemical stimuli, there are influences that increase the mechanical sensitivity of a nociceptor. Among other substances (e.g., PGs of the E type), BK is capable of sensitizing muscle nociceptors to mechanical stimuli. This process is associated with a decrease in the mechanical threshold of the receptor so that it responds to everyday mechanical stimuli, such as weak local pressure (Fig. 2-14). The receptor is still connected to nociceptive pathways and, therefore, will elicit subjective pain when activated by weak mechanical stimulation.

The sensitization of the receptor shown in Figure 2-14 was quite specific, in that the sensitivity to local pressure stimulation increased but the sensitivity to stretch and active contractions did not. Other nociceptors exhibited a preferential sensitization to stretch and contractions. This sensitization of muscle nociceptors is probably the peripheral mechanism underlying the local tenderness and the pain on movement of a pathologically altered muscle. The above data suggest that tenderness and pain during movement may be mediated by different populations of receptors. (Essential to an understanding of the nature of

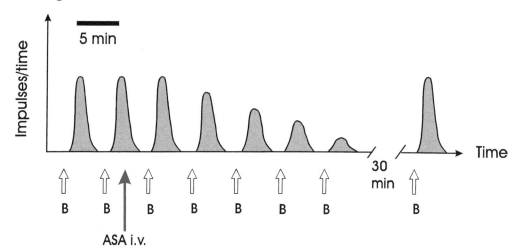

Figure 2-13. Reduction of the responses to bradykinin injections *(B)* by an intravenous injection of acetylsalicylic acid *(ASA i.v.)*. Experimental procedure and labeling are as in Figure 2-12. ASA was injected at a dose of 50 mg/kg body weight. Approximately 1 hour after administration of ASA, the magnitude of the response to bradykinin had returned to normal.

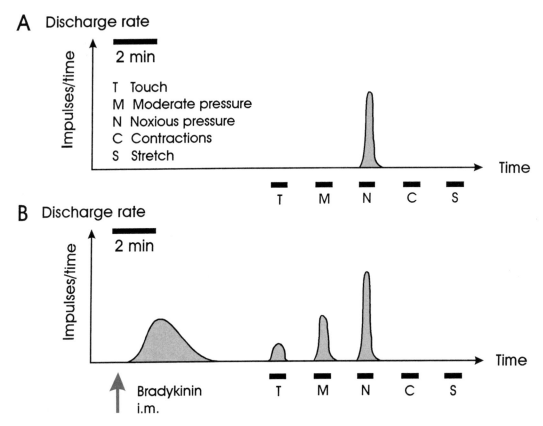

A   Discharge rate

2 min

T Touch
M Moderate pressure
N Noxious pressure
C Contractions
S Stretch

Time

T   M   N   C   S

B   Discharge rate

2 min

Time

Bradykinin
i.m.

T   M   N   C   S

Figure 2-14. Sensitization of a muscle nociceptor by bradykinin to mechanical stimuli. Bradykinin was injected intramuscularly *(bradykinin i.m.)* into the area where the receptive ending was located. **Panel A.** The receptor responded only to painful stimuli (noxious pressure). **Panel B.** Same sequence of stimuli as in **Panel A,** applied directly after bradykinin-induced activation. The receptor now behaves like a low-threshold mechanosensitive ending, in that it responds to touch and moderate pressure. These stimuli were completely ineffective before application of bradykinin. Procedure and labeling are as in Figure 2-10.

tenderness is the fact that there is also a central nervous mechanism of tenderness; see Chapter 7).

Recent data indicate that in the sensitization of nociceptors by PGE_2, a novel type of membrane channel, the tetrodotoxin-resistant (insensitive) sodium channel, is involved. Tetrodotoxin (TTX) is a powerful neurotoxin found in the Japanese puffer fish, which blocks sodium channels and thus inhibits conduction in nerve fibers. By increasing the level of cAMP in the nociceptive ending and activating protein kinase A, PGE_2 changes the TTX-resistant sodium channels so that the ion current passing through the channel is enhanced. Some evidence suggests that on a longer time scale, the number of receptors for sensitizing agents in the membrane of nociceptors increases. This applies particularly to the B_1 receptor, which is not important for the excitation of the normal ending, but in inflamed tissue the synthesis of the receptor is increased and BK now mainly acts by binding to the B_1 receptor (for a recent review on sensitization mechanisms, see Ref. 13a).

Leukotrienes (LTs) are likewise released from tissue cells under pathologic conditions, and some (e.g., LT B_4) have been shown to promote inflammatory processes and induce hyperalgesia in behavioral experiments.[105, 113, 114] Leukotriene D_4 appears to be the only LT whose influence on single muscle receptors has been tested so far.[47a, 85] The effect of this type of LT on rat muscle nociceptors was not sensitizing but desensitizing. The desensitization after infiltration of the receptive fields with 0.1 to 1.0 μg of LT D_4 expressed itself in a reduction of the response magnitude to mechanical stimulation. Whether this effect is associated with subjective hypoalgesia in humans is unknown. The increased synthesis of LTs by lipoxygenase following a drug-induced block of cyclo-oxygenase (COX-1 and COX-2) has been discussed as a mechanism that may contribute to the analgesic action of cyclo-oxygenase blockers such as ASA.[116]

Preliminary data obtained from single group IV fibers in an in vitro preparation (rat hemidiaphragm with its phrenic nerve attached [see Section B4 and Fig. 2-22]) indicate that SP in concentrations of 10 to 100 μM has an excitatory action on nociceptors but does not sensitize the receptors to mechanical stimuli.[107] In these experiments, the SP action expressed itself in an increase in background activity of the receptors. The response magnitude of the same ending to noxious mechanical stimulation, however, was not increased (Fig. 2-15). This finding clearly demonstrates that activation and sensitization of a receptive ending are independent of each other. Therefore, a nociceptor can be activated without being sensitized (this situation may lead to subjective pain without tenderness) or can be sensitized without being activated (this may lead to tenderness without spontaneous pain).

8. Free Nerve Endings in Muscle That Probably Do Not Fulfill Nociceptive Functions

Among the group III and IV muscle afferent units are many receptors that can be activated by weak deformations of the muscle (moderate local pressure, called low-threshold mechanosensitive [LTM] receptors), by physiologic stretch, or by contractions. Careful testing with a variety of mechanical stimuli in animal experiments excluded an origin of these nerve fibers in muscle spindles or tendon organs. It appears that relatively high proportions of the group III and IV units (including free nerve endings) comprise LTM receptors (Fig. 2-16, *Panel A*).[87]

This book distinguishes nociceptive and non-nociceptive receptors as two distinct populations. However, the LTM endings show larger responses to noxious

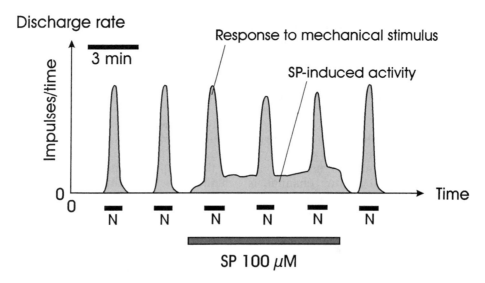

Figure 2-15. Effect of substance P *(SP)* on a single nociceptor in vitro. The receptor was stimulated with noxious local pressure *(N)* every 3 minutes and gave consistent responses to this stimulus. After the third stimulus, SP was added to the bathing solution for 9 minutes *(red bar)* so that a concentration of 100 μM SP resulted in the bath. The mechanically induced responses were not changed by SP, but the background (or resting) activity was increased as long as SP was present in the organ bath. Apparently, SP excited the nociceptor without sensitizing it, which would have produced larger responses to mechanical stimulation.

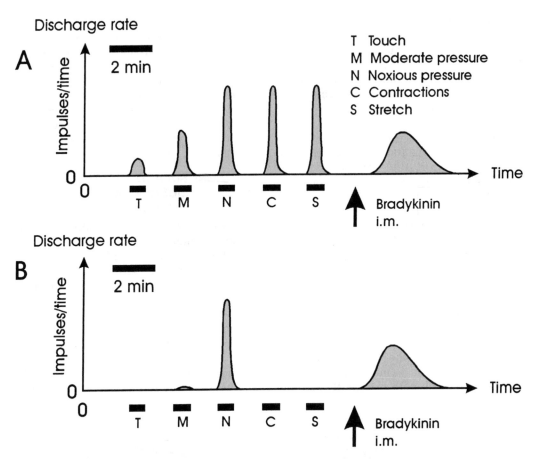

Figure 2-16. Typical discharges of a contraction-sensitive free nerve ending in the gastrocnemius muscle of the cat. **Panel A.** The non-nociceptive receptor responded in graded fashion to pressure stimulation and to active contractions and passive stretch. The force of the active contractions was adjusted to 50% maximal contraction (not painful); the stretch (6 mm) was likewise in the physiologic range. **Panel B.** Responses to the same stimuli of the nociceptor also shown in Figure 2-10. During muscle work, the receptor in **Panel A** is likely to be highly active, whereas the receptor in **Panel B** will be silent. Both receptors are excited by noxious mechanical and chemical stimuli. The responses of the contraction-sensitive receptor to noxious stimuli are considered as reflecting an activation of a non-nociceptive ending by a noxious (excessively strong) stimulus. Experimental procedure and labeling are as in Figure 2-10.

than to innocuous intensities of mechanical stimulation and thus are theoretically capable of distinguishing physiologic (innocuous) from tissue-threatening (noxious) stimuli. Such a response behavior may indicate a nociceptive function (see above). In the work of one of the authors (S.M.), the receptors were not classified as nociceptors, however, because their responses to innocuous stimuli reached a considerable percentage of the maximum discharge rate. These endings probably elicit strong central nervous effects during normal muscle activity, which is, of course, atypical for nociceptors. Non-nociceptive muscle receptors with large-diameter afferent fibers, such as muscle spindles, behave similarly, in that they exhibit a low mechanical threshold and maximum responses to noxious mechanical stimuli.

A particularly interesting subtype of non-nociceptive group III and IV muscle receptors are receptors that respond vigorously during active contractions and show an almost linear characteristic between muscle force and discharge rate.[63, 88] The existence of such "ergoreceptors" had been postulated by Kao[61] because of indirect evidence; they are supposed to mediate respiratory and circulatory adjustments during physical work. These receptors seemingly act like tendon organs, but the activity originating in tendon organs influences locomotion, not circulation.

Whether non-nociceptive group III and IV muscle receptors elicit subjective sensations is unknown. Judging from their response behavior, the LTM units could mediate pressure and force sensations from skeletal muscle and also from the tendon, where these endings are likewise present.[86] In fact, clinical experience shows that deep tissues underneath a completely denervated skin region are still sensitive to light pressure.[46]

The most frequent type found among group III units was the LTM receptor (44%), followed by nociceptive (33%) and contraction-sensitive units (23%; Fig. 2-17). Taken together, the presumably non-nociceptive units (the LTM and contraction-sensitive ones) made up approximately two thirds of the group III receptors.

In contrast to the group III units, the group IV units contained thermosensitive receptors that showed graded responses to temperature changes in the innocuous range. Among the endings with group IV afferent fibers, the nociceptive type was the most frequent (43%), and each of the other three types (LTM, contraction-sensitive, thermosensitive) occurred with the same frequency of 19%.

B. DIAGNOSIS AND TREATMENT OF LOCAL MUSCLE PAIN
1. Mechanical in Nature

Blow to Muscle. An impact to the muscle sufficiently forceful to activate nociceptors is painful. A minimal blow may activate nociceptors without causing damage to muscle fibers; a stronger blow of one knuckle impacting the deltoid muscle causes a temporarily painful lump that appears at the site of the blow and then subsides spontaneously within half an hour or so. This same phenomenon is observed when a muscle is impacted against the bone immediately postmortem.

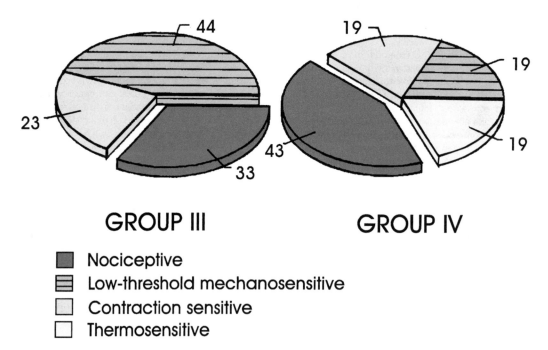

Figure 2-17. Percent distribution of receptor types among group III and IV muscle afferent units. The receptors are grouped according to the diameter of their afferent fibers: *group III*, thin myelinated; *group IV*, unmyelinated.

The pain associated with this phenomenon indicates that muscle nociceptors have been temporarily activated. Often, the pain outlasts the noxious stimulus. This may be the result of afterdischarges in nociceptors following a strong activation or of the release of substances from the activated nociceptive ending (e.g., SP). The cause of the transient swelling has not been clearly resolved; possibly it is local tissue edema plus activation of sarcomeres by release of calcium from damaged sarcoplasmic reticulum. Because this is a transient, self-limited condition, it requires no treatment.

Impacts that bruise the muscle and cause bleeding within the muscle belly result in local swelling, tenderness, and increased warmth that may remain for days and can be associated with a hematoma that may not appear as an ecchymosis for several days. The obvious evidence of tissue destruction and noninfectious inflammatory reaction indicates the release of substances that are capable of sensitizing nociceptors.

The immediate application of cold to and the elevation and support of the injured part help to reduce inflammatory reactions. In this simple situation, reducing these reactions expedites healing and increases comfort. In a day or two, after the initial local reaction to the trauma has subsided, application of warmth to the skin of the affected region and gentle use of the muscles facilitate tissue repair.

Rupture. A momentary overload that causes rupture (tearing) of the muscle or its tendon has been described for the pectoralis major,[76] peroneal,[18] gastrocnemius,[34, 78] plantaris, tibialis posterior,[24, 48] and extensor digitorum longus muscles.[101]

At the time a muscle ruptures, the patient is likely to be aware of a ripping or tearing sound and, in the case of muscles but not of tendons (see below), acute onset of local pain immediately followed by circumscribed swelling and tenderness. Several days later, local or distant ecchymosis may appear as a result of bleeding at the site of muscle tear. On examination, the deficit in muscle bulk or lack of palpable continuity of the tendon can often be identified at the site of the tear. The site will likely remain tender for a considerable time. In the case of tendon ruptures, the patient may not have noticed or may not remember the initial event. If the tibialis anterior tendon is torn, the patient may present with a complaint of the foot no longer fitting the shoe or of difficulty going up and down stairs.[48]

The pain of a ruptured muscle arises for the same reasons as from a blow to the muscle, but with more bleeding and tissue disruption. The latter will generally result in more ruptured blood vessels and the release of more sensitizing substances. As with a muscle bruise, a ruptured muscle is generally treated symptomatically to reduce inflammatory reaction and then to promote healing. It is rarely repaired surgically. In the case of a ruptured tendon, especially in the ankle region, however, surgical repair may be critically important to avoid muscle imbalance and serious disturbance of ambulation.

Hematoma. An occasional but distressing complication of anticoagulation therapy is a large, loculated, spontaneous, intramuscular hematoma. The iliopsoas muscle seems particularly vulnerable[124] and can develop a hematoma following minor trauma.[37] In these cases, the hematoma causes swelling, local pain, and tenderness, and can seriously compromise femoral nerve function. The diagnosis can be confirmed by ultrasound scanning or computed tomography.

Postexercise Muscle Soreness. Excessive or unaccustomed eccentric (lengthening) contractions cause postexercise muscle soreness. It commonly develops following unaccustomed descent from a mountain climb, lifting weights up and down, or any vigorous sport activity. Soreness and stiffness appear between 8 and 24 hours following unusual activity that requires lengthening contractions, peaks during the first day or two of discomfort, and usually resolves in 5 to 7 days. The muscle becomes slightly swollen, tender to palpation, restricted in stretch range of motion because of pain, and painful when voluntarily contracted with more than minimal effort.

The specific vulnerability of muscles to eccentric work (lengthening contractions) as compared with concentric work relates to the well-established difference in mechanical efficiency. Mechanical efficiency of concentric work in one study averaged barely 19%. During eccentric work, however, efficiency sometimes exceeded 100%, based on the energy expended and analysis of expired air.[66a] The muscle is able to exert more force with less effort, readily overloading the muscle structure.

In recent years, the blood chemistry and histologic changes associated with postexercise muscle soreness have been well studied. Blood lactic acid was unchanged following a bout of eccentric exercise. Most blood chemistry changes peaked within the first 24 hours following exercise, generally well before the peak intensity of muscle soreness. These changes included increases in plasma interleukin-1, total thiobarbituric acid-reactive substances, lactic dehydrogenase, serum creatine phosphokinase, aspartate aminotransferase, and serum glutamicoxaloacetic transaminase. Conversely, two commonly accepted indicators of muscle damage—the concentration of plasma creatine kinase and the muscle uptake of radioisotope technetium-99m pyrophosphate—did not peak until 5 or 6 days following the exercise. This was well beyond the peak of muscle soreness and stiffness.

Biopsies of human muscles exposed to exhausting eccentric exercise showed no abnormality of fiber organization or regeneration at the cellular level. Electron microscopic studies of changes at the subcellular level, however, showed characteristic changes. Severe disorganization of the striation pattern appeared within an hour following exercise and persisted for at least 3 days. Immediately following exercise, nearly half of the myofibrillar Z bands (which connect one sarcomere to the next) showed generalized broadening and streaming (scattered severe broadening). Some Z bands were totally disrupted. The sarcomeres associated with the affected Z bands were either excessively contracted or disorganized and out of register with the remaining Z bands. Seven days following exercise, much recovery had occurred in most studies. In one study of unusually severe eccentric exercise, myofibrillar necrosis, inflammatory cell infiltration, glycogen depletion, and lack of myofibrillar regeneration persisted for 10 days.[96a]

Immunocytologic examination for the intermediate filament protein, desmin, revealed abundant longitudinal desmin extensions and strongly autofluorescent granules, representing an increased synthesis of desmin and restructuring of the cytoskeletal system in the region of the Z bands. These changes peaked at 3 days, close to the time of maximum soreness.

Several studies of resting EMG activity after strenuous eccentric exercise showed no increase in average electrical activity in the exercised muscles through the first 3 days, during the peak of soreness. Thus, neither the shortening of the muscle nor its painfulness is attributed to muscle spasm.[8, 56, 57]

The above histochemical studies indicate that the primary lesion in postexercise soreness is disruption of the myofibrillar structure caused by mechanical overload rather than by metabolic disturbances. The tenderness and pain during movement are probably caused by a sensitization of muscle nociceptors. The sensitization is likely caused by substances that are released from the damaged tissue during the repair process. In this regard, the soreness resembles a sterile inflammation. Accumulation of lactate, as assumed previously, does not appear to play a role in the pain of postexercise soreness. This notion is supported by the finding that lactate is not an effective stimulant for muscle nociceptors.[66]

The course of postexercise soreness is remarkably unresponsive to therapeutic intervention. Most studies have shown that anti-inflammatory drugs provide little or no relief. This indicates that PGs are not involved in the sensitization of nociceptors in a sore muscle. Because PGE_2 may be important in muscle repair, PG blockers such as aspirin may be not only useless but also detrimental to restoration of the damaged contractile elements. Although gentle stretching of the muscle toward restoration of its normal stretch range of motion may temporarily ameliorate the degree of soreness, in a controlled study it had no effect on the overall course of muscle soreness.[93] (This topic was recently reviewed in more detail.[70, 124])

Local Trigger Point Tenderness. The tenderness to palpation located at a trigger point (TrP) site is usually a surprise to patients who have been unaware of it. The pain for which they seek relief was referred from this hyperirritable TrP in the muscle and is commonly associated with referred tenderness in the pain reference zone, which further confuses the picture.

The TrP is located at the point of maximum sensitivity along a palpable taut band in the muscle. A highly specific palpation technique is needed to locate the taut band. The taut bands of active TrPs characteristically respond to snapping palpation at the TrP with a local twitch response in muscles that are sufficiently superficial and accessible to this palpation technique. Pain caused by TrPs is dealt with in more detail in Chapter 8.

Repetitive Strain Injury. Repetitive strain, cumulative trauma, and overuse syndrome are common descriptors used to identify a group of patients who suffer from occupational myalgia. It is believed that the muscle pain is induced by muscular activity at work that is at or near their muscles' tolerance to the manner in which they perform the work. The many names used to describe this condition reflect the relative emphasis placed on the two basic activities responsible for the problem. One is holding the muscle in a relatively fixed position, often under load, for prolonged periods. The other is a repetitive movement that gives the muscle incomplete recovery time between movements.

Much frustration and confusion arise regarding the specific cause of the muscle pain, the appropriate terminology, and questions about the validity of the patient's distress. Despite the fact that the two conditions that produce muscle overload in occupational myalgia are well known to activate and perpetuate TrPs, papers dealing with this group of myalgias consistently ignore a possible TrP role. Fortunately, the emphasis placed on improved ergonomic practices is part of the appropriate management of TrPs. Practitioners who identify and address the TrP origin of the pain, when present, help the patient to a more rapid and thorough recovery. TrPs are reviewed in more detail in Chapter 8.

Painful Contractions of Normal Muscle. Voluntary contraction of an ischemic muscle becomes painful in approximately 1 minute and, if the ischemia is sufficient, becomes extremely painful. This pain is mediated almost exclusively by group IV (unmyelinated) nociceptive fibers (see Section B4 in this chapter). Conversely, there is little experimental evidence that muscle contraction without ischemia is painful. Sustained contraction of only 10% of maximum voluntary contraction for up to 1 hour can be pain-free. Sustained contraction of 30 to 40%, however, impairs circulation. During bicycle exercise, maximum blood flow occurs between 50[123] and 70%[14] of maximum workload. Beyond that degree of effort, the muscle begins to develop a degree of relative ischemia.

It is important here to clearly distinguish between muscle pain and muscle fatigue. Fatigue is measured as progressive reduction in force of maximum voluntary contraction and reduction in median frequency of the EMG. Although it takes more effort to activate a fatigued muscle, that alone does not make movement painful. Conversely, if the movement or position becomes painful with continued effort, the pain is likely to be described as fatigued, which it may or may not be if the muscle is measured for fatigue objectively.

The converse situation, hypoxia without muscle contraction, can become painful if the hypoxia produces algogenic substances that sensitize or excite local nociceptors. In experimental situations, one can see hypoxia-induced loss of nerve membrane potential sufficient to reach excitation threshold and initiate action potentials in nociceptors.

2. Metabolic Problems

Compromise of the energy supply for muscular contraction can cause muscle fatigue and pain. Usually, metabolic inadequacies that compromise energy supply are most likely to contribute to muscle pain indirectly by acting as aggravating and perpetuating factors to TrPs. A number of metabolic deficiencies cause sufficient impairment of muscle metabolism that they are primary causes of muscle pain. Two examples are McArdle's disease and hypothyroid disease.

McArdle's Disease.   McArdle's disease is a classic enzyme-deficiency disease. It is a genetic deficiency of myophosphorylase that seriously compromises glycolytic metabolism in the muscle. Type II fibers depend primarily on this type of metabolism. Pain for one individual tends to be proportional to the amount of exercise but may show a second-wind relief with continued effort.[102] Carnitine palmitoyltransferase deficiency shows a similar clinical picture but is caused by compromise of oxidative metabolism in the muscle mitochondria.

A distinctive feature of these diseases is the development of muscle contracture (activation of the muscle contractile mechanism without motor unit action potentials). In both conditions, failure of adequate recovery of calcium by the sarcoplasmic reticulum is implicated. This calcium recovery problem is the same mechanism that is thought to be involved in the formation of myofascial TrPs.

Hypothyroid Disease.   Abnormally low thyroid function is associated with muscle pain. This pain is attributable to an inadequate supply of energy for muscle contraction, since muscles are primarily energy engines and a primary function of thyroid hormone is the control of cellular metabolism.

3. Inflammatory Conditions

Experimentally Induced Inflammation. Data on the behavior of muscle receptors in inflamed muscle are available from the cat and rat. In these animals, an experimental myositis can be induced by infiltrating the triceps surae or other muscles with carrageenan, a sulfated polysaccharide. The carrageenan-induced myositis is thought to be a neurogenic inflammation mediated by the release of SP and other agents from nociceptive afferent units (see Section A4 in this chapter). In the knee joint of the rat, SP has been shown to have strong inflammatory actions.[69] In the case of a myositis, the inflammatory function of SP is questionable because of the reported low concentration of this peptide in skeletal muscle.

A few hours after a carrageenan injection, the muscle exhibits all signs of a myositis (hyperemia, edema, infiltration by polymorphonuclear leukocytes).[5] These changes are known to be associated with the release of vasoneuroactive substances, which appear in an inflamed rat paw in a temporal order, namely, 5-HT and histamine first (up to 1.5 hours after the carrageenan injection), then BK, and finally PGs (more than 2.5 hours after carrageenan).[23]

In the cat and rat, the inflammation-induced changes in the response behavior of slowly conducting muscle afferent units are qualitatively the same, although quantitative differences exist. The main effect of an inflammation on group III and IV muscle receptors appears to be an increase in resting activity. Both the proportion of units exhibiting resting discharge and the mean discharge frequency were higher in inflamed muscle.[5, 21]

A typical feature of the resting discharge was its irregular, often intermittent nature, with phases of bursting activity alternating with long periods of silence (Fig. 2-18). Such discharges are likely to cause (spontaneous) pain if they occur in nociceptive afferent units. An increased resting discharge was present not only in high-threshold mechanosensitive (HTM; presumably nociceptive) units but also in receptors responding to innocuous pressure. In inflamed tissue, the latter ones probably comprise both true LTM receptors and sensitized (originally high-threshold) units.

Another inflammation-induced change in the response behavior of muscle receptors was an increase in the proportion of receptors responding to weak mechanical stimuli. In normal muscle of the cat, approximately 80% of the group IV units required noxious pressure for activation; this proportion dropped significantly in inflamed muscle. A possible reason for this change is a sensitization of nociceptive (originally HTM) units, which have a lowered mechanical threshold in inflamed muscle and respond to weak stimuli such as innocuous local pressure. In Figure 2-19, a HTM (presumably nociceptive) unit is shown that lowered its mechanical threshold from noxious to innocuous pressure during development of the myositis. As the receptor is still connected to nociceptive spinal pathways, its activation by innocu-

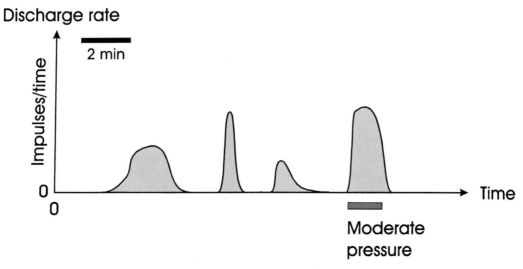

Figure 2-18. Background (resting) discharge of a free nerve ending in inflamed muscle. The recording was obtained from a group III unit whose receptive ending was situated in the carrageenan-inflamed gastrocnemius muscle of a cat. The intermittent nature of the ongoing discharges in the beginning of the recording is typical.[5] Notice that the peak frequency of the background discharge is approximately equal to that of the mechanically induced response at the end of the recording. Such an ongoing activity in a nociceptive unit may elicit the spontaneous pain of myositis or, if it occurs in non-nociceptive receptors, dysesthesia.

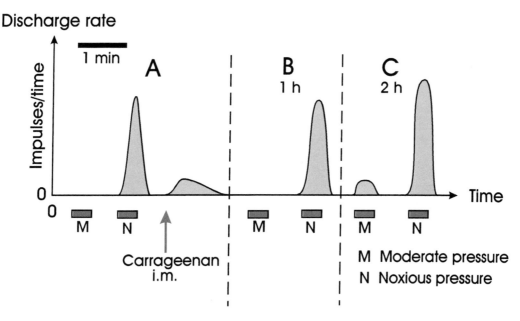

Figure 2-19. Sensitization to mechanical stimuli of a single nociceptor during the transition from normal to inflamed muscle. **Panel A.** Intact muscle before induction of the inflammation. The unit can be activated by noxious local pressure only and is also weakly excited by the intramuscular injection of carrageenan, which was used to induce the inflammation. **Panel B.** One hour after injection of carrageenan, the receptor still exhibits its normal sensitivity to local pressure, because the inflammation has not yet fully developed. **Panel C.** Two hours after injection of carrageenan, the receptor has lowered its mechanical threshold into the innocuous range and responds to moderate pressure. The activation of a nociceptive ending by weak stimuli may lead to the tenderness (and pain during movement) of an inflamed muscle.

ous stimuli will now elicit pain. This mechanism offers an explanation for the tenderness of inflamed muscle (and the pain during movements). Apparently, the tenderness is mainly caused by sensitization of group IV receptors, as the average mechanical threshold of group III units did not change significantly. In contrast, spontaneous pain and dysesthesias are probably caused by activity in group III units, as these were the only ones that showed a significant increase in resting activity in inflamed muscle.[5]

Irregular activity in the LTM (non-nociceptive) receptors might be responsible for the dysesthesias that often accompany a myositis and sometimes are the prominent subjective symptom.[19] In inflamed muscle, a true LTM receptor cannot be distinguished from a sensitized HTM unit that has become low-threshold. Therefore, the only way of telling how LTM receptors are influenced by a myositis is to record the

activity of such an ending during the transition from intact to inflamed muscle. Figure 2-20 shows an example of an LTM receptor recorded over a 3-hour period before and after induction of the myositis. Notice the increase in resting activity and the lowering in mechanical threshold from moderate pressure (innocuous deformation of the muscle) to touch (moving an artist's brush over the surface of the muscle).

The inflammation-induced sensitization of muscle receptors is probably caused by the release of vasoneuroactive substances from the inflamed tissue. Experimental evidence shows that PGs are involved in this process: Intravenous administration of ASA (known to block PG synthesis) strongly reduces the activity of group IV receptors in inflamed muscle.[21] Figure 2-21 shows a receptor in inflamed muscle that had a low mechanical threshold and a relatively high level of resting activity before injection of ASA. Approximately 30

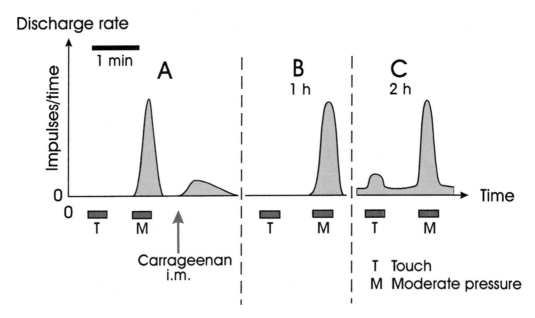

Figure 2-20. Inflammation-induced sensitization of a group IV non-nociceptive ending.[5] **Panel A.** Intact muscle. The receptor responds to moderate (innocuous) pressure stimulation but not to touching the surface of the muscle. Infiltration of the muscle with carrageenan leads to a transient discharge of low frequency. **Panel B.** One hour after injection of carrageenan, the receptor still has its original low-threshold mechanosensitive properties. **Panel C.** Two hours after injection of carrageenan, the receptor has acquired background activity and responds to touching the surface of the muscle. The increased activity of non-nociceptive endings in an inflamed muscle may be responsible for the dysesthesias that often accompany the pain of myositis.

Discharge rate

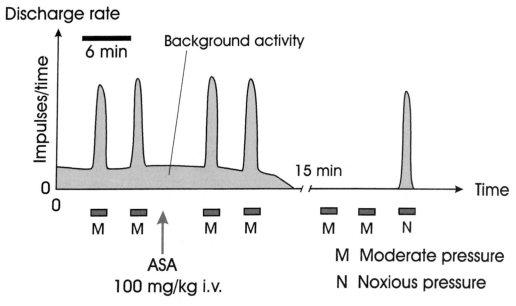

Figure 2-21. Reduction by acetylsalicylic acid (ASA) of the inflammation-induced activity of a free nerve ending.[21] In the beginning of the recording, the receptor exhibited background activity and responded twice to moderate (innocuous) pressure stimulation. Approximately 5 minutes after intravenous injection of ASA, the background activity started to decrease, but the mechanical threshold was unchanged. Half an hour later, the background activity was gone, and the receptor had a high mechanical threshold; i.e., the ending had regained the typical properties of a nociceptor. By abolishing the background activity and mechanical sensitization of nociceptors, ASA may alleviate the spontaneous pain and tenderness of inflamed muscle.

minutes after the injection, the resting activity was gone and the mechanical threshold was in the noxious range. In this case, administration of ASA abolished the sensitization of the ending and restored the typical properties of a nociceptor, namely, a lack of resting discharge and a high mechanical threshold. Other receptors, however, showed only a reduction in resting activity following administration of ASA, instead of a complete absence. Apparently, many sensitizing substances are acting simultaneously on the receptors, with ASA being capable of removing the influence of PGs only.

Another inflammatory substance of interest is SP. It seems that in the course of a neurogenic inflammation, SP can be released from nerve endings independent of their electrical activity.[49] The neuropeptide induces the release of histamine from tissue mast cells, which in turn may dilate muscular blood vessels (the vasodilating action of histamine in inflamed tissue is a matter of debate, however[4, 15, 49]).

Other substances probably involved in the induction and maintenance of inflammatory processes are CGRP and neurokinin A.[127] The results of a more recent study suggest that the local release of nitric oxide may be involved in the vasodilation of a carrageenan-induced inflammation.[52] The action of these latter substances on nerve endings in muscle is not yet established.

Myositis Including Infections and Infestations. The term "myositis" means inflammation of muscle, but it has two different forms. Most cases are infective and of bacterial pyogenic origin, commonly *Staphylococcus aureus*, which produces a classic inflammatory reaction. The muscle is tender and painful because of sensitization of muscle nociceptors (see Section A7 in this chapter). A much less common source of inflammation in the muscle is a parasitic infestation. Only one is likely to cause appreciable muscle pain: trichinellosis or trichinosis caused by *Trichinella spiralis* and acquired by eating inadequately cooked, infested pork or pork products, bear, or walrus meat.[50] After the ingested larvae mate, the gravid female burrows deep into the intestinal mucosa and discharges 500 to 1500 larvae, starting 1 to 6 weeks following infection, and continues for 2 to 4 weeks. Only larvae that reach muscle survive and increase in size approximately 10-fold over succeeding weeks, reaching 1.0 mm in diameter, which is visible with the naked eye.

Only heavily infected individuals develop recognizable symptoms of acute enteritis (abdominal discomfort and diarrhea) a day or two after ingestion. One to two weeks later, acute onset (severe cases) of fever, muscle pain and tenderness, weakness, malaise, bilateral periorbital edema, and headache follow. Sublingual, retinal, and subconjunctival petechiae and hemorrhage may be seen, sometimes with a macular, petechial, or urticarial rash. Diagnosis is most commonly made by a titer of 1 to 5 or more in the bentonite flocculation test. Since false-positives can occur, a positive reaction to one of the other four available tests is recommended. The skin test does not distinguish between past and present infection. Muscle biopsy results may be positive as early as the second week, but muscle biopsy is rarely required.[50]

Early treatment of the immature intestinal worms is effective, if detected, and advisable up to 6 weeks after infection. After that, treatment is symptomatic. Eating only well-cooked pork and pork products assures prevention.

Conversely, polymyositis is a rheumatologic disease that characteristically shows progressive proximal limb and neck muscle weakness, elevated muscle enzymes, inflammatory changes on muscle biopsy, and characteristic needle EMG abnormalities. It is considered an autoimmune disease with marked parallels to systemic lupus erythematosus and with paraneoplastic features. Many authors give the impression that muscle pain and tenderness is a variable and only moderately important symptom.

One article,[51] however, pointed out that pain and tenderness depend strongly on how rapidly the disease develops. Patients who present with a duration of around 4 weeks describe intense and unremitting pain and have exquisite tenderness in proximal and trunk musculature. Patients who present with symptoms that have fluctuated over a period of months have a modicum of muscle pain that they describe as soreness, aching, or cramping. Muscle pain and tenderness are not included among the symptoms characteristic of polymyalgia patients who present with a slowly progressing disease, often without skin involvement or other stigmata of autoimmune disease.

4. Vascular Impairment

Effects of Hypoxia on Muscle Receptors in Vitro. Some data on the behavior of single muscle receptors in ischemic muscle in vivo are available (see below, next section), but these data have the general disadvantage that they were obtained in the living animal, wherein the oxygen tension at the receptor site is usually unknown and cannot be controlled quantitatively.

For studies of the influence of a defined degree of hypoxia on the discharges of muscle receptors, an in vitro preparation is better suited. An example is the rat hemidiaphragm-phrenic nerve preparation. The preparation consists of a phrenic nerve together with one half of the diaphragm that is innervated by the nerve. The tissue is removed quickly from an anesthetized animal and mounted in a lucite chamber containing an organ bath for the diaphragm and an oil pool for the nerve. In this preparation, all of the physiologic parameters (temperature, ionic composition of the bathing solution, and the pressure of oxygen [pO_2] and carbon dioxide [pCO_2] in the organ bath) can be exactly controlled. The diaphragm containing the receptors is so thin that the gas tension at the receptor site is nearly identical with that in the bathing solution.

With the use of sharpened watchmaker's forceps, small filaments can be split from the phrenic nerve in the oil pool and put over a wire electrode for recording the action potentials of single fibers and thus single receptors. In the experiments that yielded the following results, fibers were classified as unmyelinated group IV units, if they conducted at less than 2.5 m/s, and as group III units, if they conducted at a velocity between 2.5 and 30 m/s. As pointed out above, most of the receptors formed by these fibers are probably free nerve endings.

The short conduction distance prevented exact determination of the conduction velocity of fast fibers (groups I and II). The identification of these units relied on their response behavior. Receptors were classified as primary endings of muscle spindles (supplied by Ia fibers) if they had a resting activity (discharges without mechanical stimulation) and displayed a marked differential behavior to stretching of the diaphragm. Differential behavior means that the receptor responded to a mechanical stimulus of maintained stretch with a strong initial discharge that slowly leveled down to the final impulse frequency. Secondary endings from muscle spindles (supplied by group II fibers) lacked this differential behavior; they are not addressed in this section.

Mechanical pressure stimulation of the endings in the diaphragm was performed with an artist's brush and a set of von Frey hairs that had been calibrated by using an analytic scale. Putting the tips of the hairs on the diaphragm with slight pressure so that the hairs bent identified the force being exerted on the muscle. Group III and IV units were classified as LTM, if they were clearly excited by touching or slightly stroking the diaphragm with the brush, and as HTM or nociceptive, if they required firm pressure with the handle of the brush or "stabbing" with the hairs of the brush to be excited. The borderline between LTM and HTM receptors corresponded to a von Frey threshold of approximately 0.7 p (p = pond; 1 p is the force a mass of 1 g exerts under the influence of earth's gravity). In this case, the force was exerted with a von Frey hair that was calibrated by putting its tip vertically on a scale and pushing downward until the hair bent. The force required for bending the hair is read off the scale. When the hair is pressed with its tip on the diaphragm until it bends, it exerts approximately the same pressure. The stimulating pressure of such a hair is rela-tively high because its tip is almost punctate. In the organ bath, hypoxia was induced by gassing it with 95% N_2 and 5% CO_2, resulting in a pO_2 of approximately 20 mm Hg. Normally, the bath was gassed with carbogen (95% O_2 plus 5% CO_2), resulting in a pO_2 of 390 mm Hg.

Responses of Free Nerve Endings in the Diaphragm to Hypoxia. Most of the group III and IV units were excited by prolonged hypoxia in the organ bath. This excitation occurred irrespective of the mechanical threshold of the endings; i.e., LTM and HTM units responded in a similar way to hypoxia. An example is shown in Figure 2-22. The afferent group IV fiber had two receptive fields in the diaphragm (*hatched area* in Figure 2-22A). The mechanical threshold of the left receptive field, determined with von Frey hairs, was between 0.7 and 1.3 p, while that of the right receptive field was between 1.4 and 1.5 p. The receptor was silent in the absence of experimental stimulation; it did not respond to innocuous mechanical stimulation. Because of its response behavior, the ending was classified as nociceptive. After more than 10 minutes of hypoxia, it started to fire and exhibited an intermittent pattern of discharge with high-frequency bursts alternating with periods of a low-frequency discharge (Fig. 2-22, *Panel B*).

This type of discharge is typical of a nociceptor in a pathologic environment; it was also observed in nociceptive endings in inflamed muscle. The relatively high frequency of the hypoxia-induced discharge is likely to cause pain in an awake animal. The increase in discharge rate is not a sign of irreversible damage to the receptor, since it could be abolished (restored to normal) by regassing the bath to normal oxygen tension. The mechanical thresholds of many of the HTM receptors decreased during hypoxia. In some cases, the von Frey threshold dropped from more than 1 p, which is clearly noxious, to less than 0.7 p, which is normally in the innocuous range. This means that hypoxia must be considered a sensitizing factor for nociceptors: Under hypoxia, they can be excited by innocuous mechanical stimuli. In the living and awake organism, this sensitization is likely to cause tenderness.

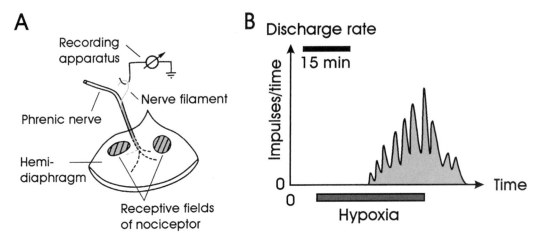

Figure 2-22. Excitation of a nociceptive nerve ending by hypoxia in vitro. **Panel A.** Rat hemidiaphragm-phrenic nerve preparation. From the phrenic nerve, small filaments are dissected and put over a wire electrode for recording of discharges in single nerve fibers. The hatched areas (light red) on the diaphragm are the two receptive fields whose mechanical stimulation at noxious intensities excited the group IV fiber under study. **Panel B.** Response to hypoxia of the nociceptive ending whose receptive fields are shown in **Panel A**. The period of hypoxia (oxygen tension approximately 20 mm Hg) is marked by the red bar underneath the abscissa. After approximately 10 minutes of hypoxia, the receptor was excited and continued discharging for approximately 30 minutes.

Effects of Hypoxia on Muscle Spindles.

Because most of the muscle spindles studied had a resting discharge, both excitations and depressions could be studied. The responses of muscle spindles to hypoxia were rather homogeneous, in that the majority (8 of 13 tested) fell silent after a few minutes of hypoxia. An example is shown in Figure 2-23. The Ia afferent being recorded had a regular resting discharge. Hypoxia in the bath led to complete silence in the afferent fiber after approximately 5 minutes. Restoration of normal pO_2 was followed by a sudden reappearance of the discharge of the receptor. A second period of hypoxia approximately 10 minutes after the first one had the same effect, except that the unit stopped firing earlier (after approximately 2 minutes of hypoxia). When the oxygen supply was normalized again, the unit resumed its resting activity, but the discharge rate now showed fluctuations that are not normal in muscle spindle afferents. Apparently, the two periods of hypoxia had damaged the ending to such a degree that it did not recover completely afterward. The other spindle afferents, which did not exhibit the complete depression shown in the figure, either were not affected or were weakly activated by hypoxia.

From these experiments, it is apparent that the main effect of a severe hypoxia on primary endings of a majority of muscle spindles is a depression or cessation of their discharge. This depression probably has two central nervous actions: (1) It reduces the excitatory drive on homonymous α-motor neurons (which have monosynaptic connections with Ia afferents) and therefore is a relaxing factor for the muscle, and (2) it will impair motor coordination, since, during the depression of the spindle discharges, the motor centers do not receive the information on muscle length that they need to coordinate movements.

Collectively, the data obtained from the in vitro preparation suggest that severe hypoxia of a muscle causes muscle pain and tenderness by exciting or sensitizing free nerve endings and causes impairment of motor coordination by depressing muscle spindle primary endings.

Responses of Free Nerve Endings in Muscle to Ischemia and Ischemic Contractions. *Effects of Ischemia Without Contractions.* Interruption of the blood supply to a resting extremity for prolonged periods of time (20 minutes) is not painful[73] and does not evoke cardiovascular reflexes.[120] Ischemia alone is likewise not an effective stimulus for slowly conducting muscle afferent units unless it lasts for long periods of time. Ligation of an artery to a resting muscle for 5 minutes in anesthetized cats did not activate muscle group III and IV receptors.[88]

Following a longer-lasting complete interruption of the blood supply (experimentally induced by circulatory arrest), most of the slowly conducting muscle afferent units developed a bursting background activity 15 to 60 minutes after onset of ischemia. The increase in activity lasted for periods of several minutes up to half an hour, then the units fell silent and could no longer be activated by electrical stimulation of the muscle nerve.[84] The latter finding indicates that the ischemia affected not only the receptive ending but also the afferent fiber. The lack of energy associated with the ischemia possibly led to a progressive depolarization of the axonal membrane, which caused transient activation when the membrane potential approached threshold potential and later produced a block of the action-potential generating system when the

membrane potential decreased further. BK is probably involved in nociception from an ischemic muscle. The kinin is released from plasma proteins during ischemia[38, 95, 118] and, because of its strong action on nociceptors, likely contributes to ischemic pain.

In humans, examples of muscle pain caused by ischemia are acute cases of compartment syndrome, which is characterized by increased pressure (resulting, for example, from inflammation or hematoma) in a muscle ensheathed by a tight fascia. The high intrafascial pressure leads to occlusion of blood vessels in the muscle. An additional factor for the elicitation of pain under these circumstances probably is the mechanical stimulation of nociceptors sensitized by the hypoxia and/or the release of BK and other endogenous substances.

Ischemic Contractions. If a muscle in awake humans is forced to contract under ischemic conditions, pain develops within approximately 1 minute.[73] Bessou and Laporte[7] were the first to show that during ischemic contractions, muscle group IV afferent units are activated. They recorded the compound action potential of many

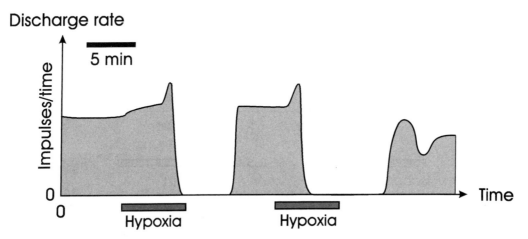

Discharge rate

Figure 2-23. Effects of hypoxia on a muscle spindle primary ending in vitro. The data were obtained from a preparation as shown in Figure 2-22**A**. Prior to hypoxia, the receptor had a regular discharge frequency typical for this type of ending. After approximately 4 minutes of hypoxia (*red bar* underneath the *abscissa*) at an oxygen tension of 20 mm Hg, the discharge became irregular and stopped suddenly. It recovered approximately 3 minutes after restoration of the oxygen supply. After the second period of hypoxia, the discharge failed sooner and the recovery was incomplete. The receptor now exhibited an irregular discharge frequency. Apparently, the receptor was damaged by the prolonged hypoxia.

group IV fibers simultaneously from intact GS muscle nerves in cats and found that a large proportion of these units became active during tetanic muscle contractions under ischemia.

Single fiber recordings from group III and IV muscle receptors yielded a relatively small population of units (approximately 10%) that reacted in a way that suggested an involvement in the mediation of ischemic pain.[88] The receptors were not, or were only weakly, activated during contractions without arterial occlusion but showed strong excitations when the same amount of muscle work was repeated under ischemic conditions (Fig. 2-24).

The time course of the activation was similar to that of the pain induced in human volunteers performing ischemic contractions.[73] After the onset of the contractions before the receptor activity rose, there was a delay of almost 1 minute, and after the contractions had been discontinued but the ischemia had been maintained,

the discharge frequency remained at an elevated level. All the receptors exhibiting strong reactions to ischemic contractions were group IV units; group III receptors were not, or were only minimally, affected.[64, 97] Therefore, the pain of intermittent claudication may be an example of muscle pain that is exclusively or predominantly caused by activity in nonmyelinated (as opposed to thin myelinated) nociceptive fibers.

Most of the group III and IV receptors tested with ischemic contractions did not react at all, although the ischemic stimulus was extremely strong (the contractions were continued until the muscle was no longer capable of maintaining its contractile force). An example is shown in Figure 2-25. The receptor recorded had a thin myelinated afferent fiber; its discharge frequency rose in a graded fashion with increasing forces of contraction. The contraction-induced responses started at a low percentage of maximal contraction

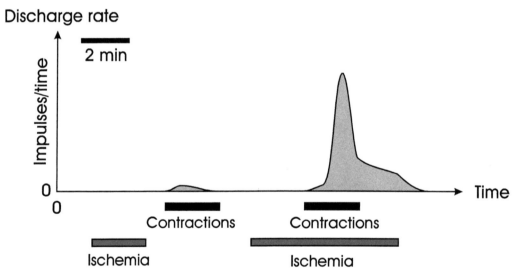

Figure 2-24. Response of a muscle nociceptor to ischemic contractions. Ischemia alone caused no activation. The first period of contractions was performed in the absence of ischemia; the receptor showed a small activation during the contractions. The second period of contractions was performed during ischemia produced by clamping the muscle artery approximately 2 minutes before the contractions started. After approximately 1 minute of ischemic contractions, the impulse activity of the receptor rose steeply and reached a relatively high frequency of discharge. The ischemia was maintained for approximately 1.5 minutes after the end of the contractions. During this ischemic period, the receptor's activity remained at an elevated level and returned to normal (in this case, to 0) only after the blood supply of the muscle had been restored.

ऑčněളের

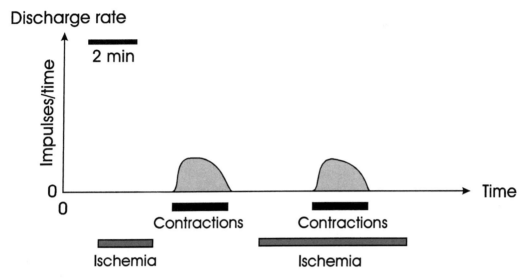

Figure 2-25. Response behavior of a contraction-sensitive group III receptor during ischemic contractions. The stimulation procedure was the same as that used for testing the nociceptor in Figure 2-24. The receptor gave no response to ischemia alone but responded clearly to contractions without ischemia. The contractions during ischemia did not elicit a greater response than was elicited without ischemia; i.e., the ischemia did not affect the excitability of the receptor. The difference in behavior between the receptors shown in Figures 2-24 and 2-25 is striking: Whereas the nociceptor in Figure 2-24 was strongly excited by ischemic contractions, the non-nociceptive receptor in Figure 2-25 was not influenced by this painful condition.

force; therefore, the receptor is likely to be highly active during normal muscular activity and for this reason cannot be considered nociceptive. In support of this assumption, the receptor's responses to contractions were not changed when the contractions were repeated under ischemic (noxious) conditions; i.e., in its response behavior the receptor was unable to distinguish between a physiologic (nonpainful) and a noxious (painful) stimulus. These data underline the high degree of specificity of free nerve endings.

The mechanisms underlying the pain of intermittent claudication are still a matter of controversy. Many substances have been and are still considered as causal factors, and no single stimulus that could elicit all aspects of the pain is known to exist. The proposed mechanisms include accumulation of acidic metabolites such as lactate,[94] potassium ions,[45] or the lack of oxidation of metabolic products.[103] In light of more recent data, lactate cannot be considered a major factor in ischemic muscle pain because (1) it is relatively ineffective in activating muscle nociceptors and (2) patients with McArdle's disease, who cannot produce lactate as the result of an enzyme deficiency, tend to have strong anginal and skeletal muscle pain during contractions.[109] A combined action of lactate with other substances cannot be excluded, however.

As stated above, BK is likely involved in ischemic pain. In contrast to lactate, phosphate, and potassium ions—all of which elicit excitations of muscle group III and IV afferent units only if present in high concentrations (in the high millimolar range, which are probably unphysiologic)—BK activates the endings at high micromolar concentrations.[66]

Recent data indicate that CGRP may also be involved in nociception during ischemia: The neuropeptide has been shown to be released from ischemic heart muscle, with BK enhancing the release.[32] Arachidonic acid likewise has been shown to increase in cat muscle during static contractions.[110] In view of the fact that during exhausting work the pH inside the muscle may drop to 6.0 to 6.6[13, 112] and that a low pH is a powerful sensitizing factor for cutaneous nociceptors,[121] an ischemia-induced increase in hydrogen ion concentration may contribute to ischemic pain. Potassium ions, which leave the contracting muscle fiber and accumulate in the extracellular fluid during ischemia,[47] are another pain-promoting factor. In 1931, Lewis and co-workers[73] rejected the theory that lack of oxygen elicits the pain of intermittent claudication; they proposed a physicochemical mechanism ("factor P") as the cause of ischemic muscle pain. We now know that the situation is more complicated than that. In a muscle that performs ischemic contractions, an unknown but presumably large number of chemical and physical factors are continuously changing.

As to the mechanisms of receptor activation during ischemic contractions, the analysis of the time course of temperature and force during the contractions showed that thermal and mechanical changes can be largely excluded as stimulating factors. A speculative interpretation is that the ischemia-induced decrease in pO_2 or pH releases BK, PGE_2, and potassium ions,[45, 54, 125] which sensitize muscle nociceptors so that they respond to the force of contraction. When the contractions are discontinued under maintained ischemia, a basal level of receptor activation (see Fig. 2-24) and pain persists because of the high intramuscular concentration of chemical stimulants.

A clinical finding supporting the assumption that BK (probably together with PGs) is a major factor for the promotion of the pain of intermittent claudication is that treatment with a proteinase inhibitor, which prevents the release of BK from its precursor molecule kallidin, prolongs the distance patients with intermittent claudication are able to walk without pain.[22]

Data obtained from patients indicate that the intensity of ischemic muscle pain depends on three factors, namely, frequency of contraction, force of contraction, and the duration of time during which the contractions continue.[90] Of these, contraction force was found to be of minor, and contraction frequency of major, importance.

Intermittent Claudication. Intermittent claudication of the lower extremities results from aortoiliac occlusive disease. Lower extremity deep-tissue pain occurs after walking a predictable distance and is relieved by several minutes' rest. It is a good example of muscle pain resulting from the combination of muscle activity and hypoxia that is caused by ischemia.

Femoral and distal pulses are usually diminished or absent. Pulses may be present at rest only to disappear with the increased blood flow required by exercise.[27] With progression of the disease, rest pain and gangrene may develop. This is another example wherein sufficient sustained hypoxia without muscle activity can be painful. Likely causes are release of algesic substances (e.g., BK) associated with blood or blood vessels and the lowered pH in the ischemic muscle.[53]

Methods for accurate assessment of arterial insufficiency include arteriography, which directly visualizes the vascular tree, and a Doppler laser or ultrasound probe, which reveals blood flow. The ankle/brachial blood pressure index is a simple and useful measure that relates to the cause of the muscle pain. The highest opening systolic pressure of the three ankle arteries is divided by the higher of the two brachial systolic pressures. A value of more than 1 is normal. Values of 0.6 to 0.9 are typical of claudication, 0.3 to 0.6 of rest pain, and below 0.3 of incipient or actual gangrene. A significant decrease in this index following treadmill exercise confirms claudication.

Medical management starts with the most important single factor—stop smoking if a smoker. It also includes weight reduction in the obese and control of heart failure, hypertension, and diabetes when applicable, but β-blocking drugs should be avoided to prevent further compromise of peripheral circulation. Selective progressive exercise of the most affected muscles within limits of comfort can increase pain-free range of walking. Some patients will need vascular surgery.

One differential diagnosis of intermittent claudication is pseudoclaudication, a poorly defined source of deep-tissue pain that is loosely associated with sciatica. Arcangeli et al.[3] noted that patients with occlusion of the common iliac or internal iliac artery were likely to have TrP phenomena in the gluteus medius (which can give a sciatica-like referred pain pattern) and tensor fasciae latae muscles. In some of these patients, walking tolerance was related more to the severity of the TrPs than to the decrease in blood flow. Inactivation of the TrPs and a regular stretching exercise of the muscles that were harboring these TrPs can markedly improve the pain symptoms of these patients.[124]

Compartment Syndrome. A compartment syndrome develops when a muscle is surrounded by an unyielding fascial and bony (or other nondistensible) enclosure and increases the amount of enclosed content for some reason, such as edema, hematoma, or infection. The increased compartment pressure tends to occlude blood flow. The resulting hypoxia can increase extravasation and aggravate the situation. If neglected, this vicious cycle can progress to necroses of the muscles and nerves within the compartment. Well-recognized lower extremity compartment syndromes are the anterior compartment, which includes the tibialis anterior muscle, and the deep posterior compartment, which includes the tibialis posterior and flexor digitorum longus muscles.[124] If the condition develops during exercise, continued contractions of the ischemic muscle can become painful and remain painful until the pressure is relieved surgically.

When the nondistensible compartment is formed by a cast around a limb for treatment of a fracture, the ischemia may develop in the absence of muscular contraction. In this case, pain does not develop as early, leaving a narrower margin of safety between the onset of pain and the onset of irreparable tissue damage.

5. Drug-Induced and Chemically Induced Myalgia

The eosinophilia-myalgia syndrome is an interesting example of a condition first considered to be a drug-induced myalgia induced by the drug tryptophan but later appeared to be a chemical contaminant of the tryptophan, which had resulted from the manufacturing process.[77] The disease was first identified in the United States in 1989 and made more than 1500 people ill and caused 37 deaths by June 1993. The cause was traced to batches of tryptophan produced by a Japanese company. The tryptophan contained six contaminants associated with eosinophilia-myalgia syndrome. The clinical and pathologic findings in this disease bear a striking resemblance to those of the toxic oil syndrome that occurred in Spain in 1981. More than 20,000 people were affected, with 839 deaths. In this case, the contaminant was aniline remaining in aniline-denatured rapeseed oil. The severe myalgia, in this case, appeared later in the illness, approximately 8 weeks following onset.

REFERENCES

1. Abrahams VC: Group III and IV receptors of skeletal muscle. *Can J Physiol Pharmacol* 64:509–514, 1986.
2. Andres KH, von Düring M, Schmidt RF: Sensory innervation of the Achilles tendon by group III and IV afferent fibers. *Anat Embryol* 172:145–156, 1985.
3. Arcangeli P, Digiesi V, Ronchi O, et al.: Mechanisms of ischemic pain in peripheral occlusive arterial disease. *Advances in Pain Research and Therapy, Volume 1.* Edited by Bonica JJ, Albe-Fessard D. Raven Press, New York, 1976 (pp. 965–973).
4. Barnes PJ, Brown MJ, Dollery CT, et al.: Histamine is released from skin by substance P but does not act as the final vasodilator in the axon reflex. *Br J Pharmacol* 88:741–745, 1986.
5. Berberich P, Hoheisel U, Mense S: Effects of a carrageenan-induced myositis on the discharge properties of group III and IV muscle receptors in the cat. *J Neurophysiol* 59:1395–1409, 1988.
6. Besson JM, Chaouch A: Peripheral and spinal mechanisms of nociception. *Physiol Rev* 67:67–186, 1987.
7. Bessou P, Laporte Y: Activation des fibres afférentes amyéliniques d'origine musculaire. *Compt Rend Soc Biol (Paris)* 152:1587–1590, 1958.
8. Bobbert MF, Hollander AP, Huijing PA: Factors in delayed onset muscular soreness of man. *Med Sci Sport Exercise* 18:75–81, 1986.
9. Brimijoin S, Lundberg JM, Brodin E, et al.: Axonal transport of substance P in the vagus and sciatic nerves of the guinea pig. *Brain Res* 191:443–457, 1980.
10. Brock LG, Eccles JC, Rall W: Experimental investigations on the afferent fibres in muscle nerves. *Proc R Soc Lond B* 138:453–475, 1951.
11. Buck SH, Walsh JH, Yamamura HI, et al.: Neuropeptides in sensory neurons. *Life Sci* 30:1857–1866, 1982.

12. Burgess PR, Perl ER: Cutaneous mechanoreceptors and nociceptors. *Handbook of Sensory Physiology, Volume II (Somatosensory System)*. Edited by Iggo A. Springer, New York, 1973 (pp. 29–78).

13. Caldwell PC: Intracellular pH. *Int Rev Cytol* 5:229–277, 1956.

13a. Cesare P, McNaughton P: Peripheral pain mechanisms. *Curr Opin Neurobiol* 7:493–499, 1997.

14. Clausen JP, Lassen NA: Muscle blood flow during exercise in normal man studied by the ^{133}Xenon clearance method. *Cardiovasc Res* 5:245–254, 1971.

15. Coderre TJ, Basbaum AI, Levine JD: Neural control of vascular permeability: interactions between primary afferents, mast cells, and sympathetic efferents. *J Neurophysiol* 62:48–58, 1989.

16. Coffman JD: The effect of aspirin on pain and hand blood flow responses to intra-arterial injection of bradykinin in man. *Clin Pharmacol Ther* 7:26–37, 1966.

17. Damas J, Deby C: Sur la libération des prostaglandines et de leurs précurseurs, par la bradykinine. *Archs Int Physiol Biochim* 84:293–304, 1976.

18. Davies JA: Peroneal compartment syndrome secondary to rupture of the peroneus longus: a case report. *J Bone Joint Surg* 61:783–784, 1979.

19. DeVere R, Bradley WG: Polymyositis: its presentation, morbidity and mortality. *Brain* 98:637–666, 1975.

20. Devor M, Wall PD, McMahon SB: Dichotomizing somatic nerve fibers exist in rats but they are rare. *Neurosci Lett* 49:187–192, 1984.

21. Diehl B, Hoheisel U, Mense S: The influence of mechanical stimuli and of acetylsalicylic acid on the discharges of slowly conducting afferent units from normal and inflamed muscle in the rat. *Exp Brain Res* 92:431–440, 1993.

22. Digiesi V, Bartoli V, Dorigo B: Effect of a proteinase inhibitor on intermittent claudication or on pain at rest in patients with peripheral arterial disease. *Pain* 1:385–389, 1975.

23. DiRosa M, Giroud JP, Willoughby DA: Studies of the mediators of the acute inflammatory response induced in rats in different sites by carrageenan and turpentine. *J Pathol* 104:15–29, 1971.

24. Downey DJ, Simkin PA, Mack LA, et al.: Tibialis posterior tendon rupture: a cause of rheumatoid flat foot. *Arthritis Rheum* 31:441–446, 1988.

25. Duggan AW, Hendry IA, Morton CR, et al.: Cutaneous stimuli releasing immunoreactive substance P in the dorsal horn of the cat. *Brain Res* 451:261–273, 1988.

26. von Düring M, Andres KH: Topography and ultrastructure of group III and IV nerve terminals of the cat's gastrocnemius-soleus muscle. *The Primary Afferent Neuron*. Edited by Zenker W, Neuhuber WL. Plenum Press, New York, 1990 (pp. 35–41).

27. Edwards JD, Brewster DC: Aortoiliac disease, Chapter 7.6.1. *Oxford Textbook of Surgery, Volume 1*. Edited by Morris PJ, Malt RA. Oxford University Press, New York, 1994.

28. Engel AG: *Myology: Basic and Clinical, Volume 1*. Ed. 2. Edited by Engel AG, Franzini-Armstrong C. McGraw-Hill, New York, 1994.

29. Ferreira SH: Prostaglandins, aspirin-like drugs and analgesia. *Nature New Biol* 240:200–203, 1972.

30. Ferreira SH, Moncada S, Vane JR: Potentiation by prostaglandins of the nociceptive activity of bradykinin in the dog knee joint. *Br J Pharmacol* 50:461, 1974.

31. Fock S, Mense S: Excitatory effects of 5-hydroxytryptamine, histamine and potassium ions on muscular group IV afferent units: a comparison with bradykinin. *Brain Res* 105:459–469, 1976.

32. Franco-Cereceda A, Saria A, Lundberg JM: Differential release of calcitonin gene-related peptide and neuropeptide Y from the isolated heart by capsaicin, ischaemia, nicotine, bradykinin and ouabain. *Acta Physiol Scand* 135:173–187, 1989.

33. Franz M, Mense S: Muscle receptors with group IV afferent fibres responding to application of bradykinin. *Brain Res* 92:369–383, 1975.

34. Froimson AI: Tennis leg. *JAMA* 209:415–416, 1969.

35. Gamse R, Posch M, Saria A, et al.: Several mediators appear to interact in neurogenic inflammation. *Acta Physiol Hung* 69:343–354, 1987.

36. Gasser HS, Grundfest H: Axon diameters in relation to the spike dimensions and the conduction velocity in mammalian A fibers. *Am J Physiol* 127:393–414, 1939.

37. Giuliani G, Poppi M, Acciarri N, et al.: CT scan and surgical treatment of traumatic iliacus hematoma with femoral neuropathy: case report. *J Trauma* 30:229–231, 1990.

38. Gomazkow OA: Das Kallikrein-Kinin-System bei Myokardischämie und Herzinfarkt — Experimentelle Untersuchungen. *Ischämie—Morphologie, Biochemie, Experimentelle Parmakologie, Klinik und Therapie*. Edited by Gross D, et al. Schattauer-Verlag, Stuttgart, 1975 (pp. 101–112).

39. Gottschall J, Zenker W, Neuhuber W, et al.: The sternomastoid muscle of the rat and its innervation. Muscle fiber composition, perikarya and axons of efferent and afferent neurons. *Anat Embryol* 160:285–300, 1980.

40. Grigg P, Schaible H-G, Schmidt RF: Mechanical sensitivity of group III and IV afferents from posterior articular nerve in normal and inflamed cat knee. *J Neurophysiol* 55:635–643, 1986.

41. Guzman F, Braun C, Lim KS: Visceral pain and the pseudoaffective response to intra-arterial injection of bradykinin and other algesic agents. *Arch Int Pharmacodyn* 136:353–384, 1962.

42. Häbler HJ, Jänig W, Koltzenburg M: Activation of unmyelinated afferent fibres by mechanical stimuli and inflammation of of the urinary bladder in the cat. *J Physiol* 425:545–562, 1990.

43. Hagbarth K-E, Hägglund JV, Nordin M, et al.: Thixotropic behaviour of human finger flexor muscles with accompanying changes in spindle and reflex responses to stretch. *J Physiol* 368:323–342, 1985.

44. Handwerker HO, Kilo S, Reeh PW: Unresponsive afferent nerve fibres in the sural nerve of the rat. *J Physiol* 435:229–242, 1991.

45. Harpuder K, Stein I: Studies on the nature of pain arising from an ischemic limb. *Am Heart J* 25:429–448, 1943.

46. Head H, Rivers WHR, Sherren J: The afferent nervous system from a new aspect. *Brain* 28:99–115, 1905.

47. Hnik P, Holas M, Krekule I, et al.: Work-induced potassium changes in skeletal muscle and effluent venous blood assessed by liquid ion-exchanger microelectrodes. *Pflügers Arch* 362:85–94, 1976.

47a. Hoheisel U, Mense S: Leukotriene D4 depresses the mechanosensitivity of group III and IV muscle receptors in the rat. *Neuroreport* 5:645–648, 1994.

47b. Hoheisel U, Mense S, Scherotzke R: Calcitonin gene-related peptide-immunoreactivity in functionally identified primary afferent neurones in the rat. *Anat Embryol* 189:41–49, 1994.

48. Holmes GB Jr, Cracchiolo A III, Goldner JL, et al.: Current practices in the management of posterial tibial tendon rupture. *Contemp Orthop* 20:79–108, 1990.

49. Holzer P: Local effector functions of capsaicin-sensitive sensory nerve endings: involvement of tachykinins, calcitonin gene-related peptide and other neuropeptides. *Neuroscience* 24:739–768, 1988.

50. Hoskins DW: Trichinellosis (Trichinosis). *Cecil Textbook of Medicine.* Ed. 17. Edited by Wyngaarden JB, Smith LH. WB Saunders, Philadelphia, 1985 (pp. 1825–1826).

51. Hudgson P, Peter JB: Inflammatory disorders of muscle. Classification. *Clin Rheum Dis* 10:3–8, 1984.

52. Ialenti A, Ianaro A, Moncada S, et al.: Modulation of acute inflammation by endogenous nitric oxide. *Eur J Pharmacol* 211:177–182, 1992.

53. Issberner U, Reeh PW, Steen KH: Pain due to tissue acidosis: a mechanism for inflammatory and ischemic myalgia? *Neurosci Lett* 208:191–194, 1996.

54. Jennische E, Hagberg H, Haljamäe H: Extracellular potassium concentration and membrane potential in rabbit gastrocnemius muscle during tourniquet ischemia. *Pflügers Arch* 392:335–339, 1982.

55. Jensen K, Tuxen C, Pedersen-Bjergaard U, et al.: Pain and tenderness in human temporal muscle induced by bradykinin and 5-hydroxytryptamine. *Peptides* 11:1127–1132, 1990.

56. Jones DA, Newham DJ, Clarkson PM: Skeletal muscle stiffness and pain following eccentric exercise of the elbow flexors. *Pain* 30:233–242, 1987a.

57. Jones DA, Newham DJ, Obletter G, et al.: Nature of exercise-induced muscle pain. *Advances in Pain Research and Therapy, Volume 10.* Edited by Tiengo M, et al. Raven Press, New York, 1987b (pp. 207–218).

58. Jose PJ, Page DA, Wolstenholme BE, et al.: Bradykinin-stimulated prostaglandin E_2 production of endothelial cells and its modulation by antiinflammatory compounds. *Inflammation* 5:363–378, 1981.

59. Ju G, Hökfelt T, Brodin E, et al.: Primary sensory neurons of the rat showing calcitonin gene-related peptide immunoreactivity and their relation to substance P, somatostatin-, galanin-, vasoactive intestinal polypeptide- and cholecystokinin-immunoreactive ganglion cells. *Cell Tissue Res* 247:417–431, 1987.

60. Juan H: Mechanisms of action of bradykinin-induced release of prostaglandin E. *Naunyn-Schmiedeberg's Arch Pharmacol* 300:77–85, 1977.

61. Kao FF: An experimental study of the pathway involved in exercise hyperpnoea employing cross-circulation techniques. *The Regulation of Human Respiration.* Edited by Cunningham DJC, Lloyd BB. Blackwell, Oxford, 1963 (pp. 461–502).

62. Kaufman MP, Iwamoto GA, Longhurst JC, et al.: Effects of capsaicin and bradykinin on afferent fibers with endings in skeletal muscle. *Circ Res* 50:133–139, 1982.

63. Kaufman MP, Longhurst JC, Rybicki KJ, et al.: Effects of static muscular contraction on impulse activity of groups III and IV afferents in cats. *J Appl Physiol* 55:105–112, 1983.

64. Kaufman MP, Rybicki KJ, Waldrop TG, et al.: Effect of ischemia on responses of group III and IV afferents to contraction. *J Appl Physiol* 57:644–650, 1984.

65. Keele CA: Excitants of pain receptors. *Acta Neuroveg* 28:392–404, 1966.

66. Kniffki K-D, Mense S, Schmidt RF: Responses of group IV afferent units from skeletal muscle to stretch, contraction and chemical stimulation. *Exp Brain Res* 31:511–522, 1978.

66a. Komi PV, Kaneko M, Aura O: EMG activity of the leg extensor muscles with special reference to mechanical efficiency in concentric and eccentric exercise. *Int J Sports Med (8 Suppl)* 1:22–29, 1987.

67. Kumazawa T: The polymodal receptor—a gateway to pathological pain. *Progress in Brain Research, Volume 113.* Edited by Kumazawa T, et al. Elsevier, Amsterdam, 1996 (pp. 3–18).

68. Kumazawa T, Mizumura K: Thin-fibre receptors responding to mechanical, chemical and thermal stimulation in the skeletal muscle of the dog. *J Physiol* 273:179–194, 1977.

69. Lam FY, Ferrell WR: Mediators of substance P-induced inflammation in the rat knee joint. *Agents Actions* 31:298–307, 1990.

69a. Lawson SN, Crepps BA, Perl ER: Relationship of substance P to afferent characteristics of dorsal root ganglion neurones in guinea pig. *J Physiol* 505:177–191, 1997

70. Layzer RB: Muscle pain, cramps, and fatigue, Chapter 67. *Myology, Volume 2.* Ed. 2. Edited by Engel AG, Franzini-Armstrong C. McGraw-Hill, New York, 1994 (pp. 1754–1768).

71. Le Greves P, Nyberg F, Terenius L, et al.: Calcitonin gene-related peptide is a potent inhibitor of substance P degradation. *Eur J Pharmacol* 115:309–311, 1985.

72. Lembeck F, Holzer P: Substance P as neurogenic mediator of antidromic vasodilation and neurogenic plasma extravasation. *Naunyn-Schmiedeberg's Arch Pharmacol* 310:175–183, 1979.

73. Lewis T, Pickering GW, Rothschild P: Observations upon muscular pain in intermittent claudication. *Heart* 15:359–383, 1931.

74. Lindahl O: Experimental skin pain induced by injection of water-soluble substances in humans. *Acta Physiol Scand* 51(Suppl 179):1–90, 1961.

75. Lloyd DPC: Neuron patterns controlling transmission of ipsilateral hind limb reflexes in cat. *J Neurophysiol* 6:293–315, 1943.

76. Marmor L, Bechtol CO, Hall CB: Pectoralis major muscle: function of sternal portion and mechanisms of rupture of normal muscle: case reports. *J Bone Joint Surg* 43A:81–87, 1961.

77. Mayeno AN, Gliech GJ: Eosinophilia-myalgia syndrome and tryptophan production: a cautionary tale. *Trends Biotechnol* 12:346–352, 1994.

78. McClure JG: Gastrocnemius musculotendinous rupture: a condition confused with thrombophlebitis. *South Med J* 77:1143–1145, 1984.

79. McMahon SB, Lewin GR, Anand P, *et al.*: Quantitative analysis of peptide levels and neurogenic extravasation following regeneration of afferents to appropriate and inappropriate targets. *Neuroscience* 33:67–73, 1989.

80. McMahon SB, Sykova E, Wall PD, *et al.*: Neurogenic extravasation and substance P levels are low in muscle as compared to skin in the rat hindlimb. *Neurosci Lett* 52:235–240, 1984.

81. Mense S: Nervous outflow from skeletal muscle following chemical noxious stimulation. *J Physiol* 267:75–88, 1977.

82. Mense S: Sensitization of group IV muscle receptors to bradykinin by 5-hydroxytryptamine and prostaglandin E_2. *Brain Res* 225:95–105, 1981.

83. Mense S: Reduction of the bradykinin-induced activation of feline group III and IV muscle receptors by acetylsalicylic acid. *J Physiol* 326:269–283, 1982.

84. Mense S: Auslösende Faktoren des Muskelschmerzes unter besonderer Berücksichtigung der Ischämie. *Schmerztherapie bei ischämischen Krankheiten, Schmerzstudien 9*. Edited by Maier C, Wawersik J. Fischer, Stuttgart, 1991 (pp. 45–56).

85. Mense S, Hoheisel U: Influence of leukotriene D_4 on the discharges of slowly conducting afferent units from normal and inflamed muscle in the rat. *Pflügers Arch* 415(Suppl 1R):105, 1990.

86. Mense S, Meyer H: Response properties of group III and IV receptors in the Achilles tendon of the cat. *Pflügers Arch* 389:R25, 1981.

87. Mense S, Meyer H: Different types of slowly conducting afferent units in cat skeletal muscle and tendon. *J Physiol* 363:403–417, 1985.

88. Mense S, Stahnke M: Responses in muscle afferent fibres of slow conduction velocity to contractions and ischaemia in the cat. *J Physiol* 342:383–397, 1983.

89. Mense S, Light AR, Perl ER: Spinal terminations of subcutaneous high-threshold mechanoreceptors. *Spinal Cord Sensation*. Edited by Brown AG, Réthelyi M. Scottish Academic Press, Edinburgh, 1981 (pp. 79–86).

90. Mills KR, Newham DJ, Edwards RHT: Force, contraction frequency and energy metabolism as determinants of ischaemic muscle pain. *Pain* 14:149–154, 1982.

91. Mitchell JH, Schmidt RF: Cardiovascular reflex control by afferent fibers from skeletal muscle receptors. *Handbook of Physiology, Section 2: The Cardiovascular System, Volume III: Peripheral Circulation and Organ Blood Flow, Part 2*. Edited by Shepherd JT, Abboud FM. American Physiological Society, Bethesda, MD, 1983 (pp. 623–658).

92. Molander C, Grant G: Spinal cord projections from hindlimb muscle nerves in the rat studied by transganglionic transport of horseradish peroxidase, wheat germ agglutinin conjugated horseradish peroxidase, or horseradish peroxidase with dimethylsulfoxide. *J Comp Neurol* 260:246–255, 1987.

93. Molea D, Murcek B, Blanken C, *et al.*: Evaluation of two manipulative techniques in the treatment of postexercise muscle soreness. *JAOA* 87:477–483, 1987.

94. Moore RM, Moore RE, Singleton AO: Experiments on the chemical stimulation of pain-endings associated with small blood vessels. *Am J Physiol* 107:594–602, 1934.

95. Nakahara M: The effect of a tourniquet on the kinin-kininogen system in blood and muscle. *Thromb Diathes Haemorrh* 26:264–274, 1971.

96. New HV, Mudge AW: Calcitonin gene-related peptide regulates muscle acetylcholine receptor synthesis. *Nature* 323:809–811, 1986.

96a. O'Reilly KP, Warhol MJ, Fielding RA, *et al.*: Eccentric exercise-induced muscle damage impairs muscle glycogen repletion. *J Appl Physiol* 63:252–256, 1987.

97. Paintal AS: Functional analysis of group III afferent fibres of mammalian muscles. *J Physiol* 152:250–270, 1960.

98. Paintal AS: A comparison of the nerve impulses of mammalian nonmedullated nerve fibres with those of the smallest diameter medullated fibres. *J Physiol* 193:523–533, 1967.

99. Perl ER: Afferent basis of nociception and pain: evidence from the characteristics of sensory receptors and their projections to the spinal dorsal horn. *Pain*. Edited by Bonica JJ. Raven Press, New York, 1980 (pp. 19–45).

100. Perl ER: Pain and nociception. *Handbook of Physiology, Section 1, The Nervous System, Vol. III, Part 2*. Edited by Darian-Smith I. American Physiological Society, Bethesda, 1984 (pp. 915–975).

101. Perlman MD, Leveille D: Extensor digitorum longus stenosing tenosynovitis. *J Am Pediatr Med Assoc* 78:198–199, 1988.

102. Pernow BB, Havel RJ, Jennings DB: The second wind phenomenon in McArdle's syndrome. *Acta Med Scand* 472(Suppl):294–307, 1967.

103. Pickering GW, Wayne EJ: Observations on angina pectoris and intermittent claudication in anaemia. *Clin Sci* 1:305–325, 1933–1934.

104. Pierau F-K, Fellmer G, Taylor DCM: Somatovisceral convergence in cat dorsal root ganglion neurones demonstrated by double-labelling with fluorescent tracers. *Brain Res* 321:63–70, 1984.

105. Piper PJ: Formation and actions of leukotrienes. *Physiol Rev* 64:744–761, 1984.

106. Reinert A, Mense S: Inflammatory changes in the density of neuropeptide-containing nerve endings in the skeletal muscle of the rat. *Pflügers Arch* 422 (Suppl 1):R62, 1993.

106a. Reinert A, Kaske A, Mense S: Inflammation-induced increase in the density of neuropeptide-immunoreactive nerve endings in rat skeletal muscle. *Exp Brain Res* 121:174–180, 1998.

107. Reinert A, Vitek M, Mense S: Effects of substance P on the activity of high- and low-threshold mechanosensitive receptors of the rat diaphragm in vitro. *Pflügers Arch* 420(Suppl 1):R47, 1992.

108. Richmond FJR, Anstee GCB, Sherwin EA, *et al.*: Motor and sensory fibres of neck muscle nerves in the cat. *Can J Physiol Pharmacol* 54:294–304, 1976.

109. Rodbard S: Pain associated with muscular activity. *Am Heart J* 90:84–92, 1975.

110. Rotto DM, Massey KD, Burton KP, *et al.*: Static contraction increases arachidonic levels in gastrocnemius muscles of cats. *J Appl Physiol* 66:2721–2724, 1989.

111. Ryu PD, Gerber G, Murase K, *et al.*: Calcitonin gene-related peptide enhances calcium current of rat dorsal root ganglion neurons and spinal excitatory synaptic transmission. *Neurosci Lett* 89:305–312, 1988.

112. Sahlin K, Harris RC, Nylind B, *et al.*: Lactate content and pH in muscle samples obtained after dynamic exercise. *Pflügers Arch* 67:143–149, 1976.

113. Samuelsson B: Leukotrienes: mediators of immediate hypersensitivity reactions and inflammation. *Science* 220:568–575, 1983.

114. Samuelsson B, Dahlén S-E, Lindgren JÅ, *et al.*: Leukotrienes and lipoxins: structures, biosynthesis and biological effects. *Science* 237:1171–1176, 1987.

115. Sandoz PA, Zenker W: Unmyelinated axons in a muscle nerve. Electron microscopic morphometry of the sternomastoid nerve in normal and sympathectomized rats. *Anat Embryol* 174:207–213, 1986.

116. Schweizer A, Brom R, Glatt M, *et al.*: Leukotrienes reduce nociceptive responses to bradykinin. *Eur J Pharmacol* 105:105–112, 1984.

117. Sicuteri F: Vasoneuroactive substances and their implication in vascular pain. *Research and Clinical Studies in Headache, Volume 1.* Edited by Friedman AP. Karger, New York, 1967 (pp. 6–45).

118. Sicuteri F, Franchi G, Fanciullacci M: Bradichinina e dolore da ischemia. *Settim Med* 52:127–139, 1964.

119. Stacey MJ: Free nerve endings in skeletal muscle of the cat. *J Anat* 105:231–254, 1969.

120. Staunton HP, Taylor SH, Donald KW: The effect of vascular occlusion on the pressor response to static muscular work. *Clin Sci* 27:283–291, 1964.

121. Steen KH, Reh PW, Anton F, *et al.*: Protons selectively induce lasting excitation and sensitization to mechanical stimulation of nociceptors in rat skin in vitro. *J Neurosci* 12:86–95, 1992.

122. Szolcsányi J: Selective responsiveness of polymodal nociceptors of the rabbit ear to capsaicin, bradykinin and ultra-violet irradiation. *J Physiol* 388:9–24, 1987.

123. Tonnesen KH: Blood-flow through muscle during rhythmic contraction measured by [133]Xenon. *Scand J Clin Lab Invest* 16:646–654, 1964.

124. Travell JG, Simons DG: Myofascial pain and dysfunction. *The Trigger Point Manual, Volume 2. The Lower Extremities.* Williams & Wilkins, Baltimore, 1992 (p. 607).

125. Uchida Y, Ueda H: Kininogen and kinin activity during local ischemia in man. *Jpn Heart J* 10:503–508, 1969.

126. Vane JR: Inhibition of prostaglandin synthesis as a mechanism of action for aspirin-like drugs. *Nature New Biol* 231:232–235, 1971.

127. Wallengren J, Håkanson R: Effects of substance P, neurokinin A and calcitonin gene-related peptide in human skin and their involvement in sensory nerve-mediated responses. *Eur J Pharmacol* 143:267–273, 1987.

128. Weddell G, Harpman JA: The neurohistological basis for the sensation of pain provoked from deep fascia, tendon, and periosteum. *J Neurol Psychiatry* 3:319–328, 1940.

129. Zenker W, Sandoz PA, Neuhuber W: The distribution of anterogradely labeled I-IV primary afferents in histochemically defined compartments of the rat's sternomastoid muscle. *Anat Embryol* 177:235–243, 1988.

CHAPTER 3
Neuropathic Muscle Pain

SUMMARY: **Neuropathic muscle pain** is caused by a lesion or dysfunction of nerve fibers in dorsal roots or spinal (cranial) nerves. Often, such pain resulting from nerve injury is felt in the innervation territory of the nerve in the sense of **projected pain**. The mechanisms leading to neuropathic pain are multifold. They can include **impulse generation** in nociceptive fibers at the site of the lesion, **cross excitation** of nociceptive fibers by non-nociceptive ones in the dorsal root ganglion, and **disinhibition of spinal neurons** because of a lack of activity in thick myelinated fibers.

A frequent cause of neuropathic pain is a mechanical lesion of a peripheral nerve by trauma or **entrapment** (pain resulting from nerve injury). If nerve fibers are severed, their proximal ends inevitably sprout and form a **neuroma**. In these cases, phantom pain can originate in the neuroma itself, in the dorsal root ganglion, or in disinhibited central nervous neurons. A lesion or dysfunction of a nerve root likewise can give rise to muscle pain (**radiculopathy**). A frequent cause of this pain is a herniated disc. A **peripheral neuropathy** is more likely the result of degenerative and metabolic diseases (e.g., diabetes). These diseases often lead to **demyelination** of thick fibers or to axonal loss of small fibers.

The **complex regional pain syndrome** (CRPS; formerly called **reflex sympathetic dystrophy**) is included in this chapter. The pain is often felt in large body regions without any topical relationship to innervation territories of nerves or dermatomes. The frequent associations of autonomic disturbances point to an involvement of the sympathetic nervous system, but the exact nature of this involvement is unclear.

Neuropathy is defined as "a disturbance of function or pathologic change in a nerve."[42] This means that in neuropathic pain, the peripheral nervous system itself is the source of pain. Generally, two situations leading to neuropathic pain can be distinguished, namely, (1) mechanical or other lesions of primary afferent neurons eliciting pathologic activity in their fibers (if nociceptive fibers are affected, projected pain occurs), and (2) degeneration or destruction of nerve fibers or cells, leading to a change in the pattern of electrical activity in afferent nerve fibers.

In many cases, pain resulting from nerve injury is caused by a mechanical lesion of afferent nerve fibers or by a whole peripheral nerve at a site between the receptive ending and the site of termination in the spinal cord. Often, the mechanical lesion is caused by compression of a nerve or a plexus by bony structures (e.g., a narrow intervertebral foramen), which disturbs the propagation of action potentials along the nerve fibers.

Based on the severity of the lesion, the effect on the function of the nerve fiber can show a broad spectrum of dysfunctions. Weak irritations are likely to cause paresthesia or pain only during movement (when additional mechanical forces act on the nerve), whereas stronger and persistent pressure will depolarize the nerve membrane to threshold, thus initiating action potentials (and pain) continuously at the site of the lesion. If the pressure increases further, the membrane of the nerve fibers becomes "leaky" and permanently depolarized. Such a long-lasting depolarization is inevitably followed by a block of conduction in the affected nerve. Sometimes, a patient will perceive this block as an alleviation of pain, but in reality, less pain means acute danger to the formerly active nerve fibers because of imminent destruction. In these cases, the interrupted nerve fibers will sprout and form neuromas.

Normally, the neuropathic lesion of a spinal nerve occurs at a site where afferent fibers from the skin and deep tissues are mixed (e.g., in the intervertebral foramen). Accordingly, the pain a patient feels is a mixture of cutaneous and deep pain. Pure muscle pain resulting from a neuropathic lesion is rare because most muscle nerves—which contain only fibers supplying muscle—are short and leave the spinal nerve relatively close to the muscle, where a neuropathic lesion is unlikely to occur.

After an amputation, action potentials can originate at the severed nerve stump where a neuroma forms. If the active fibers in the neuroma are nociceptive, the patient will feel pain in that (amputated) region formerly supplied by these fibers (phantom pain). Thus, this type of phantom pain is a special form of projected pain that has to be distinguished from local or referred pain. Referred pain is caused by activation of somatotopically inappropriate spinal neurons and is felt in a region remote from the lesion; local pain is caused by activation of nociceptive nerve endings in the periphery and is felt at the lesion site.

Nerve fiber activation in a neuroma or nerve stump represents only one of several possible causes of phantom pain. In fact, that mechanism is relatively less frequent than was earlier believed. Other mechanisms include hyperexcitability of neurons in the dorsal horn and thalamus or neuroblastic changes in the processing of the nociceptive information at the spinal or cortical level.[14, 35]

In dorsal roots, likewise, afferent fibers from the skin and deep tissues are mixed. Therefore, compression or another lesion of a dorsal root (radiculopathy) will cause pain similar to that caused by a lesion of a spinal or cranial nerve (peripheral neuropathy). A clinical example of the pain of radiculopathy is pain in the innervation territory of the sciatic nerve caused by compression of lumbosacral dorsal roots (sciatica).

In peripheral neuropathy, the dysfunction occurs as a sequel of other diseases (e.g., diabetes, alcoholism) and affects the entire course of a spinal or cranial nerve or nerves. Typically, the pain is a mixed pain from deep and cutaneous tissues and is felt in the innervation territory of the affected nerve. Because of the many mechanisms involved in the generation of neuropathic pain (see Section A), however, the clinical manifestations are also variable.

Keep in mind that the distinction between peripheral and central nervous causes of neuropathic pain is largely arbitrary. In view of recent data on neuroplasticity,[14, 30] every peripheral nerve lesion is usually likely to be followed by changes in the central nervous system (CNS). Similarly, central nervous alterations will lead to changes in the function of the peripheral nervous system.

An example of a disorder with uncertain relationship between central and peripheral components is CRPS, formerly called "reflex sympathetic dystrophy." Originally, an increase in the so-called sympathetic tone was assumed to be the basic mechanism of this pain. The recently developed technique of microneurography, which allows recordings of single fiber activity in patients, has disproved this hypothesis, however. Although an involvement of the sympathetic system is obvious, the exact nature of the contribution of sympathetic efferent activity to this type of pain is still a matter of discussion.

A. MECHANISMS INVOLVED IN THE PAIN OF NERVE INJURY

When a nerve is damaged in such a way that action potentials are initiated at the site of the lesion, the potentials propagate in the direction of both the spinal cord and the receptive ending. The central nervous centers cannot distinguish between these action potentials and those originating at the receptive ending. The activity in the damaged fiber is interpreted by the centers as originating at the receptive ending; accordingly, pain is felt in that region. If a whole nerve is affected, the pain will be felt in the innervation territory of that nerve (projected pain).

A prominent example of mechanically induced projected pain is the pain and paresthesia in the hypothenar region following a bump to the ulnar nerve at the elbow. Because in this case the bump also activates efferent motor fibers, the hand and forearm muscles supplied by the ulnar nerve perform a visible twitch.

Nerve lesions and diseases that frequently lead to neuropathic pain are mechanical trauma, entrapment, inflammation, degenerative demyelination, alcoholism, and diabetes. Four mechanisms of pain generation can be distinguished, not all of which have been proven to exist in patients.

1. Pain Elicited by Impulses Originating at the Site of the Lesion

Nerve injury is capable of directly depolarizing the nerve membrane to threshold and producing action potentials at the site of the lesion. If the impulse activity is originating in non-nociceptive afferent fibers, paresthesia or dysesthesia will ensue. If nociceptive afferents are activated, pain will dominate. Of course, efferent fibers also can be activated. This may lead to fasciculations of motor units or autonomic changes distal to the lesion.

2. Cross Excitation and Cross Talk

When the electrical insulation of individual fibers in a nerve is destroyed or impaired, discharges in one fiber can influence the electrical activity in neighboring fibers in two ways, namely, by cross excitation or by cross talk.[20]

Cross Excitation. Cross excitation occurs at sites of mechanical nerve lesions or in the dorsal root ganglion and is characterized by indirect interaction between neighboring fibers. Activity in one fiber increases the discharges in the other one, but there is no one-to-one transmission in the sense that one action potential in one fiber induces an action potential in the other (i.e., the pattern of the induced activity is independent of the original one). Moreover, single action potentials are ineffective in inducing cross excitation; a minimal level of activity in the active fiber is required for the effect to occur.

Cross Talk. Cross talk is present predominantly in neuromas (see below) and differs from cross excitation in that single impulses in one fiber are sufficient to influence or elicit activity in a neighboring one (i.e., continuous activity is not necessary to induce cross talk) and a one-to-one transmission exists from one fiber to another at a fixed latency. The prerequisite for cross talk appears to be the presence of ephapses. Ephapses are synapse-like close appositions between neighboring fibers that may provide direct electrical coupling (Fig. 3-1D). Ephapses have been proven to exist in neuromas but not at the site of nerve lesions.

3. Cross Excitation at the Site of the Lesion

Under normal conditions, a certain proportion of fibers in a spinal nerve (e.g., the Ia fibers from muscle spindles) have resting activity. Under the conditions of cross

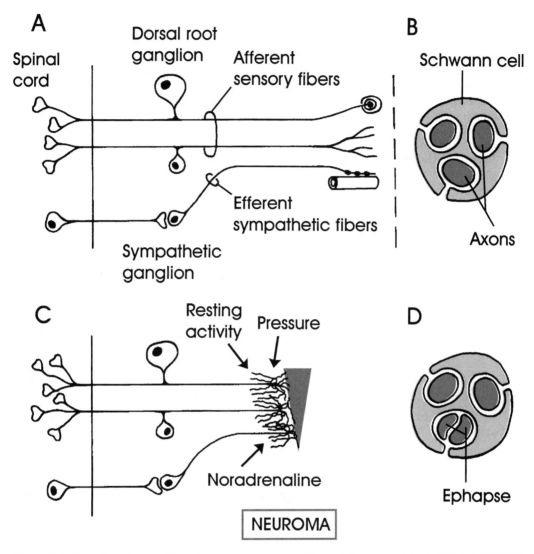

Figure 3-1. Properties of nerve fibers in a neuroma. **A.** Normal arrangement of fibers in a peripheral nerve. **B.** Cross section through a normal bundle of unmyelinated fibers, all of which are ensheathed by a single Schwann cell. **C.** Same nerve fibers as in panel **A,** after transection of the nerve. A neuroma has formed proximal to the site of axotomy. The sprouting fibers in the neuroma develop resting activity and sensitivity to weak pressure stimuli and catecholamines. **D.** Cross section through a fiber bundle in the neuroma shows ephapse formation, i.e., close appositions between axons without intervening Schwann cell sheaths. The ephapses are the sites where action potentials in one axon can depolarize the neighboring axon to threshold and thus elicit impulses in that axon (cross talk). (Modified after Jänig W: Pathophysiology of nerve following mechanical injury. *Proceedings of the 5th World Congress on Pain, Pain Research and Clinical Management, Volume 3.* Edited by Dubner R, Gebhart GF, Bond MR. Elsevier, Amsterdam, 1988 (pp. 89–108).)

excitation in a peripheral nerve, the resting activity in these normal fibers can influence neighboring damaged fibers, so that the latter ones become active. If this mechanism occurs in nociceptive fibers, pain may ensue.

4. Cross Excitation in the Dorsal Root Ganglion

When a nerve is injured, electrical activity can originate both at the site of the lesion and in the dorsal root ganglion. It is well known that a lesion of a peripheral nerve leads to morphologic changes in the ganglion, e.g., shrinking of cell bodies or even cell death. Other major effects are that the proportion of cells with resting activity increases in the presence of a peripheral lesion and that cross excitation between cells of the ganglion can occur under these circumstances.[20] The lesion-induced resting discharge in ganglion cells has been shown to be mediated by nitric oxide.[65] Apparently, the electrical properties of the cell bodies in the ganglion can be altered by a peripheral lesion to an extent that they can be excited by activity in neighboring cells.

Figure 3-2 shows a partial lesion of a spinal nerve with the skin innervation spared. In this case, many fibers are assumed to be interrupted, but it is conceivable that the mechanism described below can also be triggered by a continuous mechanical irritation of the nerve that

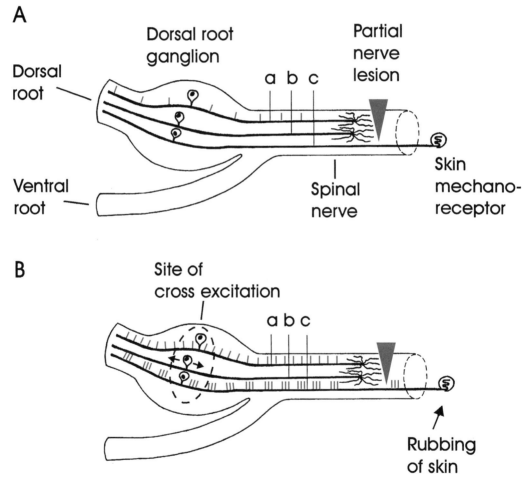

Figure 3-2. Cross excitation in a dorsal root ganglion. **A.** Partial lesion of a nerve distal to the ganglion. In this figure, fibers to the skin are assumed to be unaffected by the lesion. One of the axotomized afferent fibers (fiber *a*) has developed resting activity as a sequel of the axotomy. **B.** Rubbing of the skin excites the intact mechanosensitive skin afferents, which influence the axotomized fibers by cross excitation in the ganglion. Thus, the resting activity in fiber *a* is increased, and fiber *b* may develop resting activity that propagates from the ganglion in the direction of both the neuroma and the spinal cord. Prolonged pressure on a nerve that destroys some of the fibers can elicit the same events as shown here for a partial nerve lesion.

elicits action potentials at the site of the lesion. In the absence of afferent activity from the skin in the intact fiber (fiber *c* in Fig. 3-2*A*), there is no resting activity in severed fiber *b* and only little activity in severed fiber *a*. Rubbing the innervated skin (Fig. 3-2*B*) not only excites cutaneous afferent fiber *c* but also increases the resting activity in fiber *a* and may elicit impulses in silent fiber *b*. The action potentials that originate in the ganglion by cross excitation will propagate in the direction of both the lesion and the spinal cord.

If the origin of the potentials is the cell body, the impulses in fiber *a*, which had resting activity from the beginning, will increase the frequency in the central branch of the neuron but will collide with the afferent potentials in the peripheral branch. The afferent action potentials in fiber *b* will elicit sensations in the CNS, while the unimpeded efferent (antidromic) ones may influence the events at the lesion site by releasing biologically active substances.

In the patient, cross excitation is probably associated with at least three sensory disturbances:

Mislocalization of a stimulus. Since the activity spreads from one fiber to other fibers mediating sensations from other parts of the body, the patient mislocalizes a stimulus.

Allodynia. Since the activity in nonnociceptive fibers can be transmitted to nociceptive ones, pain can be elicited by a weak stimulus that activates only low-threshold mechanosensitive receptors.

Hyperpathia. Because of the multiplication of afferent activity that takes place in cross excitation, normal stimuli can lead to strong sensations with long-lasting aftersensations. The latter effect is probably the result of afterdischarges that can be observed in afferent fibers following cross excitation.

Findings from animal experiments indicate that after axotomy of the sciatic nerve, the electrical properties of cells in the dorsal root ganglion change, so that electrical stimulation of sympathetic efferent fibers can elicit activity in the ganglion.[19] Such an effect cannot be induced by sympathetic activity in normal ganglion cells (for effects of sympathetic activity on muscle pain, see Section E). Electrical stimulation of ventral roots was followed by an increase or by suppression of activity in the ganglion; this effect could be abolished by the α-adrenoreceptor antagonist, phentolamine. Single impulses in sympathetic fibers were ineffective, with no one-to-one transmission of activity (cross talk) from sympathetic fibers to cells of the dorsal root ganglion. The effects had a long latency of many seconds and substantial afterdischarges. Many of the cells that responded to sympathetic stimulation also showed cross excitation or cross afterdischarges following high-frequency stimulation of neighboring afferent fibers.

The functional coupling between sympathetic efferent fibers and afferent units might explain why neuropathic pain is often enhanced in stressful situations. If this coupling takes place in fibers subserving muscle pain, it would help to explain the influence of psychologic stress on muscle pain (see Section E).

5. Induction of Pain as a Result of a Lack of Activity in Thick Myelinated Fibers

Some evidence (mainly from clinical observations) suggests that interruption of afferent activity in thick myelinated (nonnociceptive) fibers may cause pain in the absence of noxious stimuli. Such an interruption may occur as a sequel of a degenerative demyelination of thick fibers.

One widely held explanation for this type of pain is that the balance between activity in thick and thin afferent fibers is disturbed under these conditions, with the dominating activity in thin fibers leading to pain. The problem with this concept is that with this type of pain there is no indication of impulse activity in nociceptive fibers. In fact, the pain-inhibiting action of activity in thick fibers at the spinal level is well proven (segmental inhibition) and is discussed in Chapter 7. The mechanism of segmental inhibition can function, however, only if impulse activity is present in nociceptive fibers. Under these conditions, input via thick myelinated fibers can only reduce the pain elicited by activity in nociceptive fibers. Recordings of the impulse activity of single nociceptors in humans and experimental animals (see Chapter 2) have shown that nociceptors are silent in the absence of a noxious stimulus. Therefore, the concept of a balance between continuous activity in nociceptive and non-nociceptive fibers must be considered questionable.

Other possible explanations for the pain following demyelination of non-nociceptive fibers are that the demyelination leads to ectopic activity in nociceptive afferent fibers or that the lack of activity in non-nociceptive fibers means functional deafferentation and leads to increased excitability or disinhibition of central nociceptive neurons.

B. NEUROMA

1. Influence of an Experimental Neuroma on the Activity in Afferent Nerve Fibers

Formation of a neuroma is the normal reaction to transection by every nerve fiber in spinal and cranial nerves. Clinically, neuroma formation following an incomplete transection is probably more frequent, but in animal experimentation a complete axotomy (nerve transection) is the preferred lesion.

A neuroma consists of nerve sprouts, fibroblasts, and fibrocytes, as well as proliferating Schwann cells.[33] The most striking feature of axotomized nerve fibers in a neuroma is that they develop ectopic resting activity (Fig. 3-1B).[64] The term "ectopic" means that the discharges originate at an abnormal location, i.e., not at the receptive ending (in the case of an afferent fiber) or in the soma of a motor neuron or postganglionic autonomic cell.

In an experimental neuroma of a spinal nerve, the proportion of A and C fibers that have abnormal resting activity varies with the species investigated and the time that elapsed after the axotomy (from a few percent to more than 30%).[33, 43] The activity has an irregular pattern and exhibits short, high-frequency bursts. This activity is likely to elicit sensations in an awake organism, with the bursts being particularly effective at central synapses. If the resting discharges occur in nociceptive fibers, they will elicit pain, and if they occur in non-nociceptive fibers, they will elicit paresthesia or dysesthesia.

Originally, this resting activity in the fibers of a neuroma was considered to be responsible for phantom sensations and phantom pain, i.e., for pain that was felt in an amputated limb. More recent data emphasize the relevance of changes in central neurons for phantom pain. Apparently, in most patients with phantom pain, central neurons are sensitized.[35] In these cases, little activity from a neuroma can lead to pain, or pain can occur in the absence of afferent activity. An important factor that may enhance the pain in amputees is that the non-nociceptive nerve impulses that normally reach the spinal cord are abolished because of the complete interruption of the nerves that supplied the amputated limb.

Another feature of nerve fibers in a neuroma is their mechanosensitivity. In a rat neuroma, 5 to 8% of the C fibers and up to 27% of the A fibers developed a sensitivity to mechanical stimuli; i.e., weak mechanical stimulation of the neuroma led to increased activity in the fibers.[43] The mechanosensitivity of axotomized fibers in a neuroma is probably the basis for the clinical Tinel sign. The mechanosensitivity varies with time; in other words, the above figures are valid only for a certain period of time in a given species (in one case, 22 to 30 hours after axotomy in the rat).

Axotomized nerve fibers also can develop chemosensitivity to catecholamines, particularly noradrenaline. Apparently, noradrenaline released from sympathetic efferent fibers in the neuroma can bind to α-receptors on afferent fibers. As a sequel, the afferent fibers are either excited or sensitized.[18, 51] This mechanism may be clinically important because it provides a positive feedback loop for the pain originating in a neuroma. The loop consists of nociceptive afferent fibers that increase the activity in sympathetic efferent fibers, which in turn release noradrenaline and activate nociceptive fibers in the neuroma. The feedback mechanism could explain why the phantom pain in some patients with neuromas is enhanced under conditions that are assumed to be associated with increased sympathetic efferent activity (mental or physical stress).

Another way of influencing fibers in a neuroma is that sympathetic efferent fibers release noradrenaline, which in this case binds to α_2-receptors on the same population of sympathetic efferent fibers. This triggers a cascade of events in these fibers that finally leads to the synthesis of prostaglandins of the E and I types. The prostaglandins belong to the types that have strong sensitizing properties on nociceptors (see Chapter 2). If these events take place in nociceptive fibers, pain can be elicited or enhanced.

A special feature of axotomized fibers in a chronic neuroma is the development of ephaptic cross talk, as compared with cross excitation described earlier. Normally, all axons in a nerve are completely ensheathed by Schwann cell processes. The sheath provides electrical insulation, and therefore, transmission of an action potential from one axon to a neighboring axon cannot occur. In a chronic neuroma, close appositions between axons that lack an insulating sheath (Fig. 3-1D) have been found.

Ephaptic transmission has been proven to exist between afferent fibers only; i.e., against general belief, there was no cross talk between efferent sympathetic and afferent nociceptive fibers.[20] For the development of pain states, the cross talk may nevertheless be important, particularly if a nerve is only partially severed. Then the target is partially reinnervated, and afferent activity from one nociceptor in the target tissue can be transmitted by ephapses in the neuroma to many nociceptive fibers. Thus, nociceptive activity is multiplied and can cause strong pain. This spread of excitation can also occur proximal to a neuroma because here ephapses have regularly been found.[33] In this case, the increased "resting" activity in a neuroma is the source of the afferent impulses that are multiplied.

Clinically, the neuroma can be excluded as a source of pain in amputees by mechanically stimulating the stump. If the patient's pain cannot be reproduced by this maneuver, the stump neuroma is unlikely to cause the pain.

This rather complicated picture of the situation in a neuroma is still a simplified one, since it ignores the changes outside the neuroma that contribute to neuroma pain. It is well known that after axotomy many cells in the dorsal root ganglion express the neuropeptides, galanin (GAL) and vasoactive intestinal polypeptide, which normally are not present in detectable amounts in these cells.[67] The sequelae of these changes for pain sensations are still unknown. They may be related to the occurrence of ectopic resting activity in the dorsal root ganglion, which is present in rats several days after axotomy.[19] Other changes following axotomy are death of neurons in the dorsal root ganglion and alterations of the anterograde and retrograde axonal transport in the axotomized fibers. Axotomy of a peripheral nerve also leads to marked changes in cells of the spinal dorsal horn. From experiments on cats and rats, it is well known that transection of a spinal nerve is followed by a considerable synaptic reorganization of the dorsal horn within a few days or even hours.[7, 30] After several days of deafferentation, neurons in the medial dorsal horn, which normally are driven by input from distal parts of a limb, acquire new input from the proximal limb. Thus, the entire dorsal horn is functionally "rewired" following a peripheral lesion.

2. Neuroma in Patients as a Cause of Muscle Pain

A neuroma is likely to form following a nerve injury that interrupts the continuity of nerve fibers. The proximal stump of the nerve, especially of sensory fibers, develops sprouts, not all of which find a suitable Schwann cell pathway. Many are physically blocked, causing a tangled web of homeless nerve endings.[15] As pointed out above, these endings become highly excitable and are responsive to minimal stimuli. Some may respond with discharges only during application of pressure, others may respond with a continuous discharge throughout the application of pressure, and some can exhibit a continuous discharge without external stimulation.[17] The latter would account for spontaneous unprovoked pain. The tendency to develop neuromas is highly variable from one person to the next.

Severing a peripheral nerve always results in the development of some degree of neuroma.[15] The site reaches maximum sensitivity in approximately 2 weeks; then the sensitivity fades but retains some degree of increased sensitivity indefinitely. Because muscle nociceptors are formed by A-δ and C fibers—the fibers that are most prone to develop neuroma[17]—and because the pain is often perceived as deep tissue pain, nociceptive fibers from muscle are likely to contribute to this pain when a nerve carrying these afferents is disrupted.

Frequently, connective tissue trigger points (TrPs) located in surgical scars behave as if they were small neuromas that developed from severed fine sensory nerves. They respond to analgesic injections when the injection is adequately localized into the highly circumscribed site of sensitivity.

C. RADICULOPATHY

Pain associated with a lesion or dysfunction of a nerve root commonly has a deep aching quality that is a deep tissue pain characteristic of pain arising from muscle. It also frequently includes other characteristics, such as sharp, stabbing, shooting sensations that are not so characteristic of myogenic pain.[21] In conducting numerous cervical discectomies under local anesthesia, Murphey et al.[45, 46] reported that touching the damaged root produced severe pain in the arm but that normal cervical roots elicited only electrical sensations. The pain response from the damaged root can be accounted for by predepolarization of the fine afferent nerve fibers (including nociceptive afferents from deep tissues), so that the additional mechanical stimulus initiated a series of action potentials. The electrical sensations from normal nerves would fit the relatively increased responsiveness of normal large myelinated nerve fibers to mechanical stimulation, compared with fine nerve fibers.

It is the experience of practitioners acquainted with myogenic sources of muscle pain such as TrPs that patients suffering from myofascial pain of TrP origin commonly arrive with the diagnosis of radiculopathy that did not meet operative criteria or was the basis of an unsuccessful operation. The referred pain patterns of muscles such as the scaleni, gluteus minimus, and piriformis closely mimic the pain expected of a radiculopathy. This is not helped by the fact that dermatomal territories show marked individual variation,[21] as do myogenic referred pain patterns.[57a, 63] A definitive differential diagnosis thus is of utmost importance to the patient.

Radiculopathy usually includes loss of sensation, in addition to pain, and often (but not necessarily) motor involvement that is identifiable by needle electromyography. Sensory radiculopathy may be detected by more sophisticated sensory nerve studies, including sensory-evoked potentials. The TrPs can be identified by the appropriate physical examination (see Chapter 8). TrPs may account for the pain in many patients diagnosed as having pseudoradiculopathy, which is often another way of saying, "It looks like radiculopathy but isn't, and I don't know what it is."

D. PERIPHERAL NEUROPATHY

In many cases, peripheral neuropathy occurs as the result of diseases such as diabetes, alcoholism, and amyloidosis. The pain of peripheral neuropathy may be spontaneous or evoked by an activity or stimulus. Spontaneous pain is commonly described as deep aching in the extremities and as a superficial stinging, prickling, or burning pain. Sometimes, it is described as shock-like and lancinating.[55]

Two pathologic processes are observed: axonal loss, often in small fibers, or demyelination of thick fibers. In axonal loss, the missing axons will not generate action potentials unless they have sprouting stumps that are hypersensitive, which is not usually the case. The loss of central stimulation from the missing small nociceptive nerve fibers, however, can induce neuroblastic changes that are algogenic, as described in Chapter 7. Demyelination is known to cause loss of conduction of action potentials, instead of serving as a source of them. Conversely, the loss of input via thick myelinated fibers may cause pain resulting from a deafferentation mechanism. In less severe cases, partial demyelination may not block but may change impulse conduction in thick myelinated fibers. This may explain paresthesias and dysesthesias, which are common in peripheral neuropathy.

The same differential diagnostic principles apply to peripheral neuropathy as to radiculopathy, described above.

E. COMPLEX REGIONAL PAIN SYNDROME (REFLEX SYMPATHETIC DYSTROPHY)
1. Basic Science Aspects

As exemplified in Chapter 6, the available experimental data concerning the contribution of sympathetic efferent activity to muscle pain are controversial.

Data obtained from receptors in a rat hemidiaphragm-phrenic nerve preparation in vitro have shown that adrenaline increases the resting discharge in HTM (high-threshold mechanosensitive, presumably nociceptive) receptors and sensitizes them to mechanical stimulation. Particularly susceptible to adrenaline were endings that were kept under the influence of a continuous noxious mechanical stimulus.[37] Hypoxia likewise sensitized some of the diaphragmatic receptors. These results support the assumption that nociceptors in a damaged muscle may be directly activated and/or sensitized by efferent sympathetic activity. A new aspect is that sympathetic postganglionic fibers in pathologically altered tissue are able to release prostaglandin E_2 (PGE_2), which in turn may sensitize nociceptors.[5]

Data obtained from patients point in the same direction, namely, that sympathetic efferent activity may enhance muscle pain under special circumstances. For example, a stellate blockade in fibromyalgia patients has been shown to relieve the pain.[6] In that situation, the sympathetic influence on peripheral nerve endings and blood vessels is not simply the result of increased frequency in postganglionic fibers; in fibromyalgia patients at least, microneurographic data do not show sympathetic overactivity.[25]

The pain-relieving effect of a stellate block in fibromyalgia is hard to understand. Theoretically, the block would be useful if the pain of fibromyalgia was caused by (catecholamine-induced) sensitization of nociceptors. As discussed in Chapter 8, however, the most likely reason for fibromyalgia is a central nervous dysfunction that should not be readily influenced by blocking a peripheral ganglion. Possibly, the block removes an additional sensitizing factor that enhances the pain locally.

Evidence in the literature indicates that sympathetic activity may be involved indirectly in muscle pain by increasing the electrogenic component of muscle tone. The increase in tone is assumed to be caused by sympathetically induced activation of the intrafusal muscle fibers of the muscle spindle. It is questionable, however, if the increase in muscle spindle input brought about by this mechanism is sufficient to increase the mechanical tension of a muscle or to induce muscle contractions via the monosynaptic stretch reflex (for a review of this aspect, see Ref. 27).

One interesting concept states that in cases of reflex sympathetic dystrophy (see Section E2 below), the pain is caused not by an increased sympathetic outflow but by a supersensitivity of vessels and/or nerves to sympathetic transmitter substances.[22] Results from animal experiments support this assumption by showing that following a partial nerve lesion, nociceptors of the skin become sensitive to efferent sympathetic activity and noradrenaline.[54]

Both nerve endings and afferent C fibers appear to be sensitive to catecholamines. In rabbits, efferent sympathetic activity has been shown to inhibit conduction in unmyelinated afferent fibers, probably by depolarizing the axonal membrane.[57] The clinical significance of this finding is hard to assess; in cases of chronic pain, the persistent depolarization of nociceptive C fibers could enhance the pain, since the membrane potential is closer to electrical threshold. This situation could lead to an increased excitability or even to instability of the afferent fiber. Conversely, a long-lasting and strong depolarization is likely to block conduction; therefore, the direction of the action of catecholamines on the afferent fiber (depression or increased excitability) will depend on the degree and duration of the depolarization.

When considering possible effects of sympathetic efferent activity on nociception from muscle, keep in mind that the functional organization of sympathetic fibers to muscle is different from that of postganglionic fibers to skin. Therefore, both subsystems can react differently under the influence of an adverse stimulus. For instance, the sympathetic activity in a muscle nerve can rise and that in a skin nerve can remain unchanged during immersion of a hand in ice water.[26] Therefore, the term "sympathetic tone" for describing the overall activity in the sympathetic nervous system is not useful.

2. Clinical Aspects

In the 1950s, the group of symptoms that behaved clinically as though they depended on abnormal sympathetic nervous system activity was included in the generic term "reflex sympathetic dystrophy." By the beginning of the 1990s, it became clear that this term was an oversimplification. It was officially replaced[42] by the noncommittal term **"complex regional pain syndrome (CRPS),"** which the authors defined as including CRPS type I, which had no known neurologic lesion to account for the pain, and CRPS type II, which was associated with partial injury of a nerve. No other clinical feature clearly distinguishes these two conditions, and in either case, the patient may have the symptoms of sympathetically maintained pain or of sympathetically independent pain. This complicated subject is of interest here because the essential pain feature commonly includes deep aching (muscle and other deep tissue) pain and/or burning pain, particularly in an extremity. In addition to muscle pain, both CRPS types I and II characteristically show disabling motor disturbances.

Clinical characteristics of CRPS include (1) pain that is intermittent or continuous and often exacerbated by physical or emotional stressors; (2) sensory changes that include hyperesthesia to any modality and allodynia in response to light touch, thermal stimulation (cold or warm), deep pressure, or joint movement; (3) sympathetic dysfunction observed as vasomotor or sudomotor instability in the involved limb; (4) edema of either the pitting or brawny type that may or may not respond to dependency and elevation of the limb; and (5) motor dysfunctions that may include tremor, dystonia, loss of strength, and

loss of endurance of the affected muscle groups.[10, 66] In cases of sympathetically maintained pain, sympatholytic interventions may provide temporary or permanent pain relief.[42] As emphasized in Jänig's summary of our current state of knowledge on this subject,[34] there are more questions than answers.

One of the unexplored, and promising, facets of CRPS type I (by far the most common) is the contribution of myofascial TrPs. In many patients, seen by a number of astute clinicians, a CRPS seemed to dispose to the development of TrPs in the affected musculature. Frequently, inactivation of the TrPs markedly improved, if not relieved, the symptoms, especially if the intervention occurred within a month or so of onset. This may be another example of the strong two-way interaction between an active TrP and the autonomic nervous system, a subject that is in need of experimental investigation. A more direct (and treatable) involvement of muscles in some of these patients may be as yet unrecognized.

F. MANAGEMENT

With the correct diagnosis properly documented, it was hoped that an understanding of the various neuropathic mechanisms responsible for the condition would make specific treatment possible. Indeed, specific antagonists are available for pain mediators like substance P, glutamate, prostaglandins, and growth factors, but clinical uses for them have not always followed the expected course. It should be possible to restore needed balance to the process of nociception (balancing pronociceptive and antinociceptive forces). Unfortunately, with only a few exceptions, specific therapies for painful neuropathic conditions, which were predicted theoretically, have remained elusive. In most cases, the most successful therapies are medical (as opposed to surgical), nonspecific (as opposed to focusing on modulating responses to a specific nociceptive receptor), and largely empiric.

Before embarking on the description of medical therapy for neuropathic pain, note that surgery can occasionally be helpful. When compressive neuropathy, exemplified by spinal stenosis or radiculopathy (vertebral spurs, extruded disc fragments, growth of a mass in a closed space), is responsible for the symptoms, surgery can be dramatically effective. Usually, however, such a reversible cause cannot be identified.

Often, the most successful medical regimens for reduction of pain, improved quality of life, and return to work involve integrated, multimodal intervention programs. The components of such approaches involve reassurance, education, and alleviation of affective symptoms, motivation, exercise, and medications. Perhaps the most common reason for failure of therapy for chronic pain is a naive dependence on medication alone to solve the problem.

Reassurance must be based on educating the affected person, must be realistic, and must be as hopeful as possible, because a positive attitude is clearly important to the hard work of rehabilitation. There is reason for optimism despite the dismal record of a 2% return to work among beneficiaries of U. S. Social Security Administration disability funding.[12] A controlled clinical trial was conducted in Texas and involved people who had been troubled by low back pain for at least 2 years and who had been off work for at least 1 year.[39] After participating in a 3-week work rehabilitation program, 87% of the subjects in the active intervention group had returned to work and were still on the job 2 years later. Only 41% of the untreated group had successfully returned to work.

The role of the affective-emotional component in perpetuating the symptoms of chronic pain is still controversial. Conversely, few would argue that when depression or anxiety is present, there should be active efforts to alleviate the affective symptoms. Short-term therapy with a nighttime dose of a tricyclic antidepressant medication, such as amitriptyline at 10 to 50 mg, may be sufficient to improve sleep and reduce the severity of the mood disorder. An anxiolytic drug, such as alprazolam 0.25 to 1.0 mg or clonazepam 0.5 to 1.0 mg, at bedtime may be sufficient to ward off the sense of doom associated with financial concerns resulting from physical impairment. When the mood disturbance or thought disorder is more serious or suicide ideation is present, psychiatric consultation is indicated. A confident, proactive, positive approach on the part of the health care team can be supportive to a patient at risk of lacking adequate motivation.

Physical exercise is valuable to any restorative program. Besides providing cardiovascular fitness, exercise provides confidence and appears to raise the endogenous serotonin levels (Geel, Russell, unpublished data). An example of a useful aerobic exercise is for the patient to walk in place while standing in water at about breast level. The patient walks at a slow comfortable warm-up pace with swinging arms for 5 minutes and then increases the pace until shortness of breath is experienced. The patient then slows the pace until again comfortable and then increases the pace to shortness of breath. Next, the patient slows to a comfortable pace to finish out a full 20 minutes. Maintaining this kind of program three times per week can go a long way to restoring cardiovascular fitness. Its best advantages include aerobic involvement of the upper extremities and minimal weight bearing on lower extremity joints, which may be compromised by arthritis or injury. Other active interventions of proven value include performance of work-like activities in a work-like environment to give the worker confidence in the skills needed for success.

Medications used with some success in people with chronic painful neuropathy include analgesics, anesthetics, sedative hypnotics, anticonvulsants, and opioids.

Non-narcotic oral analgesics, such as aspirin (650 mg PO qid), acetaminophen (1,000 mg PO tid), ibuprofen (800 mg PO tid), or naproxen (500 mg PO tid), can provide relief from moderately severe pain. The dosage of acetaminophen should be reduced by approximately 50% for patients with liver cirrhosis. The dosages of the nonsteroidal anti-inflammatory drugs (NSAIDs) may need to be reduced in the elderly or in those with recognized renal disease. The new NSAID, ketorolac (short course of 10 mg PO tid or a single IV or IM dosage of 15 to 60 mg), can be as effective as a narcotic. Tramadol (50 to 100 mg qid) is a centrally acting, non-narcotic analgesic that can be viewed as providing the combined analgesic action of a tricyclic antidepressant and a mild μ-opioid agonist.

Local injection of an anesthetic agent at the site of a myofascial TrP or even in the region of a small neuroma where cross excitation is occurring may be beneficial, even if transient.

For the treatment of a neuroma, it may be appropriate to use a long-acting agent (e.g., bupivacaine 0.25 or 0.5%, a dose of 5 mL containing 12.5 to 25.0 mg). It may provide more persistent relief (8 to 12 hours) than can be achieved by the shorter-acting agents exemplified by lidocaine (1.5 or 2.0%, a dose of 5 mL containing 75 to 100 mg).

For treatment of myofascial TrPs in skeletal muscle, bupivacaine should be avoided because it may be myotoxic[32, 48] or even neurotoxic.[8] Lidocaine 1.0% is appropriate for injection of myofascial TrPs when repeated passes with injection of less than 0.1 mL at each site is the typical procedure. The addition of epinephrine to the anesthetic is contraindicated.[57] The chief advantage of the injection of an anesthetic (compared with dry needling when needling is sufficiently precise to elicit local twitch responses) is the reduction of postinjection soreness. There is no known evidence that anesthetics that have a longer duration than lidocaine are of any advantage for the injection of TrPs. If a longer-acting anesthetic is considered necessary, etidocaine has exhibited little or no myotoxicity, compared with bupivacaine.[16] When injecting in an area of an inflamed tendon, bursa, or ligament sheath, some clinicians use a small amount of corticosteroid (microcrystalline triamcinolone hexacetonide or crystalline betamethasone) with the anesthetic agent.

Some oral sedative hypnotics are beneficial in patients with a number of neuropathic and other chronic pain conditions. The tricyclic antidepressant drugs, amitriptyline (10 to 50 mg qhs) or imipramine (10 to 50 mg qhs), can improve the quality of sleep with minimal daytime drowsiness. The analgesic effect may be related to the inhibition of serotonin reuptake in the interneural synapse.

At least two anticonvulsant drugs have been found to reduce the severity of pain in patients with trigeminal neuralgia and a variety of peripheral neuropathic conditions. Carbamazepine therapy can be used to decrease the intermittent, sharp, stabbing, burning pain symptoms associated with diabetic neuropathy and postherpetic neuralgia. Dosage should begin low, i.e., 100 mg qhs, then 100 mg bid, but may increase to 800 mg/day in divided doses. The effective dosage range for phenytoin is 200 to 400 mg/day. Because many potential adverse effects are associated with either of these agents, the health care provider must be familiar with them.

Carbamazepine has been found to be beneficial in diabetic-uropathic neuropathy,[68] for the lightning pains of tabes dorsalis,[2, 23, 24] for amyloid neuropathy,[4] for the pain of thiamine deficiency,[59] for the pain of Morton's neuroma,[29] in more than 30% of patients with trigeminal neuralgia,[62] for intractable neurogenic pain,[50] for phantom limb pain,[49] and for the pain associated with multiple sclerosis.[31] In a 4-week, randomized, double-blind crossover trial involving 15 patients with central poststroke pain, amitriptyline appeared to be more effective than carbamazepine in reducing pain severity.[38] Unfortunately, carbamazepine also produced a greater number of side effects, requiring dosage reduction.

The use of opioid agonists for chronic pain is still controversial. They seem to be safe for acute pain and are well justified in terminal malignancy, but concern exists regarding their use in treatment-resistant myogenous pain. Every effort should be made to identify the cause of the pain first, especially if it is caused by fibromyalgia or TrPs.

Generally, opioid agonists taken to relieve pain (not for their psychic effects) are not associated with progressive physical dependency (addiction). When these drugs are taken to relieve pain, the patient usually functions better at work and in social settings. When they are taken for psychic effects, these improvements are not noted. The treating physician should monitor patient behavior to confirm the purpose for which the patient is taking the opioid. When such agents are needed for moderately severe pain on a short-term basis or for recurrent use at a frequency less than three occasions per week, it may be appropriate to use codeine (15 to 30 mg PO) or hydrocodone (2.5 to 5.0 mg PO per dose compounded with aspirin or acetaminophen).

When analgesia is needed on an emergency basis for acute exacerbation of a chronically painful condition, propoxyphene or propoxyphene compounded with a non-narcotic analgesic, such as acetaminophen, would probably not be more effective than ketorolac. Morphine (10 to 30 mg IM or IV), meperidine (50 to 100 mg IM or PO), or levorphanol (2 to 12 mg IV or IM or 4 to 24 mg PO) may be appropriate in rare instances.

CRPS type I[61] may require new approaches. Strategies in the past have focused on the administration of systemic corticosteroids,[28] intermittent use of sympathetic ganglionic blockade,[36] or even surgical intervention. More recent evidence suggests that conservative therapy with a small array of medications should be the initial treatment of choice. The recommended medications include a calcium channel blocker, nifedipine[47]; an α-adrenergic blocker, phenoxybenzamine[47]; an anticonvulsant, gabapentin[41]; and a bisphosphonate, alendronate.[1] Use of one or more of these medications can be dramatically beneficial in patients with this condition. This seems particularly true for patients with relatively early and mild disease.[47]

G. MORE ABOUT THE MEDICATIONS

The following descriptions of representative medications were abstracted from standard reference services.[3, 40, 48a, 58] They provide useful data about the medications listed above. For ease in finding a given agent, they are listed alphabetically in eight categories and then by generic name. It is the responsibility of the health care provider to appropriately apply this information to a given patient or clinical situation. Most of the listed medications require careful monitoring for continued benefit and adverse effects.

1. α-Adrenergic Blockers

Generic Name: *phenoxybenzamine*
Brand Name: Dibenzyline
  Dosage: In adults, treatment should begin with 10 mg bid and increase by 10 mg qod to a maximum of 20 to 40 mg per dose bid or tid.
  Action: The onset of action is slow—over a period of hours—but once complete it is persistent for 3 to 4 days. The effect is mediated by a noncompetitive blockade of α-adrenergic receptors but does not affect β-adrenergic receptors. Cutaneous, splanchnic, and renal blood flow are increased, but cerebral and skeletal muscle blood flow are generally unchanged.
  Side Effects: Common problems include nasal congestion, miosis, postural hypotension, orthostatic dizziness, and palpitations.
  Considerations: In treatment of CRPS, the earlier in the course that treatment can begin, the more likely it is to be effective. Most of the men treated with this drug experienced impotence, but it was not a common cause for discontinuing the drug. Problems that did prompt discontinuation included orthostatic dizziness, nausea, and diarrhea.

2. Analgesics

Generic Name: *acetaminophen (paracetamol)*
Brand Name: Tylenol
  Dosage: 325 to 650 mg every 4 hours with fluid.
  Action: The analgesic effect of acetaminophen is believed to be comparable with aspirin, but there is little or no anti-inflammatory effect with acetaminophen. The combination of acetaminophen with aspirin offers little advantage, but the combination of acetaminophen with a low-dose opioid, such as codeine, appears to provide analgesic synergy. The plasma half-life is 1 to 3 hours.
  Side Effects: In a therapeutic, short-term dosage, acetaminophen is less toxic than aspirin because it is less likely to cause dyspepsia and blood loss or interfere with therapeutic anticoagulation. Dose-dependent hepatic necrosis is the most serious acute toxic effect associated with overdosage and is potentially fatal. Chronic ingestion of large dosages, especially in combinations with other agents, is hazardous to the kidney, the liver, and marrow production. The risk of hepatotoxicity is increased by coadministration of anticonvulsants or isoniazid.
  Considerations: When analgesia without an anti-inflammatory effect is desired, this agent is useful. Avoid chronic ingestion and coingestion with alcohol. The relative benefit/risk ratio should be reassessed after 10 days of therapy.

Generic Name: *acetylsalicylic acid*
Brand Name: Bayer Aspirin, Ecotrin, ZORprin
  Dosage: 325 to 650 mg every 4 hours with food or fluid.

Action: The analgesic effect of aspirin is believed to result from inhibition of prostaglandin synthesis by acetylating cyclo-oxygenase in the periphery, but actions in the CNS and directly on white blood cells may be contributory. There is no evidence for tachyphylaxis with time. In small dosages the elimination half-life is only 2 to 3 hours, but in high dosages it can extend to 15 to 30 hours.

Side Effects: The most common adverse events relate to gastrointestinal tract toxicity, resulting in dyspepsia, gastric ulceration, and bleeding. Patients may lose up to 10 mL of blood daily with resultant iron deficiency anemia.

Considerations: Despite its long history of medical usage, few analgesic preparations exhibit analgesic efficacy superior to aspirin. In patients who tolerate it, the analgesic effect is usually quite good and the cost is low. Some clinicians believe that it may be tolerated better in buffered, enteric-coated, or sustained-release forms. The relative benefit/risk ratio should be reassessed after 10 days of therapy and periodically thereafter.

Generic Name: *ketorolac tromethamine*
Brand Name: Toradol
   Dosage: Acute IV or IM dosage 30 to 60 mg, or 30 mg every 6 hours, not to exceed 120 mg/day. Oral dosage 10 to 20 mg every 4 to 6 hours with food or fluid, not to exceed 40 mg/day. For geriatric patients or those weighing less than 50 kg, the dosage should be reduced by at least 50%.
   Action: The analgesic effect is comparable with aspirin by similar mechanisms. The plasma half-life is 4 to 6 hours in healthy persons but may be longer in those with renal disease and in geriatric patients.
   Side Effects: With parenteral therapy, there may be pain or local bleeding at the site of injection. The most frequent adverse effects associated with short-term use involve the gastrointestinal tract and the nervous system. The risk of serious gastric lesions may be less with parenteral therapy than with oral therapy. CNS effects can include somnolence, dizziness, and headache, but stimulation, including seizures, can occur. Potentially serious hepatic, renal, hematologic, cardiovascular, and cutaneous effects have been reported.
   Considerations: The main advantage with this drug is its availability in parenteral form for use in severe headache or other acute pain, in which it can substitute for opioid analgesics. The relative benefit/risk ratio should be reassessed after 5 days of therapy and periodically thereafter.

Generic Name: *naproxen, naproxen sodium*
Brand Name: Naprosyn, Anaprox, and Aleve (over the counter in the United States)
   Dosage: 250 mg, 375 mg, or 500 mg every 8 to 12 hours with food or fluid.

Action: The analgesic effect is comparable with that of aspirin and occurs by similar mechanisms, except that the antiplatelet effects with naproxen are reversible. Naproxen may be more effective than aspirin for dysmenorrhea. Its plasma half-life is 10 to 20 hours.
   Side Effects: The most frequent adverse effects involve the gastrointestinal tract (gastritis, peptic ulceration, bleeding, perforation, and diarrhea), but the frequency and severity of these effects may be less than with aspirin and more than with acetaminophen. Peptic ulceration can occur *de novo* or can be exacerbated. Taking naproxen with food, or concomitant use of misoprostol at 200 µg qid, can reduce the risk of gastric mucosal injury. CNS effects can include dizziness, headache, confusion, aseptic meningitis, and tinnitus. Potentially serious gastric, hepatic, renal, hematologic, and cutaneous effects can occur.
   Considerations: Coadministration with other analgesic agents should be avoided, but coadministration with amitriptyline has been found useful in some pain states. The relative benefit/risk ratio should be reassessed after 10 days of therapy and periodically thereafter.

3. Anesthetics

Generic Name: *bupivacaine*
Brand Name: Marcaine, Sensorcaine, Bupivacaine
   Dosage: With or without epinephrine, the total dosage of bupivacaine per day should not exceed 400 mg (approximately 160 mL of 0.25%, 80 mL of 0.5%, or 53 mL of 0.75% solution). The smallest dose and the lowest concentration required to produce the desired effect should be used.
   Action: Bupivacaine blocks the generation and conduction of impulses through all nerve fibers: sensory, somatomotor, and autonomic. The elimination half-life of bupivacaine ranges from 1.5 to 5.5 hours in adults. The onset of anesthesia after local injection occurs in 2 to 10 minutes and lasts for up to 7 hours. Coadministration with epinephrine may prolong the duration of anesthesia.
   Indication: Local infiltration for nerve block is a typical use in patients with regional or neuropathic pain. Because bupivacaine appears to be toxic to skeletal muscle cells,[32, 48] its use for treating myofascial TrPs cannot be recommended. Curiously, bupivacaine may be useful in regenerating muscle that has become atrophic after denervation.[32]
   Side Effects: As noted above, bupivacaine can be toxic to skeletal muscle cells. Periodic aspiration should be exercised to avoid unintended intravenous injection, which can cause serious CNS and cardiovascular effects. Contained preservatives (e.g., sodium metabisulfite) can induce allergic or anaphylactic reactions, especially in asthmatic patients.

Considerations: Bupivacaine's main advantage over lidocaine for nerve block, and perhaps for treatment of neuroma, is its longer duration of action. Because the onset of action of lidocaine is more rapid than that of bupivacaine, combining them may be of value when rapid action is indicated. Bupivacaine is not recommended for injecting muscle TrPs.

Generic Name: *etidocaine hydrochloride*
Brand Name: Duranest
   Dosage: For peripheral nerve block and soft tissue injection with or without epinephrine, a dose of 5 to 40 mL (50 to 400 mg) is considered adequate. The lowest concentration and the smallest total dose required to produce the desired effect should be used.
   Action: Etidocaine blocks the generation and conduction of impulses through all nerve fibers (sensory, somatomotor, and autonomic). The mechanism may be a blockade of calcium-binding sites. The duration of action is long, ranging from 4.5 to 13 hours.
   Indication: Local infiltration for nerve block is a typical use in patients with regional or neuropathic pain. Etidocaine is a "long-acting" anesthetic agent and seems to exhibit little or no myotoxicity, compared with bupivacaine.[16] Therefore, it can be combined with a rapidly acting agent, such as lidocaine, for soft tissue injection, which specifically will or incidentally may involve contact with skeletal muscle.
   Side Effects: As noted above for bupivacaine, periodic aspiration should be accomplished to avoid unintended intravascular injection, which can cause CNS and cardiovascular effects. Rarely, even small doses can adversely influence cardiac function. Epinephrine can cause anxiety, palpitations, dizziness, tachycardia, angina, hypertension, pulmonary edema, and ventricular fibrillation. Contained preservatives (e.g., sodium metabisulfite) can induce allergic or anaphylactic reactions, especially in asthmatic patients.
   Considerations: Etidocaine's main advantage over lidocaine for nerve block, and perhaps for treatment of neuroma, is its longer duration of action. It appears to exhibit little or no myotoxicity, so it can be considered relatively safer than bupivacaine for soft tissue injection but is not recommended for myofascial TrP injections. Because the onset of action of lidocaine is more rapid than that of etidocaine, combining them may be of value when rapid action is indicated.

Generic Name: *lidocaine hydrochloride*
Brand Name: Lidocaine, Xylocaine
   Dosage: Solutions ranging in concentration from 0.5 to 4.0% are available for parenteral injection, with or without epinephrine. The total dosage should not exceed 4.5 mg/kg in adults.

   Action: Like other anesthetic agents, lidocaine blocks the generation and conduction of impulses through all nerve fibers (sensory, somatomotor, and autonomic). The mechanism may be a blockade of calcium-binding sites.
   Indication: Local infiltration for nerve block is a typical use in patients with regional or neuropathic pain. Lidocaine is appropriate for use in injecting myofascial TrPs in skeletal muscle. The duration of action in the absence of epinephrine is only approximately 90 minutes.
   Side Effects: As with other local anesthetic agents, care should be exercised to avoid unintended intravenous injection, which can cause CNS and cardiovascular effects. Rarely, even small doses can adversely influence cardiac function.
   Considerations: Lidocaine's main advantage over bupivacaine is that lidocaine seems to be less toxic for skeletal muscles and has a shorter duration of action for situations in which that is desired. Combining lidocaine with epinephrine or a longer-acting anesthetic agent (bupivacaine, etidocaine, or tetracaine) can prolong the duration of anesthesia. Epinephrine is contraindicated when injecting TrPs. The durations of action of these agents are approximately 4 to 7 hours, 4 to 13 hours, and 1 to 3 hours, respectively. Etidocaine and tetracaine seem not to exhibit the myotoxicity observed with bupivacaine.[16] A good combination regimen is lidocaine with etidocaine (1:4, v:v).

4. Anticonvulsants

Generic Name: *carbamazepine*
Brand Name: Tegretol, Epitol, Carbamazepine
   Dosage: For trigeminal neuralgia, begin with 100 mg PO bid and gradually increase to a maximum of 1.2 g/day in 2 to 3 divided doses. Maintenance dosage may range from 200 mg/day to 1.2 g/day but usually ranges from 400 to 800 mg/day.
   Action: Carbamazepine is structurally related to the tricyclic antidepressants, such as amitriptyline. Like phenytoin, carbamazepine reduces synaptic transmission within the trigeminal nucleus. It also exhibits sedative, antidepressant, and muscle relaxant actions. It is absorbed slowly from the gastrointestinal tract. Steady-state plasma levels may not be reached for 2 to 4 days. Therapeutic levels range from 3 to 14 µg/mL. The plasma half-life ranges from 8 to 72 hours, with the major source of metabolism being the liver. Carbamazepine can induce liver microsomal enzymes to enhance its own metabolism and that of other drugs.
   Indication: The main indications are seizure disorders (generalized, partial complex), trigeminal neuralgia, and neurogenic pain (especially lightning pains of tabes dorsalis).
   Side Effects: As with phenytoin, many potential adverse effects are associated with use of carbamaze-

pine. They can include CNS effects (such as confusion, blurred vision, dizziness, insomnia, headache), cardiovascular system effects (such as tachycardia, arrhythmias, atrioventricular block), gastrointestinal tract effects (such as nausea, vomiting), hepatic effects (such as toxic hepatitis), genitourinary system effects (such as urinary retention, renal failure, impotence), effects on the skin (such as photosensitive reactions, urticaria), lymphatic system effects (localized or generalized lymphadenopathy, serum sickness), effects on the blood (such as thrombocytopenia, leukopenia, granulocytopenia), musculoskeletal system effects (myalgia, arthralgia, muscle cramps), and endocrine system effects (such as hyponatremia, inappropriate antidiuretic syndrome). A complete blood cell count, liver function tests, and renal function tests should be evaluated prior to initiating therapy and periodically thereafter. Carbamazepine should be used with caution in combination with other anticonvulsants, calcium channel blocking agents, erythromycin, doxycycline, psychotherapeutic agents, and warfarin because of crossed effects on metabolism.

Considerations: Carbamazepine has the potential to be helpful in many neuropathies, but the risk of adverse events is also high. It is more likely than phenytoin to be helpful in those disorders.

Generic Name: *clonazepam*
Brand Name: Klonopin
Dosage: When used for periodic leg movements during sleep, 0.5 to 2.0 mg qhs may be effective. Notice that the dosage is lower than is indicated for anxiety or panic. Although parenteral forms are available, oral therapy is the usual route of administration for treatment of pain, sleep, and movement disorders.

Action: The mechanism associated with benefit is uncertain, but the anxiolytic or sedating effects may be responsible. There is evidence that benzodiazepines cause skeletal muscle relaxation by facilitating the inhibitory action of γ-aminobutyric acid in the brain or spinal cord. The duration of benefit from a single dose may be up to 8 hours.

Indication: The main uses of this drug have been in the treatment of petit mal seizures and as concomitant therapy for seizures resistant to other agents alone. It has been used with benefit in patients with akinetic or myoclonic seizures.

Side Effects: The most frequent untoward effects associated with short-term use of clonazepam are similar to those of other benzodiazepine drugs. CNS effects can be sedation, abnormal mentation, nightmares, dysarthria, and extrapyramidal reactions. Chronic usage can contribute to dependency. Acute discontinuation of large dosages can result in breakthrough seizures.

Considerations: Administration at night for myoclonic movements offers the potential additional benefit of improved sleep for patients with chronic pain. There may be synergy with other analgesic drugs. The relative benefit/risk ratio should be reassessed after 2 to 3 months of therapy because dependency may occur. When discontinuation of chronic therapy is indicated, the dosage should be tapered down at a rate of approximately 0.5 mg every 3 days.

Generic Name: *phenytoin*
Brand Name: Dilantin, Phenytoin
Dosage: Initial therapy can begin with 100 mg bid to tid. Chronic therapy often requires 300 mg every morning.

Action: The principal mechanism of action is by a reduction of the post-tetanic potentiation of synaptic transmission and/or by a reduction of nerve conductance. This raises the seizure threshold. Rapid absorption from the gastrointestinal tract is associated with peak plasma levels at 1 to 3 hours from a single oral dosage of 100 mg, while extended-release capsules give peak levels at 4 to 12 hours. Phenytoin is metabolized primarily by the liver and is excreted in the urine as the glucuronide (60 to 75%). The average plasma half-life is approximately 22 hours, but it may range from 7 to 42 hours.

Indication: Proven uses include seizure disorders of generalized type and partial complex type, cardiac arrhythmias, migraine headache, and trigeminal neuralgia. Phenytoin can be used for the treatment of other types of neuralgia.

Side Effects: A package insert states that "if a new clinical problem develops during phenytoin therapy, the phenytoin is the cause until proven otherwise." Most patients tolerate (are relatively free of side effects) blood levels of less than 25 µg/mL. Between 25 and 30 µg/mL, nystagmus, ataxia, and diplopia may develop. Above 30 µg/mL, drowsiness, lethargy, and coma may develop. Slow metabolizers are unusually susceptible to side effects, even at low dosages. There are common side effects in the CNS (such as confusion, blurred vision, dizziness, insomnia, headache, dyskinesia, chorea, tremor), gastrointestinal tract (such as nausea and vomiting), liver (toxic hepatitis), skin (such as gum hyperplasia, hypertrichosis, morbilliform rash), lymphatic system (such as localized or generalized lymphadenopathy, pseudolymphoma, lymphoma), blood (such as thrombocytopenia, leukopenia, granulocytopenia, pancytopenia, macrocytosis, megaloblastic anemia responsive to folic acid therapy), skeletal system (osteomalacia resulting from interference with vitamin D metabolism), and endocrine system (hyperglycemia, increased insulin requirement in diabetics, hyperosmolar-nonketotic coma).

Considerations: This drug would probably be used for neuropathic pain only after more conservative and safer remedies have proven unsuccessful or inadequate. Carbamazepine is used for this indication more often than is phenytoin. Confusion may arise during treatment of neuropathy because neuropathy is a reported side effect of long-term (>5 years) treatment with phenytoin.[44, 56, 60]

5. Calcium Channel Blockers

Generic Name: *nifedipine*
Brand Name: Short-acting: Procardia 10 mg or 20 mg; Adalat 10 mg or 20 mg; Long-acting: Procardia XL 30 mg, 60 mg, 90 mg; Adalat 30 mg, 60 mg, 90 mg.

Dosage: Begin therapy with a short-acting drug at 10 mg tid or with a long-acting drug at 30 mg once daily. Dosage can be increased as indicated over a period of a few days to 90 mg/day of the short-acting drug in divided dosages or as a single morning dosage of the long-acting form.

Action: The drug is believed to inhibit ion-control gating mechanisms of the calcium channel and to interfere with the release of calcium from the sarcoplasmic reticulum. By doing so, it inhibits contraction of cardiac and smooth muscle. As a result, coronary and systemic arteries become dilated.

Side Effects: The list of possible side effects is long, but the drug is usually well tolerated. Headache was the main side effect that interfered with therapy for CRPS patients. In patients receiving the drug for treatment of hypertension, common side effects included an increase in the frequency or severity of angina, orthostasis, weakness, peripheral edema, and syncope. Gastrointestinal distress, including constipation, diarrhea, cramping, flatulence, and bleeding, has also been attributed to the drug. Hematologic manifestations included blood cytopenias and purpura.

Considerations: Careful consideration of the benefit/risk ratio should be evaluated at intervals. The potential risks may be heavily offset by benefits toward reducing the severity of the pain symptoms and by the substantial physical dysfunction associated with CRPS.

6. Corticosteroids

Generic Name: *triamcinolone hexacetonide*
Brand Name: Aristospan

Dosage: Depending on the clinical situation (e.g., the intensity of the inflammation) and on the size of the tissue area to be treated, triamcinolone hexacetonide 0.1 mL of 5 mg/mL to 2 mL of 20 mg/mL can be administered intralesionally.

Action: Triamcinolone is used principally as an anti-inflammatory or immunosuppressant agent. It has virtually no mineralocorticoid activity. The hexacetonide microcrystalline preparation is used for intralesional or intra-articular injection, usually along with a local anesthetic such as 1% lidocaine. The crystalline suspension is intended to provide a longer duration of local action of the corticosteroid effect. One important mechanism of corticosteroid action in inflammation may be inhibition of phospholipase-A_2–mediated cleavage of arachidonic acid from internal cellular membranes. That action would then limit local availability of substrate for cyclo-oxygenase and peroxidase production of proinflammatory prostaglandins.[9, 53]

Indication: Local injection of triamcinolone is provided to reduce local inflammation or pain mediated by locally released inflammatory mediators, including prostaglandins.

Side Effects: Repeated injections of depot corticosteroid can have the effect of suppressing the hypothalamic-pituitary-adrenal axis. Local depot corticosteroid injected near bone can decrease local bone density and injected near tendons or ligaments can weaken them, increasing their risk of rupture. A subcutaneous corticosteroid depot can cause local fat necrosis with dimple formation.

Considerations: The mixed microcrystalline preparation of corticosteroid is provided to prolong the local effect of the glucocorticoid. Rarely, the crystals of corticosteroid can induce an acute local inflammatory reaction analogous to that induced by pathologic crystals such as monosodium urate, calcium pyrophosphate, hydroxyapatite, or even cholesterol crystals.

Generic Name: *betamethasone (acetate/sodium phosphate)*
Brand Name: Celestone Soluspan

Dosage: Depending on the clinical situation (e.g., the intensity of the inflammation) and on the size of the tissue area to be treated, betamethasone 0.1 mL to 2 mL of 6 mg/mL can be administered intralesionally.

Action: Betamethasone is used principally as an anti-inflammatory or immunosuppressant agent. It has virtually no mineralocorticoid activity. The mixed (acetate and sodium phosphate) microcrystalline salt preparation is used for intralesional or intra-articular injection along with a local anesthetic such as 1% lidocaine. For other properties, see Section G6, triamcinolone hexacetonide.

Indication: Local injection of betamethasone is provided to reduce local inflammation or pain mediated by locally released prostaglandin inflammatory mediators.

Side Effects: See triamcinolone hexacetonide.
Considerations: See triamcinolone hexacetonide.

7. Narcotics

Generic Name: *codeine (methyl morphine)*
Brand Name: Codeine Phosphate (oral, injection)

Dosage: Usual oral dosage for treatment of moderately severe pain is 30 mg every 4 hours.

Action: Codeine is a μ-opioid agonist, which exerts its analgesic effect by binding to and activating the μ-opioid receptor in the spinal cord and brain.

Codeine and its salts are well absorbed following oral administration or parenteral injection. The oral preparation is approximately two thirds as effective as the same dosage given parenterally. The onset of action by either route of administration is apparent in approximately 15 to 30 minutes and is maintained for 4 to 6 hours. The analgesic action appears to be enhanced by coadministration with the non-narcotic analgesics, acetaminophen (e.g., Tylenol with Codeine) or aspirin (e.g., Empirin with Codeine), and may be further augmented (especially for headache) by addition of caffeine and butalbital (e.g., Fiorinal with Codeine).

Indication: It is appropriate to use this agent for the relief of mild to moderate acute pain in adults. The concern with chronically painful conditions of any kind is that physical dependency will result from regular use. The resultant escalation of the dosage necessary to achieve relief from pain ultimately requires an even more painful withdrawal. Moreover, prolonged and regular intake of the mixed preparations is likely to cause drug-induced headache. Therefore, their use should be discontinued after a short period of time, or simple analgesics, such as ASA, should be taken.

Side Effects: Other than dependency, small dosages of codeine exhibit minimal side effects. Early adverse effects can include dysphoria and nausea. Large dosages can cause respiratory depression by binding to the μ_2-receptor or by cross-reacting activation of the κ- or δ-opioid receptors. There may be interference with the normal response to rising plasma carbon dioxide tension. The cough reflex can be suppressed sufficiently to limit expectoration of pulmonary secretions. Chronic therapy will likely cause some inhibition of bowel motility with resultant constipation. Some preparations contain sulfites, which can cause allergic-type reactions, including anaphylaxis and life-threatening bronchospasm, especially in asthmatics.

Considerations: Common indications for use of opioid agonists, such as codeine, include situations in which temporary analgesia is needed for the symptomatic control of moderate to severe pain. Examples might include myocardial infarction, renal or biliary colic, acute trauma, postoperative pain, terminal cancer, or diagnostic procedures. Opioid agonists, such as codeine, can dangerously potentiate the effects of sedative hypnotics, such as alcohol, tricyclic antidepressants, and monoamine oxidase inhibitors.

Generic Name: *hydrocodone bitartrate*
Brand Name: Lortab (2.5 mg with 500 mg acetaminophen), Lorcet or Vicodin (5 mg with 500 mg acetaminophen), Lortab ASA (5 mg with 500 mg aspirin), Vicodin ES (7.5 mg with 750 mg acetaminophen)
Dosage: The usual adult dosage is 5 to 7.5 mg every 4 to 6 hours as needed for severe pain.

Action: See codeine.
Indication: See codeine.
Side Effects: See codeine.
Considerations: See codeine.

Generic Name: *levorphanol tartrate*
Brand Name: Levo-Dromoran, Levorphanol Tartrate (2 mg oral tablets), Levo-Dromoran (2 mg/mL for parenteral injection)
Dosage: The usual adult dosage of levorphanol by oral or parenteral routes is 2 mg. The smallest effective dose should be used for the shortest duration that will manage the symptoms.

Action: See codeine. Levorphanol is approximately 60-fold more potent than codeine but is less potent (by approximately 50%) than hydromorphine hydrochloride.

Indication: The main use for levorphanol is moderately severe, acute pain or terminal malignancy pain not responsive to more conservative therapy.

Side Effects: See codeine. Although levophorphanol may produce less nausea, vomiting, and constipation, it appears to produce more sedation and more smooth muscle stimulation than do equivalent analgesic doses of morphine sulfate.

Considerations: This drug is a strong analgesic available in both oral and parenteral forms. It is available for treatment of intractable pain (e.g., terminal illness). There will be few indications for this agent in the management of conditions associated with chronic pain.

Generic Name: *meperidine hydrochloride*
Brand Name: Demerol, Meperidine HCl
Dosage: The usual adult dosage is 50 to 150 mg every 3 to 4 hours. The smallest effective dose should be used for the shortest duration.

Action: Approximately 30% more potent than codeine (see codeine).

Indication: The main use for meperidine is management of moderately severe, acute spontaneous pain or surgical pain.

Side Effects: Similar to but more severe than with codeine (see codeine).

Considerations: Meperidine is now available in both oral and parenteral forms. There will be few indications for this agent in the management of chronic pain conditions.

Generic Name: *morphine sulfate*
Brand Name: Morphine Sulfate (oral tablets 15 mg, 30 mg; oral solutiond; rectal suppositories 5 mg, 10 mg, 20 mg, 30 mg; and parenteral injection).
Dosage: The usual adult dosage is 10 to 30 mg every 4 hours as needed for severe pain. The smallest effective dose should be used for the shortest period of time.

Action: See codeine.

Indication: Morphine sulfate is a strong analgesic to be used for relief of severe, acute pain or moderately severe, chronic terminal pain (e.g., terminal cancer). It is also used to treat anxiety in congestive heart failure.

Side Effects: Similar to but substantially more severe than with codeine (see codeine).

Considerations: Morphine sulfate is a potent analgesic available in a wide variety of administration forms. There will be few indications for this agent in the management of chronic pain conditions other than malignancy.

Generic Name: *propoxyphene hydrochloride*

Brand Name: Darvon (65 mg oral tablets), Darvon Compound preparations (65 mg with acetaminophen: Darvon-N, Wygesic; 65 mg with aspirin and caffeine: Darvon Compound-65 Pulvules)

Dosage: One tablet or capsule every 4 hours. The smallest effective dose should be used for the shortest duration.

Action: See codeine.

Indication: Propoxyphene can provide relief from moderately severe pain. It is not potent enough to be useful in the treatment of severe pain. Propoxyphene 65 mg alone may be a less potent analgesic than 30 mg of codeine or 650 mg of aspirin.

Side Effects: The adverse effect profile is similar to that of codeine in many respects. Propoxyphene is more likely to cause liver injury, including reversible jaundice.

Considerations: Chronic use of this agent is not easily justified. It has been willfully abused by addicts. One method used by addicts is to dissolve the pellets in a solvent and inject the resultant solution intravenously. Inadvertent intra-arterial injection can cause downstream or digital gangrene.

8. Sedative Hypnotics

Generic Name: *alprazolam*

Brand Name: Xanax

Dosage: When used for treatment of insomnia and pain in patients with fibromyalgia, the dosage is much lower than is indicated for the treatment of anxiety or panic.[52] Although parenteral forms are available, oral therapy is typically used for the treatment of pain. The dosage is 0.25 to 1.0 mg PO qhs, and, in some patients, an additional 0.25 to 0.5 mg is given every morning.

Action: The mechanism associated with benefit in fibromyalgia is uncertain, but the drug's anxiolytic or sedating effects may be responsible. There is evidence that alprazolam may increase platelet serotonin by inhibiting platelet turnover induced by platelet-activating factor.[13] There may also be direct depression of motor nerve and muscle function. The duration of benefit from a single dose may be up to 8 hours.

Side Effects: The most frequent adverse effects associated with short-term use of alprazolam are similar to the benzodiazepine drugs. CNS effects can be sedation, abnormal mentation, nightmares, dysarthria, and extrapyramidal reactions. Chronic usage may contribute to dependency, and acute discontinuation of large dosages can lead to seizures. Less common are hepatic, hematologic, and cutaneous effects.

Considerations: Administration of alprazolam at night offers the benefit of improved sleep for patients with chronic pain. There may be synergy with analgesic drugs. The relative benefit/risk ratio should be reassessed after 2 to 3 months of therapy because dependency may occur. When discontinuation of chronic therapy is indicated, the dosage should be tapered down at a rate of approximately 0.5 mg every 3 days.

Generic Name: *amitriptyline hydrochloride*

Brand Name: Elavil

Dosage: When used for insomnia or pain, the dosage is usually lower than is indicated for major depression. Although parenteral forms are available, oral therapy is typically used for treatment of pain. The dosage is usually 10 to 50 mg PO qhs.

Action: The analgesic effect is apparently independent of its antidepressant effect. The plasma half-life is 10 to 50 hours.

Side Effects: The most frequent adverse effects associated with short-term use relate to the anticholinergic effects of xerostomia, palpitations, constipation, and urinary retention. CNS effects can include somnolence, dizziness, psychosis, confusion, and even coma. Less common are hepatic, hematologic, and cutaneous effects.

Considerations: Administration at night offers the benefit of improved sleep for patients with chronic pain. There may be synergy with other analgesic drugs. The relative benefit/risk ratio should be reassessed after 2 to 3 months of therapy because tachyphylaxis may occur.

Generic Name: *imipramine hydrochloride*

Brand Name: Tofranil, Janimine

Dosage: When used for pain, the dosage is usually lower than is indicated for major depression. Although parenteral forms are available, oral therapy is usual for pain. Oral dosage is 10 to 75 mg qhs with fluid.

Action: The analgesic effect is apparently independent of its antidepressant effect. The plasma half-life is 10 to 50 hours.

Side Effects: See amitriptyline hydrochloride.

Considerations: Administration at night offers the benefit of improved sleep for patients with chronic pain. There may be synergy with other analgesic drugs. The relative benefit/risk ratio should be reassessed after 2 to 3 months of therapy because tachyphylaxis may occur at about that time.[11]

REFERENCES

1. Adami S, Fossaluzza V, Gatti D, et al.: Bisphospho-nate therapy of reflex sympathetic dystrophy syndrome. Ann Rheum Dis 56:201–204, 1997.
2. Alarcon-Segovia D, Lazcano MA: Carbamazepine for tabetic pain. JAMA 203:57, 1968.
3. Amerson AB, Wanke ML: Amitriptyline. DRUG-DEX® System. Edited by Gelman CR, Rumack BH, Hess AJ. MICROMEDEX, Englewood, CO, revised June 1997.
4. Bada JL, Cervera C, Padro L: Carbamazepine for amyloid neuropathy. [Letter]. N Engl J Med 296:396, 1977.
5. Basbaum AJ, Levine JD: The contribution of the nervous system to inflammation and inflammatory disease. Can J Physiol Pharmacol 69:647–651, 1991.
6. Bengtsson A, Bengtsson M: Regional sympathetic blockade in primary fibromyalgia. Pain 33:161–167, 1988.
7. Beylich G, Hoheisel U, Koch K, et al.: Changes in the functional organization of the dorsal horn during acute myositis and following muscle nerve axotomy. Proceedings of the 7th World Congress on Pain, Progress in Pain Research and Management, Vol. 2. Edited by Gebhart GF, Hammond DL, Jensen TS. IASP Press, Seattle, 1994 (pp. 251–264).
8. Billington L, Carlson BM: The recovery of long-term denervated rat muscles after Marcaine treatment and grafting. J Neurol Sci 144:147–155, 1996.
9. Blackwell GJ, Carnuccio R, Di Rosa M, et al.: A polypeptide causing the anti-phospholipase effect of glucocorticoids. Nature 287:147–149, 1980.
10. Boas RA: Complex regional pain syndromes: symptoms, signs, and different diagnosis, Chapter 5. Reflex Sympathetic Dystrophy: A Reappraisal. Edited by Jänig W, Stanton-Hicks M. IASP Press, Seattle, 1996.
11. Carette S, Bell MJ, Reynolds WJ, et al.: Comparison of amitriptyline, cyclobenzaprine, and placebo in the treatment of fibromyalgia. A randomized, double-blind clinical trial. Arthritis Rheum 37:32–40, 1994.
12. Chapman SL, Brena SF: Pain and litigation. Textbook of Pain. Ed. 2. Edited by Wall PD, Melzack R. Churchill Livingstone, New York, 1989 (p. 1032).
13. Chesney CM, Pifer DD, Cagen LM: Triazolobenzodiazepines competitively inhibit the binding of platelet activating factor [PAF] to human platelets. Biochem Biophys Res Commun 144:359–366, 1987.
14. Coderre TJ, Katz J, Vaccarino AL, et al.: Contribution of central neuroplasticity to pathological pain: review of clinical and experimental evidence. Pain 52:259–285, 1993.
15. Cousins M: Acute and postoperative pain. Textbook of Pain. Ed. 2. Edited by Wall PD, Melzack R. Churchill Livingstone, New York, 1989 (pp. 284–305).
16. Danko I, Fritz JD, Jiao S, et al.: Pharmacological enhancement of in vivo foreign gene expression in muscle. Gene Ther 1:114–121, 1994.
17. Devor M: The pathophysiology of damaged peripheral nerves. Textbook of Pain. Ed. 2. Edited by Wall PD, Melzack R. Churchill Livingstone, New York, 1989 (pp. 63–81).
18. Devor M, Jänig W: Activation of myelinated afferents ending in a neuroma by stimulation of the sympathetic supply in the rat. Neurosci Lett 24:43–47, 1981.
19. Devor M, Jänig W, Michaelis M: Modulation of activity in dorsal root ganglion neurons by sympathetic activation in nerve-injured rats. J Neurophysiol 71:38–47, 1994.
20. Devor M, Wall PD: Cross-excitation in dorsal root ganglia of nerve-injured and intact rats. J Neurophysiol 64:1733–1746, 1990.
21. Dubuisson D: Nerve root damage and arachnoiditis. Textbook of Pain. Ed. 2. Edited by Wall PD, Melzack R. Churchill Livingstone, New York, 1989 (pp. 544–565).
22. Drummond PD, Finch PM, Smythe GA: Reflex sympathetic dystrophy: the significance of differing plasma catecholamine concentrations in affected and unaffected limbs. Brain 114:2025–2036, 1991.
23. Ekbom K: Tegretol: a new therapy of tabetic lightning pains. Preliminary report. Acta Med Scand 179:251, 1966.
24. Ekbom K: Carbamazepine in the treatment of tabetic lightning pains. Arch Neurol 26:374, 1972.
25. Elam M, Johansson G, Wallin BG: Do patients with primary fibromyalgia have any altered muscle sympathetic nerve activity? Pain 48:371–375, 1992.
26. Fagius J, Karhuvaara S, Sundlöf G: The cold pressor test: effects on sympathetic nerve activity in human muscle and skin nerve fascicles. Acta Physiol Scand 137:325–334, 1989.
27. Grassi C, Passatore M: Action of the sympathetic system on skeletal muscle. Ital J Neurol Sci 9:23–28, 1988.
28. Grundberg AB: Reflex sympathetic dystrophy: treatment with long-acting intramuscular corticosteroids. J Hand Surg Am 21:667–670, 1996.
29. Guiloff RJ: Carbamazepine in Morton's neuralgia. Br Med J 2:904, 1979.
30. Hoheisel U, Beylich G, Mense S: Effects of an acute muscle nerve section on the excitability of dorsal horn neurons in the rat. Pain 60:151–158, 1995.
31. Honig LS, Wasserstein PH, Adornato BT: Tonic spasms in sclerosis: anatomic basis and treatment. West J Med 154:723–726, 1991.
32. Itagaki Y, Saida K, Iwamura K: Regenerative capacity of mdx mouse muscles after repeated applications of myo-necrotic bupivaine. Acta Neuropathol 89:380–384, 1995.
33. Jänig W: Pathophysiology of nerve following mechanical injury. Proceedings of the 5th World Congress on Pain, Pain Research and Clinical Management, Volume 3. Edited by Dubner R, Gebhart GF, Bond MR. Elsevier, Amsterdam, 1988 (pp. 89–108).
34. Jänig W: The puzzle of "reflex sympathetic dystrophy": mechanisms, hypotheses, open questions, Chapter 1. Reflex Sympathetic Dystrophy: A Reappraisal. Edited by Jänig W, Stanton-Hicks M. IASP Press, Seattle, 1996.
35. Jensen TS, Rasmussen P: Phantom pain and related phenomena after amputation. Textbook of Pain. Ed. 2. Edited by Wall PD, Melzack RD. Churchill Livingstone, New York, 1989 (pp. 508–521).

36. Kaplan R, Claudio M, Kepes E, *et al.*: Intravenous guanethidine in patients with reflex sympathetic dystrophy. *Acta Anaesthesiol Scand* 40:1216–1222, 1996.

37. Kieschke J, Mense S, Prabhakar NR: Influence of adrenaline and hypoxia on rat muscle receptors in vitro. *Prog Brain Res* 74:91–97, 1988.

38. Leijon G, Boivie J: Central post-stroke pain—a controlled trial of amitriptyline and carbamazepine. *Pain* 36:27–36, 1989.

39. Mayer TG, Gatchel RJ, Mayer H, *et al.*: A prospective two-year study of functional restoration in industrial low back injury. *JAMA* 258:1763, 1987.

40. McEvoy GK, Editor: *AHFS Drug Information.* American Society of Health-System Pharmacists, Bethesda, MD, 1996.

41. Mellick GA, Mellick LB: Reflex sympathetic dystrophy treated with gabapentin. *Arch Phys Med Rehab* 78:98–105, 1997.

42. Merskey H, Bogduk N: *Classification of Chronic Pain: Descriptions of Chronic Pain Syndromes and Definitions of Pain Terms.* IASP Press, Seattle, 1994.

43. Michaelis M, Blenk K-H, Jänig W, *et al.*: Development of spontaneous activity and mechanosensitivity in axotomized afferent nerve fibers during the first hours after nerve transection in rats. *J Neurophysiol* 74:1020–1027, 1995.

44. Mochizuki Y, Suyehiro Y, Tanizawa A, *et al.*: Peripheral neuropathy in children on long-term phenytoin therapy. *Brain Dev* 3:375, 1981.

45. Murphey F: Sources and patterns of pain in disc disease. *Clin Neurosurg* 15:343–350, 1968.

46. Murphey F, Simmons JCH, Brunson B: Ruptured cervical discs, 1939 to 1972. *Clin Neurosurg* 20:9–17, 1973.

47. Muizelaar JP, Kleyer M, Hertogs IA, *et al.*: Complex regional pain syndrome (reflex sympathetic dystrophy and causalgia): management with the calcium channel blocker nifedipine and/or the alpha-sympathetic blocker phenoxybenzamine in 59 patients. *Clin Neurol Neurosurg* 99:26–30, 1997.

48. Nosaka K: Changes in serum enzyme activities after injection of bupivacaine into rat tibialis anterior. *J Appl Physiol* 81:876–884, 1996.

48a. Olin BR, Editor in Chief: *Facts and Comparisons.* Facts and Comparisons, St. Louis, 1992.

49. Patterson JF: Carbamazepine in the treatment of phantom limb pain. *South Med J* 81:1100–1102, 1988.

50. Rapeport WG, Rogers KM, McCubbin TD, *et al.*: Treatment of intractable neurogenic pain with carbamazepine. *Scott Med J* 29:162–165, 1984.

51. Roberts WJ: A hypothesis on the physiological basis for causalgia and related pains. *Pain* 24:297–311, 1986.

52. Russell IJ, Fletcher EM, Michalek JE, *et al.*: Treatment of primary fibrositis/fibromyalgia syndrome with ibuprofen and alprazolam. A double-blind, placebo-controlled study. *Arthritis Rheum* 34:552–560, 1991.

53. Russo-Marie F, Paing M, Duval D: Mechanism of glucocorticoid-induced inhibition of prostaglandin synthesis. *Agents Actions Suppl* 4:49–62, 1979.

54. Sato J, Perl ER: Adrenergic excitation of cutaneous pain receptors induced by peripheral nerve injury. *Science* 251:1608–1610, 1991.

55. Scadding JW: Peripheral neuropathies. *Textbook of Pain.* Ed. 2. Edited by Wall PD, Melzack R. Churchill Livingstone, New York, 1989 (pp. 522–534).

56. Selhorst JB, Kaufman B, Horwitz SJ: Diphenylhydantoin-induced cerebellar degeneration. *Arch Neurol* 27:453, 1972.

57. Shyu BC, Olausson B, Huang KH, *et al.*: Effects of sympathetic stimulation on C-fibre responses in rabbit. *Acta Physiol Scand* 137:73–84, 1989.

57a. Simons DG, Travell JG, Simons LS: *Travell & Simons' Myofascial Pain and Dysfunction: The Trigger Point Manual, Volume 1. Upper Half of Body.* Ed. 2. Williams & Wilkins, Baltimore, 1999.

58. Siston DW, Special Projects Editor: *Physicians Desk Reference.* Medical Economics, Montvale, NJ, 1997.

59. Skelton WP, Skelton NK: Neuroleptics in painful thiamine deficiency neuropathy. *South Med J* 84: 1362–1363, 1991.

60. So EL, Penry JK: Adverse effects of phenytoin on peripheral nerves and neuromuscular junction: a review. *Epilepsia* 22:467–473, 1981.

61. Stanton-Hicks M, Jänig W, Hassenbusch S, *et al.*: Reflex sympathetic dystrophy: changing concepts and taxonomy. *Pain* 63:127–133, 1995.

62. Taylor JC, Brauer S, Espir MLE: Long-term treatment of neuralgia with carbamazepine. *Postgrad Med J* 57:16–18, 1981.

63. Travell JG, Simons DG: *Myofascial Pain and Dysfunction. The Trigger Point Manual, Volume 2. The Lower Extremities.* Williams & Wilkins, Baltimore, 1992.

64. Wall PD, Gutnick M: Ongoing activity in peripheral nerves: the physiology and pharmacology of impulses originating from a neuroma. *Exp Neurol* 43:580–593, 1974.

65. Wiesenfeld-Hallin Z, Hao J-X, Xu X-J, *et al.*: Nitric oxide mediates ongoing discharges in dorsal root ganglion cells after peripheral nerve injury. *J Neurophysiol* 70:2350–2353, 1993.

66. Wilson PR, Low PA, Bedder MD, *et al.*: Diagnostic algorithm for complex regional pain syndromes, Chapter 6. *Reflex Sympathetic Dystrophy: A Reappraisal.* Edited by Jänig W, Stanton-Hicks M. IASP Press, Seattle, 1996.

67. Xu XJ, Wiesenfeld-Hallin Z, Villar MJ, *et al.*: On the role of galanin, substance P and other neuropeptides in primary sensory neurons of the rat: studies on spinal reflex excitability and peripheral axotomy. *Eur J Neurosci* 2:733–743, 1990.

68. Zarday Z, Soberman RJ: Carbamazepine in uremic neuropathy. *Ann Intern Med* 84:296, 1976.

CHAPTER 4

Pain Referred from and to Muscles

SUMMARY: Referral phenomena can pose a serious problem in the diagnosis and treatment of muscle pain because they lead to **mislocalization of the pain**. The muscle in which the pain is felt serves only as a starting point for finding the source of the pain, which is really what requires treatment.

In the basic science portion of this chapter (Section A), various mechanisms of **pain referral** are discussed. Basically, pain referral appears to result from nociceptive information taking a wrong path in the spinal cord and reaching (somatotopically) inappropriate dorsal horn neurons. An alternative explanation for pain referral is that there are dorsal root ganglion cells with branched peripheral axons that supply two different muscles. **The convergence-projection theory** of Ruch[43] still is the central concept for the explanation of referred pain. It states that a given dorsal horn neuron receives synaptic connections from two separate innervation areas (convergent input) and that the neuron induces subjective pain in only one (and always the same) area, even when it is excited from the other area. Applied to the referral of muscle pain, this would mean that a noxious stimulus in one muscle elicits pain in another muscle. Still another alternative mechanism of pain referral between muscles is that the increased activity in nociceptive afferents of a lesioned muscle releases substances from the spinal terminations of the afferents that open up new and **somatotopically inappropriate interneuronal connections**. Thus, the nociceptive information takes a wrong course in the spinal cord, and the pain is mislocalized.

In the clinical portion of this chapter (Section B), pain referred from and to muscle is addressed. Pain referral between seemingly normal muscles can be elicited in a relatively high proportion of healthy subjects (approximately one fourth). Therefore, the finding that referred pain can be elicited from a muscle site does not identify that site as a trigger point (TrP). Tender musculotendinous junctions can also refer pain to other muscles.

Pain and tenderness can be referred to muscle from joints, other muscles, and viscera and as pain originating in the central nervous system. Clinically, **referral of pain from joint to muscle** is frequent; it often occurs in muscles crossing the joint. Muscle pain referred from other muscles has the typical characteristics of deep-tissue pain and can be elicited (e.g., by focal pressure) from muscles that appear to be normal. Typical examples of **muscle pain referred from viscera** include the chest wall pain of cardiac infarction and the flank pain of renal calculi. Finally, pain can be experienced in muscle as an expression of central pain, i.e., pain caused by lesions of the central nervous system. Phantom limb pain is a prominent example of such muscle pain.

A. NEUROBIOLOGICAL BASIS OF PAIN REFERRED FROM MUSCLES

1. Referral as a Symptom of Muscle Pain

It is well established that muscle pain and tenderness, similar to visceral pain, not only is perceived at the site of a lesion but also is usually referred. If only the referred muscle pain or tenderness is present, localization of the pain source may be difficult.[52] As muscle lesions often show a typical and constant pattern of pain referral, the patterns can be used to help locate the muscle that contains the source of pain. This is particularly true of the pain caused by trigger points (TrPs). Pressure exerted on the TrP (e.g., by digital pressure) typically reproduces the pattern of referred pain the patient also perceives spontaneously.[49, 54] An example of a constant referral pattern occurs when TrPs in the upper trapezius characteristically refer the pain up the back of the neck and into the head. Therefore, this type of muscle pain is often misdiagnosed as tension-type headache.

A remarkable feature of referred muscle pain is that often it is not confined to the borders of one dermatome or myotome, although its constancy suggests that it follows fixed anatomic pathways.[54] The elegant experiments of Bogduk[5] have likewise shown that electrical stimulation of the dorsal ramus of a lumbar spinal nerve in patients leads not only to referred pain in the region supplied by the ventral ramus of the same nerve but also to pain in segments supplied by other spinal nerves. For instance, electrical stimulation of the dorsal ramus of the fourth lumbar nerve caused referred pain in the innervation territory of the femoral nerve (which originates partly from the ventral ramus L4) and in the inguinal region (which is mainly supplied by the spinal nerve L1).

Patients sometimes describe their pain as spreading from the initial focus to a larger adjacent area. Whether the mechanisms causing spread of muscle pain are different from those underlying referral is unknown. Parallels are that spread is marked only if the pain is intense, that it has a slow time course, and that spread of deep pain to the skin does not occur.[25] Possibly, referral of muscle pain to closely neighboring regions is perceived as spread.

A clinically important aspect of muscle pain is that it not only can be referred to other tissues but also can be the result of referral from other sources of pain. It has been well documented that visceral pain can be referred not only to the skin but also to skeletal muscle.[50] For instance, pain in the pectoralis muscle can accompany coronary infarction.[54]

Besides inducing spontaneous muscle pain, a visceral lesion can also induce hyperalgesia in skeletal muscle. An example of such a referred hyperalgesia in muscle is the hyperalgesia of the obliquus externus muscle in patients with calculi in the upper renal tract.[13, 57] This effect can be reduplicated in rats in which renal calculosis was experimentally induced. The animals likewise exhibited hyperalgesia (measurable as a lowering in electrical pain threshold) in the obliquus externus muscle. Interestingly, in both patients and rats there was a correlation between the number of colics and the degree of hyperalgesia; apparently, the hyperalgesia became more severe with every colic.[13] The reason for the referred muscle hyperalgesia in rats with calculosis is probably hyperexcitability of dorsal horn neurons, induced by the nociceptive input from the viscera.[14]

2. Possible Mechanisms of Pain Referral

General Considerations. As the connectivity of dorsal horn neurons with input from muscle nociceptors is similar to those involved in visceral nociception, the referral concepts developed for visceral pain (convergence-projection theory of Ruch[43] and convergence-facilitation theory by McKenzie[33]) may also apply to muscle pain. A central assumption of these concepts is that higher central nervous centers are unable to localize the peripheral lesion correctly because the information provided by neurons in lower centers (e.g., in the spinal cord) is equivocal or misleading. The reason for mislocalization of the pain source is seen in the fact that nociceptive neurons in lower centers receive convergent inputs from various tissues so that higher centers cannot identify the actual input source. All recent animal studies on dorsal horn neurons have supported this aspect of the convergence-projection theory by showing that cells driven by nociceptive afferent fibers from muscle,[18, 60] joint,[45] and viscera[8, 12] exhibit an extensive convergence from these sources, often in addition to input from the skin.

It is tempting to speculate that the dorsal horn neurons receiving convergent input, for example, from muscle and joint are responsible for the referral of muscle pain to neighboring joints,[26] but this explanation probably is too simple. Many of the neurons with muscle input have additional receptive fields (RFs) in the skin, but referral of muscle pain (experimental and pathologic) to the skin does not seem to occur.[26, 28] The assumption that the convergent cells mediate cutaneous pain does not solve the problem, because there is then no function for the deep RF; referral of skin pain to deep tissues has not been described. The statement that the neurons with RFs in both skin and muscle may be involved in the cutaneous hyperalgesia and hypoalgesia that often accompanies muscle pain[17, 50] is so general that it does not explain anything. As shown below, however, a convergent connection from two deep tissues (preferably from two muscles) can be used as the first approach to explain referral from one muscle to another.

Another relatively new problem for the understanding of referred muscle pain is the finding that dorsal horn neurons can change the size, number, and nature (high-threshold or low-threshold) of their RFs rapidly in the presence of noxious stimuli to muscle.[18, 24] Thus, the input convergence onto a given neuron is not a constant feature; it may develop acutely under the influence of a peripheral lesion. A finding supporting this view is that the stimulus-induced formation of new RFs or changes in existing RFs in animal experiments often take several minutes, during which new synaptic connections may become effective (see above). Evidence obtained in clinical studies likewise suggests that referral of deep pain may not be brought about by the use of fixed connections; referral occurs only (or predominantly) if the pain reaches

a high intensity,[50, 53] and it needs time to develop.[25] A possible interpretation of these data is that the referral of muscle pain reflects the formation of new central nervous connections and thus may be another aspect of neuroplasticity (for a recent review of referral mechanisms, see Mense[35]).

Branching of Primary Afferent Fibers. In animal experiments in which the impulse activity of single primary afferent fibers from muscle was recorded, sometimes units were encountered that had two discontinuous RFs; i.e., these fibers could be activated from two separate areas of the muscle.[37] In the deep tissues of the cat tail, primary afferent units were found that had one RF in deep somatic tissues (muscle, joint, periosteum) and another in the skin distal to the deep RF.[38] The anatomic basis of this feature probably is branching of the afferent fiber. For the following considerations, two types of branched axons must be distinguished: short terminal branches, such as those of free nerve endings in their receptive region; and fibers with long branches supplying different types of tissue, such as two different muscles or a muscle and joint. For pain referral, only the second type is important; the first type just determines the size of the RF of the afferent fiber.

The sensations elicited by activity in a primary afferent fiber, with one RF in the skin and one in deep tissues, probably depend on its central connections: If the fiber is connected to neurons mediating nociception from the skin, pain may be felt in the region of the cutaneous RF when the deep RF is stimulated.[50] This mechanism does not explain referred muscle pain, however, since pain from muscle and other deep somatic tissues is referred not to the skin but to other deep tissues.[17, 28]

An alternative assumption would be that the fiber with two RFs is connected to central neurons mediating deep pain and that referred deep pain is elicited by noxious stimulation of the cutaneous RF. This assumption is unlikely, however, since everyday experience shows that pinching the skin evokes no deep sensations. (Of course, it is also possible that these fibers with branched axons do not elicit subjective sensations at all.)

Sinclair and coworkers[50] put forward the hypothesis that action potentials originating in the deep RF of the fiber antidromically invade its cutaneous branch and release "irritating" substances from this branch via the axon reflex. The irritating substances were assumed to sensitize nociceptors in the vicinity of the antidromically invaded branch. In light of more recent findings, neuropeptides such as substance P (SP) and calcitonin gene-related peptide (CGRP) could play the role of the irritating substances. Both peptides are present in free nerve endings of skin and muscle and are released during neuronal activity. A recent study has shown that SP has an excitatory, but not a sensitizing, action on muscle nociceptors.[42] This means that SP caused the receptors to discharge action potentials but did not increase their responsiveness to other stimuli. SP, however, can liberate bradykinin (BK) and serotonin from blood constituents and histamine and prostaglandins from other tissue cells. Most of these substances do have a sensitizing action on nociceptors; thus, SP could sensitize muscle nociceptors **indirectly** by releasing other substances.

When the deep branch of the branched axon is activated by a noxious stimulus, the resulting sensitization of nociceptors around the branch in the skin may lead to the cutaneous hyperalgesia that often accompanies muscle pain.[50] In this model, the cutaneous hyperalgesia is assumed to be mediated by separate cutaneous afferents that supply the region where the superficial branch terminates. Sometimes, however, muscle pain has been described as being associated with a cutaneous hypoalgesia[5] not explained by the axon reflex. The axon reflex is likewise not an explanation for pain referred to a completely denervated body region.[11]

The hypothesis of Sinclair and coworkers requires primary afferent units with long branched axons supplying muscle and skin. Anatomic and neurophysiologic studies[10, 41] have shown that axons with long branches are relatively rare (a few percent of all afferent fibers). If in fact these fibers are involved in the referral of deep pain or

in the cutaneous hyperalgesia accompanying muscle pain, an extremely small number of units must be sufficient to elicit these effects (which is unlikely).

As muscle pain is often referred to other muscles, the branched axon theory would require the existence of primary afferent neurons that have receptive endings in two different muscles (Fig. 4-1). Under these conditions, the second-order neuron in the dorsal horn cannot identify the origin of the impulse activity. It is not clear, though, what subjective sensations a painful stimulus to muscle A in Figure 4-1 would elicit. It may cause pain in only muscle A if the pathway from muscle B is normally not active; then, higher centers will have "learned" that all activity in the primary afferent neuron is caused by stimulation of muscle A. A painful stimulus may also cause pain in only muscle B if the pathway from muscle A is normally inactive. This latter situation would reflect referral of pain from muscle A to muscle B. Pain in both muscles is also possible when both pathways are equivalent and equally busy all the time.

Thus, whereas the importance of the short terminal branches of a primary afferent unit for the local axon reflex (leading, for example, to wheal and flare around a lesion) is well documented,[21, 27] the role of the few afferents with long branches in referral and associated phenomena is questionable. As to the central effects of activity in nociceptive afferent fibers with multiple deep RFs, these fibers may contribute to the diffuse nature of muscle pain, since multiple RFs of primary afferent fibers are likely to reduce the spatial resolution of the nociceptive system.

Input Convergence on Spinal Neurons. The convergence-projection theory of Ruch[43] is still the central concept for the explanation of referred pain. This theory states that referral takes place if afferent fibers from two different sources (e.g., viscera and skin) have synaptic contacts with the same dorsal horn neuron. If the neuron is part of pathways mediating cutaneous pain, it will signal this information ("cutaneous pain") to higher centers, also, when it is activated by afferents from

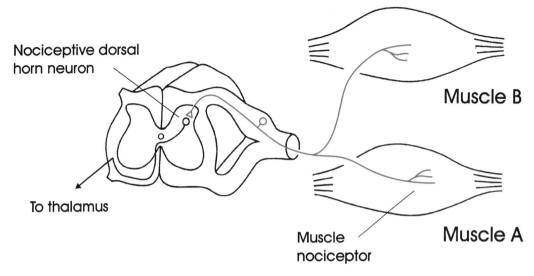

Figure 4-1. Branched axon theory of pain referral. A primary afferent neuron (red) gives rise to a peripheral axon with two long branches that terminate in nociceptors in muscle *A* and muscle *B*. As described in the text, this arrangement could, at least theoretically, explain referral of muscle pain from muscle *B* to *A* if the assumption is made that the nociceptive dorsal horn neuron mediates pain in muscle *A* irrespective of from where the neuron is activated. Thus, a noxious stimulus to muscle *B* could lead to pain perceived in muscle *A*.

viscera. As stated above, in this situation higher centers cannot identify the actual location of the lesion. According to this theory, the mislocalization of visceral pain to the skin occurs when afferent fibers from the viscera are *a priori* connected to functionally and somatotopically inappropriate neurons, namely, to cells mediating cutaneous pain from a body region remote from the visceral lesion.

In Figure 4-2, the theory has been adapted to a situation in which pain is referred from a proximal muscle to a distal one. Dorsal horn neuron *A* mediates pain from the distal muscle, and neuron *C*, located in the lateral dorsal horn, mediates pain from the proximal muscle. Neuron *B* has convergent input from both muscles and, therefore, can be excited from both muscles *A* and *B*. If neuron *B* sends its messages in the pathway that mediates pain from the distal muscle, its activation will subjectively elicit pain in the distal muscle irrespective of from where it is excited. Thus, activation of neuron *B* by nociceptors in the proximal muscle will elicit pain in the distal muscle.

Several aspects of referred pain are not explained by the convergence-projection theory. First, referral of pain requires a certain minimum intensity of pain at the site of the original lesion,[50, 53] but the spinal circuitry that Ruch's theory is based on suggests that referral should occur as soon as pain is elicited from the original lesion. Second, establishing a pathway for pain referral takes time (in the order of minutes to hours).[25, 28] Third, referral often occurs to regions outside the segment of the original lesion,[9, 25] whereas the theory postulates that input convergence occurs onto a neuron pool in the same segment. The first two points suggest that there is a dynamic component in the referral of pain; the third point indicates that a simple convergence of two afferents within the same spinal segment is not sufficient to explain referral.

Data from animal experiments, obtained in the laboratory of one of the authors (S.M.), shed new light on the convergence-projection theory and its applicability to referred pain from muscle. As to the main postulate of the theory, there is no doubt that extensive convergence exists at the spinal level. This has been shown in electrophysiologic experiments on rat and cat dorsal horn neurons that process convergent input from viscera and skin[8, 12] or from various somatic structures (skin, muscle, joint).[19, 24, 45, 60] In these experiments, the convergence expresses itself in the presence of two or more regions from which a given dorsal horn neuron can be activated. In neurons having one high-threshold mechanosensitive (HTM) RF in deep tissues, the other RF often was likewise HTM and located in the skin. This finding supports the hypothesis that neurons with convergent inputs are involved in cutaneous hyperalgesia accompanying muscle pain if two assumptions are made: First, the neuron is connected to central pathways mediating cutaneous pain; and second, there is a

continuous impulse traffic from the deep RF that sensitizes the dorsal horn neuron (in the sense of the convergence-facilitation theory of McKenzie).[33] Frequently, however, the second RF in the skin was low-threshold mechanosensitive (LTM), which does not fit in the above interpretation unless it is assumed that this type of neuron elicits cutaneous hyperesthesia instead of hyperalgesia.

An important aspect of the connections in the dorsal horn is that many anatomically existing (preformed) connections are functionally ineffective; i.e., impulse activity arriving in the presynaptic terminal has only a negligible effect on the postsynaptic neuron. One possible explanation for the lack of efficacy is that presynaptic activity causes only subthreshold synaptic potentials in the postsynaptic membrane that do

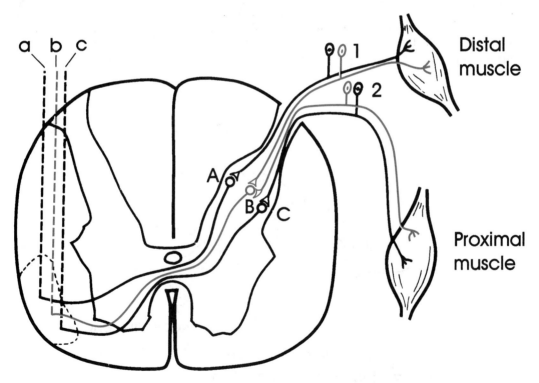

Figure 4-2. Modified convergence-projection theory of pain referral of Ruch.[43] The figure has been adapted to explain the referral of pain from a proximal to a distal muscle. Dorsal horn neuron A is activated only from the distal muscle; neuron C is activated only from the proximal muscle. Neuron B can be excited by afferents from both muscles (*red*). If the axon of neuron B has connections with higher neurons that elicit subjective pain in the distal muscle, then activation of this neuron from the proximal muscle will lead to subjective pain in the distal muscle. *a, b,* and *c* are axons of neurons A, B, and C, respectively, in the spinothalamic tract. *1* and *2* primary afferent neurons supplying the distal and proximal muscle, respectively.

not excite the postsynaptic neuron. Under certain circumstances (see below), however, these connections may become effective.

The data of several research groups indicate that the spinal terminations of a given spinal nerve extend over many segments in the spinal cord (for the gastrocnemius-soleus [GS] muscle nerve, see Refs. 36 and 47). In neurophysiologic experiments in which the electrical activity of dorsal horn neurons is recorded, however, cells can be driven from a nerve only within a few segments of the entry zone of that nerve. This finding suggests that many of the presynaptic boutons in the spinal cord are ineffective in driving dorsal horn neurons. These functionally ineffective spinal terminations probably surround the effective ones and extend over a larger distance than the latter. Such an arrangement is depicted in Figure 4-3.

The ineffective synaptic connections are by no means unimportant. On the contrary, they most likely are involved in neuroplastic changes during pathophysiologic forms of pain and, therefore, are important for the development of referral and for the transition from acute to chronic pain.

The transformation from ineffective to effective connections need not take long; it can occur within a few minutes when a strong noxious stimulus acts on nociceptors in the periphery. Such a change may lead to an increase in dorsal horn convergence by a mechanism such as is shown in Figure 4-4. Originally, the afferent fiber from muscle A had effective connections with dorsal horn neuron A only, whereas the afferent fiber from muscle B had effective connections with neuron B and subthreshold connections with neuron A. Normally, neuron A will be excited only by afferents from muscle A, and neuron B will be excited only by afferents from muscle B. After the synaptic efficacy of the connection between muscle B and neuron A has been enhanced, neuron A can also be excited by muscle B. When neuron A is activated by the formerly ineffective afferent from muscle B, however, neuron A will

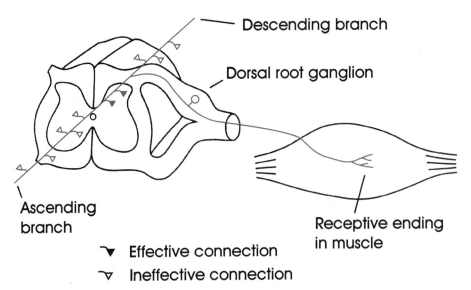

Descending branch

Dorsal root ganglion

Ascending branch

Receptive ending in muscle

▼ **Effective connection**

▽ **Ineffective connection**

Figure 4-3. Schema of the extent of the spinal projections of a single muscle afferent. After having entered the spinal cord, the afferent fiber divides into an ascending and a descending branch. Both branches have many collaterals with presynaptic terminals (boutons; shown as *triangles*). Effective synaptic connections (*filled* presynaptic boutons) with dorsal horn neurons are present mainly in a few segments close to the level of entry of the afferent fiber. Ineffective synapses (*open* presynaptic boutons) extend over a much greater distance rostrally and caudally.

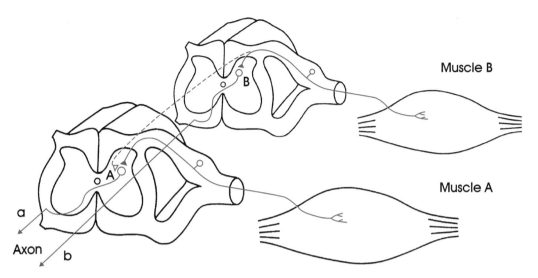

Figure 4-4. Acute formation of a convergent input by opening up a formerly ineffective connection. Muscle A has an effective (suprathreshold) connection with neuron A; muscle B has an effective connection with neuron B and an ineffective (subthreshold) connection with neuron A (*dashed line*). If the ineffective connection becomes effective, neuron A can be excited from both muscles A and B. Thus, a painful stimulus to muscle B can elicit pain in muscle A by activating neuron A (in addition to pain in muscle B that is mediated by neuron B).

still send the message "pain in muscle *A*" to higher centers. Thus, Figure 4-4 is a dynamic model of pain referral from muscle *B* to muscle *A*. The main difference to Ruch's concept is that the pathways of pain referral are ineffective in the beginning and become effective under the influence of a long-lasting and strong painful stimulus.

In animal experiments in which the activity of single dorsal horn neurons is recorded, the opening up of new connections in the dorsal horn can be recognized by two phenomena, namely, the formation of new RFs and a lowering in stimulation threshold of preexisting RFs. An example of such an experiment is shown in Figure 4-5. A rat dorsal horn neuron with an RF in the biceps femoris muscle (Fig. 4-5*A*) exhibited two new RFs 5 minutes after injection of a painful dose of BK into the tibialis anterior muscle (Fig. 4-5*B*, *left panel*). One RF appeared at the injection site, and the other appeared in the deep tissues of the dorsum of the paw. Fifteen minutes after the painful stimulus, the newly formed RFs still persisted, and the original RF exhibited a reduction of the mechanical threshold into the innocu-

ous range (merely moderate pressure stimulation was now effective; Fig. 4-5*B*, *right panel*). Since this RF had not been injected, the lower threshold must be due to a change in excitability of the dorsal horn neuron, i.e., to central sensitization. Please note that the injection was made outside the original RF of the cell; accordingly, the recorded neuron was not excited by the painful BK injection.

A likely interpretation of these findings is that a noxious stimulus somewhere in the periphery leads to widespread changes in excitability of dorsal horn neurons. In the cell shown in Figure 4-5, the excitability was increased, and formerly ineffective synaptic connections with the periphery became effective. This resulted in the formation of new RFs that had a high mechanical threshold and were located in deep somatic tissues.

Another factor influencing input convergence is the descending antinociceptive system.[2] Blocking the system by cooling the spinal cord rostral to the recording site, for example, leads to an increase in the number of RFs in dorsal horn neurons[19] (see Chapter 7). These findings demonstrate that

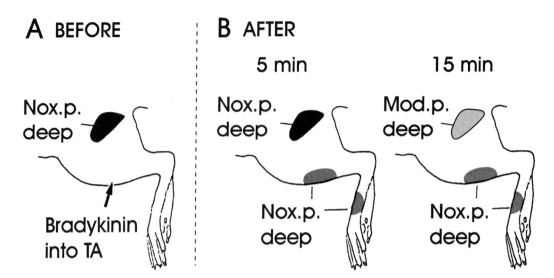

Figure 4-5. Unmasking of receptive fields (RFs) of a dorsal horn neuron by a painful stimulus to muscle. **A.** Location and size of the original RF (*black*) before the intramuscular injection of a painful dose of bradykinin (BK). The neuron responded only to noxious deep pressure stimulation (*Nox. p. deep*) of the black region in the proximal biceps femoris muscle. The *arrow* points to the injection site in the tibialis anterior muscle. **B (left panel).** Five minutes after the BK injection, the neuron could be excited from two additional RFs (*dark red*), both of which were located in deep tissues and had a high mechanical threshold. **B (right panel).** Fifteen minutes after the BK injection, the original RF (now *red*) displayed a lowering in mechanical threshold; i.e., the neuron now responded to stimulation of this region with moderate (innocuous) deep pressure (*Mod. p. deep*). (Redrawn from Hoheisel U, Mense S, Simons DG, *et al.*: Appearance of new receptive fields in rat dorsal horn neurons following noxious stimulation of skeletal muscle: a model for referral of muscle pain? *Neurosci Lett* 153:9–12, 1993.)

many of the synaptic connections in the dorsal horn are not constant in their efficacy but can be changed by various influences.

In the neuron shown in Figure 4-5, the formation of new RFs took less than 5 minutes; in other experiments, the delay between application of the noxious stimulus and appearance of new RFs was longer than 15 minutes. The newly formed RFs persisted for periods of time that by far outlasted the duration of the noxious stimulus. As stated above, one likely interpretation of these findings is that the formation of new RFs results from neuroplastic changes in the connectivity of the dorsal horn (see also Hoheisel et al.[20]).

Of course, the critical question is whether the formation of new RFs in animal experiments has anything to do with referral of muscle pain in human patients. A somewhat speculative answer to this question follows: If the discharge of a nociceptive neuron contains information on the site of the lesion, the appearance of a new RF in the tibialis anterior muscle,

distal to and remote from the original RF in the biceps femoris muscle (Fig. 4-5), means that the neuron that signals pain in the biceps femoris muscle also now transmits this information to higher centers when a noxious stimulus acts on the tibialis anterior muscle. If the additional assumption is made that activity in nociceptive neurons elicits pain, the above situation may lead to referral of muscle pain from a distal to a discontinuous proximal region; i.e., a lesion of the tibialis anterior muscle will cause pain in this area (mediated by neurons with RFs in that muscle) and pain referred to the biceps femoris muscle (mediated by neurons that have RFs in that muscle and acquire new RFs in the tibialis anterior muscle).

If we follow the same line of thinking, then the reduction of the mechanical threshold of the original RF in the biceps femoris muscle could lead to referred tenderness in that muscle. Following noxious stimulation of the tibialis anterior muscle that altered the RFs, moderate pressure stimulation of the biceps femoris muscle will cause pain because the neuron, which now has an LTM RF in that muscle, is still connected to pathways mediating muscle pain. (The other newly formed RFs had a high mechanical threshold, which means that the neuron required painful stimulation of those RFs for activation.)

The response of the neuron to weak mechanical stimulation of the originally high-threshold RF in the biceps femoris muscle most likely is an expression of central sensitization. Apparently, the noxious stimulation of the tibialis anterior muscle has increased the sensitivity of the neuron to an extent that it now responds to activation of LTM receptors. One possible interpretation of this change is that formerly ineffective synapses on the surface of the neuron that connect to low-threshold mechanoreceptors have become effective. (Often, high-threshold dorsal horn neurons have additional input from low-threshold afferents that normally is so weak that it does not activate the cell following natural stimulation of muscle receptors.) The opening up of LTM synaptic connections with nociceptive neurons is presently being discussed as a possible mechanism of secondary hyperalgesia that may lead to allodynia in pain patients (for a review on central sensitization, see Treede and Magerl[56]).

After BK injections into hindlimb muscles, approximately half of the neurons tested reacted with the formation of new RFs. All newly formed RFs had a high mechanical threshold and were situated in deep tissues (never in the skin). Apparently, only nociceptive connections from deep tissues are opened up following noxious stimulation of muscle. This may be a parallel to clinical muscle pain that is referred to other deep tissues.

The appearance of new RFs adds a dynamic component to the convergence theory with a time course similar to that of referred pain in patients. The majority of the newly formed RFs were located distal to the original ones; as exemplified above, this arrangement could provide an explanation for proximal referral. In patients and test persons, muscle pain is predominantly referred distally,[26, 48, 49, 55] although proximal referral has also been observed in patients[25, 48] and in volunteers following electrical stimulation of muscle nerve fascicles.[53]

In animal experiments, a persistent nociceptive input from muscle can be produced by inducing an experimental myositis with injections of carrageenan. This procedure leads to a histologically recognizable inflammation within 2 hours and to increased activity in nociceptors of the inflamed muscle.[3] Systematic mapping of rat dorsal horn neurons responding to electrical stimulation of peripheral nerves showed that in the course of a myositis of the GS muscle, the population of neurons that could be activated by afferents from that muscle increased in size.[4] This effect was most marked in the lateral dorsal horn of segments L4 and L5; it was associated with a rostral expansion of the input region of the muscle nerve to segment L3. The expansion to the rostrally adjacent segment demonstrates that the changes in dorsal horn connectivity are not restricted to the spinal segment of the lesion.

In rats with a myositis of the GS muscle, neurons in the lateral segment L3 not only responded to electrical stimulation of the GS nerve but also acquired mechanosensitive RFs in the GS muscle. In animals with normal GS muscle, such an input to L3 was completely absent; the main input region of the GS muscle nerve was the medial dorsal horn in segments L4 and L5. Apparently, the increase in excitability (the central sensitization) spreads within the dorsal horn.

Experimental evidence[60] indicates that the topographic arrangement of dorsal horn neurons with deep input is similar to the somatotopy of cutaneous input.[7] Therefore, an increase in the number of cells responding to GS input in the lateral dorsal horn means that neurons in this region, which originally had input from the proximal limb and mediated sensations from this region, now receive additional input from the distal limb. Under these conditions, a distal lesion could elicit referred pain in the proximal limb. The spread of the excitability to adjacent neuron populations in the dorsal horn might cause the subjective sensation of spreading or radiating pain. In the myositis model, the increase in neuronal excitability expanded into the rostrally adjacent segment. This finding may relate to the clinical observation that muscle pain is often referred (or spreads) to regions outside the segment of the original lesion.[49]

3. Possible Mechanisms Underlying Changes in Dorsal Horn Connectivity

The mechanisms underlying the above-described changes in excitability of dorsal horn neurons are largely unknown. Theoretically, an increase in neuronal excitability can result from disinhibition or facilitation of impulse transmission; both processes can take place presynaptically or postsynaptically. Since the increased excitability following BK injections occurred without the neurons being activated by the noxious stimulus (see above), post-tetanic potentiation can be excluded. The process resembles "heterosynaptic facilitation,"[59] which leads to central sensitization.

In some way, the dorsal horn changes must be associated with alterations in synaptic efficacy. As stated above, one possible mechanism would be that anatomically existing but functionally ineffective fiber connections between the spinal neurons and the periphery are unmasked by the noxious input. Such an unmasking of ineffective or latent connections has been described to occur in the dorsal horn following denervation.[58] A hypothetical neuroanatomic model that offers an explanation for the observed changes in dorsal horn excitability is shown in Figure 4-6.

The basic assumption made in Figure 4-6 is that dorsal horn neurons have two types of afferent connections with the periphery. Connections of one type have a high synaptic efficacy and are always open; i.e., activity in presynaptic terminals usually excites the postsynaptic neuron. These connections form the original RF of the neuron. Connections of the other type are of low synaptic efficacy and have only a negligible influence on the postsynaptic dorsal horn neuron. In a study on mechanosensitive afferents from the skin, Meyers and Snow[39] demonstrated the existence of such ineffective fiber collaterals. Whether nociceptive fibers likewise have such collaterals is unknown. For reasons of simplicity, no interneurons have been included in the model; this does not mean that the connections between the ineffective collaterals of the primary afferent fiber and the projecting dorsal horn neuron are monosynaptic.

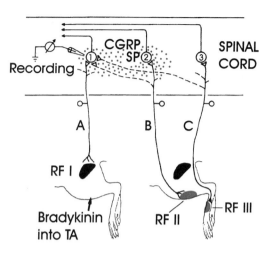

Figure 4-6. Hypothetical explanation of pain referral by acute unmasking of synaptic connections. The neuroanatomic model shown may explain the appearance of new RFs in Figure 4-5. The activity of neuron *1* was recorded with a microelectrode introduced into the spinal cord. The neuron is connected by pathway *A* to its original RF in the biceps femoris muscle (*RF I*). Synaptically effective connections are drawn as *solid lines;* ineffective (latent) connections are drawn as *dashed lines.* The injection of BK was made outside *RF I* into the tibialis anterior muscle (TA), which contains an RF of neuron 2 (*RF II*). The BK-induced excitation of nociceptive fibers of pathway *B* is assumed to release SP (and CGRP) in the dorsal horn, which diffuses (*stippling*) to neuron *1* and increases the efficacy of latent connections from pathways *B* and *C* to this cell. Now, neuron *1* can be activated from *RF II* and *RF III*.[35]

As to the changes in dorsal horn connectivity, the model shown in Figure 4-6 demonstrates the necessity of a combination of convergence and divergence to explain the observed effects. After injection of BK into the tibialis anterior muscle, neuron *1* shows convergent input from afferent pathways A, B, and C; conversely, input from pathway B diverges to neurons *1* and *2*. Whether divergence or convergence is the final reason for the mislocalization of the pain is a matter of point of view. Via the divergent collaterals, the nociceptive information reaches neurons that mediate pain sensations from body regions remote from the muscle lesion (the BK injection). Via the newly formed convergent connection with pathway B, neuron *1* receives afferent information from somatotopically inappropriate body regions.

Available experimental data are compatible with the assumption that the nociceptive information is fed into somatotopically inappropriate pathways at the level of the spinal cord. Similar changes in connectivity have also been described as occurring in the thalamus and cortex,[15] where the subjective (mis)localization of the pain is probably made.

How can the synaptic efficacy of the collaterals be increased? A possible explanation is that in the situation depicted in Figure 4-6, the noxious stimulus to muscle releases substances from the spinal terminals of nociceptive muscle afferents that enhance synaptic transmission. A candidate substance is SP, which has been shown to be present in muscle afferent fibers (together with CGRP and somatostatin[40]).

Administered iontophoretically at high concentrations in the dorsal horn, SP activates nociceptive neurons; administered at low concentrations, it leads to a long-lasting depolarization of the cell membrane.[44, 61] The depolarization is the prerequisite for abolishing the magnesium block of the N-methyl-D-aspartate (NMDA) ion channel. In the absence of the magnesium block, the channel opens and calcium ions enter the cell, which act as a second messenger.[30] Thus, many functions of the neuron, including its excitability, can be changed by SP. SP binds to receptor molecules in the cell membrane (mainly the neurokinin-1 receptor[31]); its action seems to be specific and not caused by a general influence on the membrane.

In contrast to amino acid transmitters, SP diffuses over long distances in the spinal cord after being released from the spinal terminals of primary afferent neurons. Therefore, SP can be regarded as a volume transmitter[1] that is capable of influencing large populations of neurons in the vicinity of the release site. This property may be important for the induction of the widespread changes in dorsal horn excitability during a muscle lesion; it may also be relevant for the referral of muscle pain to regions outside the myotome of the lesion. SP is not the only substance that may induce the observed effects; other neuropeptides (e.g., CGRP) and excitatory amino acids (e.g., glutamate and aspartate) are also capable of causing similar changes in dorsal horn excitability (for a review, see Coderre et al.[9]).

Parallel to these events, changes in gene expression occur in dorsal horn neurons in response to noxious stimulation. These changes lead to an increased synthesis of transcription factors, such as FOS and JUN proteins, which in turn alter the cell's metabolism for prolonged periods of time.[16]

B. CLINICAL PAIN REFERRED FROM MUSCLE

1. From Myofascial Trigger Points

The pain referred from myofascial TrPs is the best-known example of pain referred from muscle. Common referred pain patterns from TrPs were first published in 1953[54] and later in more detail.[49, 55] See Chapter 8, Section A, for more about TrPs.

2. From Other Sensitive Locations

In a study of 61 healthy normal subjects,[46] dolorimeter-applied pressure in the least sensitive location in the upper quadrant muscles evoked referred sensation in one and dysesthesia in five subjects (10% of subjects). Pressure on the most sensitive location evoked referred sensation in 54%; i.e., 26% experienced referred pain, and 28% experienced dysesthesia. This 26% corresponds to the 25% previously reported in healthy normal subjects.[51]

Similarly, Hong et al.[23] reported eliciting referred pain from 23% of control sites 4 cm from a latent TrP but from 47% of control sites for an active TrP. Therefore, finding a sensitive spot in muscle that refers pain does not, alone, identify a TrP. Hong[22] identified as sensitive loci these non-TrP sites that refer pain. The reason for this spot sensitivity in normal muscle is unexplored.

Pain induced by saline infusion of muscle produced distinct areas of local and referred pain, which usually appeared distal to the infusion site,[14a] which corresponds to the location of pain referred from TrPs.[48] Repeated sequential infusions, or infusions at four locations simultaneously, increased the size of the referred pain and its severity.[14b] Five kinds of sensory stimuli to the area of referred pain during a 900-second infusion showed modality specific and bidirectional changes that varied in time.[14c] Also, it appears that both peripheral and central mechanisms contribute to referred pain from muscle and that myelinated fibers mediate the peripheral component.[26a]

Painful stimulation with hypertonic saline infusion into pain-free muscles of fibromyalgia syndrome (FMS) patients produced an increased intensity and duration of referred pain, increased areas, and referral of pain to additional atypical locations (e.g., proximal), compared with normal subjects.[14d] Repeated stimulations of muscle (but not of skin) caused a greater increase of pain in FMS patients than in normal controls. These findings point to a central hyperexcitability specific for muscle (muscle hyperalgesia) in FMS patients.

3. From Enthesitis

No study has been found that specifically addresses the characteristics of pain referred from tender musculotendinous junctions of skeletal muscles. That musculotendinous junctions in muscles with active TrPs are tender and will produce referred pain when compressed is a clinical observation. Considering the findings noted above, this is not surprising.

C. PAIN AND TENDERNESS REFERRED TO MUSCLE

Pain and tenderness can be referred to muscle from joints, other muscles, and viscera and as pain originating in the central nervous system. This means that the complaint of muscle pain is nonspecific. As stated at the beginning of the chapter, the muscle in which the pain and tenderness is located often serves only as a starting point for finding the source of the pain, which is really what requires treatment. The examiner is more likely to be right than wrong to expect that the patient's muscular pain complaint originates elsewhere.

1. Referred From Joints

The early studies of Kellgren[26] described pain referred from joint capsules when injected with hypertonic saline. Similarly, McCall et al.[32] illustrated patterns of deep pain referred from the zygapophyseal joints between L1 and L2 and also between L4 and L5 to the lateral hips and upper thigh.

Bogduk and Simons[6] illustrated how confusingly overlapping are the referred, deep-tissue pain patterns from cervical zygapophyseal joints and the referred pain from TrPs in muscles crossing those joints. Clinically, one sees analogous patterns of pain referred from symptomatic blocked joints throughout the body. The muscles crossing involved joints are also likely to develop TrPs,[29] producing a secondary, muscle-induced pain because of the joint problem.

2. Referred From Other Muscles

The pain referred from apparently normal muscle in response to the application of focal pressure, even when there is no evidence of abnormality, is usually experienced as deep-tissue pain that includes muscles.[46] Active TrPs characteristically refer deep pain that includes muscle tissue. The typical referred pain patterns for the major muscles of the body have been presented in detail.[49, 55]

3. Referred From Viscera

Recognition of the deep-tissue referred pain patterns characteristic of diseased viscera is basic to the practice of internal medicine. Physicians are expected to recognize the referred chest wall pain of cardiac infarction, the left shoulder pain of a diseased gallbladder, and the flank pain of renal calculi, so much so, in fact, that they are prone to ignore the other common sources of referred pain to these same regions.

The visceral pathology responsible for the referred pain is commonly verified by surgery, electromyography, or imaging techniques. Since the other sources of referred pain to muscle are not so readily and clearly demonstrable, they have remained under a cloud of suspicion and neglect.

4. Referred From the Central Nervous System

Pain arising spontaneously within the central nervous system (central pain) that is experienced in deep tissues (which include muscles) is another distant source. Examples are phantom limb pain[34] and central pain experienced as a result of spinal cord injury. This topic is addressed in more detail in Chapter 7.

In summary, it appears that muscles (and related deep tissues) tend to serve as a common denominator for the expression of nociceptive input from many other tissues. It is little wonder that musculoskeletal pain has been so enigmatic and hard to understand.

REFERENCES

1. Agnati LF, Fuxe K, Zoli M, et al.: A correlation analysis of the regional distribution of central enkephalin and beta-endorphin immunoreactive terminals and of opiate receptors in adult and old male rats. Evidence for the existence of two main types of communication in the central nervous system: the volume transmission and the wiring transmission. Acta Physiol Scand 128:201–207, 1986.
2. Basbaum AI, Fields HL: Endogenous pain control system: brainstem spinal pathways and endorphin circuitry. Ann Rev Neurosci 7:309–338, 1984.
3. Berberich P, Hoheisel U, Mense S: Effects of a carrageenan-induced myositis on the discharge properties of group III and IV muscle receptors in the cat. J Neurophysiol 59:1395–1409, 1988.
4. Beylich G, Hoheisel U, Koch K, et al.: Neuroplastic changes induced in dorsal horn neurones by an experimental myositis and muscle nerve axotomy. Pflgers Archiv 422(Suppl. 1):R61, 1993.
5. Bogduk N: Lumbar dorsal ramus syndrome. Med J Australia 2:537–541, 1980.
6. Bogduk N, Simons DG: Neck pain: joint pain or trigger points? Chap. 20. Progress In Fibromyalgia and Myofascial Pain, Volume 6 of Pain Research and Clinical Management. Edited by Vaerøy H, Merskey H. Elsevier, Amsterdam, 1993 (pp. 267–273).
7. Brown PD, Fuchs JL: Somatotopic representation of hindlimb skin in cat dorsal horn. J Neurophysiol 38:1–9, 1975.
8. Cervero F: Somatic and visceral inputs to the thoracic spinal cord of the cat: effects of noxious stimulation of the biliary system. J Physiol 337:51–67, 1983.
9. Coderre TJ, Katz J, Vaccarino AL, et al.: Contribution of central neuroplasticity to pathological pain: review of clinical and experimental evidence. Pain 52:259–285, 1993.
10. Devor M, Wall PD, McMahon SB: Dichotomizing somatic nerve fibers exist in rats but they are rare. Neurosci Lett 49:187–192, 1984.
11. Doran FSA, Ratcliffe AH: The physiological mechanism of referred shoulder-tip pain. Brain 77:427–434, 1954.
12. Foreman RD, Blair RW, Weber N: Viscerosomatic convergence onto T2–T4 spinoreticular, spinoreticular-spinothalamic, and spinothalamic tract neurones in the cat. Exp Neurol 85:597–619, 1984.
13. Giamberardino MA, Vecchiet L: Visceral pain, referred hyperalgesia and outcome: new concepts. Eur J Anaesthesiol 12(Suppl. 10):61–66, 1995.
14. Giamberardino MA, Dalal A, Vecchiet L: Changes in activity of spinal cells with muscular input in rats with referred muscular hyperalgesia from ureteral calculosis. Neurosci Lett 203:1–4, 1996.
14a. Graven-Nielsen T, Arendt-Nielsen L, Svensson P, Jensen TS: Experimental pain: a quantitative study of local and referred pain in humans following injection of hypertonic saline. J Musculoskeletal Pain 5(1):49–69, 1997.
14b. Graven-Nielsen T, Arendt-Nielsen L, Svensson P, Jensen TS: Quantification of local and referred muscle pain in humans after sequential i.m. injections of hypertonic saline. Pain 69(1–2):111–117, 1997.
14c. Graven-Nielsen T, Arendt-Nielsen L, Svensson P, Jensen TS: Stimulus-response functions in areas with experimentally induced referred muscle pain—a psychophysical study. Brain Res 744(1):121–128, 1997.
14d. Graven-Nielsen T, Sörensen J, Henriksson KG, et al.: Central hyperexcitability in fibromyalgia. J Musculoskeletal Pain 7(1/2):261–271, 1999.
15. Guilbaud G: Central neurophysiological processing of joint pain on the basis of studies performed in normal animals and in models of experimental arthritis. Can J Physiol Pharmacol 69:637–646, 1991.
16. Herdegen T, Tölle TR, Bravo R, et al.: Sequential expression of JUN B, JUN D and FOS B proteins in rat spinal neurons: cascade of transcriptional operations during nociception. Neurosci Lett 129:221–224, 1991.
17. Hockaday JM, Whitty CWM: Patterns of referred pain in the normal subject. Brain 90:481–496, 1967.
18. Hoheisel U, Mense S: Long-term changes in discharge behaviour of cat dorsal horn neurones following noxious stimulation of deep tissues. Pain 36:239–247, 1989.
19. Hoheisel U, Mense S: Response behaviour of cat dorsal horn neurones receiving input from skeletal muscle and other deep somatic tissues. J Physiol 426:265–280, 1990.
20. Hoheisel U, Mense S, Simons DG, et al.: Appearance of new receptive fields in rat dorsal horn neurons following noxious stimulation of skeletal muscle: a model for referral of muscle pain? Neurosci Lett 153:9–12, 1993.
21. Holzer P: Local effector functions of capsaicin-sensitive sensory nerve endings: involvement of tachykinins, calcitonin gene-related peptide and other neuropeptides. Neuroscience 24:739–768, 1988.
22. Hong C-Z: Pathophysiology of myofascial trigger point. J Formos Med Assoc 95:93–104, 1996.
23. Hong C-Z, Chen Y-N, Twehous D, et al.: Pressure threshold for referred pain by compression on the trigger point and adjacent areas. J Musculoskeletal Pain 4(3):61–79, 1996.
24. Hu JW, Sessle BJ, Raboisson P, et al.: Stimulation of craniofacial muscle afferents induces prolonged facilitatory effects in trigeminal nociceptive brainstem neurones. Pain 48:53–60, 1992.
25. Inman VT, Saunders JB, de CM: Referred pain from skeletal structures. J Nerv Ment Dis 99:660–667, 1944.
26. Kellgren JH: Observations on referred pain arising from muscle. Clin Sci 3:175–190, 1938.
26a. Laursen RJ, Graven-Nielsen T, Jensen TS, Arendt-Nielsen L. The effect of compression and regional anaesthetic block on referred pain intensity in humans. Pain 80(1–2):257–263, 1999.

27. Lembeck F, Holzer P: Substance P as neurogenic mediator of antidromic vasodilation and neurogenic plasma extravasation. *Naunyn-Schmiedeberg's Arch Pharmacol* 310:175–183, 1979.
28. Lewis T: *Pain*. Macmillan, London, 1942.
29. Lewit K: *Manipulative Therapy in Rehabilitation of the Locomotor System*. Ed. 2. Butterworth Heinemann, Oxford, 1991.
30. MacDermott AB, Mayer ML, Westbrook GL, *et al.*: NMDA-receptor activation increases cytoplasmic calcium concentration in cultured spinal cord neurones. *Nature* 321:519–522, 1986.
31. Maggi CA, Patacchini R, Rovero P, *et al.*: Tachykinin receptors and tachykinin receptor antagonists. *J Autonom Pharmacol* 13:23–93, 1993.
32. McCall IW, Park WM, O'Brien JP: Induced pain referral from posterior lumbar elements in normal subjects. *Spine* 4:441–446, 1979.
33. McKenzie J: *Symptoms and Their Interpretation*. Shaw and Sons, London, 1909.
34. Melzack R: The gate control theory 25 years later: new perspectives on phantom limb pain, Chapter 2. *Proceedings of the 6th World Congress on Pain*. Edited by Bond MR, Charlton JE, Woolf CJ. Elsevier, Amsterdam, 1991.
35. Mense S: Referral of muscle pain. New aspects. *Am Pain Soc J* 3:1–9, 1994.
36. Mense S, Craig AD: Spinal and supraspinal terminations of primary afferent fibers from the gastrocnemius-soleus muscle in the cat. *Neuroscience* 26:1023–1035, 1988.
37. Mense S, Meyer H: Different types of slowly conducting afferent units in cat skeletal muscle and tendon. *J Physiol* 363:403–417, 1985.
38. Mense S, Light AR, Perl ER: Spinal terminations of subcutaneous high-threshold mechanoreceptors. *Spinal Cord Sensation*. Edited by Brown AG, Réthelyi M. Scottish Academic Press, Edinburgh, 1981 (pp. 79–86).
39. Meyers DER, Snow PJ: Somatotopically inappropriate projections of single hair follicle afferent fibres to the cat spinal cord. *J Physiol* 347:59–73, 1984.
40. Molander C, Ygge I, Dalsgaard C-J: Substance P-, somatostatin-, and calcitonin gene-related peptide-like immunoreactivity and fluoride resistant acid phosphatase-activity in relation to retrogradely labeled cutaneous, muscular and visceral primary sensory neurons in the rat. *Neurosci Lett* 74:37–42, 1987.
41. Pierau F-K, Fellmer G, Taylor DCM: Somato-visceral convergence in cat dorsal root ganglion neurones demonstrated by double-labelling with fluorescent tracers. *Brain Res* 321:63–70, 1984.
42. Reinert A, Vitek M, Mense S: Effects of substance P on the activity of high- and low-threshold mechanosensitive receptors of the rat diaphragm in vitro. *Pflgers Arch* 420(Suppl. 1):R47, 1992.
43. Ruch TC: Visceral sensation and referred pain. *Howell's Textbook of Physiology*. Ed. 16. Edited by Fulton JF. Saunders, Philadelphia, 1949 (pp. 385–401).
44. Sastry BR: Substance P effects on spinal nociceptive neurones. *Life Sci* 24:2169–2178, 1979.
45. Schaible H-G, Schmidt RF, Willis WD: Convergent inputs from articular, cutaneous and muscle receptors onto ascending tract cells in the cat spinal cord. *Exp Brain Res* 66:479–488, 1987.
46. Scudds RA, Landry M, Birmingham T, *et al.*: The frequency of referred signs from muscle pressure in normal healthy subjects. *J Musculoskeletal Pain* 3(Suppl 1):99, 1995. [Abstract]
47. Shortland P, Wall PD: Long-range afferents in the rat spinal cord. II. Arborizations that penetrate grey matter. *Phil Trans R Soc Lond B* 337:445–455, 1992.
48. Simons DG: Referred phenomena of myofascial trigger points, Chapter 28. *New Trends In Referred Pain and Hyperalgesia*. No. 27 in the series Pain Research and Clinical Management. Edited by Vecchiet L, Albe-Fessard D, Lindblom U, Giamberardino MA. Elsevier, Amsterdam, 1993.
49. Simons DG, Travell JG, Simons LS: *Travell & Simons' Myofascial Pain and Dysfunction: The Trigger Point Manual, Volume 1. Upper Half of Body*. Ed. 2. Williams & Wilkins, Baltimore, 1999.
50. Sinclair DC, Weddell G, Feindel WH: Referred pain and associated phenomena. *Brain* 71:184–211, 1948.
51. Sola AE, Kuitert JH: Myofascial trigger point pain in the neck and shoulder girdle. *Northwest Med* 54:980–984, 1955.
52. Staff PH: Clinical consideration in referred muscle pain and tenderness—connective tissue reactions. *Eur J Appl Physiol* 57:369–372, 1988.
53. Torebjörk HE, Ochoa JL, Schady W: Referred pain from intraneural stimulation of muscle fascicles in the median nerve. *Pain* 18:145–156, 1984.
54. Travell J, Rinzler SH: The myofascial genesis of pain. *Postgrad Med* 11:425–434, 1952.
55. Travell JG, Simons DG: *Travell & Simons' Myofascial Pain and Dysfunction. The Trigger Point Manual, Volume 2. The Lower Extremities*. Williams & Wilkins, Baltimore, 1992.
56. Treede R-D, Magerl W: Modern concepts of pain and hyperalgesia: beyond the polymodal C-nociceptor. *NIPS* 10:217–228, 1995.
57. Vecchiet L, Giamberardino MA, Dragani L, *et al.*: Referred muscular hyperalgesia from viscera: clinical approach. *Advances In Pain Research and Therapy*, Volume 13. Edited by Lipton S, et al. Raven Press, New York, 1990 (pp. 175–182).
58. Wall PD: The presence of ineffective synapses and circumstances which unmask them. *Phil Trans R Soc London B* 278:361–372, 1977.
59. Woolf CJ, Wall PD: Relative effectiveness of C primary afferent fibers of different origins in evoking a prolonged facilitation of the flexor reflex in the rat. *J Neurosci* 6:1433–1442, 1986.
60. Yu X-M, Mense S: Response properties and descending control of rat dorsal horn neurones with deep receptive fields. *Neuroscience* 39:823–831, 1990.
61. Zieglgänsberger W, Tulloch IF: Effects of substance P on neurones in the dorsal horn of the spinal cord of the cat. *Brain Res* 166:273–282, 1979.

CHAPTER 5
Pain Associated with Increased Muscle Tension

SUMMARY: Measurable sources of muscle tension include **viscoelastic tone**, **physiologic contracture** (neither of which involve electromyographic activity of the muscle), **voluntary contraction**, and **muscle spasm**, which we define as involuntary muscle contraction. The latter two conditions of muscle depend on electromyographic activity to generate the tension. Total muscle tension is most accurately measured as **stiffness**. **Thixotropy** of muscle is an ubiquitous and functionally important phenomenon that is not commonly recognized.

A clinical pain condition sometimes associated with increased muscle tension is **tension-type headache**, which is largely muscular in origin. Tension-type headache is often caused by myofascial trigger points but not by a **pain-spasm-pain cycle**, which is a physiologically and clinically untenable concept. Clinical conditions associated with painful muscle spasm include spasmodic torticollis, trismus, unnecessary muscle tension, nocturnal leg cramps, and stiff-man syndrome.

A. IDENTIFICATION OF MUSCLE TENSION

Understanding of musculoskeletal pain, and of muscle pain in particular, has been greatly hampered by poorly defined terminology that often does as much to obscure as to clarify the source of muscle tension. Commonly, two terms are used clinically to identify muscle tension: muscle tone and muscle spasm. Unfortunately, both terms are ambiguous because they are used with conceptually different meanings. One is a general, inclusive meaning, and the other is specifically limited. The specific definitions are much more useful for scientific communication. It would help greatly if authors identified clearly whether they were using a general definition or a specific definition and, if they were using a specific definition, what meaning they were ascribing to muscle tone or muscle spasm.

Muscle tension depends physiologically on two factors: the basic viscoelastic properties of the soft tissues associated with the muscle, and/or the degree of activation of the contractile apparatus of the muscle. Thus, it will be most helpful to the reader if the author makes it clear whether the term used applies to one or both of these basic sources of muscle tension.

Electromyographic (EMG) recordings identify only electrogenic contraction (i.e.,

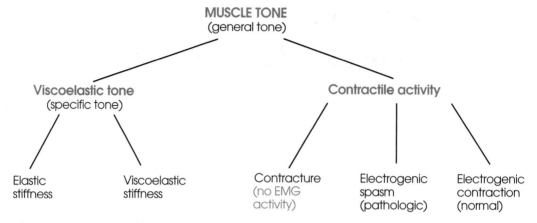

Figure 5-1. Relationship among terms commonly used to characterize muscle tension: tone, stiffness, contracture, and spasm.

contraction elicited by electrical activity of the motor nerve and muscle cell) and not endogenous contracture of the contractile apparatus of skeletal muscle, since the latter does not depend on propagated action potentials in the muscle cell. The clinical importance of making this distinction is presented in Chapter 8.

Until recently, the viscoelastic tone of resting muscle devoid of action potentials was profoundly enigmatic. Demonstration of major changes in the viscoelastic tone (i.e., of thixotropic behavior) of normal muscle opens a new and promising approach to understanding this enigma. The clinical applications of this basic phenomenon of muscle thixotropy are largely unexplored and may relate to known cytoskeletal molecules.[116a]

Figure 5-1 presents graphically the ambiguities and relationship of these terms as commonly used. The viscoelastic tone is distinguished as a separate entity when it is used in the specific sense of being independent of contractile activity. Any contractile activity is often identified as spasm when that term is used in the general sense. Contractile activity, however, may occur in three different forms:

1. *Electrogenic contraction* or *stiffness*, i.e., muscle tension coming from electrogenic muscle contraction (based on observable EMG activity) in normals who are not completely relaxed. (The term electrogenic refers to the fact that the α-motor neurons and the neuromuscular junction are active under these conditions.)
2. *Electrogenic spasm,* which specifically identifies pathologic involuntary electrogenic contraction.
3. *Contracture,* which arises endogenously within the muscle fibers independent of EMG activity.

Figure 5-1 makes it clear why "muscle tone" and "muscle spasm," used in a general sense, are frequently indistinguishable and how the muscle tension being described can come from unidentified multiple sources. This ambiguity thwarts clear understanding of the communication.

Measurements of muscle stiffness (in the physical sense of resistance to movement; see below under "Definitions Related to Muscle Tone") in relaxed subjects will include whatever is present from both major components of muscle tension: viscoelastic tone and muscular contractile activity. Monitoring the muscles for EMG activity identifies the absence, or indicates the relative importance, of electrogenic contractile activity (muscle spasm or normal electrogenic contraction). The contribution of muscle contracture is more difficult to measure separately but must be considered as a possible component to muscle stiffness. These noninvasive measures of stiffness include the effect not only of the muscles themselves but also of the soft tissues surrounding them.

Use of a high-resolution engineering approach to the measurement of objective muscle stiffness has led to surprising and fundamentally important results. Normal muscle tone shows strong thixotropic properties that are a fundamental and rarely appreciated characteristic of muscle. Recognition of the thixotropic properties of muscle helps to clarify the nature of viscoelastic tone, helps to identify some common misconceptions about it, and opens new avenues of investigation. These same sensitive, reliable measures clearly demonstrate an enigmatic but important subjective muscle stiffness that does not involve increased resistance to movement, just discomfort. The morning "stiffness" felt by patients with rheumatoid arthritis is not accounted for primarily by changes in measurable stiffness and relates more to subjective discomfort associated with movement than to a change in soft tissue viscoelastic properties.

More detailed consideration of muscle tension follows under the three headings: "Viscoelastic Tone," "Contracture (in the Physiologic Sense)," and "Muscle Spasm."

1. Viscoelastic Tone

Definitions applicable to this section are found below under "Definitions Related To Muscle Tone."

Muscle tone as applied to clinical practice is measurable as stiffness, which is the resistance to passive movement. Two kinds of stiffness can be measured: elastic and viscoelastic (Fig. 5-2). Elastic stiffness (Fig. 5-2A) is measured in terms of the distance moved. The passive movement should be performed slowly enough that viscous ef-

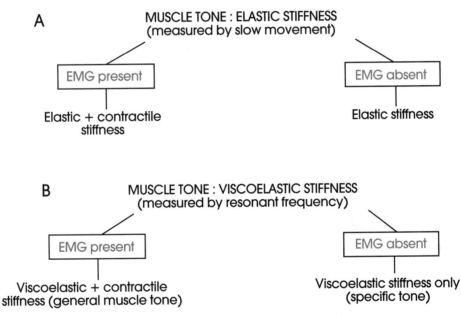

Figure 5-2. Muscle tone measured as stiffness. The presence or absence of EMG activity is critical for understanding what is being measured. **A.** Muscle tone measured as elastic stiffness, which is the resistance encountered by a force applied slowly through a given distance (force/distance). This method is suitable for measuring the rigidity of Parkinson's disease. This rigidity is more position sensitive than rate sensitive. **B.** Change in muscle stiffness measured as a change in resonant frequency. This method measures rate-sensitive changes seen in the spasticity of spinal cord-injured patients and hemiplegics. Without EMG monitoring, the contribution of muscle spasm is unclear. Thixotropy is measured as changes in viscoelastic muscle tone (stiffness) that appear following movement or change in movement; it is observed in the complete absence of EMG activity.

fects and reflex spasm are not significant components. This technique assesses the elastic properties as if the stiffness were caused only by the spring effect, as illustrated in Figure 5-3.

Viscoelastic stiffness (Fig. 5-2*B*) considers the effect of the speed of movement, which is often included in the clinical assessment of spasticity. Measurements of stiffness that include velocity are more complicated and more informative. They include the viscous and elastic components of viscoelasticity as well as inertial (weight) effects. The nonspecific common usage definition of tone is convenient because it is so inclusive, but it is dangerously ambiguous in meaning.

The specific meaning of tone as used in this book applies only to viscoelastic changes in the absence of muscle contractile activity. Any dynamic measurement of muscle stiffness includes the viscoelastic component and the effect of any contractile activity (muscle contraction) that is present. The only way one can measure just the elastic stiffness of a body segment (stiffness in the limited sense) is to ensure an absence of electrogenic contractile activity by adequate monitoring and by finding no EMG activity. Therefore, the presence or absence of EMG activity is of fundamental importance as to what is being measured. This fact is emphasized by the initial dichotomy of whether EMG activity is present or absent, as shown in Figure 5-2. Confusion results when the terms "tone" and "stiffness" are applied indiscriminately without regard to whether EMG activity is present.

Definitions Related to Muscle Tone

Elastic stiffness (physics definition): "In an elastic system: the steady force required to produce unit displacement."[105] This definition explicitly excludes rate of movement as a consideration and corresponds to the physics (and engineering) definition of elasticity, which is the resistance encountered by moving something a certain distance.

Elasticity: "The property whereby a body, when deformed, by an applied load, recovers its previous configuration when the load is removed. According to Hooke's law the stress [applied force] is proportional to the strain [resulting movement] within the elastic limit."[105] Again, velocity is not a consideration. The physical meaning of elastic stiffness is portrayed in Figure 5-3.

Stiffness (common usage; two definitions): Something that is stiff is (1) "not easily bent, rigid, inflexible" and (2) "firmer than liquid in consistency, thick or viscous."[17] The first definition concerns

A

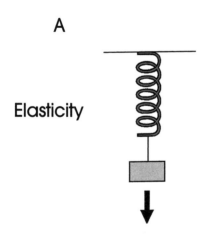

Elasticity

B

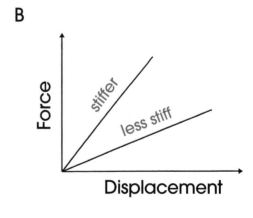

Force

stiffer

less stiff

Displacement

Figure 5-3. Elastic stiffness of an ideal spring as expressed by Hooke's law; i.e., the distance moved (displacement or strain) is proportional to the force applied (stress). The rate of application of the force is not a consideration. (Adapted from Walsh EG: *Muscles, Masses and Motion: The Physiology of Normality, Hypotonicity, Spasticity and Rigidity*. Mac Keith Press, distributed by Cambridge University Press, New York, 1992.)

simple displacement or deformation and is measured as elasticity. The second definition is measured as resistance to rate of movement (see below under "Definitions Related to Mechanical Properties of Muscle"), is a more inclusive definition, and is measured as viscoelastic stiffness.

Tone (specific, as defined in this book): Measured as elastic or viscoelastic stiffness in the absence of contractile activity.

Tone (general): Measured as elastic or viscoelastic stiffness, including any involuntary contractile activity.

Suggested Definition of Muscle Tone. Resting muscle tone (in the specific sense) is measured as the elastic and/or viscoelastic stiffness in the absence of contractile activity (motor unit activity and/or contracture).

Clinical Usage of Muscle Tone. **Hypertonia** is generally used to mean increased muscle tone for any reason. It includes a variety of conditions, such as spasticity, rigidity, dystonia, and muscular contracture.[88] Each of these conditions is associated with a particular diagnosis, but the origins and mechanisms of the increased tone may be totally different. This open-ended and diverse diagnostic approach to terminology is useful clinically but can lead to serious ambiguities and confusion. To understand the nature of muscle tone in these various conditions, it helps to use unambiguous terms relating to measurable phenomena and to their physiologic origin.

The **hypotonia** of "floppy" infants is noteworthy because it describes an enigmatic loss of normal elastic stiffness that may relate to thixotropy. Although normal resting muscle tone is usually ascribed to a lack of sufficient motor neuron activity under the control of α-motor reflexes, evidence suggests that this is not a satisfactory explanation.

It is true that patients with cerebellar lesions and monkeys with lesions of the interposed or fastigial nuclei have a decrease in tonic muscle tension (hypotonia) and a decrease in the steady background of muscle spindle afferent activity.[34] A corresponding change in extrafusal motor unit

activity has not been demonstrated, however—just assumed. The change in spindle afferent activity would result from change in tension of the intrafusal fibers, which, because of their small mass and arrangement parallel to the extrafusal muscle fibers, is unlikely to contribute directly to the change in muscle tone. An interesting speculation is that the central lesions may also directly influence the thixotropic properties of muscle, although presently no solid evidence is available in this regard.

Similarly, it is widely assumed that the pathways modulating stretch reflexes (e.g., the pontine and medullary reticulospinal tracts)[93] are responsible for resting muscle tone. For reasons described below, however, this mechanism is not a credible source of the resting elastic tone of muscle. Disturbance of these pathways would affect the control of movement.

Walsh[115] eloquently reviewed the common misconception in the medical literature that resting muscle tone depends on a low-level tonic discharge of motor neurons to muscles, resulting in a gentle tonic contraction. Walsh reviewed the historic facts that the concept was introduced by Waller in 1896, based on an irrelevant frog experiment reported by Brondegeest in 1860. When the Sherrington school in Oxford later equated the stretch reflex to tone, the concept became embedded. Unfortunately, the fact that their studies of spinalized animals are applicable to paraplegic or quadriplegic (but not to intact) human beings is commonly overlooked.

Efforts to find EMG evidence of resting muscle tone in normal subjects have failed.[3, 15, 91] Needle EMG studies are a sensitive and reliable method of detecting any α-motor neuron activity that would be responsible for that source of muscle tone. The activation of one neuron activates one motor unit, which activates 500 or more muscle fibers in most postural muscles. Thus, the electrical activity of 1 motor unit is readily observed from any location within a diameter of approximately 1 cm in most postural skeletal muscles. In addition, sensitive resonant frequency studies of changes in muscle stiffness before and after anesthesia[63, 64] showed no reduction in tone as a result of surgical anesthesia.

Therefore, the elastic tone of normal resting muscle must be caused by its viscoelastic properties in the absence of muscle contractile activity. Clinically, one can examine a body segment for resistance to movement sufficiently slowly that the speed of movement does not affect the result (static evaluation of elastic stiffness), or one can assess how much force is required to make the segment move at different speeds (dynamic evaluation of general stiffness). This distinction is applied effectively in the clinical evaluation of patients with spastic cerebral palsy.[63]

The **compliance** (compressibility) of a muscle is assessed clinically by pressing a finger into it or by squeezing it between the fingers to determine how easily it is indented and how "springy" it is. The less easily it is indented and the more it tends to return to its original shape, the more stiff (elastic) it is. The speed of application of the pressure is not included as a determining factor in this assessment of hypotonia and hypertonia.

The **limitation of range of motion** of a muscle is estimated clinically by slowly extending the muscle until it reaches a barrier of increasing tension. This barrier has the effect of shortening the muscle. The test is usually done slowly enough to eliminate rate of movement as a factor in the results. This test alone fails to distinguish among increased viscoelastic tension, spasticity, physiologic contracture, and fibrosis. When this test shows increased range of motion (hypermobility), it is sometimes interpreted as decreased muscle tone. This interpretation alone is unreliable, however, because hypermobility can also be caused by laxity of ligamentous and capsular connective tissue elements.

The more general **flapping test** is performed by grasping the fingertips of the extended arms and rhythmically shaking them up and down to see how loose or how stiff the musculature of each extremity is. With progressively more rapid movements, the examiner can estimate the resonant frequency of each limb. Proximal-distal and bilateral differences are noted. This dynamic test is useful for assessing hypotonia and hypertonia by estimating general muscle stiffness.

Measurements of Muscle Tone. The **pendulum** test (Wartenberg test[117]) is performed with the relaxed patient sitting on the edge of the table and his or her legs hanging freely over the edge. The examiner lifts both of the patient's legs to the horizontal position (knees straight) and then releases them, observing their movement as they swing freely. Figure 5-4*A* illustrates that normally a leg swings in smoothly decreasing sinusoidal arcs. In Figure 5-4*B*, the overreactive reflex stretch responses of spastic muscles reduce the number and smoothness of oscillations of an affected limb and may interrupt the first swing before it can complete its initial downward phase. In muscular hypotonia (Fig. 5-4*C*), additional smoothly decreasing arcs continue for a prolonged period of time.

Several authors[2, 10, 55] have attempted to instrument this test to make it more quantitative. Walsh[115] reviewed a number of these efforts. This gravity-driven approach has the advantage of simplicity but is restricted to testing a few muscles around the knee and provides only one source of force (gravity). The contribution made by the mass of the calf is so variable among subjects and is so hard to estimate that absolute standards have poor resolution.

Compliance measured with a simple handheld compliance meter provides a quantitative estimate of the information obtained by pressing on or squeezing the muscle. A commercially available spring-loaded compliance meter of this type simultaneously measures the surface indentation in millimeters and the force in kilograms applied to a 1-cm² footplate.[30] This device can easily provide a rough estimate of muscle elasticity. However, the results are an ambiguous combination of skin, subcutaneous, and muscle compliance. They are generally useful only when the measurements are comparative readings, e.g., bilaterally or as a series of readings at the same site.

Motor-driven testing devices are more complicated, but can provide a much wider range of test conditions and more sophisticated analysis. These devices lend themselves to the control and measurement of velocity, which permits separate identifica-

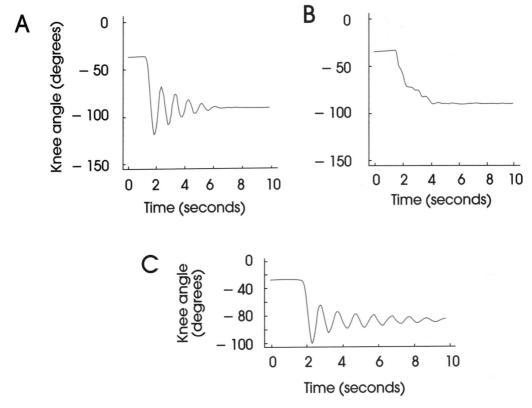

Figure 5-4. Recordings of the pendulum (Wartenberg) test. **A.** Normal oscillations. **B.** Reduced oscillations in a patient with Parkinson's disease. **C.** Prolonged oscillations characteristic of hypotonia.

(Adapted from Walsh EG: *Muscles, Masses and Motion: The Physiology of Normality, Hypotonicity, Spasticity and Rigidity.* Mac Keith Press, distributed by Cambridge University Press, New York, 1992.)

tion of additional measures: viscosity, damping, resonant frequency, and thixotropy. See "Definitions Related to Mechanical Properties of Muscle" below for definitions of related terms.

Definitions Related to Mechanical Properties of Muscle

Mechanical impedance: The resistance to motion produced by the interaction of elasticity, momentum, and viscosity. It concerns rate of movement. To a physicist or engineer, it is "the ratio of the (complex) force acting on a given mechanical device to the resulting linear velocity in the direction of the force. The units are mechanical ohm or (N s m^{-1})," which are Newton seconds per meter.[105] This linear form of the definition is readily converted to the rotational

form. Then, the force is applied as torque, as described by Lakie and Walsh.[115] Systems that have impedance show the characteristic of resonance.

Viscosity: "The resistance to fluid flow, set up by shear stresses within the flowing liquid."[105] See damping in Figure 5-5.

Resonance: Resonance of an oscillatory system is "the marked increase in the amplitude of oscillation . . . when the system is subjected to an impressed frequency that is the same [as] (or very close to) the natural frequency of the system."[105] Resonance is measured as the frequency of minimum resistance to movement. (See velocity trace in Figure 5-7.) In mechanical systems, resonance occurs at the frequency at which elasticity balances momentum and the only resistance to motion comes from viscosity.

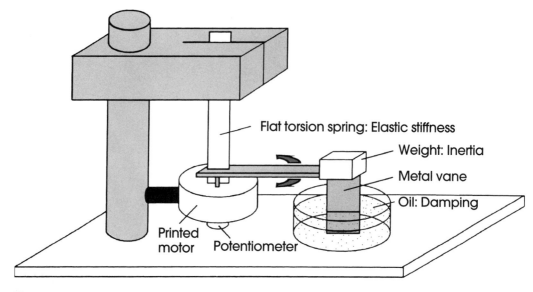

Figure 5-5. Model demonstrating the principle of resonance as measured by Walsh.[115] The printed circuit motor is coupled to a flat torsion spring that provides elastic stiffness. Inertia is imparted by the weight fixed to the lever. Damping (viscosity) is provided by a vane moving in oil. At resonance, the effect of inertia balances the effect of elastic stiffness, and there is minimum resistance to movement of the lever (provided only by the damping effect of viscosity). (Adapted from Walsh EG: *Muscles, Masses and Motion: The Physiology of Normality, Hypotonicity, Spasticity and Rigidity.* Mac Keith Press, distributed by Cambridge University Press, New York, 1992.)

It is convenient to think of this resistance to motion as viscoelastic stiffness. The resonant frequency is sensitive to small changes in the viscoelastic stiffness of soft tissues. This frequency increases nearly as the square of stiffness.

Thixotropy: A "property shown by many gels of liquefying on being shaken and of reforming on standing."[105] This loss of resistance to movement can also occur in response to stirring.

Stiffness Measured as Resonant Frequency. Measuring changes in resonant frequency of a limb segment permits accurate measurement of relatively small changes in the viscoelastic stiffness of that segment if EMG activity is absent. For example, a violin string produces a tone at its resonant frequency, which is tuned by adjusting its tension (viscoelastic stiffness). Figure 5-5 schematically presents the principles involved when measuring the resonant frequency of the soft tissues of a limb segment. The torsion spring provides elastic stiffness that corresponds to the elastic part of the viscoelastic component of resis-

tance to movement. The weight corresponds to the inertia imparted by the mass of the tissues. The vane in oil provides the damping, which corresponds to the viscous part of the viscoelastic component. The motor is controlled to perform sinusoidal movements and drives the system at progressively faster frequencies. As the weight reaches the end of a sinusoidal excursion, the energy of the system is stored as potential energy in the torsion spring, and as the weight passes the neutral position, the energy is stored in the weight as kinetic energy.

At speeds slower than resonance, the mechanical impedance increases because of increasing importance of the effect of mass. At speeds greater than resonance, the mechanical impedance increases because of increasing importance of the effect of elasticity. The proportion of the mechanical impedance caused by viscosity does not depend on the speed of movement. Resonance occurs at the speed at which the potential energy stored by the elastic component exactly matches the kinetic energy supplied by the mass component as they trade energy back and forth. At resonance, all of the mechanical impedance comes from viscosity. The accuracy of this use of resonant frequency as a measure of change in viscoelastic stiffness depends on little or no change in the mass or viscosity of the structures between test conditions.

Walsh and associates employed a printed circuit motor to apply a finely controlled, constant-amplitude alternating (sine-wave) torque to the hand at the wrist joint (Fig. 5-6). The motor provided smooth, precise control of the force input so that they could control the rate of oscillation while measuring the resultant amplitude and acceleration of hand movement.[115] They measured

EMG activity to ensure that there was no electrogenic contractile component involved. By smoothly doubling the rate of oscillation approximately every 3 seconds through several octaves, changes in resonant frequency were clearly revealed and measurable, as shown in Figure 5-7. Change in resonant frequency is a sensitive and accurate method of measuring changes in muscle stiffness. As demonstrated mathematically,[115] the resonant frequency increases as the square of the increase in stiffness. Therefore, a threefold increase in stiffness produces a ninefold increase in resonant frequency.

At resonant frequency, the energy required for moving the system is minimal.

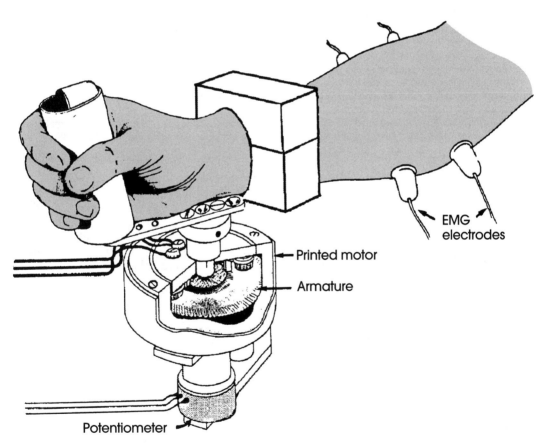

Figure 5-6. Application of a printed circuit motor for dynamic measurements of resistance to movement and rate of movement at the wrist. The printed circuit motor is shown in cutaway form. Its shaft is aligned with the axis of rotation at the wrist. The two halves of the block of plastic stabilize the forearm to permit precise measurement of hand motion. The hand is passively moved by the motor in an oscillatory sinusoidal pattern. Suction cup electrodes provide for electromyographic recordings, and a potentiometer records hand movement (displacement). (Reproduced with permission from Walsh EG: *Muscles, Masses and Motion: The Physiology of Normality, Hypotonicity, Spasticity and Rigidity*. Mac Keith Press, distributed by Cambridge University Press, New York, 1992.)

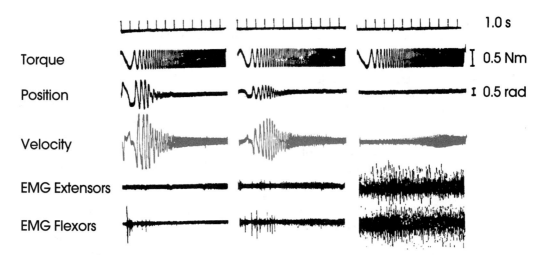

Figure 5-7. Marked increase in the resonant frequency of the musculature at the wrist. This resulted from increased stiffness as a result of voluntary cocontraction of the flexor and extensor muscles. The frequency of constant force (torque) oscillations applied in flexion and extension was smoothly and steadily increased through several octaves, starting at approximately 1 Hz. The resonant frequency corresponds to the maximum-amplitude excursions of velocity, which is the first derivative of position. The EMG traces show the nearly complete lack of electrical activity in the relaxed record (*left*), a slight increase in resonant frequency with minimal voluntary contraction of the forearm muscles (*middle*), and a marked increase in resonant frequency with strong voluntary cocontraction of the forearm flexor and extensor muscles (*right*). Time is in seconds (s), torque is in Newton meters (Nm), and position is in radians (rad). (Adapted from Walsh EG: *Muscles, Masses and Motion: The Physiology of Normality, Hypotonicity, Spasticity and Rigidity*. Mac Keith Press, distributed by Cambridge University Press, New York, 1992.)

Interestingly, birds use their wings at resonant frequency and thus save energy. Because of their smaller mass, the wings of small birds have a higher resonant frequency than the wings of large birds.

Thixotropy. A number of materials, such as paint, tomato ketchup, and human blood, show the property of thixotropy. When first stirred or poured, thixotropic substances resist stirring or movement. After initial movement, their viscosity decreases, often precipitously. The resistance to movement depends strongly on the preceding history of movement. The same kind of instrumentation described above for measuring resonant frequency is well suited to measuring the surprisingly marked thixotropic property of human muscle, as illustrated in Figure 5-8. An increase in torque for two or three cycles caused a large reduction in the resistance to movement, recognizable in the larger amplitude of the movement after the torque had been adjusted to its original strength. The figure shows a more than threefold increase, indicating a reduction to one third of the initial resistance to motion. The reduced muscle stiffness persisted as long as motion persisted, but it returned to its previous state, sometimes quickly (in approximately 1 second, as seen here) and sometimes after a much longer time (e.g., 2 or 3 minutes).[40] Walsh[115] noted that EMG monitoring showed no evidence that could account for these changes in the resistance to motion. This conclusion was further substantiated by the failure of neuromuscular blocking drugs to affect the thixotropic effect. This change in the viscoelastic properties of muscle is attributed primarily to changes in effective viscosity, probably between sliding filaments.

The work of Lakie et al.[65] was substantiated in principle by Hagbarth and colleagues,[40] who observed similar thixotropic effects, using a smaller printed motor to drive the metacarpophalangeal joint of the index finger in relaxed normal subjects. The test force was applied only toward extension, and they found that voluntary contraction of the flexors produced a reduction in muscle stiffness similar to passive extension of the finger. Lakie and col-

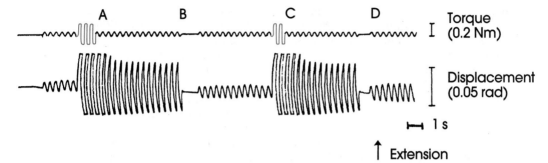

$\uparrow$ Extension

Figure 5-8. Thixotropic effect (reduced resistance to movement) caused by a large increase in the force (torque) applied for three cycles *(red part of upper trace)*. The reduction in elastic stiffness (measured as displacement, *lower trace*) at **A** persisted despite immediate return of the torque to its original level. A brief, three-cycle interruption of passive wrist motion at **B** restored the stiffness to its original level, which again responded to two cycles of increased torque at **C**, essentially as it had responded previously at **A**. A briefer, two-cycle interruption of movement at **D** failed to fully return the musculature to its original state of looseness. This temporary loss of muscular tone in response to a sudden, brief increase in its activity is an example of thixotropy, which expresses the effect of movement history on muscle stiffness. During this test, no EMG activity was present. Torque is measured in Newton meters, displacement in radians, and time in seconds. (Adapted from Walsh EG: *Muscles, Masses and Motion: The Physiology of Normality, Hypotonicity, Spasticity and Rigidity*. Mac Keith Press, distributed by Cambridge University Press, New York, 1992.)

leagues[65] observed no difference in flexion or extension responses but applied force symmetrically in both flexion and extension movements instead of in only one direction. Hagbarth *et al.*[40] also observed, with cessation of movement, a longer persistence of thixotropic effects than did Lakie and colleagues—several minutes compared with several seconds.

In a subsequent study, Lakie and Robson[62] explored in more detail the rate of recovery of thixotropic stiffening with rest. They found a threefold increase after 10 minutes that continued at a declining rate that could still be detected 24 to 30 hours later. Thixotropic time constants can cover a considerable range. Many factors that might influence them, such as age and psychologic status, are unexplored.

An important application of thixotropy is the practice of athletes of warming up prior to strenuous exercise. This releases accumulated thixotropic muscle stiffness. Conversely, the high viscosity of a resting muscle (e.g., of the erector spinae) can help maintain a given posture without expenditure of energy.

The most widely accepted explanation for thixotropy of muscles is a tendency for the actin and myosin filaments to stick together when inactive for a period of time.[40, 115] More recent data, however, indicate that changes in myoplasmic viscosity and connectin filaments may be of greater importance.[80a]

Clinical Applications. The exact origin of muscle tone not dependent on motor unit activity remains enigmatic. Even more enigmatic is soft tissue pain related to movement that is not associated with an increased, objectively demonstrable stiffness. The identification of thixotropy, a fundamental property of muscle that has been largely unrecognized, opens a path to a new way of thinking of muscle tone, with new tools to explore its enigmas. A clearer and more realistic understanding of the sources of painful muscle tone should contribute to improved clinical management of that pain.

Stiffness Based on Resonant Frequency. Authors have tried to demonstrate increased resistance to passive motion associated with the morning stiffness of patients with rheumatoid arthritis. Previous studies have given conflicting results with measurement of the metacarpophalangeal joint.[45, 119, 121] Using the sensitive resonant frequency technique at the wrist, Walsh *et al.*[116] examined seven female patients with rheumatoid arthritis, all of whom had early morning stiffness lasting for 20 to 360 minutes, usually for 2 or 3 hours. They were examined at some time between 9:00 a.m. and noon. For moderate to small forces of torque, the patients had lower resonant frequencies than did controls. Damping, in absolute terms, occurred less in the patients, indicating less instead of more stiffness in patients than in controls.

The morning stiffness of rheumatoid arthritis apparently has a major subjective component. The patient feels as if it will hurt if the member is moved rapidly or through more than a limited range of motion.

The common stiffness of old age, after periods in a fixed position (when traveling), may well be another example of subjective stiffness, but the magnitude of its viscoelastic stiffness component has not been measured.

The gradual and enigmatic loss of muscle tone as one falls asleep may be an example of thixotropy influenced by nervous system effects and needs to be studied by measuring viscoelastic stiffness changes through this period with adequate EMG monitoring.

Thixotropy. The marked (up to 10-fold) thixotropic decrease in muscle stiffness, when the muscle is suddenly mobilized, greatly helps to explain how one is able to stand without sustained postural muscle EMG activity, except for only occasional minimal corrective bursts of activity to maintain balance,[4] and then start to move with little restriction. The resting tone of muscle can include a significant thixotropic component, which could result in variable measurements of compliance, depending on how rapidly and how often the measurements were made.

Considering how enigmatic common pain-related changes in muscle stiffness are, the possibility that the stiffness is related to thixotropic phenomena of various time constants, some possibly developing in hours and not minutes, deserves serious research consideration.

2. Contracture (in the Physiologic Sense)

Physiologists use the term "contracture" specifically to describe endogenous shortening of the muscular contractile apparatus in the absence of EMG activity initiated by anterior horn cells[20] (see Figure 5-1).

Confusingly, the same term, "contracture," is commonly used by clinicians to describe fibrotic remodeling (shortening) of connective tissue that may include joint capsules and ligaments and reduction in the number of sarcomeres. These changes can occur when a muscle remains in a shortened position for a prolonged period of time.[71] This condition also lacks EMG activity, but for a different reason. When using the term "contracture," authors should state clearly which definition applies.

Suggested Definition of Contracture. Physiologic contracture (or rigor) is a state of muscle contractile activity unaccompanied by electrical activity.[66]

Clinical Usage of Contracture. A number of clinical examples of EMG-free muscle contractures that are painful are well known, but relatively uncommon, genetic abnormalities. Some are more painful than others. Painfulness seems to relate to an imbalance between increased energy demand and reduced energy supply. Genetic abnormalities are of two types: those that result in excessive release of calcium from the sarcoplasmic reticulum, and those that cause impaired uptake of calcium by the sarcoplasmic reticulum.

Examples of excessive calcium release are **myoedema** and the **rippling muscle syndrome**.[66] Myoedema is EMG-free mounding of the muscle following percussion caused by nonpropagated local contracture of the muscle. It is seen in some individuals with normal muscle relaxation and is a common postmortem phenomenon. Percussion of the muscles of persons with rippling muscle syndrome initiates a rolling wave of contraction that spreads laterally across the muscle in both directions. Both conditions are attributed to an exaggerated release of calcium from the sarcoplasmic reticulum in response to mechanical deformation. An ongoing exaggerated release of calcium from the sarcoplasmic reticulum could also explain the palpable taut bands found in some normal muscles and in close association with myofascial trigger points (TrPs).

Conversely, patients with myxedema resulting from hypothyroidism experience painful muscle spasms during exercise. This is associated with slow muscle relaxation caused by slow uptake of calcium by the sarcoplasmic reticulum. Calcium uptake is also impaired by genetic enzyme deficiencies that impair either glycolytic or aerobic energy metabolism of the muscle. As a result of accumulation of this calcium, these individuals are subject to muscle contractures associated with exercise that may be painful and that are relieved by rest. Examples include deficiencies in muscle phosphorylase, debrancher enzyme, phosphofructokinase, phosphoglycerate kinase, and lactate dehydrogenase. The precise mechanism of contracture in McArdle's syndrome is unresolved,[66] but it is classified as a myophosphorylase deficiency (glycogenosis type V).[22]

Much more common, and of major significance to the differential diagnosis of painful conditions of muscle, is the enigmatic phenomenon of palpable taut bands so closely associated with one of the commonest causes of musculoskeletal pain—myofascial TrPs. Although it has not been unequivocally proven that palpable taut bands are the result of muscle fibers in regional contracture, the explanation fits clinical observations. For example, the marked reduction in the tenseness of the taut band immediately after effective inactivation of a TrP in that band makes the release of contracture by restoration of more normal function of the calcium channels in the sarcoplasmic reticulum a likely explanation (see Chapter 8, Section D3).

Measurement of Contracture. The more uniformly distributed total muscle contracture of the metabolic disorders is readily measured as increase in stiffness by measuring increased elastic stiffness (the force/displacement ratio) or by measuring increased viscoelastic stiffness (increased resonant frequency), as described above under "Definitions Related to Muscle Tone" and "Definitions Related to Mechanical Properties of Muscle." Tissue compliance, the reciprocal of elastic stiffness (deformation in millimeters per force in kilograms), is another way of measuring the effect of muscle contracture.

Although the taut bands of TrPs involve only a part of the muscle and are surrounded by normally loose muscle tissue, a quantitative indication of their relative stiffness can be obtained with a handheld compliance meter.[30] This measurement also includes stiffness of subcutaneous tissue, which has been noted clinically as trophedema,[39] and observed as thickening when measured by ultrasound.[114]

3. Muscle Spasm

When examiners automatically classify any tense muscle as being in spasm, the clinically important distinction between muscle contraction and muscle contracture is lost. See Figure 5-1.

Suggested Definition of Muscle Spasm. EMG activity that is not under voluntary control and is not dependent on posture. It may or may not be painful.

Clinical Usage of Muscle Spasm. Including pain as a necessary part of the definition of spasm[59] complicates efforts to distinguish spasm from other forms of increased muscle tension and seriously complicates the measurement of spasm.

By including any abnormal increase in palpable muscle tension as spasm,[60] the definition of spasm becomes hopelessly enmeshed with the definition of muscle tone. Such a broad definition compromises the usefulness of both terms for scientific communication.

Spasticity is a clinical term commonly applied to muscle spasm observed in conditions such as hemiplegia, brain injury, or spinal cord injury. It is associated with hyperactive tendon jerks and other stretch reflexes that are caused by lesions of the premotor areas or their outflow.[33] Resistance to passive movement of a limb increases with increased speed of movement. Sufficiently rapid movements may elicit clonus. The reduced threshold of the stretch reflex results from increased excitability of the monosynaptic pathway itself.[33] In patients with spinal cord injury, a muscle spasm may be initiated by any afferent input to that portion of the spinal cord, indicating a loss of supraspinal inhibitory influence on the α-motor neurons.[23] Thus, spasticity can be thought of as occurring at the spinal level because of loss of supraspinal inhibition.

When spasticity is tonic (sustained) and not just a response to rapid stretch, as occurs in some cases of central nervous system (CNS) damage, it is much more likely to be painful and may require serious consideration of spasmolytic procedures, such as drug therapy, motor point block, or selective injection of motor endplate zones with botulinum A toxin (BTx).

Rigidity is distinctly different from spasticity and has a different nervous system etiology, although its effects are also caused by muscle spasm (involuntary contraction). It is characterized clinically as "stiffness or inflexibility"[74] that appears early and progresses in Parkinson's disease. Because this rigidity is caused by imbalance between the direct and indirect pathways of the basal ganglia and is characterized by cocontraction of antagonist muscles,[115] it can be considered a muscle spasm of supraspinal origin.

Walsh reviewed and illustrated the results of rate-sensitive measurements of patients with Parkinsonian rigidity,[115] including records of cog wheeling, which is an early symptom that resembles tremor and may become apparent only when the patient partially stiffens the limb. Walsh[115] also illustrated the later dystonic stage of Parkinson's disease, showing the continuous cocontraction of antagonistic muscle groups, sometimes described as rigor. He summarized Webster's report of records in which rigidity almost disappeared as the patient became drowsy and which was strongly enhanced by alerting reactions. These observations correlate with the clinical phenomenon of locomotor freezing when the patient is confronted with a challenging ambulatory obstacle.[87]

Although many standard texts make no mention of pain as a symptom characteristic of Parkinson's disease, multiple locations of musculoskeletal pain are sometimes associated with advanced disease and marked muscular involvement as described above.[61] The advanced stage of sustained cocontraction that is associated with a flexed posture results from chronic spasm.[5] This stage would be expected to become painful because of sustained contraction with muscles held in a shortened position.

Clinically, muscle **contraction** is properly associated with EMG activity of the muscle fibers and may be initiated voluntarily via anterior horn cell activity or by electrical stimulation.

A muscle **cramp** is commonly considered to be a painful muscle spasm, such as nocturnal leg cramps,[66] which could serve as a useful clinical definition. Painful but EMG-free contracture as observed in McArdle's syndrome is also called a cramp,[9] but it actually is a contracture (in the physiologic sense). The cause of the cramp pain in most cases may be that, as observed electromyographically,[81] only parts of the muscle are cramping. The resulting shearing forces between cramping and normal muscle are likely to activate nociceptors mechanically.

Measurement of Spasm. If muscle spasm is, by definition, muscle contraction caused by EMG activity, then it can be measured in terms of EMG activity and in terms of increased muscle stiffness caused by electrogenic spasm. The measurement of muscle stiffness was considered under muscle tone. The use of muscle stiffness as a measure of spasm is valid only to the extent that other non-EMG sources of stiffness have been eliminated or accounted for quantitatively.

The EMG activity can be measured by needle electrodes or by surface electrodes, which record activity from a relatively large sample of the muscle (and often some activity from adjacent muscles). Monopolar needle electrodes monitor a more restricted region of activity within the muscle than does surface EMG and, therefore, are subject to greater danger of sampling error because of functional compartmentalization of the muscle, unless that degree of specificity is desired. Coaxial, bipolar, and single-fiber needle electrodes sample successively smaller regions of muscle activity.

Spasticity has been studied in terms of EMG activity produced by reflex responses as a function of motor-driven flexion or extension of the body segment[118] or as the response to various frequencies of applied oscillatory movement.[12] In these studies, the investigators usually recorded the amount of force required to move the body segment a predetermined distance. Using EMG monitoring and controlled displacement velocities, Thilmann et al.[107] recently demonstrated that the mechanism of spastic hypertonus at the elbow of hemiparetic patients was caused much more by pathologic increases in reflex gain than by reduction in the threshold of the stretch reflexes. Walsh and associates explored another approach, that of measuring the distance and velocity imparted to the segment by a carefully controlled, predetermined force, using a special printed circuit motor for high-precision results.[115] This engineering approach to the measurement of tone helps greatly to distinguish the contributions of elasticity, viscosity, and mass. The results have been well worth the extra effort.

The amount of spasm can be estimated quantitatively by measuring the EMG activity present in the relaxed subject. This is now commonly accomplished by full-wave rectifying of the potentials and then smoothing (averaging) them to obtain a curve that indicates the amount of spasm as time progresses. Alternatively, the activity can be averaged through a set interval to obtain a single value that indicates the amount of spasm during that period.

B. CLINICAL CONDITIONS WITH PAINFUL INCREASED MUSCLE TENSION

At least half of patients seen by most practitioners for muscle pain cannot be assigned a specific diagnosis.[80, 99] Low back pain is a symptom, not a diagnosis. This section addresses specifically some of the clinical confusions responsible for this state of affairs.

1. Tension-Type Headache

The Problem. The International Headache Society[82] recently designated the term "tension-type headache" (T-TH) to include a number of commonly used terms, including tension headache, muscle contraction headache, psychomyogenic headache, stress headache, ordinary headache, and psychogenic headache. That there may be myogenic and psychogenic factors of variable importance is generally recognized. The terms listed above reflect this recognition but also reflect a serious lack of agreement on what to call it.

Many definitions of this sort of headache depend primarily on the clinical history with little or no concern for physical findings. The International Association for the Study of Pain publication, *Classification of Chronic Pain*,[77] distinguishes "acute tension headache" from "tension headache: chronic form (scalp muscle contraction headache)." The former diagnosis has no physical findings associated with it, while the latter may or may not include tenderness of the pericranial and/or nuchal muscles. The pathology is unresolved, and increased muscle activity is *sometimes* demonstrable on EMG.[77] This semantic controversy continues.[86, 101]

Muscle tenderness of head and neck muscles is closely associated with T-TH in many studies, but EMG activity appears to be unrelated to the symptoms of T-TH. Why this discrepancy? One study[43] showed that muscle tenderness was positively correlated with severity of T-TH, but in the same subjects, EMG was not related to severity. Lous and Olesen[70] found that nearly all of 13 patients with muscle contraction headache (now called T-TH) had tender pericranial muscles (masseter, 92%; sternocleidomastoid, 92%; temporalis, 76%; lateral pterygoid, 70%; frontalis, 0%). Frequently, the site of pain complaint, however, was not where the tenderness was observed in the muscles. They did not report examining the muscles for specific TrP characteristics (see Chapter 8), so a likely source of the pain was not considered. The lack of tenderness of the frontalis muscle is not surprising. Although it is often the site of pain *referred* from pericranial myofascial TrPs, it is rarely the source.[103a, 110]

Sakai and associates[96] reported that compared with controls, two muscle groups in T-TH patients showed significantly increased stiffness (reciprocal of compliance): a 40% increase in the trapezius muscles, and a 15% increase in the posterior neck muscles. Without EMG monitoring and palpation of the stiff muscles for TrPs, there is no way of knowing if the increased tension came from taut bands associated with TrPs or from muscle spasm.

It was originally assumed that muscle spasm (involuntary contraction) was responsible for the pain and that relaxing the pericranial muscles would relieve it. Repeated, well-controlled efforts have failed to confirm increased EMG activity of the head and neck muscles in patients with T-TH.[85, 98] Peterson *et al.*[85] examined five muscles and were perplexed by the site-specificity of findings. In an editorial in 1991, Olesen and Jensen[83] emphasized that increased EMG activity did not account for the muscle tenderness and pain of T-TH. Some other explanation must be found. Unconvincing theories abound.

Proposed Solution. As so often happens with enigmas, the answer may lie at hand and is simply being overlooked. Jaeger[49] and Simons *et al.*[103a] illustrated how referred pain patterns of TrPs in pericranial muscles (temporalis, sternocleidomastoid, upper trapezius, and suboccipital) can produce a clinical picture of T-TH. Figure 5-9 illustrates the sternocleidomastoid component of that composite pain pattern.

Other authors have implicated TrPs as a major cause of several kinds of headache, especially headaches associated with tender pericranial muscles.[19, 32, 94] Jaeger *et al.*[50] found, in 14 tension headache sufferers, a significant ($P < 0.01$) correlation between the usual pain level and tenderness (by pressure algometry), but only in the TrPs specific to the predicted pattern of referral for each patient. In Bonica's *The Management of Pain,* three authors[26] state, "Myofascial syndrome with trigger points must be assumed to be an element of the clinical picture of any patient presenting with facial and other head pain until it has been ruled out by systematic search of the musculature."

Myofascial TrPs fit nicely the characteristics that have made T-TH so enigmatic.[103a] The palpable taut band makes the muscle feel tense but is NOT associated with propagated action potentials observable as EMG activity. Minute loci of the TrP itself, however, show extremely localized electrical activity,[102, 103] which is apparently abnormal endplate potentials.[102a] The tension of the *taut band* results from stretch exerted by endogenous muscle contracture, not contraction. The TrP is

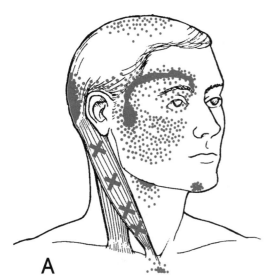
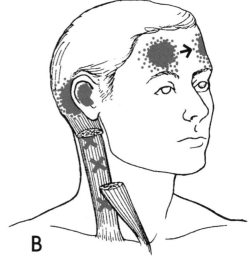

Figure 5-9. Referred pain patterns (*red stippling*) with location of corresponding trigger points (Xs) in the right sternocleidomastoid muscle. **A.** Trigger points in the sternal (superficial) division. **B.** Trigger points in the clavicular (deep) division. (Reproduced with permission from Simons DG, Travell JG, Simons LS: *Travell & Simons' Myofascial Pain and Dysfunction: The Trigger Point Manual, Volume 1. The Upper Half of the Body.* Ed. 2. Williams & Wilkins, Baltimore, 1999.)

exquisitely tender to palpation and usually causes pain referred to another location. The pain caused by TrPs is often intermittent, as the ebb and flow of life stresses modulate the activity level of the TrP. If TrPs are active enough, the pain becomes continuous.[109] As TrPs are allowed to become chronic in the presence of uncorrected perpetuating factors, the TrPs tend to propagate, causing more extensive involvement both of the CNS and of other muscles (see Chapter 8).

Psychologic stress often aggravates T-TH pain.[42, 97] The observations that psychologic stress intensifies both TrP pain and the electrical activity at active loci of TrPs fit both clinical experience[111] and experimental evidence.[76]

When patients with symptoms of T-TH are effectively treated for the TrPs that are causing their pain, the results[36, 46] can save the patients much misery and the health care system much expense.

There are good reasons why this important diagnosis has been overlooked. Unless the examiner is aware of the diagnosis and looks for the TrPs, it will be missed or misconstrued. A specific TrP examination technique that is rarely included as part of a routine physical examination is needed; it requires both training and experience.[47a, 102] A limited number of talented clinicians have been able to learn how to examine effectively for TrPs only from available publications; qualified training opportunities are limited. Only recently have a number of publications reported the critical research needed to identify the most appropriate diagnostic criteria and the importance of examiner skill (see Chapter 8, Section B4).

Differential Diagnosis. The majority of T-TH episodes occur in the course of an active day and never come to the attention of a physician because they respond to conservative measures, such as changes in position, rubbing the neck, or taking an over-the-counter analgesic.

When physicians are confronted with more severe and recalcitrant symptoms, careful assessment is indicated. Diagnostic considerations can include radiculopathy, arthritis (atlantoaxial articulation, subaxial facet joint, temporomandibular joint), or nonarticular pain (myofacial pain syndrome, temporomandibular disorders, or fibromyalgia syndrome). Poor posture can cause muscle pain when it projects the head forward for long periods of time while reading or watching television with a large pillow under the head. The resultant symptoms can be similar to those experienced with fatigue resulting from inadequate quantity or quality of sleep. A persistent headache can be the first sign of an inflammatory process, such as sinusitis, dental abscess, or giant cell arteritis. Intracranial masses, such as abscess or neoplasia, usually present with localizing neurologic signs but may be atypical early in their course. Finally, more distal problems, such as adhesive capsulitis of a shoulder joint or a compression neuropathy such as carpal tunnel syndrome, can cause splinting of the cervical musculature, resulting in headache. Most of these possibilities can be confirmed or excluded on the basis of a careful history and inexpensive clinical testing.

Medications. The most typical lay treatment for intermittent mild T-TH is oral ingestion of an over-the-counter analgesic. Advertisements in the public media are replete with claims and testimonials to indicate that one brand name analgesic is superior to another for this application. Examples include acetylsalicylic acid, acetaminophen, ibuprofen, and naproxen. Available dosages tend to be relatively low and fairly safe when used occasionally. When the problem is due to a nonarticular syndrome, such as myofascial pain syndrome or temporomandibular disorder, the active TrP areas can be treated with standard spray and/or stretch and injection techniques. Patients with fibromyalgia syndrome are treated for concurrent TrPs and given a graduated exercise program with oral medications. Acute therapy may warrant parenteral Toradol or even a narcotic, but these should be avoided for chronic treatment. Low oral dosages of a tricyclic sedative, such as amitriptyline, and of benzodiazepine anxiolytic drugs, such as alprazolam, have found utility in prophylaxis of fibromyalgia headache for periods of time up to 3 months. Longer periods of treatment with these drugs may result in tachyphylaxis.

A brief summary of the features of representative therapeutic agents follows. For more complete drug information, the reader should also seek original reference sources.

Generic Name: *aspirin (acetylsalicylic acid)*
Brand Name: Bayer Aspirin, Ecotrin, ZORprin
  Dosage: 325 to 650 mg every 4 hours with food or fluid.
  Action: The analgesic effect is believed to result from inhibition of prostaglandin synthesis by acetylating cyclo-oxygenase in the periphery, but an action in the CNS may be contributory. There is no evidence for tachyphylaxis with time. In small dosages, the elimination half-life is only 2 to 3 hours, but in high dosages it can extend to 15 to 30 hours.
  Side Effects: The most common events relate to the gastrointestinal tract, with dyspepsia, gastric ulceration, and bleeding. Patients may lose up to 10 mL of blood daily with resultant iron deficiency anemia. Other concerns include decreased renal blood flow, hepatic transaminitis, tinnitus, pulmonary edema, platelet dysfunction, skin eruptions, and hypersensitivity reactions.
  Considerations: Despite its long history in medicine, few if any analgesic preparations have been found to be superior to aspirin for analgesic efficacy. In patients who tolerate it, the analgesic effect is usually good and the cost is low. Some clinicians believe that it may be tolerated better in buffered, enteric-coated, or sustained-release forms. The relative benefit/risk ratio should be reassessed after 10 days of therapy.

Generic Name: *acetaminophen (paracetamol)*
Brand Name: Tylenol
  Dosage: 325 to 650 mg every 4 hours with fluid.
  Action: The analgesic effect is believed to be fairly comparable with that of aspirin, but there is little or no anti-inflammatory effect. A combination with aspirin offers little advantage, but a combination with low-dose opioids, such as codeine, appears to provide analgesic synergy. The plasma half-life is 1.25 to 3 hours.
  Side Effects: In therapeutic short-term dosages, acetaminophen is less toxic than aspirin because it is less likely to cause dyspepsia or blood loss or to interfere with therapeutic anticoagulation. Chronic ingestion of large dosages, especially in combination with other agents, can hazard the kidney, liver, and marrow production. Dose-dependent hepatic necrosis is the most serious acute toxic effect associated with overdosage and is potentially fatal.
  Considerations: Avoid chronic ingestion and co-ingestion with chronic use of alcohol. The relative benefit/risk ratio should be reassessed after 10 days of therapy.

Generic Name: *ibuprofen (p-isobutylhydratropic acid)*
Brand Name: Motrin, Advil, Nuprin
  Dosage: 400 mg every 4 hours with food or fluid.
  Action: The analgesic effect is comparable with aspirin by similar mechanisms except that the antiplatelet effects are reversible. Ibuprofen may be more effective than aspirin for dysmenorrhea. The plasma half-life is 2 to 4 hours.
  Side Effects: The most frequent adverse effects involve the gastrointestinal tract, but the frequency and severity may be less than with aspirin and more than with acetaminophen. CNS effects can include dizziness, headache, confusion, aseptic meningitis, and tinnitus. Potentially serious hepatic, renal, hematologic, and cutaneous effects can occur.
  Considerations: Coadministration with other analgesic agents should be avoided. The relative benefit/risk ratio should be reassessed after 10 days of therapy.

Generic Name: *ketorolac tromethamine*
Brand Name: Toradol
  Dosage: Acute IV or IM dosage 30 to 60 mg, or 30 mg every 6 hours, not to exceed 120 mg/day. Oral 10 to 20 mg every 4 to 6 hours with food or fluid, not to exceed 40 mg/day. For geriatric patients or those weighing less than 50 kg, the dosage should be reduced by at least 50%.
  Action: The analgesic effect is comparable with aspirin by similar mechanisms. The plasma half-life is 4 to 6 hours in healthy individuals but may be longer in patients with renal disease and in geriatric patients.
  Side Effects: The most frequent adverse effects associated with short-term use involve the gastrointestinal tract and the nervous system. CNS effects can include somnolence, dizziness, and headache, but stimulation, including seizures, can occur. The risk of serious gastric lesions may be less with parenteral than with oral therapy. There may be pain or local bleeding at the injection site. Potentially serious hepatic, renal, hematologic, cardiovascular, and cutaneous effects can occur.
  Considerations: The main advantage with this drug is its availability in parenteral form for use in severe headache or other acute pain in which it can substitute for opioid analgesics. The relative benefit/risk ratio should be reassessed after 5 days of therapy.

Generic Name: *amitriptyline*
Brand Name: Elavil
  Dosage: When used for pain, the dosage is usually lower than is indicated for major depression. Although parenteral forms are available, oral therapy is usual for pain. Oral dosage is 10 to 75 mg qhs with fluid.

Action: The analgesic effect is apparently independent of its antidepressant effect. The plasma half-life is 10 to 50 hours.

Side Effects: The most frequent adverse effects associated with short-term use relate to anticholinergic effects, such as xerostomia, palpitations, constipation, and urinary retention. CNS effects can include somnolence, dizziness, psychosis, confusion, and even coma. Less common are hepatic, hematologic, and cutaneous effects.

Considerations: Administration at night offers the benefit of improved sleep for patients with chronic pain. There may be synergy with other analgesic drugs. The relative benefit/risk ratio should be reassessed after 2 to 3 months of therapy because tachyphylaxis may occur.

Generic Name: *tramadol*
Brand Name: Ultram

Dosage: For oral therapy in adults with severe pain, begin with 50 to 100 mg to test tolerance of side effects like dizziness and nausea. Maintenance dosage may be up to 400 mg/day in divided doses at 4- to 6-hour intervals. Dosage must be reduced in patients with compromised renal or hepatic function.

Action: This drug is unique in that its analgesic properties depend on both a μ-opiate agonist effect and an inhibition of biogenic amine uptake receptors for serotonin and norepinephrine. Metabolism of tramadol produces a product that is even more potent as an analgesic in animals than is the parent compound. The duration of analgesia from a single dose is approximately 3 to 6 hours.

Side Effects: The most frequent adverse effects associated with short-term use are dizziness, somnolence, nausea, constipation, dry mouth, sweating, and pruritus. At usual dosages, the risk of cardiovascular effects (hypotension, syncope, tachycardia) and respiratory depression is low. Tramadol may enhance the risk of seizures, thus a combination with other drugs that lower the seizure threshold represents a risk. Tramadol may also potentiate the effects of CNS depressant drugs. Even though tramadol has true opiate agonist action and can exhibit both tolerance and dependence, the abuse potential is sufficiently low that it is not subject to the United States Federal Controlled Substances Act of 1970.

Considerations: Administration of the initial dosage at night may improve sleep while avoiding adverse symptoms of nausea and dizziness. The relative benefit/risk ratio should be reassessed after 2 to 3 months of therapy because tolerance and dependency may occur.

Generic Name: *alprazolam*
Brand Name: Xanax

Dosage: When used in patients with fibromyalgia, the dosage is lower than is indicated for anxiety or panic. Although parenteral forms are available, oral therapy is usual for pain. Oral dosage is 0.25 to 1.0 mg qhs and, in some patients, 0.25 to 0.5 every morning.

Action: The mechanism associated with benefit in fibromyalgia is uncertain, but the drug's anxiolytic or sedating effects may be responsible. There is evidence that benzodiazepines cause skeletal muscle relaxation by facilitating the inhibitory action of γ-aminobutyric acid (GABA) in the brain or spinal cord. There may also be direct depression of motor nerve and muscle function. The duration of benefit from a single dose may be up to 8 hours.

Side Effects: The most frequent adverse effects associated with short-term use are similar to the benzodiazepine drugs. CNS effects can be sedation, abnormal mentation, nightmares, dysarthria, and extrapyramidal reactions. Chronic usage may contribute to dependency, and acute discontinuation of large dosages can lead to seizures. Less common are hepatic, hematologic, and cutaneous effects.

Considerations: Administration at night offers the benefit of improved sleep for patients with chronic pain. There may be synergy with analgesic drugs. The relative benefit/risk ratio should be reassessed after 2 to 3 months of therapy because dependency may occur. When discontinuation of chronic therapy is indicated, the dosage should be tapered down at a rate of approximately 0.5 mg every 3 days.

2. Painful Muscle Spasm

This section examines a number of conditions that are attributed to *painful muscle spasm*. Why sustained muscular contraction is painful is reviewed in Chapter 2, Section B4. In most cases, the decisive factor seems to be that the muscle becomes ischemic and releases pain-producing substances. The reason for the ischemia is that the muscle compresses its own blood vessels if it contracts at a force above a certain level (approximately 30% of maximal contraction force). Another possible explanation for the pain of muscle spasm is that only parts of the muscle contract and become overloaded under these conditions, even though the contraction force of the muscle as a whole is small. This section also considers some conditions characterized by muscle spasm that may or may not be painful, as well as painful conditions in which the pain is erroneously attributed to spasm that, in fact, may not be present.

A previous section ("Muscle Spasm") considers common usage of the term "spasm" and ways of measuring it. Muscle spasm, as used in this book, is involuntary muscle contraction determined by appropriate EMG monitoring of the muscle.

Differential Diagnosis. *Pain-Spasm-Pain Misconception.* We are all familiar with the fact that prolonged sustained contraction of muscle becomes painful. The commonly accepted dictum that muscle pain causes spasm of the same muscle, which in turn causes more pain, etc., is not substantiated by critical analysis. Commonly, the painful muscle, even though it may feel tense, shows *no* EMG activity. Not all muscle spasm (identified electromyographically) is painful.

Ernest Johnson, editor of the *American Journal of Physical Medicine and Rehabilitation* and author of a well-recognized textbook on electrodiagnosis,[53] wrote an enlightening editorial entitled "The Myth of Skeletal Muscle Spasm."[54] In it, he summarized overwhelming evidence that the commonly accepted practice of considering muscle spasm as synonymous with muscle pain is erroneous but has been strongly reinforced by drug companies. Johnson said that in the absence of an appropriate diagnosis, physicians use this convenient diagnosis of muscle spasm (often made without an adequate physical examination) to justify billing a third-party payer.

This misconception (of a pain-spasm-pain cycle) is strongly reinforced by the misunderstanding of motor reflexes that Walsh[115] discussed in connection with the confusion concerning muscle tone (see earlier in this chapter). The mythical explanation is passed on from author to author[56]: Pain increases motor neuron activity, which induces increased motor neuron activity that is responsible for spasm (EMG activity), and spasm causes more pain to perpetuate the cycle. Unfortunately for this theory, there is usually *no* EMG activity, and when there is, its timing and intensity do not correlate with the pain. In addition, clinical and physiologic studies indicate that muscle pain tends to inhibit, not facilitate, voluntary and reflex contractile activity of the same muscle (see Chapter 6, Section A).

A study of human subjects[72] showed that reflexly induced muscle spasm from painful stimulation of **viscera** occurred immedi-

ately, but pain did not develop until approximately 1 hour later. The pain appears to be a more slowly developing response to the sustained reflex spasm. A more recent study using ambulatory tape recordings related amount of movement, EMG activity, and pain levels.[100] Movement and EMG activity correlated highly when the subjects were pain free but not when they were in pain. These authors also observed a delay between muscle activity and pain, with increased muscle tension preceding pain. This lack of correlation between muscle pain and increased EMG activity applies as well to the low back pain literature[1, 69, 79] as it does to the headache literature (see Section B1 earlier in this chapter).

When involuntary EMG activity (spasm) is present in patients who complain of pain, one cannot assume that the spasm is causing the pain. Sufficient spasm can cause pain, and in that case, the amount of spasm and pain will correlate closely; but something other than the muscle pain is causing the spasm. A group of nine patients who complained of low back pain and who had palpable paraspinal muscle "spasm" showed some EMG activity nearly continuously during the night.[29] A spasm-pain-spasm vicious cycle was assumed to relate the two findings. Five of the patients were diagnosed as having myofascial pain caused by TrPs. A growing body of evidence suggests that TrPs can induce muscle spasm in muscles other than that harboring the TrP[25]; the taut bands associated with the TrPs would contribute to the palpable findings, the pain, and the variable degree of spasm measured. The other four patients were identified as suffering from low back strain, which was not defined and which might have been articular dysfunction. Ligamentous strain, articular dysfunction, and TrPs can induce muscle spasm in associated muscles. All three of these conditions can be inherently painful in the presence or absence of secondarily induced muscle spasm.

Spasmodic Torticollis. Spasmodic torticollis is characterized by muscle spasms that may be tonic (relatively continuous), phasic (episodic), or tremulous (shaking)[21] and can be extremely painful. Because drugs and/or physiotherapy provide adequate relief to only a minority of suffer-ers,[67, 106, 113] the next choice is usually BTx injections into the muscle; this is expensive and only temporarily effective for most people. Failing that, surgery may be suc-cessful.

Etiology. No one cause of spasmodic torticollis is generally recognized, but ex-perimental evidence indicates it is likely a central disturbance of motor control. The amplitude of the intracranial N30 somato-sensory potential evoked by median nerve stimulation was abnormally decreased, more so in patients with spasmodic torti-collis than in patients with Parkinson's disease. This indicates that the lesion involves the basal ganglia or their connec-tions with the supplementary motor area.[73]

Nerve conduction velocity measure-ments between the sternocleidomastoid muscle and the intracranial portion of the spinal accessory nerve were compared with those across the portion of the nerve undergoing microvascular decompression for spastic torticollis. Slowed conduction was observed in only the *central* segment in 9 of the 12 patients who had unilateral symptoms and in all 5 patients with bilat-eral symptoms.[95] Evaluation of visuospa-tial function indicated discrete dysfunction of the striatal-frontal circuits in a subgroup of patients.[68]

Based on polymyographic recordings, the muscles most commonly involved in rotational spastic torticollis with regard to the direction of chin deviation were the contralateral sternocleidomastoid and/or the ipsilateral splenius muscle. The contra-lateral splenius muscle was overactive in approximately one third of these patients; rarely, the contralateral trapezius muscle was involved. Retrocollis was caused by bilateral splenius activity, and laterocollis was caused by overactivity of all recorded muscles on that side of the neck.[21] This surface EMG monitoring is useful for mak-ing a more specific, functional diagnosis and for guiding treatment.

In children, acute torticollis often is the result of a reflex muscle spasm arising from an inflammatory process. The most common causes are upper respiratory in-fection, sinusitis, otomastoiditis, cervical adenitis, and retropharyngeal abscess or cellulitis. Torticollis was associated with subluxation of the atlantoaxial joint in four patients.[8]

Treatment. The most satisfactory non-surgical treatment is injection of the spastic muscles with BTx. Most patients have less pain (65%[6] to 84%[89]) and a similar im-provement in posture. Half of the patients experienced improved tremor and range of motion.[6] Injection with BTx also improved pain and involuntary movement in three cases of tardive dystonia.[57]

Not everyone responds positively to BTx injection. Ten percent[37] to fifteen per-cent[89] of patients with torticollis developed BTx resistance on repeated injections. At least 4% of 559 patients treated with BTx developed antibodies to it. Responding patients require treatment again in a few weeks to several months, depending on how thoroughly endplate function is de-stroyed and how quickly the muscle fibers are reinnervated.[37]

Transient side effects include fatigue, dysphagia, neck weakness, hoarseness, and local pain.[6, 89] Because BTx acts by com-pletely inactivating acetylcholine release at the neuromuscular junction, it follows that the more specifically the neuromuscular junctions of the spastic muscle are injected, the more effective the injection will be and the fewer the side effects.

The importance of thoroughness is con-firmed by the significantly improved clini-cal results obtained when multiple (instead of single) points were injected in each muscle.[7] The value of greater specificity of injection was confirmed by the signifi-cantly greater number of patients who experienced marked improvement and the significantly greater magnitude of improve-ment when EMG guidance was used to ensure that the injection was being given in the involved muscle by having the patient voluntarily contract the muscle to be in-jected.[18] A needle specifically for this purpose is manufactured by Nicolet Bio-medical Instruments (P.O. Box 4287, Madi-son, WS 53711-0287, USA).

Clinical results were similarly improved when the desired muscle was located for BTx injection by monopolar needle stimu-lation.[92] Because motor endplates in the endplate zone are the desired targets, additional specificity would be realized by identifying them specifically. One can locate the endplate zone (previously called the motor point) by electrically stimulating superficial muscles through the skin,[58] by looking for endplate potentials,[84] or by observing the initial negative polarity of motor unit action potentials.[11] To do the latter, one can ask the patient to do a minimal voluntary contraction and then observe the background motor unit activity. Only action potentials that are recorded from a muscle fiber within 1 mm of the endplate show a steep and purely negative onset.[11] Action potentials originating farther from the endplate have a positive first deflection.

When it was considered necessary to perform surgery for spasmodic torticollis, microvascular decompression was reported as a nondestructive method. Of 17 patients who were followed for at least 5 years, 65% were reported cured, and 20% were reported improved with minimum spasm.[52]

Trismus. Trismus is defined as a firm closing of the jaw resulting from tonic spasm of the muscles of mastication.[75] An example of trismus is lockjaw caused by tetanus infection. In practice, the term is commonly applied not only to restricted opening of the mouth because of muscle spasm but also to fibrotic contractures and/or adhesions. Mouth opening restricted by fibrotic contractures encounters a hard, sharply defined, highly reproducible barrier, and reaching the barrier may not be painful. The muscles will likely be relatively slack unless they are in spasm. When the opening is restricted by muscles in spasm, serious attempts to open the mouth and to chew are painful. The muscles in this case always evidence EMG activity and exhibit uniform tension throughout the muscle. When the mouth is opened fully passively, the endpoint caused by spasm is painful, softer (more compliant), and less clearly defined and is more variable than that of fibrosis.

Trismus caused by muscle spasm may be the result of trauma, such as mandibular fractures[35] or of acute inflammation caused by tissue injury during surgical procedures.[112] Muscle spasm may occur after

sustained opening of the patient's mouth for dental treatment.[49] All of these muscle stresses may activate myofascial TrPs that contribute to the patient's pain and delay return of normal function (see Chapter 8). Medications, such as Compazine and Stelazine or other major tranquilizers, may cause muscle spasm.[49]

Widespread injection of the spastic muscles with 0.5 or 1% procaine or lidocaine produces temporary relief by blocking neural transmission. As the initiating stimulus that causes the reflex spasm subsides, the muscle tends to relax. Jaw use within pain-free limits is then strongly encouraged. As the painfulness of active movement of the jaw decreases, gradual *active* stretching with simultaneous application of counterstimulation or injection as described above facilitates prompt restoration of normal function. Neglect can lead to permanent restriction of mouth opening.[49]

Unnecessary Muscle Tension. Unnecessary muscle tension is a confusing intermediate between muscle contraction that is beyond voluntary control (spasm) (see Chapter 5, Section A3) and viscoelastic tension that shows no EMG activity (see Chapter 5, Section A1). This unintentional muscle contraction at times can itself cause pain and can seriously influence other sources of muscle pain, such as TrPs. This unwitting muscular contraction, which is amenable to voluntary control (sometimes requiring biofeedback assistance), is commonly identified clinically as muscle tension due to situational stress.[90]

Confusion in terminology and understanding of muscle tension is aggravated by the fact that this increased motor unit activity is involuntary in the sense that the person is not consciously causing it. With effort and appropriate assistance or guidance, however, it can be voluntarily eliminated. Unwarranted assumptions as to the psychologic nature of its origin further cloud the issue (see Chapter 5, Section B2).

Another reason this concept of muscle tension is a gray area is that some patients, with appropriate help and training, have been able to exercise a degree of "voluntary" influence over an organic brain dysfunction of motor control. Patients with spastic torticollis, which originates in motor control pathways of the brain, were significantly improved either by EMG feedback training or by relaxation training with graded neck exercises.[51]

Another study[41] showed that with the use of biofeedback techniques, children could be trained to maintain a predetermined baseline level of EMG activity. This was done because, before training, their usual baseline fluctuations were annoyingly large for experimental purposes.

Three sources of unnecessary muscle activity (tension) are well recognized: (1) psychologic distress or anxiety, (2) overload from sustained contraction or repetitive activity, and (3) inefficient (untrained) use of muscles.

Situational Psychologic Distress. Emotional distress and anxiety are normally expressed through increased muscular activity. We say that someone is "uptight," reflecting an apparent increase in muscular tension. Activity of the facial muscles often reveals a person's emotional reaction to a situation. It is this kind of muscular activity, not primarily for body movement, that has been the focus of attention in the use of EMG feedback techniques.

Muscle Overload. Common causes of muscle overload are poor posture, poor positioning, poor workstation arrangement, and inappropriate patterns of muscle use. These factors are now recognized as sources of chronic musculoskeletal pain.[78] Muscles are intolerant of sustained contraction or of monotonously repetitive movements. When the demands of such activity exceed muscle tolerance, muscle function decompensates, often painfully. With the advent of computer terminals, individuals spend long hours in nearly the same position, doing the same thing repetitively. Until recently, little attention was paid to the muscle pain that resulted.

The rapidly developing discipline of ergonomics is dedicated to providing a work situation that provides optimal trunk and limb support and placement of work materials. A goal of ergonomics is to minimize unnecessary motor activity, especially repetitive and sustained muscle contraction. This unnecessary muscle overload, by definition, is not spasm but is a potent cause of painful muscles.

The nomenclature of the literature concerned with the problem of muscle overload in the workplace concentrates on the stress condition without an adequate understanding of the cause of the pain. For the most part, three issues are addressed: the cumulative nature of the stress or trauma, the repetitive nature of the activity, and overuse. The need to reduce stress is appropriately emphasized, but to most authors, the mechanism by which the stress causes the pain remains enigmatic. The immediate problem in these overload conditions concerns *muscle dysfunction* that is demonstrated by surface EMG testing recordings.[44] The muscles were rarely examined for the source of pain.

A review of 56 occupational myalgia papers published between 1990 and 1995 and indexed in MEDLINE showed that 28 (one half) of them were concerned with the repetitive nature of the activity, most commonly identified as *repetitive strain injury*[38] with variants: *repetitive motion injury*, *studies of repetitive motion*, *repetitive strain disorder*, *repetitive motion disorder*, and *repetitive use injury*. The mushrooming of occupational computer use has brought with it a virtual epidemic of repetitive strain injury of the upper quarter of the body.[108]

A second group of 20 papers emphasized the cumulative nature of the problem. It was identified 18 times as *cumulative trauma disorder*,[14] once as *cumulative stress disorder*, and once as *cumulative trauma illness*.

The third group of seven papers referred to the *overuse syndrome*. And one author called it *overuse injury syndrome*.[31]

Most of these authors concentrated their diagnostic attention on neurologic causes, tendinitis, biopsychosocial dysfunction, and central disturbance of nociception, but rarely on muscles. With this variety of terms and unresolved cause of the pain, it is little wonder that half of the doctors responding to a 1995 questionnaire felt there was no genuine organic condition corresponding to their understanding of repetitive strain injury.[24] Based on the diverse definitions offered by the responding physicians, the authors of the survey concluded that so many completely different meanings are applied to this condition that it is medically (and legally) meaningless.

There are a number of separate (but often related) causes for the pain. Causes include fatigue caused by demands that exceed the tolerance of that muscle, sustained contraction with hypoxia, and unrecognized TrPs that are initiated and aggravated by these conditions. Acute pain that persists eventually becomes chronic pain that is processed in the brain differently. Acute pain activates sensory centers in the brain and has little effect on emotion, whereas chronic pain has a strong action on centers concerned with emotion[47] (in this case, suffering). Prevention of the pain in the first place or early and effective intervention can pay big dividends to the sufferer and to the health care system. Much can be gained by concentrating on why the muscles are hurting and by focusing treatment on the cause of the pain.

Inefficient Use. Inefficient (unnecessary) use of muscles is best illustrated by the differences in the way a novice and a skilled athlete use muscles to perform the same activity. At any given moment during a movement, the skilled athlete uses ONLY those muscles that are required. As soon as a muscle is no longer needed, it immediately relaxes. Muscles that need not be involved remain relaxed. The result is a smooth, rhythmic, graceful movement. The novice, on the other hand, recruits muscles unnecessarily. This produces much wasteful cocontraction of antagonists and allows muscles to continue to contract when no longer needed. The additional muscular activity contributes to fatigue and to stiff and awkward movements. The difference in the use of muscles becomes painfully apparent when one observes a mixed group of novice and skilled skaters at a rink.

One form of inefficient use of muscles is the failure to relax fully following voluntary contraction. Subjects with work-related trapezius myalgia retained a significantly higher level of muscle tension between contractions, compared with normal controls.[28] Abnormal failure to relax was also seen during alternating movements in muscles with TrPs as they became fatigued.[48]

Nocturnal Leg Cramps. The topic of nocturnal leg cramps (sometimes called calf cramps or systremma) was fully reviewed recently,[66, 111] thus it is summarized briefly here. Clinically, these cramps most commonly occur in the gastrocnemius muscle (also in other leg muscles) and have an explosive onset when one is sitting quietly or sleeping. The contraction, which is visible, is extremely painful and may leave soreness and swelling. It tends to be restricted to one muscle or one functional muscle group. Contraction may wax and wane in different parts of the muscle. Cramps are likely to occur when the muscle has remained for some time in the shortened position. Cramps are often induced by voluntarily contracting the muscle in the shortened position.

Studies indicate that the common leg cramp is of neuromuscular origin. Common leg cramps are characterized by motor unit action potentials and probably originate in the intramuscular portion of motor nerve terminals,[20] which is also an anatomic site of myofascial TrPs.[102, 103a] Sometimes, cramps are associated with fasciculations and lower motor neuron disease. Most people with frequent fasciculations have frequent muscle cramps, but the reverse is not true. Also, fasciculations are not characteristic of TrPs. Leg cramps also may result from changes in extracellular fluid produced by rapid dehydration (e.g., diuretic therapy), by hemodialysis, and by electrolyte imbalance.[66]

Effective relief is usually obtainable by passively stretching the muscle. Actively stretching the cramping muscle by voluntarily contracting its antagonist is usually more effective with this addition of reciprocal inhibition but can also induce cramp in the antagonistic muscle. Many individuals are helped by walking for relief. Frequently, muscles prone to this type of cramping have identifiable latent or active TrPs. When the TrPs are inactivated (see Chapter 8, Section E1) and suppressed by *daily*, slow stretching exercises, the cramps are less likely to recur and often cease.

In a variant of muscle cramps (cramp-fasciculation syndrome), the fasciculations and evoked potentials were also abolished by regional application of curare (which inactivates the motor endplates) but not by nerve block. Carbamazepine therapy was considered helpful.[104]

Stiff-Man Syndrome. This rare condition has recently been reviewed.[66] The term is a misnomer; women are equally affected.[27] Diagnostic criteria include slowly progressive stiffness of the axial and proximal limb muscles; intermittent painful muscle spasms that are spontaneous (or that are triggered by sensory stimulation, emotion, movement, or passive stretching of the muscle); positive EMG findings (including at rest); and suppression of EMG activity by sleep, anesthesia, myoneural block, or nerve block.[27, 66] Muscle histology is normal. Symptoms begin with intermittent aching and tightness of axial limb muscles, followed by continuous board-like stiffness that interferes with mobility. The muscle spasms can become severe enough to fracture the neck of the femur.[16] Despite this, in one patient the condition was still diagnosed as psychogenic. Stiff-man syndrome is of spinal or brainstem origin and shows evidence of being an autoimmune disease.[13, 66, 120]

Medications. This section has dealt with a group of disorders whose common theme is muscle spasm; in reality, however, the separate entities are more different than similar. Because the pathophysiologic mechanisms responsible for these conditions are apparently different, it should come as no surprise that a single treatment is not effective for all. In fact, the drugs typically considered to be muscle relaxants are often of little benefit in true muscle spasm except as they provide the sedation that allows centrally mediated relaxation.

The current treatment of choice for spasmodic torticollis is BTx injections strategically placed in skeletal muscle, as discussed above. Trismus is often successfully treated by local injections of anesthetic agents, such as lidocaine or procaine, into affected skeletal muscle. Unnecessary muscle tension, which includes the effects of psychologic distress, muscle overload, and inefficient use, may involve the use of sedative hypnotic drugs to relieve tension and facilitate sleep. Conversely, the emphasis should be on posture principles, taking breaks to stretch fatigued muscles, and recognizing the signs of mechanical muscle pain before the symptoms become chronically fixed.

The medications presented in the following list have been advocated for the relaxation of skeletal muscle in situations such as surgery, assisted ventilation, or ambulatory muscle spasm.

Skeletal muscle relaxant drugs can include centrally and peripherally acting agents. The peripherally acting agents tend to be in the neuromuscular blocking group, while the more centrally acting agents are more frequently orally administered sedatives.

Most of the peripherally acting agents (except for dantrolene sodium) are poorly adsorbed from the gastrointestinal tract and are not dependably distributed from intramuscular injection; thus they are usually administered intravenously. They can be divided into depolarizing agents (e.g., succinylcholine) and nondepolarizing agents (e.g., tubocurarine chloride, gallamine triethiodide, vecuronium bromide). These agents are used primarily as part of an anesthetic program during surgery or for immobilization during intubated passive respiration. Only one of the peripherally acting agents (BTx) is profiled.

The centrally acting agents are widely marketed as muscle relaxant drugs but actually exert their benefits more through sedation than through direct relaxation of contracted skeletal muscle.

Generic Name: *botulinum A toxin*
Brand Name: Not in *AHFS Drug Information* 1996
  Dosage: See above text (p. 118).
  Action: See above text (p. 118).
  Side Effects: Transient side effects include fatigue, dysphagia, neck weakness, hoarseness, and local pain.[6, 89] Because BTx acts by completely inactivating acetylcholine release and destroying the neuromuscular junction, it follows that the more specifically the neuromuscular junctions of the spastic muscle are injected, the more effective will be the injection and the fewer the side effects.

Generic Name: *quinine sulfate*
Brand Name: Quinamm, Quindane, Quiphile
  Dosage: 200 to 300 mg PO at bedtime.

Action: The mechanism of the quinine effect on skeletal muscle is still unclear. It is believed to increase the tensile response of muscle to a single maximum stimulus, but it also increases the refractory period of the muscle by a direct action on the muscle fiber. It may affect the distribution of calcium within muscle fibers. Quinine has been used for years to manage nighttime leg cramps, but controlled clinical trials have failed to prove it significantly better than placebo. As of February 1995, the United States Food and Drug Administration (FDA) no longer considers it useful for that indication, and thus it has been dropped from many institutional formularies.

Side Effects: Hypersensitivity reactions may take the form of a rash, edema, or airway obstruction. A classical effect is cinchonism manifested by tinnitus, headache, nausea, and visual disturbances. Quinine is contraindicated in pregnancy because of potential teratogenic effects.

Considerations: Coadministration with cardiac glycosides, such as digoxin, can decrease the renal clearance of the glycoside and result in cardiotoxicity.

Generic Name: *clonazepam*
Brand Name: Klonopin
Dosage: When used for periodic leg movements during sleep, 0.5 to 2.0 mg qhs may be effective. Notice that the dosage is lower than is indicated for anxiety or panic. Although parenteral forms are available, oral therapy is usual for pain.

Action: The mechanism associated with benefit is uncertain, but the drug's anxiolytic or sedating effects may be responsible. There is evidence that benzodiazepines cause skeletal muscle relaxation by facilitating the inhibitory action of GABA in the brain or spinal cord. There may also be direct depression of motor nerve and muscle function. The duration of benefit from a single dose may be up to 8 hours.

Side Effects: The most frequent untoward effects associated with short-term use are similar to those of other benzodiazepine drugs. CNS effects can be sedation, abnormal mentation, nightmares, dysarthria, and extrapyramidal reactions. Chronic usage can contribute to dependency, and acute discontinuation of large dosages can lead to seizures.

Considerations: Administration at night offers the benefit of improved sleep for patients with chronic pain. There may be synergy with analgesic drugs. The relative benefit/risk ratio should be reassessed after 2 to 3 months of therapy because dependency may occur. When discontinuation of chronic therapy is indicated, the dosage should be tapered down at a rate of approximately 0.5 mg every 3 days.

Generic Name: *levodopa-carbidopa*
Brand Name: Sinemet
Dosage: Must be titrated and adapted to each clinical situation and individual patient. For the treatment of Parkinson's syndrome, the dosage of levodopa should not exceed 8000 mg/day, and the optimal level of carbidopa is 70 to 100 mg/day. For the treatment of nocturnal myoclonus, a single tablet of 25 mg carbidopa or 100 mg levodopa has been used at bedtime, but controlled clinical studies are needed to formally test its efficacy. For the treatment of anoxic myoclonus, combinations of carbidopa with either levodopa or oxitripan (L-5-hydroxytryptophan) have been used, but efficacy is unproved.

Action: Parkinson's syndrome results from a decrease in dopamine effect in the CNS. Levodopa readily crosses the blood-brain barrier and is enzymatically converted to dopamine. Carbidopa inhibits the peripheral decarboxylation of levodopa without affecting its conversion to dopamine in the CNS. Thus, carbidopa increases the amount of levodopa available to the brain from a given oral dose. Carbidopa also inhibits peripheral decarboxylation of L-5-hydroxytryptophan (available as oxitriptan) to 5-hydroxytryptamine. Some of the effects of carbidopa may relate to central serotonin functions. The mechanism of the levodopa-carbidopa effect on nocturnal myoclonus is not known. It may relate to the relative relationship of dopamine to serotonin or simply to sedative properties.

Side Effects: Most of the side effects of levodopa are dose-related and reversible with dosage reduction. The combination of carbidopa with levodopa reduces the frequency of systemic adverse effects but does not reduce central adverse effects of levodopa. The most prominent central effects are involuntary movements, such as bruxism, grimacing, chewing, protrusions of the head, or rhythmic motions of the head. Psychologic manifestations may include affective manifestations, alterations in mood, and behavioral disturbances. Troublesome palpitations or cardiac arrhythmias can be averted in some patients by coadministration of a β blocker, such as propranolol. Periodic monitoring of blood counts and liver function tests is indicated. Rapid reduction of dosage should be avoided because it can induce a neuroleptic malignant-like syndrome. Levodopa is contraindicated in angle-closure glaucoma, post-myocardial infarction with arrhythmias, peptic ulceration, and certain psychiatric disorders.

Considerations: Carbidopa is available alone as Lodosyn in 25 mg tablets. Similarly, levodopa (100 to 500 mg) is available separately as Dopar or Larodopa.

Generic Name: *diazepam*
Brand Name: Valium, Valrelease
Dosage: Should be individualized. For oral treatment of muscle spasticity, initial dosage may be 2.5 mg at bedtime, advanced to 2.0 to 10.0 mg daily in 3 or 4 divided doses.

Action: The mechanism responsible for the antianxiety effects of the benzodiazepines is primarily related to its CNS effects. These drugs bind avidly to receptors in the brain for which the natural ligand is unknown. An interaction between that site, GABA, and chloride influences the function of chloride channels in the brain. The mechanism by which the benzodiazepines influence skeletal muscle spasm may be more localized in the spinal cord. There is also evidence that they may have some direct effects at the myoneural junction. There may also be analgesic properties.

Side Effects: The most common adverse effect is sedation, but amnesia, headaches, vivid dreams, dysarthria, paradoxic agitation resulting from disinhibition, dry mouth and other anticholinergic effects, impotence, metallic taste, urticaria, rash, and hypotension may also occur.

Considerations: Chronic dosage can cause some tendency to dependence, thus the dosage should be tapered down rather than being suddenly discontinued. Hazardous interactions with alcoholic beverages must be avoided.

Generic Name: *cyclobenzaprine hydrochloride*
Brand Name: Flexeril

Dosage: Usual dosage for muscle spasm is 20 to 40 mg daily in 2 to 4 divided doses for no more than 3 weeks. In fibromyalgia, the dosage is 5 to 10 mg qhs.

Action: This sedating CNS depressant resembles the tricyclic antidepressants both structurally and pharmacologically. The mechanism of its influence on skeletal muscle is central; it has no direct local action on skeletal muscle. Like the tricyclic antidepressants, this agent is serotonergic, noradrenergic, and anticholinergic. Its elimination half-life is 1 to 3 days.

Side Effects: The main symptoms are drowsiness, dry mouth, and dizziness. It may contribute to blurred vision, confusion, tiredness, tachycardia, hypotension, nausea, constipation, weight gain, rash, urticaria, and even anaphylaxis. As with other agents with anticholinergic activity, caution should be used with angle-closure glaucoma and urinary retention.

Considerations: Controlled clinical studies have indicated that this agent is effective for the treatment of fibromyalgia syndrome, but that condition is not among the indications listed by the FDA. There may be value in providing 1-month "holidays" from therapy with all serotonin uptake inhibitors, approximately every 3 months, to maintain effectiveness. It is certainly possible that the effectiveness in fibromyalgia comes principally from its sedative effect, countering the patient's insomnia.

Generic Name: *carisoprodol*
Brand Name: Soma

Dosage: 350 mg tid and at bedtime.

Action: The activity of carisoprodol is primarily on the CNS, since it has little or no direct action on skeletal muscles, including the neuromuscular junction. It may disconnect central pain perception without interfering with peripheral pain reflexes. The onset of action after oral administration is approximately 30 minutes and lasts up to 4 to 6 hours, with a plasma half-life of approximately 8 hours.

Side Effects: The main adverse effect is drowsiness, but other CNS effects may include irritability, headache, affective symptoms, vertigo, and tremor.

Considerations: Dosage of carisoprodol may need to be reduced in patients with liver or renal insufficiency. Chronic administration of large dosages can predispose to a withdrawal complex with abrupt discontinuation.

Generic Name: *baclofen*
Brand Name: Lioresal

Dosage: Oral dosage for muscle spasm must be individualized. Initially, dosages of 5 mg tid to qid can be increased every 3 to 5 days to a maximum of 80 mg/day. Discontinuation should not be abrupt, but dosage reduction can follow the same pattern as the initiating dosage.

Action: The mechanism of baclofen is incompletely understood. It is a structural analog of GABA, coupled to a phenylethylamine moiety. It appears that the main mode of action is inhibition of afferent signal transmission in the spinal cord because there is little penetration of the blood-brain barrier. There is evidence for both antinociceptive action and inhibition of motor neuron-related muscle spasticity. Indications for use of oral baclofen include muscle spasticity of spinal cord origin associated with multiple sclerosis and other cord injuries. Unapproved uses for baclofen include Huntington's choreiform movements, spasticity of cerebral lesions, stiff-man syndrome, and rheumatic diseases. The onset of action after oral administration is approximately 2 hours, and its plasma half-life is 2.5 to 4 hours.

Side Effects: The most common adverse effect is drowsiness; thus operation of mechanical equipment may be hazardous. Other effects may involve the sensory organs, seizure exacerbations, mood disturbances, and anticholinergic-like symptoms. Caution should be exercised when treating patients with seizure disorders, equipment operators, peptic ulcer patients, and psychotic individuals. Withdrawal of this drug too rapidly can cause hallucinations, seizures, and recurrence of muscle spasms.

Considerations: Compared with 30 mg of diazepam daily, 60 mg of baclofen daily has been found to be equipotent in reducing painful spasticity but is less sedating. The dosage should be reduced in patients with renal insufficiency.

Generic Name: *dantrolene sodium*
Brand Name: Dantrium

Dosage: Individualize dosage as tolerated until optimal benefit without side effects. Initial oral dosage is 25 mg once daily. It can be increased progressively to 25 mg two to four times daily and then to 400 mg/day in divided dosages. If benefit is not achieved within 45 days, the dosage should be tapered down and discontinued.

Action: This drug is partially (35%) adsorbed orally and directly affects skeletal muscle by inhibiting the release of calcium from the sarcoplasmic reticulum. It has little or no effect on the functions of cardiac or smooth muscle. Beneficial effects often take 1 week before becoming evident. Plasma half-life is approximately 9 hours.

Side Effects: There are serious adverse effects associated with long-term therapy with dantrolene, including development of a seizure disorder, fatal hepatotoxicity, and serositis (pleural effusions, pericarditis). In most cases, the abnormalities resolve with discontinuation of the drug, but especially worrisome is the fact that the hepatotoxicity can be idiosyncratic and irreversible.

Considerations: Careful monitoring of the liver function tests should be performed, and the dosage should be modified on the basis of the findings. The drug should be used cautiously in patients who operate machinery and in patients with severely impaired heart disease, chronic obstructive lung disease, or liver disease.

Generic Name: *methocarbamol*
Brand Name: Robaxin
Dosage: Must be individualized. The usual initial oral dosage is 1.5 gm four times per day for 2 to 3 days. Maintenance dosage is 4 to 4.5 gm daily in four divided doses.
Action: This drug is a CNS sedative with skeletal muscle relaxant effects. The mechanism of the effect on skeletal muscles is not known, but there is no direct effect on the muscle. Serum half-life is 0.9 to 1.8 hours.
Side Effects: The most frequent problems are drowsiness, dizziness, and lightheadedness. Other effects may include blurred vision, headache, fever, nausea, anorexia, adynamic ileus, metallic taste, syncope, bradycardia, and hypotension.
Considerations: Urinary excretion of methocarbamol can falsely elevate both urinary 5-hydroxyindolacetic acid and vanillylmandelic acid by some methodologies.

Generic Name: *orphenadrine citrate*
Brand Name: Norflex [Norgesic + aspirin, caffeine]
Dosage: Orally 100 mg bid.
Action: This drug has central atropine-like effects on central motor centers or on the medulla. It also has some antihistaminic effects but is stimulatory when diphenhydramine would be sedating.
Side Effects: The main side effects are those associated with anticholinergic actions, such as dry mouth, urinary retention, blurred vision, drowsiness, increased intraocular pressure, palpitation, CNS stimulation, and insomnia.
Considerations: There may be an additive stimulatory effect of this agent with propoxyphene.

Generic Name: *valproic acid*
Brand Name: Depakene, Depakote
Dosage: Must be carefully and slowly adjusted to individual needs. Initial dosage could be 15 mg/kg daily and can be increased by 5 to 10 mg/kg daily at weekly intervals until symptoms are controlled or until adverse events become limiting. Blood levels considered therapeutic are 50 to 100 µg/mL.
Action: This drug is an anticonvulsant but has been observed to reduce the chorea and tardive dyskinesia in patients on antipsychotic drug therapy. It probably influences skeletal muscle spasticity in a manner similar to baclofen. It inhibits GABA transferase, allowing for a greater central effect of GABA.
Side Effects: The most common problems are gastrointestinal intolerance, which may be less with the sodium salt than with the acid form. It can cause hepatic failure resulting in death. It can be sedating or can lead to anxiety, confusion, depression, or agitation. Oddly, ammonia may be elevated even in the absence of apparent hepatotoxicity. It can suppress marrow function, resulting in loss of any or all blood cellular elements, but it can also interfere with the second phase of platelet aggregation.
Considerations: Concomitant administration with other central depressants, such as phenobarbital or alcohol, can result in oversedation.

3. Muscle Stiffness

The increasing muscle stiffness characteristic of aging is painful only in the sense that it reduces the pain-free range of motion and the maximum rate of movement, most noticeable following prolonged inactivity. It is one of those common, non-life-threatening conditions that has been neglected as a subject of serious research, even though it apparently causes much geriatric disability and musculoskeletal dysfunction.

The slow, stiff gait of many elderly people results from the cumulative effect of their not making the effort to retain full range of motion. They increasingly restrict activity to stay within the comfort zone. Two common phenomena may be related: the palpable taut bands of TrPs in muscle, and the increased muscular stiffness with advancing age.

Differential Diagnosis. This rather benign condition must be distinguished from the pain of progressive peripheral joint osteoarthritis, silent ankylosing spondylitis, progressive osteopenia, capsular contraction of the ligaments about a peripheral joint, endocrine disease such as hypothyroidism, a vitamin deficiency such as B_{12} with concomitant neuropathy, radiculopathy, spinal stenosis resulting from degenerative or hypertrophic spine disease, muscular infestations such as trichinosis, and a paraneoplastic syndrome. A thorough history, physical examination, and laboratory assessment should identify the characteristic features of these conditions.

Treatment. The most valuable modalities for the management of stiffness in the elderly is a daily gentle muscle-stretching program supplemented with proper diet, physical exercise, and adequate rest. The problem in some cases is that poor sleep predisposes to fatigue, which leads to inactivity and progressive weakness. When physical exertion is initiated, it is poorly planned, unaccustomed, and potentially damaging. Some of the sedating muscle relaxant medications presented above can be used at night to enhance sleep and occasionally during the day in low dosage to relieve pain associated with exertion. The rest is dependent on good advice about how to restore physical mobility and on compliance by the elderly person.

REFERENCES

1. Arena JG, Sherman RA, Bruno GM, et al.: Electromyographic recordings of low back pain subjects and non-pain controls in six different positions: effect of pain levels. *Pain* 45:23–28, 1991.
2. Bajd T, Vodovnik L: Pendulum testing of spasticity. *J Biomed Eng* 6:9–12, 1984.
3. Basmajian JV: New views on muscular tone and relaxation. *Can Med Assoc J* 77:203–205, 1957.
4. Basmajian JV, Deluca CJ: *Muscles Alive*. Ed. 5. Williams & Wilkins, Baltimore, 1985.
5. Berlit P (Ed.): *Klinische Neurologie, Eine Einführung.* VCH, Weinheim, 1992 (pp. 216–221).
6. Boghen D, Flanders M: Effectiveness of botulinum toxin in the treatment of spasmodic torticollis. *Eur Neurol* 33:199–203, 1993.
7. Borodic GE, Pearce LB, Smith K, et al.: Botulinum A toxin for spasmodic torticollis: multiple vs single injection points per muscle. *Head Neck* 14:33–37, 1992.
8. Brendenkamp JK, Maceri DR: Inflammatory torticollis in children. *Arch Otolaryngol–Head Neck Surg* 116:310–313, 1990.
9. Brooke MH, Patterson V, Kaiser K: Hypoxanthine and McArdle disease: a clue to metabolic stress in the working forearm. *Muscle Nerve* 6:204–206, 1983.
10. Brown RA, Lawson DA, Leslie GC, et al.: Does the Wartenberg pendulum test differentiate quantita-

tively between spasticity and rigidity? A study in elderly stroke and Parkinsonian patients. *J Neurol Neurosurg Psychiatry* 51:1178–1186, 1988.
11. Buchthal F, Guld C, Rosenfalck P: Innervation zone and propagation velocity in human muscle. *Acta Physiol Scand* 35:175–190, 1955.
12. Burke D, Gillies JD, Lance JW: Hamstrings stretch reflex in human spasticity. *J Neurol Neurosurg Psychiatry* 34:231–235, 1971.
13. Chen BJ: [Clinical analysis of 30 cases of stiff-man syndrome]. Chung-Hua Shen Ching Ching Shen Ko Tsa Chih. *Chinese J Neurol Psychiatry* 25:363–365, 385, 1992.
14. Childre F, Winzeler A: Cumulative trauma disorder: a primary care provider's guide to upper extremity diagnosis and treatment. *Nurse Pract Forum* 6:106–119, 1995.
15. Clemmesen S: Some studies on muscle tone. *Proc R Soc Med* 44:637–646, 1951.
16. Cohen L: Stiff-man syndrome. Two patients treated with diazepam. *JAMA* 195:222–224, 1966.
17. *Collins English Dictionary*, Ed. 3. Harper Collins, Glasgow, 1991 (p. 1517).
18. Comella CL, Buchman AS, Tanner CM, et al.: Botulinum toxin injection for spasmodic torticollis: increased magnitude of benefit with electromyographic assistance. *Neurology* 42:878–882, 1992.
19. Dejung B, Angerer B, Orasch J: Chronische Kopfschmerzen [Chronic headaches]. *Physiotherapie* 12:121–126, 1992.
20. Denny-Brown D: Clinical problems in neuromuscular physiology. *Am J Med* 15:368, 1953.
21. Deuschl G, Heinen F, Kleedorfer B, et al.: Clinical and polymyographic investigation of spasmodic torticollis. *J Neurol* 239:9–15, 1992.
22. DiMauro S, Tsujino S: Nonlysosomal glycogenoses, Chapter 59. *Myology, Vol. 2*. Ed. 2. Edited by Engel AG, Franzini-Armstrong C.. McGraw-Hill, New York, 1994 (pp. 1554–1576).
23. Dimitrijevic MR, Nathan PW: Studies of spasticity in man. 3. Analysis of reflex activity evoked by noxious cutaneous stimulation. *Brain* 91:349–368, 1968.
24. Diwaker HN, Stothard J: What do doctors mean by tenosynovitis and repetitive strain injury? *Occup Med* 45(2): 97–104, 1995.
25. Donaldson CCS, Skubick DL, Clasby RG, et al.: The evaluation of trigger-point activity using dynamic EMG techniques. *Am J Pain Manage* 4:118–122, 1994.
26. Dworkin SF, Truelove EL, Bonica JJ, et al.: Facial and head pain caused by myofascial and temporomandibular disorders, Chapter 40. *The Management of Pain*. Edited by Bonica JJ. Lea & Febiger, Philadelphia, 1990 (pp. 727–745).
27. Editorial: Stiff-man syndrome. *JAMA* 201:105, 1967.
28. Elert J, Dahlqvist SR, Almay B, et al.: Muscle endurance, muscle tension and personality traits in patients with muscle or joint pain—a pilot study. *J Rheumatol* 20:1550–1556, 1993.
29. Fischer AA, Chang CH: Electromyographic evidence of paraspinal muscle spasm during sleep in patients with low back pain. *Clin J Pain* 1:147–154, 1985.

30. Fischer AA: Clinical use of tissue compliance meter for documentation of soft tissue pathology. *Clin J Pain* 3:23–30, 1987.

31. Fry HJ: The treatment of overuse injury syndrome. *Md Med J* 42:277–282, 1993.

32. Gerwin RD: The clinical assessment of myofascial pain, Chapter 5. *Handbook of Pain Assessment.* Edited by Turk DC, Melzack R. Guilford Press, New York, 1992 (pp. 61–70).

33. Ghez C: Posture, Chapter 39. *Principles of Neural Science.* Ed. 3. Edited by Kandel ER, Schwartz JH, Jessell TM. Elsevier, Amsterdam, 1991 (pp. 596–607).

34. Ghez C: The cerebellum, Chapter 41. *Principles of Neural Science.* Ed. 3. Edited by Kandel ER, Schwartz JH, Jessell TM. Elsevier, Amsterdam, 1991 (pp. 626–646).

35. Gonzalez AJ, Sakamaki H, Hatori M, *et al.*: Evaluation of trismus after treatment of mandibular fractures. *J Oral Maxillofacial Surg* 50:223–228, 1992.

36. Graff-Radford SB, Reeves JL, Jaeger B: Management of chronic head and neck pain: effectiveness of altering factors perpetuating myofascial pain. *Headache* 27:186–190, 1987.

37. Greene P, Fahn S, Diamond B: Development of resistance to botulinum toxin type A in patients with torticollis. *Movement Dis* 9:213–217, 1994.

38. Guidotti TL: Occupational repetitive strain injury. *Am Fam Phys* 45:585–592, 1992.

39. Gunn CC, Milbrandt WE: Early and subtle signs in low-back sprain. *Spine* 3:267–281,1987.

40. Hagbarth K-E, Hägglund JV, Nordin M, *et al.*: Thixotropic behaviour of human finger flexor muscles with accompanying changes in spindle and reflex responses to stretch. *J Physiol* 368:323–342, 1985.

41. Harver A, Segreto J, Kotses H: EMG stability as a biofeedback control. *Biofeedback Self Reg* 17:159–164, 1992.

42. Hatch JP, Moore PJ, Borcherding S, *et al.*: Electromyographic and affective responses of episodic tension-type headache patients and headache-free controls during stressful task performance. *J Behavior Med* 15:89–112, 1992.

43. Hatch JP, Moore PJ, Cyr-Provost M, *et al.*: The use of electromyography and muscle palpation in the diagnosis of tension-type headache with and without pericranial muscle involvement. *Pain* 49:175–178, 1992.

44. Headley BJ: Physiologic risk factors. *Management of Cumulative Trauma Disorders.* Edited by Sanders M. Butterworth-Heineman, London, 1997 (pp. 107–128).

45. Helliwell PS, Howe A, Wright V: Lack of objective evidence of stiffness in rheumatoid arthritis. *Ann Rheum Dis* 47:754–758, 1988.

46. Hendler N, Kozikowski JG, Schlesinger R, *et al.*: Diagnosis and treatment of muscle tension headaches. *Pain Manage* 4:33–41, 1991.

47. Hsieh JC, Belfrage M, Stone-Elander S, *et al.*: Central representation of chronic ongoing neuropathic pain studied by positron emission tomography. *Pain* 63:225–236, 1995.

47a. Hsieh C-Y, Hong C-Z, Adams AH, *et al.*: Interexaminer reliability of the palpation of trigger points in the trunk and lower limb muscles. *Arch Phys Med Rehabil* 81:258–264, 2000.

48. Ivanichev GA: [*Painful Muscle Hypertonus-in Russian*]. Kazan University Press, Kazan, 1990 (pp. 46–47).

49. Jaeger B: Differential diagnosis and management of craniofacial pain, Chapter 11. *Endodontics.* Ed. 4. Edited by Ingle JI, Bakland LK. Williams & Wilkins, Baltimore, 1994 (pp. 550–607).

50. Jaeger B, Reeves JL, Graff-Radford SB: A psychophysiological investigation of myofascial trigger point sensitivity vs. EMG activity and tension headache. *Cephalalgia* 5(Suppl. 3):68, 1985.

51. Jahanshahi M, Sartory G, Marsden CD: EMG biofeedback treatment of torticollis: a controlled outcome study. *Biofeedback Self Reg* 16:413–448, 1991.

52. Jho HD, Jannetta PJ: Microvascular decompression for spasmodic torticollis. *Acta Neurochir* 134:21–26, 1995.

53. Johnson EW (Ed.): *Practical Electromyography.* Ed. 2. Williams & Wilkins, Baltimore, 1988.

54. Johnson EW: The myth of skeletal muscle spasm [Editorial]. *Am J Phys Med* 68:1, 1989.

55. Kasdon DL, Abromovitz JN: Neurosurgical approaches. *The Practical Management of Spasticity in Children and Adults.* Edited by Glenn MB, Whyte J. Lea & Febiger, Philadelphia, 1990.

56. Katz WA, Dube J: Cyclobenzaprine in the treatment of acute muscle spasm: review of a decade of clinical experience. *Clin Therapeut* 10:216–228, 1988.

57. Kaufman DM: Use of botulinum toxin injections for spasmodic torticollis of tardive dystonia. *J Neuropsychiatr Clin Neurosci* 6:50–53, 1994.

58. Kimura J: *Electrodiagnosis in Diseases of Nerve and Muscle,* Vol. 2. FA Davis, Philadelphia, 1989.

59. Kraus H: Treatment of myofascial pain. *Current Therapy in Physiatry.* Edited by Ruskin A. WB Saunders, Philadelphia, 1984 (pp. 623–658).

60. Kraus H, Fischer AA: Diagnosis and treatment of myofascial pain. *Mt Sinai J Med* 58:235–239, 1991.

61. Kunze K: Krankheiten der Basalganglien, Kap. 6. *Lehrbuch der Neurologie.* Edited by Kunze K. Georg Thieme Verlag, Stuttgart, 1992 (pp. 376–379).

62. Lakie M, Robson LG: Thixotropic changes in human muscle stiffness and the effects of fatigue. *Q J Exp Physiol* 73:487–500, 1988.

63. Lakie M, Walsh EG, Wright GW: Wrist compliance. *J Physiol* 295:98–99, 1979.

64. Lakie M, Tsementzis ST, Walsh EG: Anesthesia does not (and cannot) reduce muscle tone? *J Physiol* 301:32P, 1980.

65. Lakie M, Walsh EG, Wright GW: Resonance at the wrist demonstrated by the use of a torque motor: an instrumental analysis of muscle tone in man. *J Physiol* 353:265–285, 1986.

66. Layzer RB: Muscle pain, cramps, and fatigue, Chapter 67. *Myology,* Vol. 2. Ed. 2. Edited by Engel AG, C. Franzini-Armstrong C. McGraw-Hill, New York, 1994 (pp. 1754–1768).

67. Lee MC: Spasmodic torticollis: medical and botulinum A toxin treatment. *Yonsei Med J* 33(4):289–293, 1992.

68. Leplow B, Stubinger C: Visuospatial functions in patients with spasmodic torticollis. *Percept Motor Skills* 78(3 Pt 2):1363–1375, 1994.

69. Letchuman R, Deusinger RH: Comparison of sacrospinalis myoelectric activity and pain levels in patients undergoing static and intermittent lumbar traction. *Spine* 18:1361–1365, 1993.

70. Lous I, Olesen J: Evaluation of pericranial tenderness and oral function in patients with common migraine, muscle contraction headache and "combination headache." *Pain* 12:385–393, 1982.

71. Lusskin R, Grynbaum BB: Spasticity and spastic deformities. Contracture by fibrosis, Chapter 38. *Rehabilitation Medicine.* Edited by Goodgold J. CV Mosby, St. Louis, 1988 (pp. 531–551).

72. Mac Lellan AM, Goodell H: Pain from the bladder, ureter and kidney pelvis. *Proc Assoc Res Nerv Mental Dis* 23:252, 1943.

73. Mazzini L, Zaccala M, Balzarini C: Abnormalities of somatosensory evoked potentials in spasmodic torticollis. *Movement Dis* 9:426–430, 1994.

74. McDonough JT Jr. (Ed.): *Stedman's Concise Medical Dictionary Illustrated.* Ed. 2. Williams & Wilkins, Baltimore, 1994 (p. 893).

75. McDonough JT, Jr. (Ed.): *Stedman's Concise Medical Dictionary Illustrated.* Ed. 2. Williams & Wilkins, Baltimore, 1994 (p. 1054).

76. McNulty WH, Gevirtz RN, Hubbard DR, *et al.*: Needle electromyographic evaluation of trigger point response to a psychological stressor. *Psychophysiology* 31:313–316, 1994.

77. Merskey H, Bogduk N: *Classification of Chronic Pain.* Ed. 2. IASP Press, Seattle, 1994.

78. Middaugh SJ, Kee WG, Nicholson JA: Muscle overuse and posture as factors in the development and maintenance of chronic musculoskeletal pain. *Psychological Vulnerability to Chronic Pain.* Edited by Grezesiak R, Ciccone D. Springer Publishing, New York, 1994.

79. Miller DJ: Comparison of electromyographic activity in the lumbar paraspinal muscle of subjects with and without chronic low back pain. *Phys Ther* 65:1347–1354, 1985.

80. Mills KR, Edwards RHT: Investigative strategies for muscle pain. *J Neuro Sci* 58:73, 1983.

80a. Mutungi G, Ranatunga KW: The viscous, viscoelastic and elastic characteristics of resting fast and slow mammalian (rat) muscle fibers. *J Physiol* 496(3):827–836, 1996.

81. Norris FH Jr, Gasteiger EL, Chatfield PO: An electromyographic study of induced and spontaneous muscle cramps. *Electroencephalogr Clin Neurophysiol* 9:139–154, 1957.

82. Olesen J (Chairman): Headache Classification Committee of the International Headache Society. Classification and diagnostic criteria for headache disorders, cranial neuralgias and facial pain. *Cephalgia* 8(Suppl. 7):1–96, 1988.

83. Olesen J, Jensen R: Getting away from simple muscle contraction as a mechanism of tension-type headache. [Editorial]. *Pain* 46:123–124, 1991.

84. Ottaviani LB, Childers MK: Localization of the neuromuscular junction through needle electromyography. *Arch Phys Med Rehabil* 76:1045, 1995.

85. Peterson AL, Talcott GW, Kelleher WJ, *et al.*: Site specificity of pain and tension in tension-type headaches. *Headache* 35(2):89–92, 1995.

86. Pfaffenrath V, Isler H: Evaluation of the nosology of chronic tension-type headache. *Cephalalgia* 13(Suppl. 12):60–62, 1993.

87. Poeck K: Krankheiten der Stammganglien, Kap. 11. *Neurologie.* Springer-Verlag, Berlin, 1990 (p. 342).

88. Poewe W: The clinical spectrum of spastic syndromes. *Spasticity: The Current Status of Research and Treatment.* Edited by Endre M, Benecke R. Parthenon Publishing, Park Ridge, NJ, 1989.

89. Poewe W, Schelosky L, Kleedorfer B, *et al.*: Treatment of spasmodic torticollis with local injections of botulinum toxin. One-year follow-up in 37 patients. *J Neurol* 239:21–25, 1992.

90. Rachlin ES: Trigger point management, Chapter 7. *Myofascial Pain and Fibromyalgia: Trigger Point Management.* Edited by Rachlin ES. Mosby, St. Louis, 1994 (pp. 143–360).

91. Ralston HJ, Libet B: The question of tonus in skeletal muscle. *Am J Phys Med* 32:85–92, 1953.

92. Roggenbuck DJ, Yablon SA: Suboptimal response of index distal phalanx spasticity following treatment with botulinum toxin A: indications for precise muscle localization with needle stimulation. *Arch Phys Med Rehabil* 76:1070, 1995.

93. Role LW, Kelly JP: The brain stem: cranial nerve nuclei and the monoaminergic systems, Chapter 44. *Principles of Neural Science.* Ed. 3. Edited by Kandel ER, Schwartz JH, Jessell TM. Elsevier, Amsterdam, 1991 (p. 692).

94. Rosen NB: Myofascial pain: the great mimicker and potentiator of other diseases in the performing artist. *Md Med J* 42:261–266, 1993.

95. Saito S, Moller AR, Jannetta PJ, *et al.*: Abnormal response from the sternocleidomastoid muscle in patients with spasmodic torticollis: observations during microvascular decompression operations. *Acta Neurochir* 124:92–98, 1993.

96. Sakai F, Ebihara S, Akiyama M, *et al.*: Pericranial muscle hardness in tension-type headache. A non-invasive measurement method and its clinical application. *Brain* 118(Pt 2):523–531, 1995.

97. Sandrini G, Antonaci F, Pucci E, *et al.*: Comparative study with EMG, pressure algometry and manual palpation in tension-type headache and migraine. *Cephalalgia* 14:451–457, 1994.

98. Schoenen J, Gerard P, De Pasqua V, *et al.*: EMG activity in pericranial muscles during postural variation and mental activity in healthy volunteers and patients with chronic tension type headache. *Headache* 31:321–324, 1991.

99. Serratrice G, Gastaut JL, Schiano A, *et al.*: A propos de 210 cas de myalgies diffuses. *Sem Hop Paris* 56:1241, 1980.

100. Sherman RA, Arena JG, Searle JR, *et al.*: Development of an ambulatory recorder for evaluation of muscle tension-related low back pain and fatigue in soldiers' normal environments. *Mil Med* 156:245–248, 1991.

101. Silberstein SD: Tension-type headaches. *Headache* 34:S2–S7, 1994.

102. Simons DG: Clinical and etiological update on myofascial pain from trigger points. *J Musculoskeletal Pain* 4:93–121, 1996.

102a. Simons DG: Do endplate noise and spikes arise from normal motor endplates? *Am J Phys Med Rehabil* 79: 2000 (accepted for publication).

103. Simons DG, Hong C-Z, Simons LS: Prevalence of spontaneous electrical activity at trigger spots and control sites in rabbit muscle. *J Musculoskeletal Pain* 3:35–48, 1995.

103a. Simons DG, Travell JG, Simons LS: *Travell & Simons' Myofascial Pain and Dysfunction: The Trigger Point Manual, Volume 1. The Upper Half of the Body.* Ed. 2. Williams & Wilkins, Baltimore, 1999.

104. Tahmoush AJ, Alonso RJ, Tahmoush GP, *et al.*: Cramp-fasciculation syndrome: a treatable hyper-excitable peripheral nerve disorder. *Neurology* 41:1021–1024, 1991.

105. Thewlis J: *Concise Dictionary of Physics.* Ed. 2. Pergamon Press, Oxford, 1979 (pp. 111, 214, 285, 311, 318, 336, 353).

106. Thiel A, Dressler D, Kistel C, *et al.*: Clozapine treatment of spasmodic torticollis. *Neurology* 44:957–958, 1994.

107. Thilmann AF, Fellows SJ, Garms E: The mechanism of spastic muscle hypertonus. Variation in reflex gain over the time course of spasticity. *Brain* 114:233–244, 1991.

108. Thompson JS, Phelps TH: Repetitive strain injuries. How to deal with "the epidemic of the 1990's." *Postgrad Med* 88:143–149, 1990.

109. Travell JG: Chronic myofascial pain syndromes. Mysteries of the history, Chapter 6. *Myofascial Pain and Fibromyalgia, Advances in Pain Research and Therapy, Vol. 17.* Edited by Fricton JR, Awad EA. Raven Press, New York, 1990.

110. Travell JG, Simons DG: *Myofascial Pain and Dysfunction: The Trigger Point Manual, Volume 1.* Williams & Wilkins, Baltimore, 1983.

111. Travell JG, Simons DG: *Myofascial Pain and Dysfunction: The Trigger Point Manual, Volume 2. The Lower Half of the Body.* Williams & Wilkins, Baltimore, 1992.

112. Troullos ES, Hargreaves KM, Butler DP, *et al.*: Comparison of nonsteroidal anti-inflammatory drugs, ibuprofen and flurbiprofen, with methylprednisolone and placebo for acute pain, swelling, and trismus. *J Oral Maxillofacial Surg* 48:945–952, 1990.

113. van Herwaarden GM, Anten HW, Hoogduin CA, *et al.*: Idiopathic spasmodic torticollis: a survey of the clinical syndromes and patients' experiences. *Clin Neurol Neurosurg* 96:222–225, 1994.

114. Vecchiet L, Dragani L, de Bigontina P, *et al.*: Experimental referred pain and hyperalgesia from muscles in humans, Chapter 19. *New Trends in Referred Pain and Hyperalgesia,* No. 27 in the series Pain Research and Clinical Management. Edited by Vecchiet L, Albe-Fessard D, Lindblom U, Giamberardino MA. Elsevier, Amsterdam, 1993 (pp. 239–249).

115. Walsh EG: *Muscles, Masses and Motion: The Physiology of Normality, Hypotonicity, Spasticity and Rigidity.* Mac Keith Press, distributed by Cambridge University Press, New York, 1992.

116. Walsh EG, Wright GW, Powers N, *et al.*: Biodynamics of the wrist in rheumatoid arthritis—the enigma of stiffness. *Proc Inst Mech Eng* 203:197–201, 1989.

116a. Wang K: Titin/connectin and nebulin: giant protein rulers of muscle structure and function. *Adv Biophys* 33:123–134 (1996).

117. Wartenberg R: Pendulousness of the legs as a diagnostic test. *Neurology* 1:18–24, 1951.

118. Webster DD: Quantitative measurements of L-dopa therapy in Parkinson's disease. *Neurology* 20:376–377, 1970.

119. Wright V, Johns RJ: Physical factors concerned with the stiffness of normal and diseased joints. *Bull Johns Hopkins Hosp* 106:215–231, 1960.

120. Young W: The stiff-man syndrome. *Br J Clin Pract* 20(10):507–510, 1966.

121. Yung P, Unsworth A, Haslock I: Measurement of stiffness in the metacarpophalangeal joint: the effects of physiotherapy. *Clin Phys Physiol Measure* 7:147–156, 1986.

CHAPTER 6
Reflexly Mediated and Postural Muscle Pain

SUMMARY: In many cases, muscle pain attributed to muscle reflexes is actually caused by **pain referral** from other sources. Vicious cycles in the sense of the **pain-spasm-pain** concept have not been proven to exist. Under experimental conditions, an *acute* painful stimulus to a muscle has varying (excitatory or inhibitory) effects on the α-motor neurons that supply the painful muscle; a *longer-lasting* noxious stimulus is likely to inhibit the neurons. In γ-motor neurons, activation occurs in response to an acute painful stimulus, but in animal experiments this activation has been shown to change to an inhibition if the stimulus persists for a longer period of time (hours). Collectively, the available data indicate that **a chronic painful muscle is reflexly turned off, not on.** Associated spasms most likely do not occur in the painful muscle but in other muscles.

Reflexes from joints can induce spasm in muscles, often in those muscles that cross the affected joint. It is well known, however, that under certain conditions a lesioned joint can also **reflexly inhibit** muscles acting on that joint.

In some cases, permanent activation of central nervous motor pathways as a reaction to psychic stress may cause symptoms that can be misinterpreted as motor reflexes.

The influence of **sympathetic reflexes** on muscle pain is still a matter of discussion. Probably, there is a certain influence of sympathetic activity on muscle pain, particularly in chronic cases, but this influence does not appear to be reflex in nature.

A frequent phenomenon is **reflex muscle spasm from diseased viscera,** for example, from cardiac infarction, appendicitis, renal colic, and acute pancreatitis. These spasms may activate trigger points (TrPs), which can lead to persistent pain.

Low back pain is often assumed to result from reflexes originating in the local muscles, but this is unlikely because the painful back muscles are not in spasm. Frequent causes of low back pain probably are myofascial or ligamentous TrPs and tears of muscle fibers caused by muscle imbalance and overload.

Muscle imbalance and **poor posture** are often combined. In some cases, a skeletal abnormality is the reason for muscle imbalance. Maintained awkward positions can cause extremely strong pain after a few minutes. The sources of this pain most likely are the ligaments and joint capsules that are under continuous tension.

The presence of TrPs in dysfunctional or neighboring muscles has to be taken into account in the diagnosis and treatment of reflexly mediated spasm and muscle pain. **TrPs can be a powerful source of spasm** and can refer pain to muscles other than those that harbor the TrPs. Conversely, increasing evidence shows that a TrP in one muscle can inhibit the function of another muscle. The weakness and inhibition of muscles in cases of muscle imbalance may well be the result of such a **TrP-induced inhibition.**

Muscle pain is often believed to result from muscle reflexes but is actually referred from other deep tissues. Referral of deep pain is a common phenomenon and must be excluded before pain caused by muscle reflexes can be seriously considered as the functional mechanism. Of course, the best way of identifying muscle reflexes is to record the electromyographic (EMG) activity. If there is involuntary EMG activity in the painful muscle, then the cause of this activity must be identified (e.g., joint dysfunction or a trigger point [TrP] in another muscle). When pain is referred to a muscle, usually EMG activity is absent in the painful target muscle. In these cases, the main problem is to find the cause and site of origin of the pain. Often, the cause is a TrP in the same muscle or in another muscle in the same region of the body. Knowledge of the patterns of pain referral from TrPs in various muscles will help to find the TrP that is causing the pain.

A. NATURE OF REFLEXLY MEDIATED MUSCLE PAIN

1. Reflexes Versus Vicious Cycles

Under physiologic circumstances, motor reflexes are completed within a fraction of a second (or a few seconds in some autonomic reflexes) and do not cause pain. For instance, a nociceptive input from the skin of an extremity leads to contraction of the flexor muscles, which move the limb away from the stimulus. Even repeated elicitation of the reflex will not produce pain in the flexor muscles, although the stimulus that caused the reflex was painful. This type of reflex and others that elicit motor responses through activation of cutaneous nociceptors are well studied and can be easily reproduced experimentally in humans and animals.

A widely held concept states that some painful conditions are caused by feedback from the effector organ of the reflex arc (the muscle) when it acts back on the receptor organ (nociceptor). Thus, a feedback loop might be formed that maintains the pain. The existence of such a loop depends on the assumption that the contraction of the muscle is painful (see Chapter 5 for a discussion of the pain-spasm-pain cycle). In fact, the neuroanatomic connections and biochemical mechanisms necessary for the formation of such a feedback loop do exist. This does not mean, however, that under pathologic conditions the loop is actually functional. From recent neuroanatomic research, it is well known that under normal circumstances many of the central nervous connections are ineffective (not open for transmission) or need additional input to activate the postsynaptic neuron. As pointed out in Chapter 5, the pain-spasm-pain cycle has to be considered an example of such a mechanism for which the neuroanatomic basis exists but which is not functional under natural conditions.

2. Alpha Reflexes: The Flexor Reflex

Normally, the flexor (or flexion) reflex occurs in response to a noxious stimulation of the skin and leads to a contraction of the flexor muscle (Fig. 6-1) and, simultaneously, to an inhibition of the antagonistic extensor muscle (Fig. 6-2). But the reflex often shows deviations from the normal pattern of flexor activation and extensor inhibition. An example is the activation of the medial gastrocnemius (MG) muscle following noxious stimulation of the skin of the heel in the rabbit.[20] (The MG muscle is a physiologic extensor,[44] although because of its retroaxial location it is considered a flexor in many anatomic textbooks.) Apparently, the pattern of muscle activation can be changed if the prevention of damage requires it. In this case, the MG muscle must contract to lift the heel off the ground

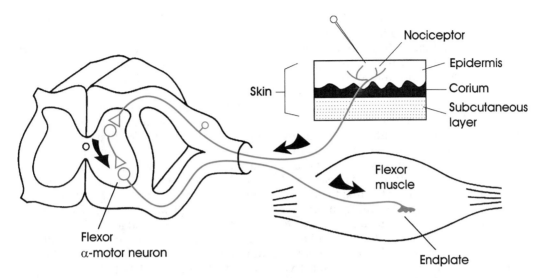

Figure 6-1. Flexor reflex arc from the skin to a flexor muscle. A noxious stimulus (a needle) excites nociceptors in the skin of an extremity. The afferent fibers of the nociceptors are connected via a chain of several neurons (so-called interneurons) to α-motor neurons of a flexor muscle of the stimulated extremity. Only one interneuron is shown in the figure (in the spinal gray matter beside the *arrow*). The reflexly induced contraction of the flexor muscle moves the stimulated skin region away from the noxious stimulus. This movement requires simultaneous inhibition of the extensor muscles of the same limb as shown in Figure 6-2.

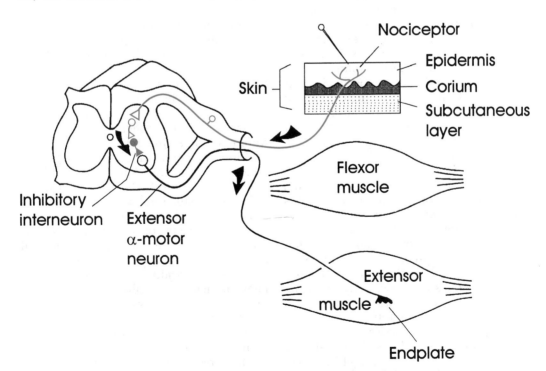

Figure 6-2. Nociceptive reflex arc from the skin to an extensor muscle. The noxious stimulus that reflexly causes contraction of the flexor muscle as shown in Figure 6-1 simultaneously inhibits the extensors of the same extremity. For reasons of clarity, the two simultaneously occurring processes are depicted separately. The excitatory interneurons in the spinal cord that mediate the flexor reflex (*open circle* and *open synaptic bouton* in the gray matter, cf. Figure 6-1) also have connections with inhibitory interneurons (*filled circle* and *filled synaptic bouton*). The inhibitory interneurons depress the activity of extensor motor neurons of the stimulated limb.

and thus withdraw it from the noxious stimulus. These data demonstrate an important aspect that is true for almost all reflexes: Even though the "wiring" of the reflex connections in the spinal cord is quite simple, the reflex can be, and normally is, modified to a great extent.

Although the occurrence of a flexor reflex on activation of cutaneous nociceptors is a common experience, the elicitation of the reflex by nociceptors in deep tissues has been less well studied. O'Leary and coworkers[81] were among the first to demonstrate that electrical stimulation of the small-diameter afferent fibers in a muscle nerve leads to a reflex contraction of flexor (and extensor) muscles. As electrical stimulation excites all nerve fibers irrespective of their function and not all of the slowly conducting muscle afferent units can be considered nociceptive,[75] experiments employing natural stimuli had to be performed to show that the nociceptors or "pressure-pain receptors" of skeletal muscle are capable of eliciting or facilitating the flexor reflex and inhibiting α-motor neurons of extensor muscles (Fig. 6-3).[82]

In 1951, Brock and coworkers[12] studied the effects of afferent volleys in muscle nerves on motor neurons and found that the actions of group II and III muscle afferents were similar, in that both elicited a flexor reflex pattern by activating flexor motor neurons and inhibiting extensor motor neurons. From these findings, the concept of the "flexion reflex afferents" (FRA) comprising group II, III, and IV fibers emerged. It must be emphasized that the concept is based on data from experiments dealing with locomotion rather than nociception. Therefore, the term "flexion reflex afferents" does not imply that the afferent units are nociceptive and the reflex is nocifensive.[26, 47] Furthermore, activation of the FRA does not necessarily elicit the reflex. Instead, the FRA must be considered as afferents that *can* elicit the flexion reflex under special circumstances.[91]

Intracellular recordings from α-motor neurons in cats have shown that input via muscle group III and IV afferent units induced by noxious chemical stimulation of the gastrocnemius-soleus (GS) muscle (an extensor) inhibits most of the GS motor

neurons, whereas flexor motor neurons are facilitated[64] (Fig. 6-3).

Most of the above studies were performed in spinalized animals. The data, therefore, cannot be directly transferred to humans with an intact neuraxis.

More recent data indicate that a short-lasting input via unmyelinated afferent fibers from muscle facilitates the flexor reflex for a long period of time and that the duration of the facilitation induced by muscle input lasts much longer than that induced by a comparable input from the skin.[108] Long-lasting reflex facilitations have also been observed following intrathecal application of substance P and calcitonin gene-related peptide.[111] Activation of the N-methyl-D-aspartate (NMDA) receptor appears to be involved in the reflex facilitation because it can be abolished by NMDA antagonists.[110]

The induction or facilitation of the flexor reflex by nociceptive afferent units from muscle is of clinical interest because these mechanisms could offer an explanation for long-lasting muscle spasms. According to the pain-spasm-pain concept, the spasms are attributed to a vicious cycle that is triggered presumably by nociceptive input from muscle: The nociceptive input elicits the flexor reflex, and the contracting muscle compresses its own vasculature and/or consumes large amounts of oxygen if the contraction is of sufficient strength and duration. Thus, the muscle is forced to perform the contractions under ischemic conditions. Ischemic contractions activate muscle nociceptors that maintain the flexor reflex (see Chapter 5).[25, 29]

Direct experimental evidence supporting this concept of a vicious cycle is missing. In fact, the available experimental evidence is contradictory to this concept. For instance, results from animal experiments indicate that a prolonged pathologic input from deep tissues abolishes the capability of C fibers from muscle to facilitate the flexor reflex for prolonged periods of time.[109]

More recent interpretations of motor reflexes at the spinal level emphasize that the flexor reflex is not a stereotyped reflex that occurs in flexor muscles every time the FRA are activated (for a review of muscle

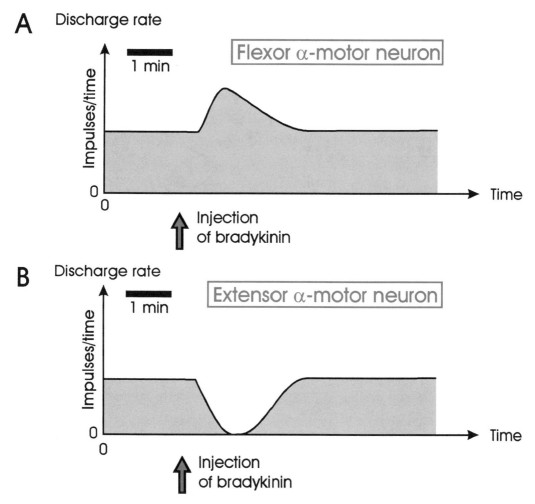

A Discharge rate

Flexor α-motor neuron

1 min

Impulses/time

0
0
Time

Injection
of bradykinin

B Discharge rate

Extensor α-motor neuron

1 min

Impulses/time

0
0
Time

Injection
of bradykinin

Figure 6-3. Responses of a flexor and an extensor α-motor neuron to painful stimulation of muscle. An intra-arterial injection of a painful dose of brady-kinin (BK) into the artery of an extensor muscle, the gastrocnemius-soleus (GS) muscle, was given to stimulate nociceptors in that muscle. Simultaneously, the impulse activity of a single α-motor neuron supplying the stimulated extensor muscle and another one supplying the antagonistic flexor muscle (the tibialis anterior) was recorded from thin filaments of the muscle nerves. **A.** Discharge rate versus time of the flexor α-motor neuron. The time of injection of BK is indicated by an *arrow*. Note that the impulse activity of the neuron increased only for a period of time that corresponds largely to the duration of the nociceptive input elicited by BK (see Chapter 2); i.e., there is no maintained activity in the sense of a vicious cycle. **B.** Discharge rate versus time of the extensor α-motor neuron. The neuron is inhibited for about the same time the flexor motor neuron is excited. These data show that a noxious stimulus to a muscle excites flexor motor neurons only transiently and inhibits the stimulated muscle if it is an extensor. Therefore, this α-reflex by itself cannot explain chronic spasm that is known to occur in both flexor and extensor muscles.

reflexes, see Ref. 91). The FRA comprise not only nociceptive afferent fibers from the skin and muscle but also non-nociceptive mechanosensitive afferents from skin, joint, and muscle (Fig. 6-4). The FRA are connected to interneurons in the spinal cord that finally make synaptic contacts with α-motor neurons. An important aspect of this pathway is that, in contrast to what their name suggests, the FRA can also inhibit flexors, in that they have alternative excitatory (*I* in Fig. 6-4) and inhibitory (*II* in

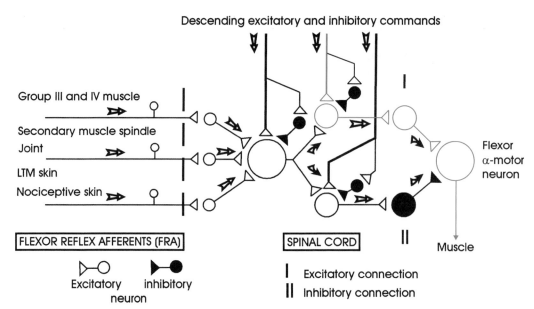

Figure 6-4. Overview of the connections between flexor reflex afferents (FRA) and a flexor α-motor neuron. Note that the reflex arc in the spinal cord contains both excitatory (*I*) and inhibitory (*II*) connections. Descending controls from higher motor centers determine whether the input from the FRA excites or inhibits the flexor α-motor neuron. The pathway for an excitatory descending command is shown in *red*. Excitatory neurons are shown as *open symbols*; inhibitory neurons are shown as *filled symbols*. (Redrawn from Schomburg ED: Spinal sensorimotor systems and their supraspinal control. *Neurosci Res* 7:265–340, 1990; and Schomburg ED: Spinal functions in sensorimotor control movements. *Neurosurg Rev 13*:179–185, 1990.)

Fig. 6-4) connections to both flexor and extensor motor neurons. The direction of their action on motor neurons is determined by descending motor pathways from higher motor centers, including the motor cortex.

For practical considerations, it is important to know that the gain of the reflex is normally very low. This means that activation of the FRA by themselves is not capable of evoking the reflex. Only if the descending excitatory (facilitating) command is strong enough can the input from the FRA activate motor neurons. By this mechanism, unwanted reflexes during passive movements or following skin contact during manipulations are avoided. Taken together, these data show that in the absence of a facilitating descending command, a nociceptive input from muscle is unlikely to cause chronic spasm via the segmental pathway, as suggested by the vicious cycle concept.

Likewise, in patients with temporomandibular dysfunction, the painful masticatory muscles have been reported to show no increased EMG activity. Instead, the force of maximal voluntary contractions of the painful muscles was reduced.[73] These data contradict the assumption that painful input reflexly drives muscles to higher activity. In their short review of pain mechanisms in masticatory muscles, Lund and coworkers[73] arrive at the conclusion that, at least for temporomandibular pain, the vicious cycle model is incorrect.

One of the crucial assumptions of the vicious cycle concept, namely, that a spastic muscle compresses its vasculature, is likewise questionable. Although there is compelling evidence that during maximal voluntary contraction (MVC) the high intramuscular pressure occludes the muscle arteries,[100] moderate degrees of static exercise (up to 30% MVC) have been shown to lead to an increase in muscle blood flow in humans[85] and experimental animals.[46] These data cannot be generalized, however, because some muscles (like the supraspinatus) show significant reductions in blood flow during static contractions of as little as 16% of MVC.[56]

3. Gamma Reflexes as a Possible Cause of Muscle Spasms

In the older clinical literature, there are reports postulating that an increased activity or excitability of the γ-motor neuron system is the reason for the rigidity of Parkinsonian patients and for the painful spasms that sometimes develop in cases of rheumatism and stiff-man syndrome.[11, 24, 77] The increased activity in γ-motor neurons is assumed to lead to a higher discharge frequency in muscle spindle afferent fibers that in turn activate α-motor neurons. By this mechanism, the same vicious cycle as described above for α-motor neurons can be triggered if the activation of the α-motor neurons is strong enough for inducing ischemic contractions (see Fig. 6-5). In view of recent data (see above), this unlikely mechanism, too, would require a simultaneous facilitating influence from higher motor centers.

Two more vicious cycles have been constructed by Johansson and Sojka.[57] The first assumes that muscular work liberates metabolic substances (potassium, lactate, and arachidonic acid) in concentrations sufficient to activate muscular group III and IV afferents, which in turn excite α-motor neurons. The second postulates that the metabolite-induced activation of group III and IV units excites γ-motor neurons, which activate muscle spindles. The secondary muscle spindle afferents have excitatory connections with γ-motor neurons, which in turn activate the secondary muscle spindle afferents.

Although the above-mentioned anatomic connections surely exist, it seems highly unlikely that they have a strong influence on the contractile state of the mus-

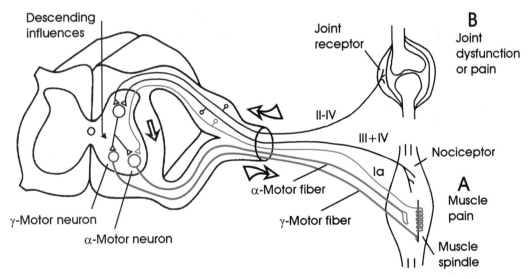

Figure 6-5. Hypothetical (and unlikely) mechanism for the development of chronic muscle spasm via activation of γ-motor neurons. The reflex contractions are supposed to be triggered by either a painful lesion of the affected muscle (**A**) or dysfunction of a neighboring joint (**B**). The afferent fibers from muscle and joint (myelinated group II and III, as well as unmyelinated group IV fibers) are assumed to activate γ-motor neurons more strongly than they activate α-motor neurons. The γ-motor neurons induce a contraction of the fine muscle fibers inside the muscle spindle. This contraction increases the activity in muscle spindle afferent fibers (Ia fibers), which excite α-motor neurons monosynaptically. The pathway from the γ-motor neuron via the muscle spindle through the α-motor neuron is shown in *red*. As stated in the text, the indicated fiber connections in the spinal cord are known to exist, but the synaptic efficacy is so low that in the absence of descending excitatory influences, the reflex is unlikely to lead to muscle contractions.

The reflex may become functional, however, when descending motor commands are present. Probably, not only input from muscle and joint but also psychic stress can lead to a tonic activation of γ-motor neurons through descending excitatory commands. This may result in static contractions even in periods without locomotor activity. (Redrawn from Berberich P, Hoheisel U, Mense S, *et al.*: Fine muscle afferent fibres and inflammation: changes in discharge behaviour and influence on gamma-motoneurons, Chapter 17. *Fine Afferent Nerve Fibres and Pain.* Edited by Schmidt RF, Schaible HG, Vahle-Hinz C. VHC, Weinheim, 1987 (pp.165–175).)

cle. One strong argument against the existence of these vicious cycles is that the normal muscle metabolites are ineffective in activating group III and IV receptors.[63]

Also in the clinical literature, the involvement of γ-motor neuron reflexes in disorders of muscle tone is not generally accepted and has been strongly objected to by other authors (for a review, see Burke[17]). The experimental support for the assumption that activation of muscle nociceptors leads to increased activity in homonymous γ-motor neurons is weak. In the literature, both excitatory and inhibitory influences of these receptors on γ-motor neurons have been reported.[2, 28, 101] Apparently, the flexor reflex concept (meaning that nociceptor activity causes contraction of flexor and inhibition of extensor muscles) cannot be applied to the γ-system.[2]

In a study in which muscle group III and IV receptors were activated by intra-arterial injections of algesic chemicals, both extensor and flexor γ-motor neurons were excited.[49] The results obtained with administrations of algesic agents are difficult to interpret, however, because the input elicited by this type of stimulation is probably not purely nociceptive.[74] The findings do not mean that muscle nociceptors generally have an excitatory action on homonymous fusimotor neurons.

To gain more insight into these mechanisms, the effects of an experimental myositis of the lateral GS muscle (LGS) on the activity of γ-motor neurons supplying the synergistic medial head (MG) were studied in animal experiments.[76] In contrast to the working hypothesis that expected an increase in γ-activity, the resting activity of the γ-motor neurons was significantly reduced during the inflammation (Fig. 6-6), and the reflex excitability of the neurons by electrical and mechanical stimulation of afferent units from the inflamed muscle was likewise inhibited. The electrical excitability of γ-motor neurons supplying the antagonistic tibialis anterior muscle was (slightly) enhanced under identical conditions, but this effect was so small that it was

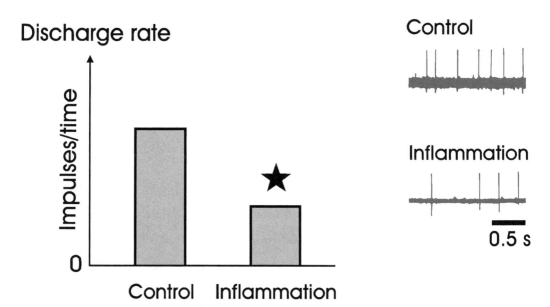

Figure 6-6. Inhibitory effect of an experimental myositis on γ-motor neurons supplying the inflamed muscle. The *ordinate* shows the mean background activity of γ-motor neurons of the medial gastrocnemius muscle. *Control*, data from animals without a myositis; *Inflammation*, data from animals in which inflammation of the lateral head of the GS muscle had been induced several hours before. The *insets* are examples of original recordings of the activity in single γ-motor neurons under control and test conditions. The *star* above the inflammation *bar* indicates $p < 0.05$. (Redrawn from Mense S, Skeppar P: Discharge behaviour of feline gamma-motoneurones following induction of an artificial myositis. *Pain* 46:201–210, 1991.)

unlikely to lead to a recognizable change in motor activity of the entire muscle.

Taken together, the results obtained from γ-motor neurons suggest that nociceptive input from an extensor muscle leads to a transient excitation of homonymous γ-motor neurons, which evolves into an inhibition when the input continues for several hours. The facilitation of the excitability of flexor γ-motor neurons observed under the same conditions is much too weak to explain muscle spasms as a result of painful alterations in the homonymous muscle. Therefore, the main sequel of a longer-lasting muscle lesion on γ-activity is inhibition of γ-fibers to the homonymous muscle.

Teleologically, the inhibition of homonymous fusimotor neurons induced by a myositis may be an advantage because it could reduce the forces acting on the damaged muscle. The inhibition clearly contradicts the assumptions of the pain-spasm-pain concept. Conversely, the observed inhibition of the γ-motor neurons may be the neurophysiologic basis of the reflex inhibition of skeletal muscle that sometimes occurs following acute trauma. Thus, if the primary source of pain is muscular, the muscle is likely to be turned off, not on (see Section A5).

In the above-described animal experiments, the postulated activation of the homonymous γ-system by a muscle lesion (Fig. 6-5) was not present. It requires either an input different from that elicited by a myositis or an additional descending command that was missing in the anesthetized animals.

It would be extremely helpful for our understanding of the mechanisms of muscle spasm if direct recordings of the γ-activity would be made in patients. The crucial experiment would be to record the impulse activity in single γ-motor neurons supplying the muscle of patients with muscle spasm. With the use of microneurographic techniques, this goal could be reached with few side effects for the patient. Such recordings would also answer the question as to what extent the data obtained from animal γ-motor neurons can be applied to patients.

In assessing the importance of motor neuron reflexes for muscle pain, keep in mind that there are regional differences. The masticatory muscles differ from locomotor ones in at least two ways:

1. There are no crossed reflexes of antagonistic muscles. Except for laterally grinding movements of the mandible, the two temporomandibular joints must open and close together.
2. The excitatory reflexes between muscle spindle primary endings and α-motor neurons are spatially more limited or missing completely.[86]

Systematic EMG measurements of muscles located around a muscle with a myofascial TrP in patients showed that the input from the TrP can induce spasm in muscles other than that harboring the TrP. An example of such a mechanism is shown in Figure 6-7: Pressing on a TrP in the infraspinatus muscle elicited spasm in the anterior deltoid muscle.[42] In this context, the muscle harboring the TrP usually contains a taut band but is not in spasm. Therefore, the above conclusion that a painful muscle is reflexly turned off rather than turned on can be extended by assuming that the painful muscle can induce spasm in other muscles. Further evidence supporting this conclusion was obtained in experiments in which chemical excitation of nociceptors in cervical paraspinal tissues (including muscle) caused increased EMG activity in neck and jaw muscles in anesthetized rats.[50]

4. Reflexes From Joints

As mentioned above, the motor neurons of a muscle can be influenced not only by afferent activity from receptors in the same or other muscles but also by receptors in neighboring joints.[35] Human and animal studies have shown that the effects of articular receptors on α-motor neurons are heterogeneous and depend on the type of receptors activated and on the location of the affected joint.

It is likely that under certain circumstances, the input from joint receptors may cause spasm in a muscle that acts on that joint. Neuroanatomic data show that at least some of the connections between joint afferents and α-motor neurons in the spinal cord are excitatory, whereas those of muscle afferents are mainly inhibitory.[91]

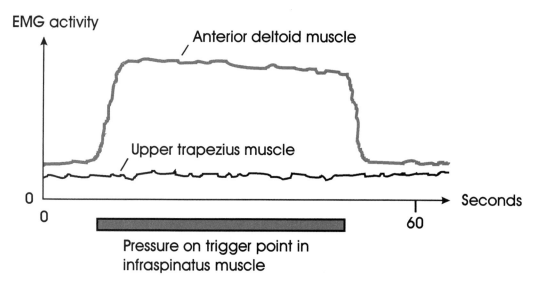

Figure 6-7. Induction of spasm in a muscle by input from a myofascial trigger point (TrP) in another muscle. The TrP was located in the infraspinatus muscle, and electromyographic (EMG) recordings were made from the anterior deltoid (*red line*) and upper trapezius (*black line*) muscle. The lines show the rectified and integrated EMG activity of both muscles. During mechanical stimulation of the TrP in the infraspinatus muscle (*red bar* underneath the *abscissa*), the EMG activity in the anterior deltoid muscle increased reflexly. The EMG of the upper trapezius muscle did not change. This latter finding indicates that the increase in EMG activity of the anterior deltoid muscle is not caused by an unspecific pain reaction by the patient. (Redrawn after Headley BJ, personal communication, 1996.)

Electrophysiologic findings indicate that electrical stimulation of articular nerves at an intensity sufficient to stimulate group III to IV fibers[36] and inflammation of the knee joint[30] facilitate the flexor reflex in neighboring muscles. Evidence also indicates that a longer-lasting increase in γ-activity may occur (at least in part of the neurons) if the site of the lesion is in a neighboring joint.[35, 41] Stimulation of knee joint nociceptors has been described to excite both α- and γ-motor neurons of flexor and extensor muscles of the hindlimb.[41]

Thus, it is conceivable that nociceptive (or non-nociceptive) input from a joint rather than from a muscle leads to a contraction in a neighboring muscle, as depicted in Figure 6-5*B*. The contraction of the muscle may put stress on the joint capsule where most of the receptors are located and thus could increase the discharges of joint receptors. Actually, injection of the small-fiber excitant mustard oil into the region of the temporomandibular joint in rats has been shown to elicit increased EMG activity in jaw muscles.[112] Even though mustard oil induces an inflammation at the site of injection that stimulates nociceptors for many hours, the increase in EMG activity persisted for less than 30 minutes. This means that the jaw muscles did not develop spasm in spite of the presence of a long-lasting noxious stimulus (i.e., *no vicious cycle occurred*).

5. Inhibitory Reflexes

For many years, clinical case reports have described muscle inhibition rather than activation as a sequel to lesions of the musculoskeletal system. An example is the Chassaignac syndrome,[19] which is characterized by an acute paralysis of the arm muscles in children following a forceful traction to the upper extremity. Such a traction may occur when adults hold a child by the hand and try to keep him or her from falling down. The primary trauma is a luxation of the head of the radius out of the annular ligament. The sudden deep pain accompanying this lesion apparently leads to a transient paralysis by inhibition of muscle function.

The mechanisms underlying reflex inhibition and reflex atrophy of muscles have been thoroughly studied in patients.[97, 99] A prominent example of such an inhibition is the weakness (and later atrophy) of the quadriceps femoris muscle following surgery of the knee joint. Experimental data show that activation of articular mechanoreceptors is sufficient for eliciting the reflex; i.e., activation of nociceptors is unnecessary. Graded reduction in the muscle's voluntary force can be induced by increasing the pressure in the joint capsule by filling it with saline.[22, 99] When small amounts of fluid are used, the maneuver is not painful.

The effect appears to result from activation of non-nociceptive mechanoreceptors in the joint capsule that are excited by the increased pressure in the joint. Filling the joint cavity with saline to which a local anesthetic has been added does not induce the weakness. This proves the reflex nature of the phenomenon. Possibly, the non-nociceptive FRA from the joint form the afferent limb of the reflex. These afferents are assumed to terminate extension movements of the joint by inhibition of the extensor muscles when the joint reaches an extreme position.[91] The reflex is not nociceptive; it is locomotor in nature and has the purpose of simultaneously stopping the extensor movement and initiating contraction of the flexors during stepping.

The reflex inhibition of the quadriceps muscle is an example of a motor reflex that by itself is not painful. A vicious cycle may develop, however, if the wasting of the muscle is so marked that instability of the knee joint results. This situation may cause increased effusion in the joint cavity and joint pain, which enhance the reflex inhibition of the muscle. The muscle becomes atrophic, not spastic. This example of a powerful inhibition of muscle activity by joint input demonstrates that a general spasm-producing effect cannot be assumed to exist for joint input.

Clinical evidence indicates that the painful malfunction of a muscle (or muscle group) may lead to overload and malfunction of another muscle, which in turn may influence a third muscle. This cascade of events has been called "chain reaction" by Lewit ("Kettenmyose" in German).[67] The exact nature of these events is still unknown. One possible mechanism may be that the overload leads to the formation of myofascial TrPs. The nociceptive input from the TrP then could inhibit the painful muscle, which in turn could overload a third muscle that has to compensate for the second muscle. Another theoretical possibility may be that the chain reaction is mediated via reflex pathways that are under the control of central nervous motor centers.

At present, no generally accepted concept seems to exist that could explain why muscles react with spasm to one lesion and with inhibition or even paralysis to another. Clinical experience suggests that static (postural) muscles tend to become hyperactive, whereas phasic (locomotor) muscles tend to become atrophic,[66] or that painful muscles are inhibited, whereas those muscles that protect the damaged muscle from painful movements become hypertonic.[15]

6. Supraspinal "Reflexes"

Another possibility for inducing involuntary muscle hyperactivity is that the spasm and EMG activity observed in some patients with muscle pain are not caused by motor reflexes in the strict sense but by a permanent activation of descending motor pathways as a reaction to psychic stress or because of poor motor control. The latter mechanism has been discussed as a cause of occupational (e.g., writer's) cramp.[27]

The practical conclusion that can be drawn from this section is that chronic muscle spasm is presumably not caused by a lesion of the spastic muscle itself, as suggested by the vicious cycle concept. The real causes of the spasm are probably located outside the muscle. They may be TrPs in other muscles, dysfunctions of neighboring joints, or disturbance of central nervous system (CNS) function. Effective treatment of the spasm should consider this possibility and should not be restricted to the spastic muscle.

7. Sympathetic Reflexes as a Possible Enhancing Factor in Muscle Nociception

The available data concerning the contribution of sympathetic efferent activity to pain in general are controversial. As far as muscle pain is concerned, an additional problem is that most studies have been performed on cutaneous pain. At the level of the primary afferent neuron, whose cell body is in the dorsal root ganglion, the bulk of the data indicate that a normal nociceptor is neither activated nor sensitized by efferent sympathetic activity.[5] Evidence shows, however, that nociceptive endings that have been sensitized by noxious stimuli may be activated by efferent sympathetic activity.[88] Whether these findings can be generalized is unclear at present because other groups arrived at a different conclusion.[94]

To date, the view prevails that painful clinical syndromes that were originally assumed to be caused by reflexes in the sympathetic nervous system (such as reflex sympathetic dystrophy) are not reflex in nature. The possible influence of sympathetic activity on muscle pain is discussed in more detail in Chapter 3, Section E.

B. DIAGNOSIS AND TREATMENT OF REFLEXLY MEDIATED MUSCLE PAIN

In the majority of an unselected group of people, the most commonly occurring type of pain is of musculoskeletal origin.[31] Most musculoskeletal pain is referred and most muscle spasm is of reflex, not local, origin. (The clinical aspects of sympathetic reflex contributions to muscle pain are not included in this section because they were considered in Chapter 3.)

In addition to pain of reflex origin, this section also calls attention to muscle spasm of reflex origin to emphasize the distinct differences. Relatively rarely does spasm that is observed in a muscle cause pain in that muscle. Both the pain and the spasm are likely to be referred from another source. As emphasized by Janda[53] and reviewed in Chapter 5, it is of fundamental importance to distinguish muscle spasm from muscle tightness. Muscle spasm is associated with motor unit action potentials observable as EMG activity that originates in the CNS. Conversely, muscle tightness is caused by contracture of the muscle fibers.

In this case, shortening of the muscle fibers originates within the muscle, in the absence of any propagated EMG activity that originated in the CNS. Either pain alone, or spasm alone, or a variable combination of both can be referred to a muscle from the same source or from different sources.

Muscle spasm originating from outside the involved muscle is usually of reflex nature. The action potentials responsible for reflex muscular contraction are propagated through one afferent pathway and through a different efferent pathway. The mechanisms described as causing referred pain do not necessarily involve separate afferent and efferent pathways. If there is an intermediate step, such as activating an algogenic TrP in the muscle, however, then the process may qualify as being reflexly mediated.

1. Reflex Muscle Pain and Spasm From Diseased Viscera

Muscular rigidity (spasm) is one of the most important clinical manifestations of deep somatic or visceral disease.[10] This section includes some common examples of pain and spasm in the skeletal muscles that originate from distressed viscera. In addition to the cardiac, appendiceal, renal, and pancreatic sources described here, many other examples are known, such as cholecystitis and peptic ulcers.

Cardiac Pain. The referred pain that results from an inadequate blood supply to the heart muscle is well known. At first, the patient is unlikely to describe a pain; rather, he or she is likely to describe a discomfort, a tightness, a constricted feeling like "a band across the chest," or "a weight on the center of the chest." The discomfort or pain is commonly felt deep to the sternum with radiation to one or both arms, to the throat and mandible, or to all of these areas.[39]

This sensory process includes a visceromotor reflex that can induce a somatic component of spasm and activate TrPs in the chest wall muscles, particularly the pectoralis major.[39] The original cardiac insult resolves, but the TrP pain, which can feel the same as the cardiac pain, often persists. This TrP phenomenon was clearly described nearly 50 years ago by Rinzler and Travell.[87] When other causes, such as muscle overload, activate these anterior chest wall TrPs that commonly refer pain to the chest and arm, the patient is likely to be diagnosed mistakenly as having a form of effort angina.[103] The confusion arises because TrP pain is often associated with muscular activity, but in this case, it is more likely due to activity of the upper rather than the lower extremities.[96]

Appendicitis. Initially, the steady referred pain of acute appendicitis appears in the epigastric or periumbilical region and is unaffected by movement.[61] As the inflammation spreads to the adjacent parietal peritoneum in the right iliac fossa, the pain becomes more sharply localized to that area, and marked reflex spasm of the lower abdominal musculature is common.[21] Persistent TrPs activated by these viscerosomatic processes can cause persistent abdominal pain long after resolution of the appendicitis. Conversely, abdominal TrPs in this region can simulate the pain of appendicitis and produce palpable increased muscle tension that has often been mistaken for appendicitis, resulting in many unnecessary appendectomies.

Acute Renal Pain.   The referred pain of renal colic, caused by distension of the kidney, pelvis, and/or ureter, is one of the most severe pains known to humans. Detailed experiments using a balloon to cause dilation demonstrated both referred pain and often splinting and spasm of the lateral abdominal and loin muscles. The pain persisted after the stimulus was removed. Some subjects developed a "side ache" that increased in intensity during the next 12 hours, possibly caused by sustained strong muscle spasm. These experiments demonstrate that visceral pain can induce spasm in skeletal muscle and that even though the painful visceral stimulus was identical in all subjects, only some of them developed painful spasm. The latter finding speaks against the existence of a simple reflex arc as a cause of the pain, because such a reflex would be expected to induce muscle spasm in all subjects. (Another example of the absence of a vicious cycle following long-lasting nociceptive input is that chronic distension of the human knee capsule with a large effusion may be relatively pain free several months after a much smaller effusion was associated with severe pain in the acute phase.[1])

The location of referred pain depends on the location of responsible tissue injury or dilated viscus, for example, to the region of costovertebral angle from the renal pelvis, to the area of the anterior superior iliac spine from the ureteropelvic segment, to the middle of Poupart's ligament from the midureter, and to the suprapubic region from the ureterovesical segment. This acute "pain" does not respond to change of position or posture. Interestingly, patients who had repeated colic because of calculi in the upper urinary tract had a lowered electrical pain threshold in the external oblique muscle of the abdomen 3 to 10 years later.[36a] This is a striking example of the so-called "pain memory" formed in the CNS in response to strong pain.

Here again, activation of TrPs in the lower abdominal musculature can contribute a significant muscular component to the total pain being experienced and can persist following relief of the blockage.

Acute Pancreatitis. Pancreatitis is a common cause of acute abdominal pain requiring hospitalization and is difficult for the patient to describe. The discomfort may be described as stabbing, burning, or boring in the region of the upper midabdomen. It also often radiates to the back in the area of the lower thoracic spine and to the chest and flanks. Patients can develop reflex skeletal muscle spasm of the abdominal and lower chest walls that is sufficiently severe to seriously inhibit ventilation of the lungs.[78]

2. Pain and Spasm Associated With Joint Disease and Dysfunction

One of the few studies reporting muscle spasm related to arthritis in human subjects also examined modulation of EMG activity associated with TrPs. The authors[13] examined 18 patients with osteoarthritis of the knee and 8 healthy controls. They divided the 18 patients into two groups and treated one group of 8 patients for TrPs in the muscles around the arthritic knee. The other group of 10 patients received intra-articular injections of an anesthetic. In all subjects, the authors recorded EMG activity with coaxial needle electrodes in the vastus medialis muscle at tense and tender muscular areas, which showed well-known TrP characteristics.

They found that stimulation of the TrP with a needle or the movement of the affected arthritic joint could cause reflex spasm of the fibers in the region of the TrP. EMG activity initiated for any reason tended to persist in the fibers close to the TrP. Whether the remainder of the muscle containing the TrPs showed these same phenomena was not reported. Inactivation of the TrPs effectively eliminated the EMG response to pressure applied to the TrP, and anesthetic injected into the arthritic joint always reduced, sometimes markedly, the EMG response to weight bearing. The following provides additional detail regarding that report.[13]

METHOD

The authors' description indicates that all EMG recordings were made with the needle electrode in the taut band of a vastus medialis TrP in a muscle that crossed an arthritic joint. All subjects were examined for EMG activity while completely relaxed in the supine position during isometric voluntary contraction of the vastus medialis and during compression of the EMG-monitored region of muscle. In addition, all patients were tested for EMG response to compression of a tender area in the arthritic knee. The EMG responses were also recorded when pressure was applied to the same locations through anesthetized skin.

The eight patients of the first group received injections of tender locations in the periarticular muscles with 0.25% bupivacaine twice a week and i.v. (intravenous) administration of lysine acetylsalicylate 0.9 g twice daily for 20 days.

In the 10 patients of the second group, EMG activity in the vastus medialis muscle was recorded when they stood only on the arthritis-free leg, on both legs, only on the arthritic leg, while bending forward, and while bending backward. The EMG responses of this group were retested after injection of an equal amount of isotonic salt solution into the arthritic knee joint and also 30 min[utes] after injecting 4 to 8 mL of 0.25 or 0.50% bupivacaine into the arthritic joint. Eight healthy controls were also examined.

RESULTS

When subjects were supine and their muscles were considered to be completely relaxed, residual EMG activity appeared in 14 of the 18 patients, but in none of the eight control subjects. Because minor positional changes achieved electrical silence in all cases of residual EMG activity, this activity would more appropriately be considered evidence of motor neuron hyperexcitability but equivocal muscle spasm. The EMG activity of voluntary contraction persisted for 2 to 30 seconds in all patients but in none of the controls, again indicating neuronal hyperexcitability of motor units in the vicinity of the TrP.

Following treatment of the first (TrP) group, the EMG test showed no involuntary activity at rest, no delay of relaxation, and no response to pressure applied in the region of the monitored TrP. One likely explanation is that the treatment inactivated TrPs that were responsible for the motor neuron hyperirritability at rest, for the persistent EMG activity following voluntary contraction, and for the motor unit activation by pressure on the TrP.

Marked EMG activity (true spasm) occurred in the vastus medialis when painful pressure was applied to the knee joint in approximately half (8/18) of the patients and, whenever present, persisted up to 30 sec[onds] following release of pressure on the knee. When the skin was anesthetized, no change in EMG was observed in response to application of pressure to either deep tissue. The response did not depend on cutaneous afferent nerves.

When the second group of patients was standing, a marked EMG response was sometimes observed in the quadriceps muscle. This electrical activity of the muscle corresponded closely to the amount of weight carried by the arthritic knee and sometimes became silent with no weight bearing. When present, the activity tended to persist following a period of weight bearing. This EMG activity was not seen in normal subjects. Thirty minutes following injection of anesthetic into the arthritic joint, the EMG activity was greatly attenuated or had disappeared at all levels of weight bearing and, if present, showed no persistence when weight bearing ceased.

Another type of joint dysfunction can also be involved in the induction of muscle pain. Clinically, it is not an easy task to distinguish between primary joint dysfunction requiring mobilization, primary muscle dysfunction, or a combination of both. A tight muscle that restricts the range of motion is also likely to compromise joint function. Although no well-established explanation for the nature of this joint dysfunction is known, it can usually be relieved by joint mobilization techniques. Lewit[68] listed four observations showing that joint dysfunction can be independent of muscle dysfunction: (1) joints such as the sacroiliac, acromioclavicular, and tibiofibular that can be restricted in motion and yet are neither moved nor opposed by muscles; (2) the presence of joint play, which is movement restriction unrelated to muscular force; (3) the effectiveness of sudden thrust maneuvers for restoring normal joint mobility that produce minimal stretching of the muscles; and (4) persistence of joint movement restriction under general anesthesia.

Denslow et al.[23] observed that paraspinal muscle spasm was consistently most marked at the same segmental level as the vertebra that was most sensitive to applied pressure.

Vernon[106] reported on a referred tenderness study of paraspinal pressure pain-threshold algometer readings at sites of circumscribed tenderness. He reported a moderate association (kappa value 0.67) with positive prone motion-palpation tests of intervertebral rotation and of anterior-posterior glide within a +1 segment range.

Schaible and Grubb[89] in their review of afferent and spinal mechanisms of joint pain noted that many authors have observed discharges in motor neurons that were elicited by electrical stimulation of articular nerves. Ramcharan and Wyke[84] demonstrated EMG responses to electrical stimulation of articular nerves. Freeman and Wyke[35] demonstrated the complete reflex. In lightly anesthetized cats, they recorded EMG activity in the gastrocnemius and tibialis anterior muscles in response to motion of the tenotomized knee joint. They observed a burst of EMG activity associated with movement of the joint. The EMG activity faded over a period of several seconds to a residual tonic electrical activity that lasted as long as the joint remained in the position that would correspond to stretch of either the tenotomized gastrocnemius or tibialis anterior muscles. This

suggests that stretch reflexes may originate from joint receptors as well as from muscle spindles.

Conversely, Bullock-Saxton et al.[16] observed referred inhibition rather than referred spasm following joint injury. At least 4 months following ankle sprain, they observed a decrease of EMG activity and delayed onset of contraction in the gluteus maximus and hamstring muscles bilaterally, compared with normal subjects.

Although the pathophysiology of pain arising in the zygapophyseal joints is still not clear, it is referred to deep tissues in patterns that strongly resemble referred pain from TrPs.[9] The issue of spasm referred from zygapophyseal joints, as it can be from TrPs, was not reported.

3. Reflex Pain and Spasm From Muscle

As noted in Chapter 5 and in Section A of this chapter, muscle spasm as the result of pain in the same muscle is an exceptional occurrence. Therefore, it should not be considered the most likely source of clinically observed spasm unless there is a demonstrable muscle disease to cause it.

Ashton-Miller et al.[3] injected 5 mL of a hypertonic (5%) saline solution into the sternocleidomastoid muscle and observed the pain response and the induced EMG activity in eight neck muscles, including the sternocleidomastoid. In addition to the pain, as reported by other investigators conducting similar experiments, they reported a statistically significant increase (1 to 2 mV, $P < 0.05$) in EMG activity. That amount of increase was functionally trivial but demonstrated the presence of reflex pathways that can produce reflex spasm in the same and other muscles from nociceptive input. Muscle spasm induced from a remote pain source (for instance, by stimulating myofascial TrPs in another muscle) revealed much larger responses (10-fold increases). This may indicate that the spasm induced by TrPs may be mediated by afferents different from those stimulated by hypertonic saline or that the presensitization of the neurons mediating TrP pain makes a difference.

4. The Enigma of Low Back Pain

The Problem. If the past approach to looking for an answer to the enigma of low back pain has led only to a recommendation for denial of the problem,[34] one must suspect that that approach is looking in the wrong direction. Sometimes, even if the thing you are looking for is right under your nose, you can overlook it because there is so much of it or because it lacks the expected shape or color. The ubiquitous pain from muscles and joints has been largely overlooked. Several (sometimes interacting) conditions can be directly responsible for the patient's pain: active myofascial TrPs, blocking of a joint that requires mobilization, and ligamentous TrPs or tears. All of these demand a high level of manual and soft tissue diagnostic skill that requires special training and much clinical experience for most practitioners. This training is not yet included in the core curricula of most primary medical training institutions, but this kind of training is officially recommended for core curricula by the International Association for the Study of Pain.[32]

The myofascial TrP sources of low back pain explain many of the enigmas associated with this pain. Osteopaths[65] and chiropractors,[69, 90] who historically have concentrated on joint dysfunctions, are becoming increasingly aware of the importance of also dealing with myofascial TrPs.

A seemingly different approach to the muscular component of low back pain concerns muscle imbalance and its correction. This issue is covered in greater detail later in this chapter (see Section 3).

Recent research studies (as yet largely unpublished) are making an increasingly strong case that myofascial TrPs likely play a much more important role in causing muscle imbalance than most of the available literature on the subject indicates. The most effective treatment approaches for correcting muscle imbalance concentrate on retention and normalization of muscular coordination and function. Simply trying to strengthen just the weak muscles is often frustratingly ineffective and may be counterproductive or even injurious. One must first understand and deal with WHY the muscles are weak.

A balanced, progressive muscle reconditioning program can be remarkably effective, especially for preventing recurring episodes of low back pain. Gundewall et al.[38] reported a poorly controlled, ran-

domized prospective study of employees at a geriatric hospital. One of the two groups was trained in an exercise program to improve back muscle strength, endurance, and coordination. They were allowed to exercise during working hours. The control group did not participate in the exercise program and received no further advice or information. After 13 months, the training group missed 28 work days because of back pain; the control group lost 155 days (P < 0.004). The training group also had significantly fewer back pain complaints. Every hour spent by the physiotherapist in training reduced work absence by 1.5 days, a cost/benefit ratio of 1:10. The value of such a program was clearly demonstrated. How much of the benefit accrued from purely muscle training effect and how much from improved management-employee relations in the training group remains unanswered, however. It is probably some of both. In either case, the cost/benefit and preventive medical value of the program is valid.

V. Janda of the Czech Republic has been a pioneer in promoting an appreciation and understanding of how clinically important muscle imbalance is. Functionally weak, inhibited muscles appear as antagonists to functionally strong, shortened, hyperexcitable muscles that are usually not in spasm. A common pattern in low back pain patients is weak gluteal muscles and strong hip flexors. Treatment starts with gentle stretch to release the tightness of the strong muscles, which, remarkably, often improves the strength and reduces the inhibition of the antagonist muscles that was present during functional activity. This likely relates to releasing TrPs in the tight muscle that are causing referred inhibition of the weak muscle.

Important in the use of muscle stretching as a treatment is an understanding of the distinction between muscle stiffness and muscle flexibility. Increased range of motion could result from either reduced stiffness (resistance to passive movement compared with the distance moved, which can be displayed as a force versus distance curve—see Chapter 5) or increased extensibility. Halbertsma et al.[38a] showed clearly that in athletes with stiff hamstring muscles, stretching the tight muscle left the shape of the stiffness curve unchanged and simply extended the end of the curve into a greater range of motion. This is the result one would expect if the cause of the stiffness were taut bands of TrPs that were released by stretch. A change in extensibility changes the shape of the curve.

Jull and Janda[58] emphasize the potential danger of a vigorous program for strengthening a weak muscle without giving due consideration to the nature of the problem. The patient is likely to achieve the exercise through compensatory recruitment of substitute muscles, which overloads them, overloads and further weakens the weak muscle, and further reinforces an abnormal function pattern. Simple "strength" measurements showing the progress of muscle groups without identifying the contribution of individual muscles during testing can easily be seriously misleading.

One clinically effective treatment approach to low back pain for the many patients who have lower body postural (ambulatory) muscle imbalance has been the use of a simple device: balance shoes.[16] A "balance" shoe is a platform sandal with a dense rubber hemisphere attached on the undersole close to the center of gravity. EMG recordings verified its effectiveness in normalizing muscle function, which was correlated with clinical improvement.

Plowman[83] summarized her analysis of the muscular component of low back pain with two major points. First, high levels of hip flexor strength and shortening are to be avoided. Second, high levels of abdominal or back extensor strength alone do NOT predispose an individual to low back pain.

Epidemiology and Management. In general, the medical community seems unaware of a satisfactory explanation for most low back pain, but it is too big a problem to ignore. Recently, Plowman[83] and Fordyce[34] summarized literature that identifies the magnitude of the problem. At some point in their lives, 60 to 80% of the entire population experience low back pain, which is a *symptom,* not a *diagnosis.* Approximately 80 to 90% of them recover within 3 days to 6 weeks. Low back pain accounts for 20 million sick days per year

in the United States alone, a staggering financial loss. Once an episode occurs, it is more likely to recur. The disabling pain persists for more than a year for 1% of those experiencing an initial episode. Less than 50% of those off work longer than 6 months ever return to the workforce. This often becomes a financial and lifestyle tragedy to the sufferer.[51]

Nachemson,[79] an orthopaedic surgeon world-renowned for his decades of research to understand the cause of low back pain, states that the pathomechanics of low back pain is unknown and that there is no satisfactory diagnosis for most of these patients. To the extent that muscles were seriously considered as the source of pain, it was generally (and erroneously) assumed that a pain-spasm-pain cycle was operative. As early as 1984, Nouwen and Bush[80] reviewed this concept and concluded that the painful back muscles were rarely in spasm. In fact, Cassisi et al.[18] in one study showed that the muscles were functionally weak.

One approach to this frustrating situation was promoted by the International Association for the Study of Pain[34] for the management of *nonspecific low back pain.* This diagnosis is suggested when the physician could find no anatomic or physiologic reason for the pain that could be established by a laboratory test or imaging procedure. The Committee Report recommends 6 weeks of conservative treatment, at which point advice ends abruptly with reassignment of the patient to the diagnosis of "activity intolerance," which is "not a medical problem." This approach assumes that activity intolerance is basically a behavior problem induced by the current system of compensation.

Needless to say, this report generated considerable controversy. Although some authors agreed with Fordyce,[70, 71, 72] others took exception. Wall[107] commented, "I disagree on scientific and ethical grounds and await a report which faces the problems of the abandoned patients." Thompson[102] pointed out that the failure of the report[34] to acknowledge myofascial pain syndrome should be recognized as a critically important oversight, which has resulted in a dangerously flawed report.

C. DIAGNOSIS AND TREATMENT OF POSTURAL MUSCLE PAIN

It is widely recognized that poor posture, musculoskeletal pain complaints, and muscle imbalance and/or weakness are commonly associated. Rarely does current literature bring closure on how these factors relate to one another with a convincing explanation of what causes what.

1. Poor Posture

The importance of poor posture in relation to musculoskeletal pain and dysfunction is widely recognized, but the reason why it hurts is not well identified. This hiatus is likely the result of the overwhelming emphasis on primary skeletal origins, with relative neglect of muscles as the primary source of the pain.

Upright and Slumped Postures. The standing upright, balanced posture illustrated in Figure 6-8 shows that, seen from behind (Fig. 6-8*A*), the body is aligned so that the spine is straight and all skeletal components are symmetrically arranged on either side of the midline. Seen from the side, the body is standing balanced and upright (Figure 6-8*B*) when the center of gravity passes through the auditory canal and the acromion and follows the midaxillary line through the midpoint of the iliac crest and the lateral epicondyle of the femur to a point approximately 2 cm posterior to the lateral condyle.[105] This posture places minimum strain on muscles and ligaments.[65]

A standing slumped (slouched) posture (Fig. 6-9) results in an excessive lumbar lordosis, an excessive dorsal kyphosis, and head-forward positioning. Normal upright posture is a balanced posture that requires no muscular effort and places no strain on ligaments to maintain it. This slumped posture requires some posterior cervical muscular effort to maintain it; otherwise, the head would fall forward. The farther forward the head, the more effort required. The thoracolumbar "S" curve depends on ligamentous tension to maintain it. One common source of this type of posture is muscle imbalance, described in detail in Section 3A below.

The seated erect and slumped postures in Figure 6-10 show that an upright posture

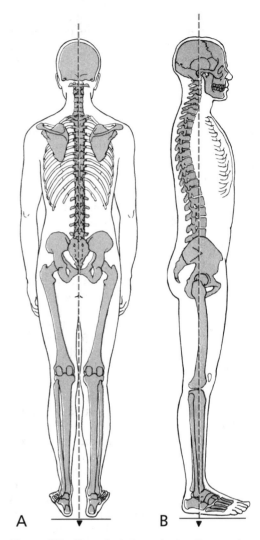

Figure 6-8. Normal, balanced standing posture. **A.** View from behind. Midline is straight and structures are arranged symmetrically. **B.** View from the right side. The *vertical line (red)* shows that the head is balanced squarely over the pelvis and that the pelvis and knees are aligned directly above the weight-bearing arch of the ankle. (Reproduced with permission from Kendall FP, McCreary EK, Provance PG: *Muscles, Testing and Function.* Ed. 4. Williams & Wilkins, Baltimore, 1993.)

(Fig. 6-10*B*) balances the head over the thorax and the thorax over the pelvis. The slumped or flexed posture of Figure 6-10*A* places the head forward of the thorax and the thorax behind the hips. The contrast between balanced and flexed, head-forward posture is well illustrated by Hiemeyer et al.[45] This poor sitting posture is similar to the upper half of the standing slumped posture in Figure 6-9. This seated position also requires sustained contraction of posterior cervical muscles to keep the head from falling forward and places strain on

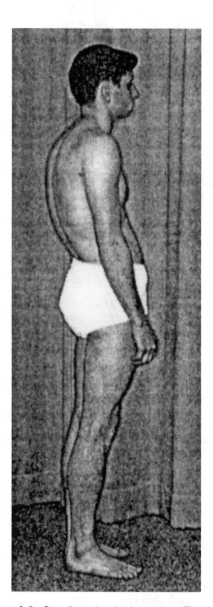

Figure 6-9. Standing slouched posture. The head and abdomen jut forward with regard to the shoulders, the center of gravity of the thorax lies behind the center of gravity of the pelvis, and the pelvis is shifted forward with regard to the ankle. This posture produces muscular and ligamentous strain. (Reproduced with permission from Brügger A: *Die Erkrankungen des Bewegungsapparates und seines Nervensystems*. Gustav Fischer Verlag, Stuttgart, 1980.)

spinal ligaments that are supporting the curve of the spine. An example of the potential value of correcting this head-forward flexed posture in fibromyalgia patients was reported in a study by Hiemeyer *et al.*[45]:

> They[45] divided into two groups 40 patients who evidenced more than 10 tender points at the 28 test sites that Yunus proposed for diagnosing primary fibromyalgia. All patients had the flexed, head-forward posture. The six patients who fell into group I showed no evidence of flexor muscle shortening when passively restored to an erect sitting posture by forward pressure at T5 in the sitting position. The same passive procedure caused the 34 group II patients pain, which was attributed to shortening of flexor muscles. Eight tender point sites in each patient were tested for change in tenderness while repositioned to an upright posture.
>
> Thirty-six (94%) of the tested tender points in group I patients were less tender in the upright position and 125 points (69%) improved in group II patients. All patients showed improvement in at least two tested points. Although the criteria for improvement were unstated, this report suggests that, at least temporarily, the improvement in posture reduced the tenderness of the fibromyalgia tender points, which usually correlates well with patient pain level and which are also often TrPs.

Asymmetric Postures.   A major source of muscle strain is skeletal asymmetry that requires compensatory muscular control to maintain an erect posture and to keep the eyes level. Many of these asymmetries have been covered in detail in previous publications.[96, 104] A good example is the chain of muscular overloads caused by a lower limb length discrepancy. The tilted pelvis requires unrelenting quadratus lumborum contraction to curve the lumbar spine to bring the rest of the body over the pelvis. Now the spine above is tilted to the other side. This tilt requires further compensation, usually of neck muscles such as the sternocleidomastoid and upper trapezius. This sustained contraction and overload facilitates the development of TrPs, which in turn cause musculoskeletal pain.

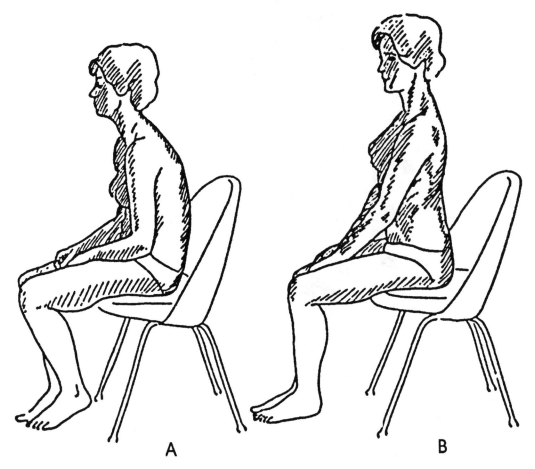

Figure 6-10. Seated postures. **A.** Flexed posture, identified by Brügger as *Sternosymphysale Belastungshaltung* (sternosymphyseal strain posture), which places a sustained load on the posterior neck muscles to support the head and on the posterior thoracic ligaments because of the excessive thoracic kyphosis. This posture also leaves anterior chest muscles in a persistently shortened position. **B.** Desirable, balanced posture that is strain-free. (Reproduced with permission from Brügger A: *Die Erkrankungen des Bewegungsapparates und seines Nervensystems.* Gustav Fischer Verlag, Stuttgart, 1980.)

The articular dysfunctions that cause body asymmetry and their correction have been a focus of attention by the osteopathic profession.[37] Kuchera[65] also includes serious consideration of the important role of TrPs, as does the chiropractic treatise by Liebenson.[69]

Awkward and Strained Postures. The previously considered postures described conditions of the body at rest. This section calls attention to postural errors related to an activity. This issue was addressed muscle by muscle by a pioneer in this field, Janet G. Travell.[96, 104] The epidemic of occupational myalgias that was aggravated by the arrival of the computer age is covered in Chapter 5, Section B. Issues such as desk and sitting arrangements to avoid unnecessarily sustained and repetitive muscular strain are finally getting the attention they deserve, with chapters dedicated to just this subject.[4, 60] Sometimes, these issues become an integral part of an entire book that emphasizes the critical role of myofascial TrPs in contributing to or causing the pain.[98]

2. Origins of Postural Pain

Ligamentous Tension. One study demonstrated the potent effectiveness of sustained ligamentous tension in the production of severe musculoskeletal pain.[40] The authors recorded the surface EMG activity of the right splenius capitis at the level of C2, the rhomboideus minor and erector spinae at the cervicothoracic junction, and the anterolateral border of the upper trapezius muscle and normalized their amplitudes to the percent of maximum voluntary effort. Ten healthy female subjects sat with the head and neck hanging down in a continuously relaxed, maximally forward-flexed position for as long as was tolerable. The steadily increasing pain levels were measured at least once every minute on a 100-mm visual analog scale (VAS). All subjects experienced pain or discomfort within 15 minutes. Subjects reached tolerance in 18 to 62 minutes at VAS levels ranging from 57 to 100 mm.

EMG levels were surprisingly low, however. Mean values increased, from essentially zero during the first 3 minutes, to mean values of from 2 to 4% of maximum contraction during the last 3 minutes of the test. The maximum value recorded at the end was 14% of maximum effort. These are gentle, nonpainful levels of contraction. Subjects reporting the most pain during the test evidenced less increase in muscle contractile activity. With few exceptions, the pain was experienced throughout the posterior half of the neck and across the shoulders above the scapular spines.[40] Evidence of voluntary effort to reduce discomfort (decrease in flexion) was not associated with any identifiable reduction. In this acute, one-time exposure to overload, restoration of normal positioning and mobility quickly ended the pain (median 6 minutes and maximum 15 minutes).

The evidence indicates that the pain was caused primarily by sustained tension on joint capsules and ligaments, not by muscle spasm. Because additional voluntary muscle contraction in this situation would only increase the ligamentous tension, it is not surprising that it did not relieve the pain. The gradually increasing, low-level EMG activity may represent reflex muscle spasm that originated in overloaded ligaments, not in the muscle.

It is a common experience that carrying a heavy load (such as an overloaded suitcase) in a hand that is hanging down by the side for more than several minutes produces increasingly intolerable shoulder pain. The lack of EMG activity in the deltoid and supraspinatus muscles[8] again identifies the ligaments rather than the muscles as the source of the pain. Changing the load to the other hand usually brings prompt relief.

Muscular Origin. Repeated reference has been made to muscle overload and muscle strain as critical factors in posturally induced musculoskeletal pain. To clinicians aware of TrPs and attentive to their patients, it is apparent both in their own personal experience and in the experience of their patients that muscles commonly develop TrPs for many reasons. These reasons include acute episodic overload, sustained contraction (especially in the shortened position), excessive repetition of the same movement, and being left in the shortened position for a period of time.[96, 104] The TrPs activated in these ways are often the missing link between the widely recognized importance of avoiding and correcting these conditions and the pain of which the patient complains. The speed and cost-effectiveness of the management and treatment of these musculoskeletal pain complaints can frequently be greatly improved if the TrP cause of the pain is recognized and dealt with as such.

3. Muscle Imbalance as a Cause of Poor Posture

The strengthening of weak muscles and work hardening to deal with loss of function because of musculoskeletal pain has become an industry in itself. As pointed out in the overview of low back pain in Section B4 of this chapter, all too often practitioners fail to identify the cause of the pain and dysfunction. This tunnel-vision treatment of a symptom rather than of the cause often produces disappointing results and can aggravate rather than relieve the primary problem. A major step forward has been Janda's recognition and electromyographic demonstration of the common pairing of weak and inhibited musculature with functionally related muscles that are abnormally tight.

Weak Muscles Versus Tight Muscles.
The visual examination for postural distortions indicative of muscle imbalance was reviewed and illustrated comprehensively for the standing posture by Vasilyeva and Lewit.[105] Conventional muscle testing[59] examines individual muscles for weakness and shortness but does not emphasize the importance of looking for paired combinations of weak and short muscles that together contribute to the same postural distortion and dysfunction. Jull and Janda[58] strongly associate muscle shortening with tightness, identified by palpably increased muscle tension. The short, tense muscles also tend to be more responsive to motor commands, responding more than expected during movement. Those authors characterized weak muscles as having a delayed and inhibited (less vigorous) response.

Janda[55] presents clinical muscle testing from the point of view of postural and functional muscular imbalance produced by sets of weak and/or tight muscles. A good example is his test for the combination of tight sternocleidomastoid muscles and weak primary anterior neck flexors. By asking the relaxed supine subject to bring the chin to the chest, the sternocleidomastoid muscles tend to elevate the head from the table without neck flexion, resulting in the chin simply jutting upward instead of rotating toward the chest.

Because patients with low back pain commonly had weak gluteus muscles, Jull and Janda[58] tested the supine patients' hip extension function by asking them to lift first one leg and then the other. They frequently electromyographically monitored the hamstrings, gluteus maximus, gluteus minimus, lumbar paraspinal muscles, and sometimes other muscles. In this test, a common set of imbalance patterns at the pelvic level was tight (shortened) hip flexors (iliopsoas and tensor fasciae latae) and weak hip extensors (gluteal muscles). At the lumbar level, the trunk flexors (abdominal wall muscles) were weak and the trunk extensors (erector spinae) were tight. The quadratus lumborum and, unexpectedly, the hamstrings tended to be tight. This combination of imbalance caused forward tilt of the pelvis, increased lumbar lordosis, and slightly increased hip flexion. The lumbar lordosis initiated a chain reaction that produced thoracic kyphosis, cervical lordosis, and a head-forward posture.

In this hip extension test, EMG testing showed that normally the hamstrings and gluteus maximus acted as prime movers, becoming active first, followed by the erector spinae. In many patients with low back pain and weak glutei, the contraction of the gluteus maximus was delayed. In the poorest (most dysfunctional) pattern, the erector spinae initiated the movement, and the delayed gluteus maximus response was weak.[58]

A comparable tight and/or weak muscle relationship is also commonly seen in musculoskeletal syndromes of the neck.[52] The muscles most likely to be tight and hyperactive are the upper trapezius, sternocleidomastoid, levator scapulae, and pectoral muscles. The muscles most likely to be weak and inhibited are lower stabilizers of the scapula (serratus anterior, rhomboids, and middle and lower trapezius muscles) and primary neck flexors (suprahyoid, mylohyoid, longus colli, and longus capitis muscles). These patients, when standing, exhibit elevation and protraction of the shoulder, rotation and elevation of the scapula, and variable winging of the scapula. This abnormal scapular posture reduces stability of the glenohumeral joint, which may require compensatory recruitment of the levator scapulae and upper trapezius muscles.[52]

Therapeutic Approaches. The previous sections have identified the need for correction of faulty posture, the need for stretching the tight muscle in the presence of muscle imbalance, and the value of coordination training.

Correction of the head-forward, flexed posture is frequently much more easily said than done. Hiemeyer et al.[45] pointed out the critical difference between those who can assume and maintain a balanced posture without discomfort and continued muscular effort and those for whom this is not possible.

In the case of those who can assume a balanced posture and maintain it in the relaxed state but just fail to do so, the problem is one of correcting a well-established bad habit. This involves behavior modification, one of the more challenging issues in medical management. The Alexander technique[6] is one example of how the patient can achieve the desired result. A simple but powerful example of how to establish more erect sitting posture is the importance of sitting back against the backrest in a chair that provides adequate lumbar support and has a seat cover that does not allow the buttocks to slide forward. A number of additional work habit corrections for head-forward posture and additional postural habit changes were summarized by Simons and Simons.[95] Fortunately, adopting new behavior patterns can be successful if approached from the point of view of adequate motivation and the judicious and often ingenious use of positive reinforcers and avoidance of a punitive approach.[33]

Those who must invoke voluntary muscular contraction to hold the desired posture have a skeletal abnormality that should be identifiable by imaging and/or a muscular imbalance, such as those mentioned above. Skeletal abnormalities such as lower limb length inequality can often be corrected by a lift.[65, 104] Articular dysfunctions require manipulation.[37, 69] Other skeletal abnormalities may need an orthopaedic solution.

The primary or major contributing cause of the poor posture is likely to be muscle imbalance. Jull and Janda[58] recommended a three-stage approach:

1. Release overactive or tight muscles to restore normal length. A recent recommendation was stretch using post-isometric relaxation and inactivation of TrPs.[54]
2. Strengthening of weak and inhibited muscles. Jull and Janda[58] noted that it is not unusual for release of the tight muscles to restore the strength and normal function of the weak muscles without further treatment. If a strengthening program is required, it is critically important to make sure that the weak muscle is gaining strength and that a pattern of substitution by other muscles is not being reinforced.

3. Establish optimal motor patterns. For patients with low back problems, retraining using a balance shoe proved clinically and electromyographically successful.[16] As pointed out above, a balance shoe is a platform sandal with a dense rubber hemisphere attached on the undersole close to the center of gravity. Walking when wearing a pair of balance shoes requires some practice and a significant increase in muscular coordination. Learning to walk in this way normalized the amplitude of EMG activity and markedly increased the rate of recruitment of gluteus medius muscle in 15 subjects with low back pain, when retested in bare feet.

The head-forward posture arising in the upper half of the body characteristically involves tight pectoral muscles, especially the pectoralis major and frequently the subscapularis muscle.

Muscular Origin of Muscle Imbalance. Mounting evidence suggests that TrPs can reflexly disturb normal muscle function in many significant ways. The muscle imbalance caused by weak and/or tight sets of muscles, which is discussed above, fits one disturbance pattern.

The taut bands associated with TrPs could account for the increased tension and shortening of the tight muscles described above.[58] These taut bands extending beyond both sides of a TrP are muscle fibers that are passively stretched by contracture of the sarcomeres of the contraction knots in the TrP (see Chapter 8). Functionally, the muscle harboring a TrP tends to be hyperexcitable and more active than normal and is slow to return to the relaxed state.[13] This change in responsiveness of the muscle could be considered a form of reflex, in the sense that afferent input from the TrP is modulating excitability of the motor neurons of the same muscle.

Conversely, the weakness of the functionally related muscle(s) may well be inhibition of weak muscles that arises from TrPs in the tense muscle. This relation is strongly suggested by the repeated observation that the weakness and delayed activation of the weak muscle is relieved by restoring the tight muscle to its normal length by using TrP treatment techniques.[58] That TrPs in one muscle may reflexly inhibit the activity of a functionally related muscle in this region has been demonstrated by Headley.[43] Weak recruitment of the gluteal muscles, identified by surface EMG, was markedly improved by inactivating TrPs in the quadratus lumborum muscle.

Unfortunately, the reflex effects of TrPs are complex. Sometimes, a TrP may be responsible for referred spasm (Fig. 6-7). Inactivation of a right soleus TrP relieved marked spasm in the right lumbar paraspinal muscles.[42] A clear example of this motor reflex activity of TrPs was observed when marked bilateral spasm of the sternocleidomastoid muscles was eliminated in one case and greatly attenuated in another by injecting and inactivating TrPs in the right and left upper trapezius and right and left supraspinatus muscles. Only one of the sternocleidomastoid muscles had an active TrP.[93]

Why TrPs would cause reflex spasm in one situation and reflex inhibition in another is not at all clear. One possibility is that the distinction between muscles prone to tightness and muscles prone to weakness, drawn by Jull and Janda,[58] may be of fundamental physiologic significance. The muscle that develops the TrP determines what reflex effect it has on functionally related muscles. If this is the case, the gluteus medius muscles may have TrPs that increase the excitability of the tight hip flexors and may even cause ongoing spasm, which could be clearly identified electromyographically. TrPs in these muscles could also account for much of the pain complaint of patients with low back pain.

Myofascial TrPs sometimes exhibit another phenomenon that might also be considered of a reflex nature and may relate to the phenomena of referred spasm and referred inhibition. Inactivation of a key TrP in one muscle can release an active satellite TrP in another muscle without any further treatment.[48] In terms of the relationships noted above, inactivation of sternocleidomastoid key TrPs inactivated digastric TrPs; inactivation of upper trapezius TrPs inactivated rhomboid minor TrPs; inactivation of lumbar paraspinal TrPs could inactivate gluteus maximus, gastrocnemius, and soleus TrPs; and inactivation of quadratus lumborum TrPs inactivated gluteus maximus TrPs and many other pairs.

The results observed from motor point blocks (which destroy endplate function and therefore also any TrP activity in the blocked region) of subscapularis muscles in seven hemiplegic patients with spasticity are another example of release of reflex inhibition in one muscle by treatment of another that may also relate to TrPs.[62] One subject showed no supraspinatus activity before treatment, but the muscle responded in all post-treatment trials. Another subject showed 100% increase in middle deltoid activity following subscapularis treatment and, in addition, appearance of activity in the supraspinatus and teres minor muscles. This focal inactivation of muscle nerve activity in the region of endplates of subscapularis muscles restored a degree of voluntary function in related functional muscles. The treatment must have inactivated afferent input from the subscapularis muscle that was inhibiting motor activity of the other muscles. Inactivating only the motor function of subscapularis motor units would not be expected to have such an effect.

REFERENCES

1. Ansell JS, Gee WF, with contributions by Bonica JJ: Diseases of the kidney and ureter, Chapter 62. *The Management of Pain.* Ed 2. Edited by Bonica JJ, Loeser JD, Chapman CR, Fordyce WE. Lea & Febiger, Philadelphia, 1990 (pp. 1232–1249).
2. Appelberg B, Hulliger M, Johansson H, *et al.*: Actions on gamma-motoneurones elicited by electrical stimulation of group III muscle afferent fibres in the hind limb of the cat. *J Physiol* 335:275–292, 1983.
3. Ashton-Miller JA, McGlashen KM, Herzenberg JE, *et al.*: Cervical muscle myoelectric response to acute experimental sternocleidomastoid pain. *Spine* 15:1006–1012, 1990.
4. Ayoub MA: Ergonomic conditions in the workplace, Chapter 48. *Handbook of Pain Management.* Ed. 2. Edited by Tollison CD. Williams & Wilkins, Baltimore, 1994 (pp. 640–666).
5. Barasi S, Lynn B: Effects of sympathetic stimulation on mechanoreceptive and nociceptive afferent units from the rabbit pinna. *Brain Res* 378:21–27, 1986.
6. Barker S: *The Alexander Technique.* Bantam Books, Toronto, 1978.

7. Basmajian JV, Deluca CJ: *Muscles Alive*. Ed. 5. Williams & Wilkins, Baltimore, 1985.

8. Berberich P, Hoheisel U, Mense S, *et al.*: Fine muscle afferent fibres and inflammation: changes in discharge behaviour and influence on gamma-motoneurons, Chapter 17. *Fine Afferent Nerve Fibres and Pain*. Edited by Schmidt RF, Schaible HG, Vahle-Hinz C. VHC, Weinheim, 1987 (pp.165–175).

9. Bogduk N, Simons DG: Neck pain: joint pain or trigger points? Chapter 20. *Progress in Fibromyalgia and Myofascial Pain, Volume 6 of Pain Research and Clinical Management*. Edited by Vaerøy H, Merskey H. Elsevier, Amsterdam, 1993 (pp. 267–273).

10. Bonica JJ, with contributions by Procacci P: General considerations of acute pain, Chapter 7. *The Management of Pain*. Ed. 2. Edited by Bonica JJ, Loeser JD, Chapman CR, Fordyce WE. Lea & Febiger, Philadelphia, 1990 (pp. 159–179).

11. Brochocki G: Die schmerzhaften Muskelkontrakturen bei rheumatischen Erkrankungen und deren Behandlung. *Praxis (Schweizerische Rundschau für Medizin)* 31:790–793, 1962.

12. Brock LG, Eccles JC, Rall W: Experimental investigations on the afferent fibres in muscle nerves. *Proc R Soc Lond B* 138:453–475, 1951.

13. Brucini M, Duranti R, Galletti R, *et al.*: Pain thresholds and electromyographic features of periarticular muscles in patients with osteoarthritis of the knee. *Pain* 10:57–66, 1981.

14. Brügger A: *Die Erkrankungen des Bewegungsapparates und seines Nervensystems*. Gustav Fischer Verlag, Stuttgart, 1980.

15. Brügger A: Neurologische und morphologische Grundlagen der sogenannten rheumatischen Schmerzen—ein Beitrag zum Verständnis der Funktionskrankheiten. *Schmerzstudien 6, Schmerz und Bewegungssystem*. Edited by Berger M, Gerstenbrand F, Lewit K. Fischer, Stuttgart, 1984 (pp. 56–79).

16. Bullock-Saxton JE, Janda V, Bullock MI: Reflex activation of gluteal muscles in walking. An approach to restoration of muscle function for patients with low-back pain. *Spine* 18:704–708, 1993.

17. Burke D: Critical examination of the case for or against fusimotor involvement in disorders of muscle tone. *Advances in Neurology, Volume 39, Motor Control Mechanisms in Health and Disease*. Edited by Desmedt JE. Raven Press, New York, 1983 (pp. 133–150).

18. Cassisi JE, Robinson ME, O'Conner P, *et al.*: Trunk strength and lumbar paraspinal muscle activity during isometric exercise in chronic low-back pain patients and controls. *Spine* 18:245–251, 1993.

19. Chassaignac CME: De la paralysie douloureuse des jeunes enfants. *Arch gén Méd 5, Ser.* I:653–669, 1856.

20. Clarke RW, Harris J, Ford TW, *et al.*: Prolonged potentiation of transmission through a withdrawal reflex pathway after noxious stimulation of the heel in the rabbit. *Pain* 49:65–70, 1992.

21. Cousins M: Acute and postoperative pain, Chapter 18. *Textbook of Pain*. Ed. 2. Edited by Wall PD, Melzack R. Churchill Livingstone, New York, 1989 (pp. 284–305).

22. DeAndrade JR, Grant C, Dixon ASJ: Joint distension and reflex muscle inhibition in the knee. *J Bone Joint Surg* 47:313–322, 1965.

23. Denslow JS, Korr IM, Krems AD: Quantitative studies of chronic facilitation in human motoneuron pools. *Am J Physiol* 105:229–238, 1947.

24. Dietrichson P: Tonic ankle reflex in Parkinsonian rigidity and in spasticity. *Acta Neurol Scand* 47:163–182, 1971.

25. Dorpat TL, Holmes TH: Backache of muscle tension origin. *Psychosomatic Obstetrics, Gynecology and Endocrinology*. Edited by Kroger WS. CC Thomas, Springfield, IL, 1962 (pp. 425–436).

26. Eccles RM, Lundberg A: Synaptic actions in motoneurones by afferents which may evoke the flexion reflex. *Arch Ital Biol* 97:199–221, 1959.

27. Edwards RHT: Hypotheses of peripheral and central mechanisms underlying occupational muscle pain and injury. *Eur J Appl Physiol* 57:275–281, 1988.

28. Ellaway PH, Murphy PR, Tripathi A: Closely coupled excitation of gamma-motoneurones by group III muscle afferents with low mechanical threshold in the cat. *J Physiol* 331:481–498, 1982.

29. Emre M, Mathies H (Eds.): *Muscle Spasms and Pain*. Parthenon, Park Ridge, NJ, 1988.

30. Ferrell WR, Wood L, Baxendale RH: The effect of acute joint inflammation on flexion reflex excitability in the decerebrate, low-spinal cat. *Q J Exp Physiol* 73:95–102, 1988.

31. Fields HL: *Pain*. McGraw-Hill, New York, 1987.

32. Fields HL (Ed.): *Core Curriculum for Professional Education in Pain*. IASP Press, Seattle, 1995 (see Ch. 19, Myofascial pain, pp. 79–81).

33. Fordyce WE: *Behavioral Methods for Chronic Pain and Illness*. CV Mosby, St. Louis, 1976.

34. Fordyce WE: *Back Pain in the Workplace: Management of Disability in Nonspecific Conditions*. IASP Press, Seattle, 1995.

35. Freeman MAR, Wyke B: Articular reflexes at the ankle joint: an electromyographic study of normal and abnormal influences of ankle-joint mechanoreceptors upon reflex activity in the leg muscles. *Br J Surg* 54:990–1001, 1967.

36. Gardner E: Reflex muscular responses to stimulation of articular nerves in the cat. *Am J Physiol* 161:133–141, 1950.

36a. Giamberardino MA: Recent and forgotten aspects of visceral pain. *Eur J Pain* 3:77–92, 1999.

37. Greenman PE: *Principles of Manual Medicine*. Ed. 2. Williams & Wilkins, Baltimore, 1996.

38. Gundewall B, Liljeqvist M, Hansson T: Primary prevention of back symptoms and absence from work. A prospective randomized study among hospital employees. *Spine* 18:587–594, 1993.

38a. Halbertsma JP, van Bolhuis AI, Goeken LN: Sport stretching: effect on passive muscle stiffness of short hamstrings. *Arch Phys Med Rehabil* 77(7): 688–692, 1996.

39. Hammermeister KE, with contributions by Bonica JJ: Cardiac and aortic pain, Chapter 54. *The Management of Pain*. Ed. 2. Edited by Bonica JJ, Loeser JD, Chapman CR, Fordyce WE. Lea & Febiger, Philadelphia, 1990 (pp. 1001–1042).

40. Harms-Ringdahl K, Ekholm J: Intensity and character of pain and muscular activity levels elicited by

maintained extreme flexion position of the lower-cervical-upper-thoracic spine. *Scand J Rehab Med* 18:117–126, 1986.

41. He X, Proske U, Schaible H-G, *et al.*: Acute inflammation of the knee joint in the cat alters responses of flexor motoneurons to leg movements. *J Neurophysiol* 59:326–340, 1988.

42. Headley BJ: Evaluation and treatment of myofascial pain syndrome utilizing biofeedback, Chapter 5. *Clinical EMG for Surface Recordings*, Vol. 2. Edited by Cram JR. Clinical Resources, Nevada City, CA, 1990 (pp. 235–254).

43. Headley BJ: Chronic pain management, Chapter 27. *Physical Rehabilitation: Assessment and Treatment.* Ed. 3. Edited by O'Sullivan SB, Schmitz TJ. FA Davis, Philadelphia, 1994.

44. Henneman E: Organization of the motor systems—a preview. *Medical Physiology*, Vol. 1. Ed. 13. Edited by Mountcastle VB. CV Mosby, St. Louis, 1974 (pp. 603–607).

45. Hiemeyer K, Lutz R, Menninger H: Dependence of tender points upon posture—a key to the understanding of fibromyalgia syndrome. *J Man Med* 5:169–174, 1990.

46. Hilton SM, Hudlická O, Marshall JM: Possible mediators of functional hyperaemia in skeletal muscle. *J Physiol* 282:131–147, 1978.

47. Holmqvist B, Lundberg A: Differential supraspinal control of synaptic actions evoked by volleys in the flexion reflex afferents in alpha motoneurones. *Acta Physiol Scand* 186(Suppl 54):1–51, 1961.

48. Hong C-Z: Considerations and recommendations regarding myofascial trigger point injection. *J Musculoskeletal Pain* 2(1):29–59, 1994.

49. Hong SK, Kniffki K-D, Schmidt RF: Reflex discharges of extensor and flexor gamma motoneurones by chemically induced muscle pain. *Pain Abstract* 1:58, 1978.

50. Hu JW, Yu X-M, Vernon H, *et al.*: Excitatory effects on neck and jaw muscle activity of inflammatory irritant applied to cervical paraspinal tissues. *Pain* 55:243–250, 1993.

51. Institute of Medicine: *Pain and Disability: Clinical Behavioral and Public Policy Perspectives.* National Academy Press, Washington, DC, May 1987.

52. Janda V: Muscles and cervicogenic pain syndromes, Chapter 9. *Physical Therapy of the Cervical and Thoracic Spine*. Edited by Grant R. Churchill Livingstone, New York, 1988 (pp.153–166).

53. Janda V: Muscle spasm—a proposed procedure for differential diagnosis. *J Man Med* 6:136–139, 1991.

54. Janda V: Muscle strength in relation to muscle length, pain and muscle imbalance, Chapter 6. *Muscle Strength*. Edited by Harms-Ringdahl K. Churchill Livingstone, New York, 1993 (pp. 83–91).

55. Janda V: Evaluation of muscular imbalance, Chapter 6. *Rehabilitation of the Spine: A Practitioner's Manual*. Edited by Liebenson C. Williams & Wilkins, Baltimore, 1996 (pp. 97–113).

56. Järvholm U, Styf J, Suurkula M, *et al.*: Intramuscular pressure and muscle blood flow in supraspinatus. *Eur J Appl Physiol* 58:219–224, 1988.

57. Johansson H, Sojka P: Pathophysiological mechanisms involved in genesis and spread of muscular tension in occupational muscle pain and in chronic musculoskeletal pain syndromes: a hypothesis. *Med Hypothesis* 35:196–203, 1991.

58. Jull GA, Janda V: Muscles and motor control in low back pain: assessment and management, Chapter 10. *Physical Therapy of the Low Back*. Edited by Twomey LT, Taylor JR. Churchill Livingstone, New York, 1987 (pp. 253–278).

59. Kendall FP, McCreary EK, Provance PG: *Muscles, Testing and Function*. Ed. 4. Williams & Wilkins, Baltimore, 1993.

60. Khalil TM, Abdel-Moty E, Steele-Rosomoff R, *et al.*: The role of ergonomics in the prevention and treatment of myofascial pain, Chapter 16. *Myofascial Pain and Fibromyalgia: Trigger Point Management*. Edited by Rachlin ES. CV Mosby, St. Louis, 1994 (pp. 487–523).

61. Kimmey MB, Silverstein FE, with contributions by JJ Bonica: Diseases of the gastrointestinal tract, Chapter 60. *The Management of Pain*. Ed. 2. Edited by Bonica JJ, Loeser JD, Chapman CR, Fordyce WE. Lea & Febiger, Philadelphia, 1990 (pp. 1186–1213).

62. Knapp L, Atchison JW, Shapiro R, *et al.*: Electromyographic and kinematic analysis of the painful hemiplegic shoulder before and after subscapularis motor point block. *Arch Phys Med Rehabil* 77:925–926, 1996.

63. Kniffki K-D, Mense S, Schmidt RF: Responses of group IV afferent units from skeletal muscle to stretch, contraction and chemical stimulation. *Exp Brain Res* 31:511–522, 1978.

64. Kniffki K-D, Schomburg ED, Steffens H: Synaptic effects from chemically activated fine muscle afferents upon α-motoneurones in decerebrate and spinal cats. *Brain Res* 206:361–370, 1981.

65. Kuchera ML: Gravitational stress, musculoligamentous strain, and postural alignment. *Spine* 9(2):463–490, 1995.

66. Lewit K: Muskelfehlsteuerung und Schmerz. *Schmerzstudien 6, Schmerz und Bewegungssystem*. Edited by Berger M, Gerstenbrand F, Lewit K. Fischer, Stuttgart, 1984 (pp. 88–97).

67. Lewit K: Chain reactions in disturbed function of the motor system. *Man Med* 3:27–29, 1987.

68. Lewit K: Management of muscular pain associated with articular dysfunction. *J Man Med* 6:140–142, 1991.

69. Liebenson C: *Rehabilitation of the Spine: A Practitioner's Manual*. Williams & Wilkins, Baltimore, 1996.

70. Loeser JD, Sullivan M: Disability in the chronic low back pain patient may be iatrogenic. *Pain Forum* 4:114–121, 1995.

71. Loeser JD, Sullivan M: On sorting out the crocks. *Pain Forum* 4:132–133, 1995.

72. Long DM: Effectiveness of therapies currently employed for persistent low back and leg pain. *Pain Forum* 4:122–125, 1995.

73. Lund JP, Donga R, Widmer CG, *et al.*: The pain-adaptation model: a discussion of the relationship between chronic musculoskeletal pain and motor activity. *Can J Physiol Pharmacol* 69:683–694, 1991.

74. Mense S: Nervous outflow from skeletal muscle following chemical noxious stimulation. *J Physiol* 267:75–88, 1977.

75. Mense S, Meyer H: Different types of slowly conducting afferent units in cat skeletal muscle and tendon. *J Physiol* 363:403–417, 1985.

76. Mense S, Skeppar P: Discharge behaviour of feline gamma-motoneurones following induction of an artificial myositis. *Pain* 46:201–210, 1991.

77. Mertens HG, Ricker K: Übererregbarkeit der gamma-Motoneurone beim "Stiff-man" Syndrom. *Klin Wochenschr* 46:33–42, 1968.

78. Mulholland MW, Debas HT, with contributions by Bonica JJ: Diseases of the liver, biliary system, and pancreas, Chapter 61. *The Management of Pain.* Ed. 2. Edited by Bonica JJ, Loeser JD, Chapman CR, Fordyce WE. Lea & Febiger, Philadelphia, 1990 (pp. 1214–1231).

79. Nachemson AL: Newest knowledge of low back pain. A critical look. *Clin Orthop* 279:8–20, 1992.

80. Nouwen A, Bush C: The relationship between paraspinal EMG and chronic low back pain. *Pain* 20:109–123, 1984.

81. O'Leary J, Heinbecker P, Bishop GH: Analysis of function of a nerve to muscle. *Am J Physiol* 110:636–658, 1935.

82. Paintal AS: Participation by pressure-pain receptors of mammalian muscles in the flexion reflex. *J Physiol* 156:498–514, 1961.

83. Plowman SA: Physical activity, physical fitness, and low back pain. *Exerc Sport Sci Rev* 20:221–242, 1992.

84. Ramcharan JE, Wyke B: Articular reflexes at the knee joint: an electromyographic study. *Am J Physiol* 223:1276–1280, 1972.

85. Richardson D: Blood flow response of human calf muscles to static contractions at various percentages of MVC. *J Appl Physiol* 51:929–933, 1981.

86. Richmond FJR, Loeb GE: Electromyographic studies of neck muscles in the intact cat. II. Reflexes evoked by muscle nerve stimulation. *Exp Brain Res* 88:59–66, 1992.

87. Rinzler SH, Travell J: Therapy directed at the somatic component of cardiac pain. *Am Heart J* 35:248–268, 1948.

88. Roberts WJ, Elardo SM: Sympathetic activation of A-delta nociceptors. *Somatosens Res* 3:33–44, 1985.

89. Schaible H-G, Grubb BD: Afferent and spinal mechanisms of joint pain. *Pain* 55:5–54, 1993.

90. Schneider MJ: Chiropractic management of myofascial and muscular disorders. *Adv Chiropract* 3:55–88, 1996.

91. Schomburg ED: Spinal sensorimotor systems and their supraspinal control. *Neurosci Res* 7:265–340, 1990.

92. Schomburg ED: Spinal functions in sensorimotor control movements. *Neurosurg Rev* 13:179–185, 1990.

93. Sella G: Personal communication, 1996.

94. Shea VK, Perl ER: Failure of sympathetic stimulation to affect responsiveness of rabbit polymodal nociceptors. *J Neurophysiol* 54:513–519, 1985.

95. Simons DG, Simons LS: Chronic myofascial pain syndromes, Chapter 44. *Handbook of Pain Management.* Ed. 2. Edited by Tollison CD. Williams & Wilkins, Baltimore, 1994 (pp. 556–577).

96. Simons DG, Travell JG, Simons LS: *Travell & Simons' Myofascial Pain and Dysfunction: The Trigger Point Manual, Vol. 1. Upper Half of Body.* Ed. 2. William & Wilkins, Baltimore, 1999.

97. Spencer JD, Hayes KC, Alexander IJ: Knee joint effusion and quadriceps reflex inhibition in man. *Arch Phys Med Rehabil* 65:171–177, 1984.

98. Starlanyl D, Copeland ME: *Fibromyalgia & Chronic Myofascial Pain Syndrome: A Survival Guide.* New Harbinger Publications, Oakland, CA, 1996.

99. Stokes M, Young A: The contribution of reflex inhibition to arthrogenous muscle weakness. *Clin Sci* 67:7–14, 1984.

100. Sylvest O, Hvid N: Pressure measurements in human striated muscles during contraction. *Acta Rheum Scand* 5:216–222, 1959.

101. Tanji J, Kato M: The long-lasting effects of cutaneous and high threshold muscle afferent volleys on semitendinosus γ-motoneurones. *Brain Res* 40:523–526, 1972.

102. Thompson E: Myofascial pain: asthma of the back and back pain in the workplace. [Letter]. *Pain* 65:111, 1996.

103. Travell J, Rinzler SH: Pain syndromes of the chest muscles: resemblance to effort angina and myocardial infarction, and relief by local block. *Can Med Assoc J* 59:333–338, 1948.

104. Travell JG, Simons DG: *Myofascial Pain and Dysfunction: The Trigger Point Manual,* Vol 2. Williams & Wilkins, Baltimore, 1992.

105. Vasilyeva LF, Lewit K: Diagnosis of muscular dysfunction by inspection, Chapter 7. *Rehabilitation of the Spine: A Practitioner's Manual.* Edited by Liebenson C. Williams & Wilkins, Baltimore, 1996 (pp. 113–142).

106. Vernon H: The role of joint dysfunction in spinal myofascial pain. *J Musculoskeletal Pain* 3(2):99–104, 1995.

107. Wall PD: Back pain in the workplace. I. [Editorial Comment]. *Pain* 65:5, 1996.

108. Wall PD, Woolf CJ: Muscle but not cutaneous C-afferent input produces prolonged increases in the excitability of the flexion reflex in the rat. *J Physiol* 356:443–458, 1984.

109. Wall PD, Coderre TJ, Stern Y, et al.: Slow changes in the flexion reflex of the rat following arthritis or tenotomy. *Brain Res* 447:215–222, 1988.

110. Woolf CJ, Thompson SWN: The induction and maintenance of central sensitization is dependent on N-methyl-D-aspartic acid receptor activation: implications for the treatment of post-injury pain hypersensitivity states. *Pain* 44:293–299, 1991.

111. Woolf C, Wiesenfeld-Hallin Z: Substance P and calcitonin gene-related peptide synergistically modulate the gain of the nociceptive flexor withdrawal reflex in the rat. *Neurosci Lett* 66:226–230, 1986.

112. Yu X-M, Sessle BJ, Vernon H, et al.: Effects of inflammatory irritant applications to the rat temporomandibular joint on jaw and neck muscle activity. *Pain* 60:143–149, 1995.

CHAPTER 7

Central Pain and
Centrally Modified Pain

SUMMARY: The major tract for all types of pain in humans is the **spinothalamic tract**. One impediment to the understanding of muscle pain is the fact that most sensory cells in the spinal cord that process information from muscle nociceptors also process input from cutaneous (and visceral) nociceptors. The mechanisms by which we are capable of distinguishing between muscle and other forms of pain are still obscure.

Input from muscle nociceptors is known to be particularly effective in eliciting **neuroplastic changes** in the spinal cord. One reaction of dorsal horn neurons to input from muscle nociceptors is a long-lasting increase in excitability (**central sensitization**). This hyperexcitability is probably associated with the opening-up of formerly ineffective synaptic connections in the spinal cord. The **opening-up of synapses** is one possible mechanism for the mislocalization of muscle pain, i.e., for referral.

The **gate-control hypothesis** has been put forward as a mechanism for the modulation of pain at the spinal level. The hypothesis is appealing, but some aspects of it are still a matter of discussion. Another circuitry with pain-inhibiting properties is the **descending antinociceptive system**, which tonically inhibits nociceptive spinal neurons. The action of the descending inhibition appears to be stronger on neurons mediating deep pain than on those mediating cutaneous pain. Therefore, a dysfunction of the inhibitory system may lead to generalized pain predominantly in deep tissues, as seen in fibromyalgia.

There are also **pain-facilitating descending pathways** in the spinal cord. Thus, the sensation of pain not only depends on the presence of a noxious stimulus but also results from complex interactions between pain-inhibitory and pain-facilitatory factors.

At the **trigeminal** level of the brainstem, the mechanisms leading to muscle pain are similar to those of the spinal cord, but the organization of motor reflexes is different at the two levels. In the **thalamus**, the parvocellular region ventral to the ventrobasal complex or the ventrobasal complex itself processes information from muscle nociceptors. The **cortical** termination of the pathway(s) for muscle pain is still unknown, as is the termination for pain in general. The anterior cingulate cortex may be of significance in this regard.

Central muscle pain can occur as a sequel to a stroke that affects the spinothalamic tract or as the result of spinal cord injury.

The **post-traumatic hyperirritability syndrome** occurs after trauma that apparently disrupts the normal function of the central nervous system (CNS). Following this event, the patients become vulnerable to minor subsequent trauma. Patients who are prone to show this reaction may have a predisposing dysfunction of their CNS that can lead to a long-lasting pain condition following an initial minor trauma.

In the past, **phantom pain** was explained as a hyperexcitability of nerve sprouts in a neuroma at the site of the amputation. Such a mechanism may exist in some patients, but the typical phantom pain is now assumed to originate in neuronal pattern generators within the CNS itself. One of the most prominent examples of central pain is **thalamic pain** that can occur following a stroke in the ventrobasal complex of the thalamus.

Modulation of muscle pain by psychologic factors has to be differentiated from **psychogenic muscle pain**. The former is defined as pain that has a peripheral origin but is modified by CNS influences, whereas psychogenic pain originates in a dysfunctional CNS and lacks a peripheral source.

A. POSSIBLE CENTRAL PATHWAYS FOR MUSCLE PAIN

1. Overview

The nociceptive information from muscle is encoded in action potentials that enter the spinal cord—or, in the case of cranial nerves, the brainstem—via nociceptive muscle afferent fibers (primary afferent fibers). The terminals of these afferents contact the second-order neurons, whose cell bodies are located in the spinal cord or brainstem, through synapses. The fibers of the second-order neurons form the ascending nociceptive tracts. The signal from the nociceptors is transmitted to these second-order neurons through the release of neurotransmitter substances. The nociceptor terminals end in presynaptic boutons that release the neurotransmitters (probably glutamate or aspartate) to activate the postsynaptic (second-order) cells. That appears to be the end of the pathway that can be considered specific for muscle pain. There is no evidence for the existence of an ascending tract that exclusively mediates muscle pain. After the first synapse, the nociceptive information from muscle is largely mixed with information from other tissues: In neurophysiologic recordings, there are almost no second-order neurons that have sole input from muscle nociceptors. The majority of neurons with input from nociceptive muscle afferents additionally process information from other receptors in other tissues. These cells form the large population of so-called convergent neurons. As all people are capable of distinguishing muscle pain from cutaneous and visceral pain, the question arises how higher centers extract the information "muscle pain" from the activity in convergent neurons.

At present, the spinothalamic tract is assumed to be the main ascending pathway for (muscle) pain in the spinal cord (Fig. 7-1). This pathway is also known to mediate cutaneous and visceral pain. Recently, a connection from the spinal cord to the ventrolateral portion of the periaqueductal gray matter (PAG) in the mesencephalon and from there to the thalamus has been described that appears to conduct information solely from nociceptors in deep tissues, including muscle.[63, 115] Further research will have to show if this tract is part of a pathway that specifically mediates pain from muscle and other deep tissues.

The next main station, which also contains the second synapse of the pain pathway, is the thalamus. Here, many terminations of the pathway are located in the lateral thalamus. These terminations appear to be associated with the sensory-discriminative component of pain. This component allows the nature, intensity, and time course of a noxious stimulus to be identified. Other pain components (emotional-affective, autonomic, motor) are mediated by other portions of the thalamus. For instance, the strong connections between the anterior thalamus and the limbic

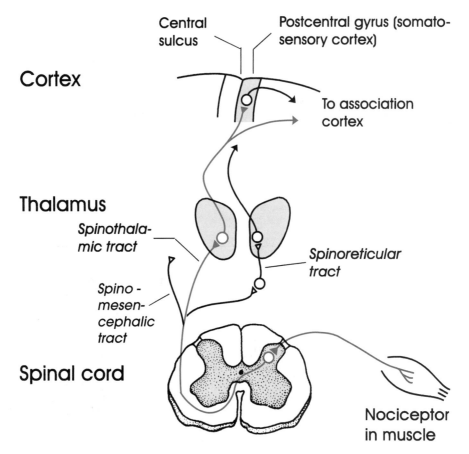

Figure 7-1. Central pain pathways. The main pathway for the mediation of muscle pain in humans is probably the spinothalamic tract, which crosses the midline near the level of entry of the nociceptive muscle afferents. The connection from the thalamus to the postcentral gyrus in the cortex may provide the sensory-discriminative aspect of muscle pain (identification of source, intensity, time course) but does not appear to be essential to account for the fact that a noxious stimulus to muscle hurts. This affective-emotional, painful aspect of muscle pain is probably mediated by cortical areas in the association cortex and in the limbic system.

The spinoreticular tract is assumed to ascend in the spinal cord both ipsilaterally and contralaterally to the painful muscle and has strong synaptic connections to the autonomic nervous system (only two of the many synapses of this tract are shown in the figure). The spinomesencephalic tract appears to be specific for deep somatic and visceral pain in the rat; its presence in humans has not yet been proven.

system as well as between the medial thalamus and the frontal cortex seem to be the basis for the affective component of pain, i.e., for the fact that a noxious stimulus hurts. This hypothesis explains why heavily traumatized patients with lesions of the frontal cortex often do not experience subjective pain, even though they are aware of their traumas and recognize the tissue lesions.

Where in the cerebral cortex the nociceptive information from muscle ends is still unknown. Evidence shows that neurons in the postcentral gyrus respond to noxious stimulation of muscle, but cells of this gyrus can be activated also by other types of noxious and innocuous stimuli. Therefore, this finding does not mean that the postcentral gyrus is the cortical area where muscle pain becomes conscious. A cortical "center" for muscle pain does not seem to exist. This also applies to pain in general: In contrast to all other sensory modalities (such as vision, hearing, mechanoreception), no region on the surface of the brain can be identified that is specialized to process muscle pain. Thus, no cortical region is known where lesions are followed by an exclusive loss of muscle pain. As outlined below, sometimes cortical lesions lead to a loss of general pain sensation, but no systematic link between the location or size of the lesion and the type and extent of the loss in pain sensation is recognizable.

2. Properties of Dorsal Horn Cells Driven by Nociceptive Input From Muscle

Location and Morphology. In the first studies dealing with slowly conducting input from muscle to dorsal horn neurons, cells receiving input from muscle group III fibers were found mainly in the neck of the dorsal horn (lamina V).[162] Later studies showed that the superficial dorsal horn (laminae I and II) likewise is an important region for nociception from deep somatic tissues[29] (Fig. 7-2). A considerable proportion of cat lamina I neurons that could be driven by noxious stimulation of muscle were found to have ascending fibers that terminate in the thalamus; i.e., they were part of the spinothalamic tract.[39] In the cat, input from slowly conducting muscle afferents is also relayed to higher centers by the spinocervical tract,[99] whose neurons of origin are located in laminae III to V (for a review of this tract, see Brown[14]). Further ascending tracts that probably convey information from deep nociceptors to higher centers are the spinoreticular tract,[61, 130] the dorsal column postsynaptic system,[3] and possibly the spinomesencephalic tract.[106, 200] For nociceptive input from neck muscles, the ventrolateral periaqueductal gray matter in the mesencepha-

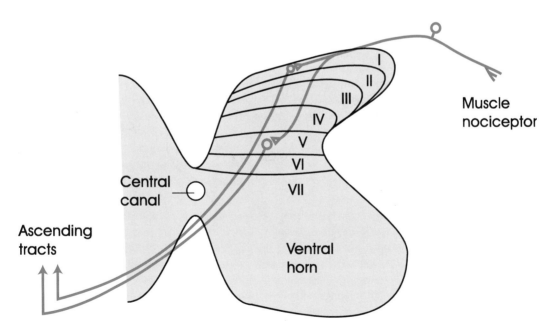

Figure 7-2. Laminae and connections of nociceptive muscle afferents in the dorsal horn of the spinal gray matter. The dorsal horn is that part of the spinal cord where most of the sensory neurons are located. Roman numerals *I* to *VII* mark the laminae after Rexed,[164] who subdivided the gray matter according to differences in size, shape, and density of neuronal cell bodies. The lamination originally had been developed for the cat but now is applied more and more to the human spinal cord.

The main synaptic connections of nociceptive muscle afferents with dorsal horn neurons are located in laminae I and V; additional ones are present in laminae II, IV, and VI. Many of the postsynaptic neurons belong to the spinothalamic tract; their axons cross the midline ventral to the central canal and ascend in the contralateral white matter, thus forming the tract.

lon appears to be an important target, whereas cutaneous nociceptors in the same region project to the lateral PAG.[115]

Similar data have been obtained from the rat and monkey. The rat spinoreticular tract has been reported to contain fibers that carry information predominantly from high-threshold (probably nociceptive) receptors in deep tissues. The cells of origin of this part of the tract are situated in the dorsolateral funiculus of the spinal cord, i.e., in the white matter (as opposed to the gray matter in the dorsal horn where sensory neuronal cell bodies are normally situated).[139] Possibly, different ascending tracts mediate the different components of pain. One finding supporting this assumption is that in the rat, there is evidence for the existence of a spinohypothalamic tract that may mediate autonomic and emotional-affective responses to pain.[18]

The location of dorsal horn cells that are probably involved in muscle pain fits well with that of primary afferent fibers from muscle nociceptors. In the few studies dealing with the spinal terminations of identified single fibers from muscle and other deep tissues, nociceptive afferent fibers have been found to form presynaptic terminals mainly in laminae I, IV, and V,[93, 144] i.e., in the same laminae in which nociceptive dorsal horn cells are located. This close spatial arrangement may be indicative of a monosynaptic connection between primary and secondary afferent neurons that mediate muscle pain.

The morphology of dorsal horn neurons processing input muscle nociceptors in muscle and other tissues seems to be diverse.[124a] In experimental animals, such as cat and rat, they include marginal cells in lamina I (Fig. 7-3), stalked cells in

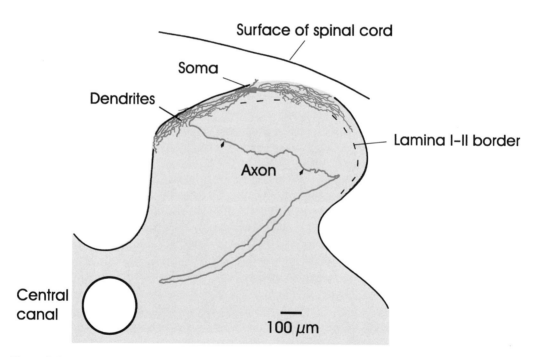

Figure 7-3. Morphology of a nociceptive marginal (Waldeyer) cell in lamina I that responded only to noxious stimulation of the muscles of the sole of the left hind paw in an anesthetized cat. The neuron was filled by intracellular injection of a dye. The soma (cell body) was located in the middle portion of lamina I, and the dendrites were distributed over almost the entire mediolateral extent of the lamina. The neuron probably belonged to the spinothalamic tract; its axon (*arrowheads*) was visible, ascending in the spinal cord approximately 200 μm within the gray matter. Its staining faded before it reached the white matter. Neurons of this type have not yet been described in the human spinal cord.

lamina II, and large multipolar cells in laminae IV to VI. The work of several groups[9, 123] has shown no clear evidence that the functional properties of a dorsal horn cell are reflected in its morphology (for reviews, see Brown[15] and Mense[141]). *Therefore, at present, dorsal horn cells mediating muscle pain cannot be recognized by their morphology.*

Response Types. *Neurons Driven Exclusively by Input From Deep Tissues.* A great proportion of dorsal horn neurons with deep input (particularly in the ventral layers of the dorsal horn) have properties of proprioceptive cells; i.e., they are dominated by input from muscle spindles and tendon organs. These cells are involved in locomotor control and are usually disregarded in the studies on deep nociception cited below.

Dorsal horn neurons responding exclusively to activation of muscle nociceptors are rare in the cat.[39] In a sample of several hundred cells with deep input studied in the laboratory of one of the authors (SM) in past years, only a few percent belonged to this type. Approximately 20% of the dorsal horn cells with deep input, however, were found to be exclusively driven by nociceptors in other deep tissues, such as joint, ligament, and tendon.[92] These neurons did not respond to innocuous mechanical stimuli but required noxious intensities of stimulation for activation. These units apparently represent a specific cell population for nociception from deep tissues, similar to the specific nociceptive cells described in studies on cutaneous nociception. In the above studies on cat dorsal horn neurons, no cell was found that had exclusive input from muscle nociceptors; nociceptive activity from muscle was processed by convergent cells that received additional input from the skin (see below). Therefore, at least in the cat, no sizable spinal pathway specific for muscle pain appears to exist.

Conversely, in a study on rat dorsal horn neurons,[209] the majority (approximately 80%) of the cells with exclusively deep input belonged to the high-threshold mechanosensitive (HTM) type, which means that they responded only to noxious mechanical stimuli (HTM deep neurons, Fig. 7-4). In contrast to the data obtained from the cat, many HTM deep neurons in the rat had receptive fields (RFs) in skeletal muscle; i.e., they could be activated by stimulating muscles. These results show that there are major species differences in the relative number of spinal neurons mediating muscle pain, and nothing is known about human dorsal horn neurons in this regard.

The remaining rat dorsal horn cells with exclusively deep input had a mechanical threshold in the innocuous range and responded strongly to weak deformation of muscle and other deep tissues (low-threshold mechanosensitive [LTM] deep neurons). The HTM deep cells, many of which had RFs in skeletal muscle, exhibited a stimulus-response function that became steeper with increasing intensity of the mechanical stimuli, whereas the response curve of LTM deep cells became flatter (Fig. 7-5). The steeper response characteristic of HTM deep neurons at high stimulation intensities may explain why muscle pain of increasing intensity, e.g., during ischemic contractions, becomes intolerable very quickly.

Neurons With Convergent Input From Receptors in Muscle and Other Tissues. It is well known that many of the dorsal horn neurons with muscle input have additional input from other sources, such as cutaneous and other deep receptors.[162] Many of these convergent cells can be excited by mechanical stimulation of small areas in both muscle and skin; i.e., they exhibit multiple (mostly two or three) separate RFs in the skin and deep tissues[92] (Fig. 7-6).

Thus, the afferent input from a large proportion of deep nociceptors appears to converge on dorsal horn neurons that can also be driven by other input sources. In contrast to cutaneous nociception, which is partly mediated by nociceptive neurons that have input exclusively from nociceptors in the skin, nociception from muscle seems to operate without dorsal horn cells that are exclusively driven by muscle nociceptors. The situation is similar to visceral nociception in which a marked viscerosomatic convergence and an almost

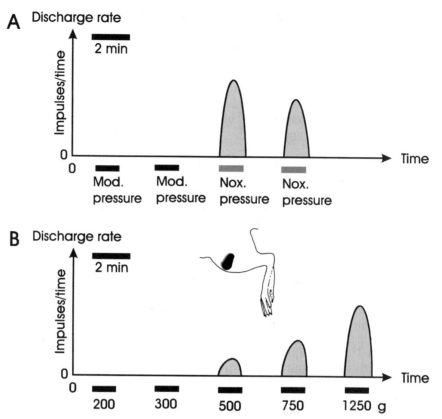

Figure 7-4. Response behavior of a high-threshold mechanosensitive (presumably nociceptive) neuron in the dorsal horn of a rat. The area from which the cell could be excited (its receptive field [RF]) was located in the biceps femoris muscle and is shown in *red* in the *inset* between panels. **A.** Responses to mechanical stimulation of the RF with moderate (*Mod.*, i.e., innocuous) and noxious (*Nox.*, i.e., painful) pressure exerted by hand with a stimulating forceps. The moderate pressure stimulus consisted of a weak deformation of the tissue, whereas the noxious stimulus was painful when applied to the hypothenar muscle of the experimenter. Note that the cell did not react to innocuous intensities of stimulation. **B.** Responses of the same neuron to mechanical stimulation of the RF with a calibrated forceps that had broadened tips 1 cm² in area. The force of stimulation is indicated in grams (*g*) underneath the *abscissa*. The 500-g stimulus was perceived as strong, marginally noxious pressure when applied to the experimenter's hypothenar muscle.

complete lack of nociceptive neurons with exclusive input from visceral nociceptors have been described.[28, 65]

Whether the HTM deep neurons alone or together with the convergent neurons are responsible for the induction of deep pain is unknown. *Input convergence from different sources does not rule out the possibility that a neuron fulfills a specific function.* In studies on dorsal horn cells with cutaneous input in monkeys, the multireceptive cells with input from various receptor classes, including nociceptors, have been reported to participate in the encoding process by which noxious stimuli to the face are perceived and identified.[52] Therefore, these neurons may mediate the sensory-discriminative component of pain that contains information on the nature, location, and duration of the noxious stimulus. In contrast, cells with exclusive input from nociceptors were assumed to mediate the affective-emotional component of pain, which is aversive and associated with suffering. The question is not settled, however; other authors have discussed the neurons with sole input from nociceptors as mediating the discriminative aspects of pain sensations.[160]

The extensive convergence at the level of the spinal neurons is one possible explanation for the poorly localized nature of muscle and other forms of deep pain. This convergence makes it difficult, however, to understand how neurons in higher central nervous centers extract the information on muscle pain from the activity of spinal neurons.

Input convergence at the spinal level is also considered to be the chief neuroanatomic basis for pain referral (see Chapter 4). Muscle pain is referred less to the skin and more to other deep somatic tissues. If the convergence concept as an explanation for pain referral is correct, referral from muscle to other deep tissues would require dorsal horn neurons with multiple RFs in deep tissues. Such neurons have been found during experiments on cats and rats[92, 209] but were few in number. Assuming that the data obtained in animals can be transferred to humans, this would mean that a small number of neurons cause a widespread phenomenon such as referred muscle pain. More recent data indicate that the number of dorsal horn cells with double or multiple RFs in muscle increases within a few hours following a muscle lesion (see below, "Behavior Under Pathologic Conditions").[94]

Because referral of muscle pain to the skin is the exception rather than the rule, the many convergent neurons with input from both muscle and skin are probably not

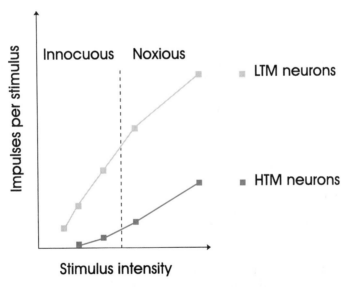

Figure 7-5. Stimulus-response curves of dorsal horn neurons processing input from deep tissues. Low-threshold mechanosensitive (*LTM*) neurons (*light red*) began to respond at low levels of innocuous intensities of stimulation and exhibited a less steep increase in their responses when strong stimuli were applied. High-threshold mechanosensitive (*HTM*) neurons (*dark red*) required strong stimuli for activa- tion. Some of them (as shown in Fig. 7-4) did not respond to innocuous stimuli at all, but in the mean values of this figure, a marginal response to strong innocuous stimuli is recognizable. This marginal response to strong innocuous stimuli is an important aspect of the function of nociceptive neurons as a warning system, which would signal the danger of tissue damage and not the presence of a lesion.

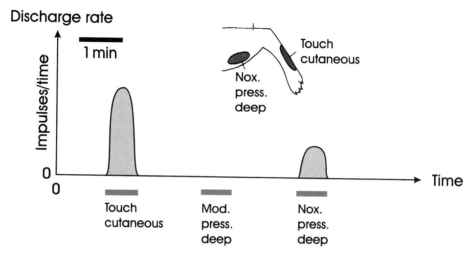

Figure 7-6. Response properties and receptive fields (RF) of a convergent neuron recorded in an anesthetized cat. The *inset* shows the two RFs (*red areas*) from which the neuron could be excited: one in the skin of the lateral aspect of the left hind paw, where touching the skin was sufficient to activate the cell (*Touch cutaneous*); and the other in the tibialis anterior muscle, where noxious pressure on the subcutaneous tissues had to be exerted to excite the neuron (*Nox. press. deep*). Pinching the skin in the latter area was ineffective. The histogram of the impulse activity shows the relatively large response of the cell to the weak touch stimulus of the skin and the small response of the same neuron to squeezing the tibialis anterior muscle. Innocuous deformation of the muscle (*Mod. press. deep*) was without effect. This indicated that the response to deep input originated in muscle nociceptors and not in the skin.

involved in the referral of muscle pain. It is more likely that these cells mediate cutaneous hypoesthesia,[73] hyperesthesia, or hyperalgesia that may accompany muscle pain. Such a function would require that the convergent cells mediate cutaneous, and not muscular, sensations. No conclusive data on this latter aspect are available.

Somatotopy in the Dorsal Horn. As described in Chapter 4, referral of muscle pain is basically a mislocalization of pain, because the referred pain is felt remote from its source. Generally, localization of a stimulus is assumed to depend on a somatotopical arrangement of central nervous neurons; i.e., each cell has afferent connections with a particular body region (its RF). A given neuron responds only if its RF is stimulated. This means that the discharge of a neuron always contains information about the site of the stimulus. With regard to the localization of muscle pain, it would be important to know whether dorsal horn neurons with deep input are somatotopically arranged.

A statistical analysis in which the proximodistal location of the RF on the hindlimb was correlated with the mediolateral location of the recording site in the dorsal horn showed that cells with deep RFs on the distal hindlimb were located medially in the dorsal horn and those with proximal RFs were located laterally.[210] If we assume that the cells with nociceptive input from deep tissues mediate deep pain, this somatotopy combined with relatively small RF sizes could form the neuroanatomic basis for a good localization of the pain, but apparently it is not used for this purpose. Possibly, the somatotopical arrangement is important for controlling local motor reflexes.

Behavior Under Pathologic Conditions. Systematic studies of the discharge behavior of dorsal horn neurons during pathologic alterations of skeletal muscle are missing. Preliminary results indicate that an acute experimental lesion (such as a myositis) leads to a raised background discharge in rat dorsal horn neurons and to an expansion of the spinal region in which cells can be driven by input from that muscle[95] (Fig. 7-7). Data obtained in rats with chronic polyarthritis,[21] in cats with acute arthritis,[174] and in rats with subacute adjuvant-induced inflammation of the subcutaneous tissues of the hindpaw[107] all point in the same direction, namely, that an inflammation of deep tissues induces an enhanced excitability in dorsal horn neurons that is expressed in increased background discharge, enlarged and/or additional RFs, enhanced responsiveness to mechanical stimuli, and increased convergence from peripheral sources (e.g., skin and deep tissues). All these changes are indications of central sensitization; i.e., the neurons have become more excitable because of sustained nociceptive input from deep tissues.

Genetic evidence indicates that the inflammation-induced increase in excitability is associated with an increased expression of the messenger ribonucleic acid (mRNA) of the immediate-early gene c-fos in the nuclei of the neurons, followed by an elevation in preprodynorphin mRNA.[48] The increased expression of immediate-early genes is known to be one of the cellular reactions to noxious stimuli. (It is not specific for noxious stimuli, however, because it also occurs in response to innocuous stimulation.) The immediate-early gene c-fos controls the synthesis of a protein (c-FOS protein) that acts as a transcription factor. The protein influences

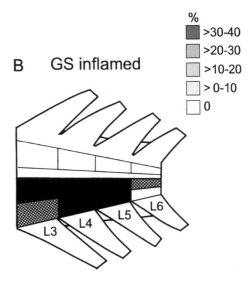
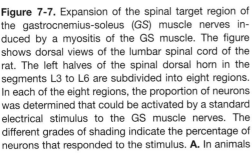
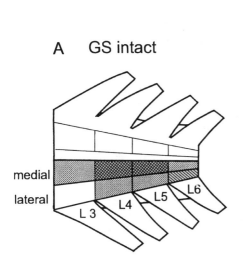

%
■ >30-40
▨ >20-30
▨ >10-20
□ > 0-10
□ 0

A   GS intact

B   GS inflamed

medial

lateral

L 3   L4   L5   L6

L3   L4   L5   L6

Figure 7-7. Expansion of the spinal target region of the gastrocnemius-soleus (*GS*) muscle nerves induced by a myositis of the GS muscle. The figure shows dorsal views of the lumbar spinal cord of the rat. The left halves of the spinal dorsal horn in the segments L3 to L6 are subdivided into eight regions. In each of the eight regions, the proportion of neurons was determined that could be activated by a standard electrical stimulus to the GS muscle nerves. The different grades of shading indicate the percentage of neurons that responded to the stimulus. **A.** In animals with intact muscle, the main target area was the medial dorsal horn in the segments L4 and L5. **B.** In animals with inflamed muscle, the population of responding neurons showed a marked expansion. This effect was most marked in the lateral dorsal horn and in the segment L3, which does not normally receive much input from the GS muscle. In the lateral L3 segment, there was a qualitative effect: In animals with intact muscle, not a single neuron responded to the standard stimulus, whereas in myositic animals, 20 to 30% did.

the production of cellular proteins and thus is capable of changing the functional properties of the cell.[47]

The increased background activity in nociceptive and other dorsal horn cells may cause the spontaneous pain and dysesthesia present in many arthritis and myositis patients. The tenderness of the inflamed tissue is probably caused not only by sensitization of peripheral nociceptors but also by sensitization of dorsal horn neurons (see section on neuroplasticity below). This central sensitization may cause tenderness and/or hyperalgesia not only by a general enhancement of excitability but also by enlargement of the RFs. A larger mean size of the RFs is likely to lead to a greater overlap between RFs and thus to an increase in the number of neurons that are excited by a given noxious stimulus.[49]

Signs of Neuroplasticity in Neurons Processing Input From Muscle Nociceptors. *Basic Mechanisms Involved in Plastic Changes of Synapses.*   Some of the synaptic processes that apparently underlie neuroplastic changes in the central nervous system (CNS) are outlined in Figure 7-8. The scheme has been developed mainly for long-term potentiation (LTP) in the hippocampus, but it is likely that similar processes occur in other places where neuroplasticity can be found. In the hippocampus, LTP represents a neuroplastic change that is characterized by a long-lasting increase in neuronal excitability following a short-lasting, high-frequency input. LTP is considered an important component of learning processes.

For the purpose of this book, the above concept has been adapted to explain pain from muscle. The data presented in the previous section show that at the spinal level neuroplastic changes occur that resemble LTP in many ways. In Figure 7-8, two basic situations have been distinguished:

1. Transient activation of an afferent pathway by a physiologic painful stimulus, such as a blow to a muscle or the tearing of a muscle. The resulting input has a low discharge frequency and a short duration; thus, it will lead to transient pain but not to long-lasting changes in neuronal responsiveness.

2. High-frequency activation by a strong, prolonged noxious stimulus, which likely leads to neuroplastic changes.

The synaptic events accompanying normal activation are depicted in Figure 7-8A: The nociceptive afferent fiber A releases glutamate as a transmitter substance. Glutamate acts on two main classes of membrane ion channels by binding to specific receptor molecules, namely, one controlled by N-methyl-D-aspartate (NMDA) receptors (the so-called NMDA channel) and channels controlled by other excitatory amino acid receptors (the non-NMDA channels). Besides glutamate receptors opening ion channels, there are also metabotropic glutamate receptors that influence the metabolism of the postsynaptic neuron. These receptors are not addressed in this chapter. Quisqualate and kainate are the main transmitter substances opening the non-NMDA channel by binding to specific receptor molecules. Binding of glutamate to the non-NMDA receptors opens the channel for positively charged small ions (mainly sodium ions), which enter the cell and depolarize the membrane (make its negative resting potential less negative). Because the depolarization brings the neuron closer to its firing threshold, the depolarization represents an excitatory postsynaptic potential. If the depolarization is large enough, the postsynaptic cell will fire an action potential; this requires the simultaneous activation of a large number of synapses.

With a certain delay, impulses will also arrive via inhibitory interneurons. In the figure, the inhibitory synapse is assumed to use γ-aminobutyric acid (GABA) as a transmitter; in the spinal cord, glycine is common for inhibiting postsynaptic neurons. The inhibitory transmitter likewise opens ion channels in the membrane by binding to receptor molecules, but in this case the ion flux leads to a hyperpolarization of the membrane, e.g., by an inward movement of negative ions. By this mechanism, the cell becomes less excitable; the synaptic potential has an inhibitory action on the postsynaptic cell (inhibitory postsynaptic potential). The hyperpolarization counteracts the depolarization and helps restore the normal resting membrane potential. One im-

A Low-frequency stimulation   **B High-frequency stimulation**

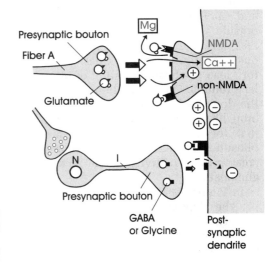

Figure 7-8. Basic synaptic events underlying plastic changes in the function of a neuron of the CNS. Such events are known to occur in the hippocampus but are probably also present in other parts of the nervous system. Two situations are shown: (**A**) low-frequency (transient) stimulation eliciting a short-lasting depolarization of the postsynaptic cell, and (**B**) high-frequency (strong) stimulation eliciting prolonged depolarization that results in plastic changes.

A. The excitatory input arrives via afferent fiber A, which releases glutamate as a transmitter. For reasons of simplicity, glutamate is assumed to bind to two types of receptor molecules only, namely, the N-methyl-D-aspartate (*NMDA*) receptors and the non-NMDA receptors (in reality, there are more receptor types for glutamate). These receptors control ion channels; i.e., binding of glutamate to the receptor molecule opens a channel protein by changing the conformation of the protein that allows ions to pass through the channel (a pore within the protein). In the absence of stimuli and during low-frequency activation, the NMDA channel is blocked by magnesium ions (*Mg*). Binding of glutamate to the non-NMDA receptors opens the associated channels, and positive ions enter the cell, leading to a short-lasting depolarization.

The depolarization is counteracted by the hyperpolarization brought about by the inhibitory interneuron I. The interneuron uses GABA or glycine as a transmitter and causes influx of Cl⁻ ions into the postsynaptic dendrite, which adds to the negative charges at the inside of the membrane. (The normal resting membrane potential of central nervous neurons is 90 mV, inside negative). **B.** During high-frequency stimulation, the depolarization of the postsynaptic membrane is large enough to remove the Mg ions from the NMDA channel. By binding to the NMDA receptor, glutamate opens the NMDA channel, and calcium ions (Ca^{++}) together with other positive ions enter the cell. Ca^{++} can activate protein kinases that phosphorylate the non-NMDA receptor proteins. This leads to a higher excitability of the non-NMDA channels.

The interneuron I becomes fatigued during high-frequency stimulation and releases less transmitter during repetitive activation. Therefore, the hyperpolarization becomes less pronounced. This is an important mechanism in maintaining the depolarization of the postsynaptic neuron. *N* indicates the nucleus of the interneuron. (Redrawn after Bliss TV, Collingridge GL: A synaptic model of memory: long-term potentiation in the hippocampus. *Nature* 361:31–39, 1993.)

portant aspect of this normal activation is that the NMDA channel is not opened. It is blocked by magnesium ions that move away from the channel only when the membrane is depolarized to a sufficient degree for a certain period of time. In the open state, the NMDA channel lets calcium ions flow into the cell.

Figure 7-8*B* shows the events at the same synapses in the presence of a strong and prolonged noxious stimulus. The frequency of the incoming action potentials via the nociceptive fiber A is so high that a persistent depolarization of the postsynaptic membrane is produced because of summation of the postsynaptic potentials. This leads to the abolition of the magnesium block; if now the glutamate molecules bind to the NMDA receptors, the channel opens and calcium ions enter the cell from the outside. The calcium ions act as second messengers; they probably activate various intracellular protein kinases, which in turn lead to phosphorylation of intracellular proteins. One possible explanation for the long-lasting increase in excitability brought about by the calcium influx is that the non-NMDA receptors are also phosphorylated. The phosphorylation increases the sensitivity of the receptors to glutamate.

In Figure 7-8B, a mechanism maintaining the depolarization has been added, namely, that the inhibitory interneuron fatigues rapidly during repetitive activation. This process is associated with a decrease in the inhibitory hyperpolarizing potentials that normally counteract the depolarization (for a review of the synaptic events, see Ref. 36).

The above model is based on data obtained from hippocampal neurons; it does not address the possible involvement of neuropeptides in neuroplastic changes. In the spinal cord, substance P (SP) released from the terminals of nociceptive primary afferent fibers may strongly influence the process because SP by itself can cause long-lasting depolarizations in dorsal horn neurons.[163, 214]

At present, it is difficult to say how strong the parallels between learning processes in the hippocampus and changes in dorsal horn excitability during chronic pain really are. The statement that the transition from acute to chronic pain in patients resembles a learning process (albeit unwanted) at the spinal and higher levels is, however, justified. In the treatment of muscle pain, the nociceptive input from muscle should be abolished as early as possible, not only to relieve the patient's pain but also to prevent the development of chronic neuroplastic changes in thea CNS.

In the long run, repeated activation of the NMDA-controlled channel will probably lead to the formation of a persistent synaptic connection with consistent transmission or to strengthening of ineffective synapses that originally elicited subthreshold excitatory postsynaptic potentials only. This mechanism is assumed to play a role in learning processes at higher levels of the CNS. For example, neurons in the striatum of male singing birds have been shown to acquire new connections this way in the process of learning their species-specific song.[150] Similar events appear to occur in cortical neurons in mammals during associative learning.[42]

In humans, central nervous plasticity may be an important factor for postoperative pain, part of which seems to result from a central change following the noxious input that is inevitably associated with surgical interventions. Local anesthesia of the operation site (in addition to general anesthesia) has been suggested as a possible means of preventing the intraoperative central sensitization.[196]

In this context, the treatment of acute muscle pain gets a new and additional meaning: Besides abolishing the pain and restoring normal function, treatment should aim at preventing the central sensitization. It is conceivable that if the treatment fails, the prolonged and repeated input from muscle nociceptors triggers events in the CNS that eventually lead to a chronic pain condition. The whole process is probably associated with morphologic changes in the CNS[186] that are reversed with difficulty.

Changes in Dorsal Horn Connectivity Following a Muscle Lesion. When noxious stimuli are applied in animal experiments, a frequent finding is that nociceptive neurons not only respond to the stimulus but also increase their sensitivity during repeated stimulation. This means that the discharge of a nociceptive cell may grow larger, even though the stimulus strength is constant. In humans, this mechanism can lead to an increase in subjective pain when the peripheral lesion is unchanged or even improving objectively. Such changes in the processing of nociceptive information usually occur following strong or long-lasting (repeated) noxious stimulation; the underlying neuronal mechanisms are often called "modulation" or "neuroplasticity."

The term "modulation" is mostly used for characterizing a change in the discharge of a neuron under the influence and in the presence of a modulating factor (e.g., a sensitizing substance). This definition implies that the neuron regains its original properties if the modulating factor is no longer present. In contrast, "neuroplasticity" describes longer-lasting alterations of neuronal properties (e.g., during development or learning processes). In animal experiments, the latter term is often used to characterize changes that outlast a triggering stimulus.

After their induction by a nociceptive input, the neuroplastic changes may become independent of the input, as has been shown in a study of the hyperexcitability (central sensitization) of rat dorsal horn neurons following the induction of an inflammation of the paw.[107] On a long-time scale, the neurons change not only their discharge behavior but also their morphologic appearance; particularly remarkable changes have been described for the form and size of synapses.[20] The transition from functional to morphologic changes may parallel the transition from acute to chronic pain. After a painful state becomes structured by morphologic changes, successful treatment will require more time to reverse the changes.

In dorsal horn neurons, neuroplastic changes require input via unmyelinated or thin myelinated afferent fibers; i.e., afferent activity in thick myelinated fibers is not sufficient. For unknown reasons, input via *muscle* C fibers is more effective than cutaneous input in inducing prolonged changes in neuronal behavior.[198] In experiments on anesthetized animals, plastic changes in dorsal horn neurons can be easily demonstrated following noxious chemical stimulation of skeletal muscle.

An example of plastic behavior of a neuron following noxious stimulation of skeletal muscle is given in Figure 7-9. The neuron had two HTM RFs, one in the gastrocnemius-soleus muscle and another one in the semitendinosus muscle. The first injection of a painful dose of bradykinin (BK) into the RF in the semitendinosus muscle led to a lowering in the mechanical threshold of the injected RF and to a large expansion of the RF size. Simultaneously, the threshold of the noninjected RF in the gastrocnemius-soleus muscle dropped to innocuous levels. The lowering in mechan-

ical threshold of the injected RF can be attributed to a BK-induced sensitization of the nociceptors in the semitendinosus muscle, but the expansion of the injected RF and the lowering in threshold of the RF in the gastrocnemius-soleus muscle suggest that the excitability of the recorded dorsal horn neuron has increased; i.e., central sensitization has occurred.

Following the second injection of BK, the lowering in threshold of the noninjected RF in the gastrocnemius-soleus muscle persisted for more than 30 minutes (at that time the recording of the neuron's activity was discontinued). This means that the BK-induced CNS effect lasted much longer than the afferent activity elicited by the intramuscular injection of the kinin, which has a duration of a few minutes, at most.[143]

The sensitization of the dorsal horn neuron in Figure 7-9 was probably induced by a strong activation of the slowly conducting afferent fibers connecting the neuron with its RFs, as fast-conducting afferent units from muscle are not excited by BK.[140] Injections of BK into muscles outside the RF of the recorded neuron showed that by such a procedure, similar changes in response behavior can be induced; approximately half of the neurons tested developed new RFs. The neurons were not excited by the BK injection; i.e., the activation of a cell was not a prerequisite for its sensitization.

The lowering in threshold of the RF in the gastrocnemius-soleus muscle can be explained by assuming that the cell that originally responded exclusively to input from nociceptive fibers is now also driven by non-nociceptive afferents. This demonstrates that, following sensitization, nociceptive central cells may respond to input from sensitive mechanoreceptors.[205] Clinically, this situation is likely to lead to allodynia.

One possible explanation for these findings is that slowly conducting muscle afferents are activated by BK and release glutamate together with neuropeptides from their terminal branches in the dorsal horn that alter the responsiveness of dorsal horn neurons. A similar hypothesis was derived from experiments in which the flexor reflex of rats was increased for prolonged periods of time following activation of muscle C fibers as a conditioning

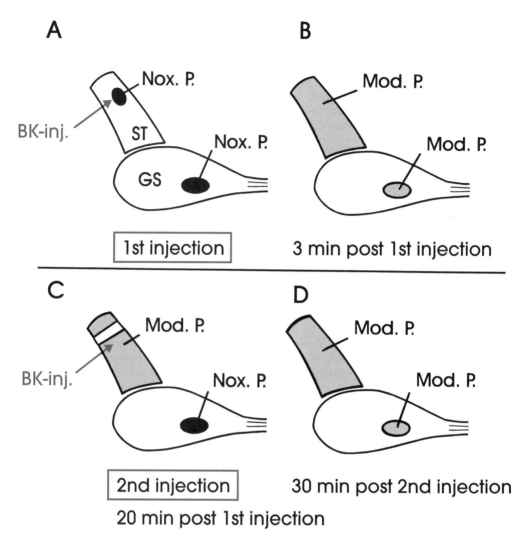

Figure 7-9. Enlargement of a bradykinin-injected receptive field (RF) and lowering in mechanical threshold of a second, noninjected RF of a dorsal horn neuron. **A.** Situation at the time and before injection of bradykinin (*BK*). The neuron had two RFs (*black*), one in the semitendinosus (*ST*) muscle and the other in the gastrocnemius-soleus (*GS*) muscle. Both had high mechanical thresholds and required noxious pressure (*Nox. P.*) stimulation to activate the cell. **B.** Three minutes after injection of a painful dose of BK into the ST muscle, the injected RF was greatly enlarged (*light red*) and had a low mechanical threshold. Stimulation of the enlarged RF with moderate (innocuous) pressure (*Mod. P.*) was sufficient to excite the neuron. The RF in the GS muscle (which surely did not come into contact with the BK solution) likewise showed a decrease in mechanical threshold. **C.** Twenty minutes after injection of BK, the time of the second injection into the ST muscle. Note that the mechanical threshold of the RF in the GS muscle had returned to its normal high value (*black*), whereas the threshold of the injected RF in the ST muscle was still lowered (*light red*). The ST now exhibited an insensitive strip (*white*) from which no response of the neuron could be elicited. **D.** Following the second BK injection, the mechanical threshold of the RF in the GS, and the entire ST muscle (*light red*) was lowered for the rest of the recording period (more than 30 minutes).

The data show that a painful stimulus to one RF of a neuron can influence the excitability of that neuron from another RF located remote from the site of the stimulus. Such a behavior is indicative of an increase in the excitability of the dorsal horn neuron, i.e., of a central sensitization. (Redrawn after Hoheisel U, Mense S: Long-term changes in discharge behaviour of cat dorsal horn neurones following noxious stimulation of deep tissues. *Pain* 36:239–247, 1989.)

stimulus.[204] Because the afferent limb of the reflex was not activated by the conditioning stimulus, the underlying mechanism was called heterosynaptic facilitation. If similar events also occur in humans, a painful lesion of a muscle could influence not only the spinal neuron pool that has synaptic connections with the site of the lesion but also neighboring neurons via the release of sensitizing substances (e.g., SP) from muscle afferents. Because the neighboring neurons normally subserve sensations from body regions remote from the lesion and now respond to input from the lesion, the afferent inflow from the lesion elicits subjective sensations from regions outside the damaged muscle. This mechanism may underlie the spread or referral of muscle pain as outlined in Chapter 4.

SP as a Possible Mediator of Central Neuroplastic Changes. Results from experiments in which SP was applied iontophoretically to dorsal horn neurons have demonstrated that this neuropeptide may be involved in the induction of neuroplastic changes by causing long-lasting depolarization in many of these cells, predominantly in nociceptive ones.[88, 163, 214] As pointed out above, the SP-induced depolarization could be an important step in triggering neuroplastic processes in that it abolishes the Mg^{++} block of the NMDA-sensitive Ca^{++} channel. Normally, the block prevents Ca^{++} ions from entering the cell (Fig. 7-8) and acting as an intracellular second messenger that induces the phosphorylation of receptor molecules and the expression of immediate-early genes such as c-fos.[43, 51, 105, 129, 151, 183]

In fact, the combined effect of SP action and NMDA-channel activation has been proposed as a possible mechanism for the sensitization of spinothalamic tract cells, which may underlie the development of hyperalgesia in patients.[46] The importance of NMDA receptor activation for the development of hyperalgesia has also been stressed in behavioral experiments in rats.[178] Evidence indicates that the release of nitric oxide from the postsynaptic cell may likewise be an important link in the pathway from NMDA receptor activation to neuroplastic changes.[67, 149]

SP-Induced Unmasking of Synaptic Connections in the Dorsal Horn. The action of SP on the responsiveness of dorsal horn neurons with input from deep tissues can be studied by superfusing the spinal cord of anesthetized rats with an SP solution and simultaneously recording the impulse activity of single cells.[97] Under the influence of the neuropeptide, some neurons acquired a new A- or C-fiber input, other cells lost an existing input, and still others showed a decrease in spike amplitude and loss of recordable neuron activity. At a concentration of 100 μM, SP affected 75% of the neurons studied, with the main effect being the unmasking of a formerly ineffective input. The unmasking of fiber connections to dorsal horn neurons may be clinically relevant, particularly if A-fiber input from LTM (non-nociceptive) receptors gains access to nociceptive dorsal horn cells. As outlined above, this situation may lead to allodynia in patients.[203, 205]

SP not only influenced the electrical excitability of the neurons but also induced marked RF changes in a large proportion of the cells tested. The SP-induced changes were comparable with those observed after intramuscular BK injections and consisted of expansions of existing RFs (Fig. 7-10) and formation of new ones. Apparently, SP opened up fiber connections between the dorsal horn neurons and the new portions of the RF.

One possible interpretation of the data is that at least some of the dorsal horn neurons possess synaptic connections that are ineffective under normal circumstances. Activation of muscle nociceptors by a strong noxious stimulus can unmask these connections (similar processes can occur following input interruption; see Wall[194]). The unmasking leads to a change in RF size and/or response properties of the cells. Comparable effects have been observed in neurons of the subnucleus caudalis and oralis of the trigeminal spinal tract nucleus, i.e., in those nuclei where afferent fibers from the head region terminate.[102] SP (probably together with calcitonin gene-related peptide)[96] is surely one of the factors capable of unmasking neuronal connections in the dorsal horn. The finding

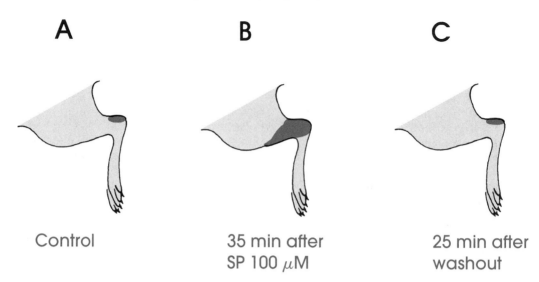

A

B

C

Control

35 min after
SP 100 μM

25 min after
washout

Figure 7-10. Changes in the size of the receptive field (RF, *dark red*) of a dorsal horn neuron induced by spinal superfusion of substance P (SP). The superfusion was performed in such a way that the exposed spinal cord (only covered by the pia mater) was continuously covered with a thin film of fluid containing SP at a concentration of 100 μM.

A. Originally (before superfusion with SP), the high-threshold RF was restricted to the calcaneal tendon; i.e., the neuron could be activated by nociceptors only in the tendon. Thirty-five minutes after the beginning of the SP superfusion (**B**), the RF of the same neuron had expanded and included the gastrocnemius-soleus, tibialis anterior, and parts of the biceps femoris muscle. This means that the neuron could now also be excited by impulses from nociceptors in these muscles. The SP effect was completely reversible, albeit with a slow time course. It took the RF 25 minutes to return to the original size (**C**).

The SP effect can be explained by assuming that the neuropeptide opened up preformed but ineffective synaptic connections between the muscles and the neuron. (Redrawn after Hoheisel U, Mense S, Ratkai M: Effects of spinal cord superfusion with substance P on the excitability of rat dorsal horn neurons processing input from deep tissues. *J Musculoskeletal Pain* 3:23–43, 1995.)

that the time course of the induction of c-fos expression and that of SP effects are similar[12] supports the assumption that SP is involved in neuroplastic changes including hyperalgesia following carrageenan-induced inflammation of deep tissues.[173]

Collectively, the above data show that in addition to a **peripheral sensitization** (of nociceptive nerve endings), there is a **central sensitization** (of CNS nociceptive neurons). Both mechanisms increase the excitability of the nociceptive system and enhance pain in patients. Usually, two clinical sequelae of central sensitization are distinguished, namely, primary and secondary hyperalgesia. The term "primary hyperalgesia" describes increased pain and allodynia in the region of a peripheral lesion and can be explained by increased excitability of damaged nociceptors and dorsal horn neurons supplying that region. Secondary hyperalgesia is present if, in addition, body regions surrounding the lesion give rise to hyperalgesic or allodynic responses. In these regions, the tissue and receptors are completely intact. The secondary hyperalgesia can be explained by assuming that hyperexcitable nociceptive dorsal horn neurons (1) have acquired effective input from regions they do not normally supply and (2) respond to innocuous input.

3. Segmental Inhibition of Dorsal Horn Neurons (Gate-Control Theory)

It is a well-established fact that activity in myelinated afferent fibers inhibits the responses of nociceptive dorsal horn neurons to noxious stimuli.[75, 197] The afferents producing this effect include thick myelinated Aβ-fibers, which supply LTM (non-nociceptive) receptors, and thin myelinated Aδ-fibers, which supply both nociceptive and non-nociceptive receptors.

This type of inhibition is often called afferent or segmental, as opposed to the descending inhibition (see below). Anyone who receives a painful blow to the shin automatically induces afferent inhibition by rubbing the skin around the painful region. The resulting input via myelinated mechanosensitive fibers, combined with a liminal activation of Aδ-nociceptors, effectively inhibits pain transmission at the spinal level.[58] Possibly, the pain-relieving action of massage treatment is also partly caused by activation of thick myelinated afferents.

In the treatment of chronic pain, the inhibition of nociceptive dorsal horn neurons by myelinated afferents is utilized by the transcutaneous electrical nerve stimulation technique, which employs stimulation of a peripheral nerve through the intact skin. The stimulating parameters can be set to high frequency and low intensity for activating predominantly myelinated fibers and thus eliciting afferent inhibition. This treatment can be beneficial in many cases of neuropathies, in which a decrease in number and activity of the thick fibers is assumed to contribute to the spontaneous pain (see Chapter 3).

In 1965, Melzack and Wall[138] put forward a theory (the gate-control hypothesis) that extended the concept of afferent inhibition by adding excitatory unmyelinated fibers to the system and including a defined neuroanatomic circuit in the spinal cord (Fig. 7-11). The unmyelinated fibers were assumed to increase the excitability of transmission cells in the spinal cord by inhibiting an inhibitory interneuron in the substantia gelatinosa of the dorsal horn, thus causing disinhibition (excitation) of the transmission neuron. The transmission cell is connected to other neurons that form the action system, which elicits a variety of responses, including pain, if the gate is open. The gate consists of the substantia gelatinosa neuron, the transmission cell, and the synapses on these cells.

The innovative aspect of the theory was that the output of the transmission cell and, therefore, the intensity of pain depend on the balance between the input via myelinated (pain-inhibiting) and unmyelinated (pain-promoting) fibers. Originally, the modulating influence of the afferent fibers was assumed to act presynaptically[138] (Fig. 7-11), but a postsynaptic action is also possible.[195] In the latter case, the transmission neuron is directly hyperpolarized by the inhibitory interneuron. It is often overlooked that in the original version, the spinal circuit is under the control of supraspinal centers that can modulate the function of the system (inhibit or increase pain).

Some of the postulations of the gate-control theory have been and still are controversially discussed (see, for instance, Ref. 175). A theoretical problem is the postulate of the existence of unmyelinated fibers that have an excitatory synapse on the output neuron and inhibitory contacts with the inhibitory interneuron. If the published schemes of the gate-control theory are taken literally, the presence of inhibitory and excitatory synaptic boutons in the same fiber violates the principle that a neuron uses either excitatory or inhibitory neurotransmitters at all of its terminals. This problem could be overcome by introducing an additional inhibiting interneuron between the unmyelinated fiber and the interneuron that inhibits the output cell, but then the theory loses some of the clarity that makes it so attractive.

An important aspect of the theory is that it explains clinical cases of nerve injury in which the predominant loss of myelinated fibers—as in some cases of neuropathy—leads to spontaneous pain. For understanding the pain-alleviating action of activity in myelinated fibers, the gate-control theory is not needed because afferent segmental inhibition gives a sufficient explanation.

4. Descending Influences on Dorsal Horn Neurons Processing Input From Deep Nociceptors

Organization of the Descending Antinociceptive System. Afferent information from muscle nociceptors is transmitted to second-order neurons in the spinal dorsal horn (probably predominantly to neurons of the spinothalamic tract[72]) and ascends in axons of that tract. The ascending axons give off collaterals that make synaptic contacts with neurons in the rostral medulla (including cells in the nucleus raphe magnus [NRM]) and in the PAG of the

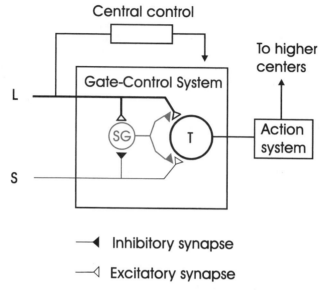

Central control

To higher centers

Gate-Control System

L

SG   T

S

Action system

◄ Inhibitory synapse

◁ Excitatory synapse

Figure 7-11. Schema of the gate-control theory of pain mechanisms. The structures in the large box are located in the gray matter of the spinal cord. L indicates large-diameter (thick myelinated) afferent fibers, and S indicates small-diameter (unmyelinated) afferent fibers. Both fiber types make synaptic contacts with inhibitory neurons in the substantia gelatinosa (*SG*) (the SG corresponds to lamina II of Rexed; see Fig. 7-2). The SG cells inhibit the transmission (*T*) cells through their presynaptic boutons (*dark red*) on the excitatory terminals of the L and S fibers. The T cells are connected to the action system. If the gate is open, the system elicits pain responses and sensations. Activity in L fibers increases the inhibition of the T cells by activating the SG neurons and closes the gate, whereas activity in S fibers reduces the inhibition (opens the gate).

The spinal gate-control system is under the influence of a central (descending) control system that can be triggered by collaterals of the large fibers. In the figure, excitatory synapses are shown as *open triangles*, and inhibitory synapses are shown as *filled black and red triangles*. Note that the schema implies that the small fibers excite the T neurons and simultaneously inhibit the SG cells. In reality, the inhibitory connection to the SG cells would require an inhibitory interneuron that is excited by the small fibers. See text for discussion. (Redrawn after Melzack R, Wall PD: Pain mechanisms: a new theory. *Science* 150:971–979, 1965.)

mesencephalon as shown in Figure 1-6. In Figure 7-12, some neurotransmitters probably used by the system are indicated (the available data on the transmitter substances are not yet complete). Theoretically, nociceptive impulses ascending the spinothalamic tract could activate the neurons in the NRM and the PAG via the collaterals, but the main excitatory input to these cells is assumed to originate in hypothalamic and cortical centers.[60] The neurons in the NRM and PAG are tonically active and produce inhibition of the spinothalamic neurons at the spinal level via multiple pathways descending in the dorsolateral spinal cord. Under normal circumstances,

the inhibition is not strong enough to completely block the spinal transmission of nociceptive signals; otherwise, there would be no pain following noxious stimulation.

There are situations, however, in which nociception is suppressed completely. For example, soldiers in combat often do not feel pain when they are wounded in action. Under these conditions, the tonic activity present in the descending antinociceptive system is enhanced by impulses originating in the hypothalamus. The hypothalamic pathway is excited as part of the CNS reaction to extreme psychic stimulation. The cells in the hypothalamus probably use endorphin (an endogenous opioid with morphine-like actions) as a transmitter. Other transmitters of the descending system are enkephalin (derived by splitting endorphin), norepinephrine, and serotonin (5-HT). The antinociceptive fibers originating in the NRM predominantly use serotonin to inhibit spinal neurons, whereas cells with origin in the nucleus ceruleus (which also belongs to the descending antinociceptive system) are mainly α-adrenergic.[6] For a recent review of the endogenous antinociceptive systems, see Sandkühler.[172]

Probably, the function of the descending antinociceptive system is to prevent nociception-induced motor reflexes such as the flexion reflex, which may interfere with

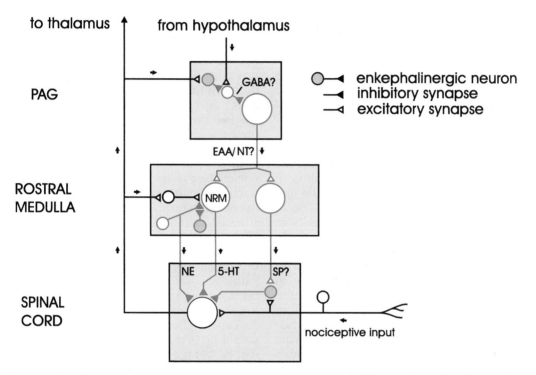

Figure 7-12. Neurotransmitters used by the descending antinociceptive system (*red structures*). As already shown in Figure 1-6, the system has three levels: (1) the periaqueductal gray matter (PAG) in the mesencephalon, from where the descending pathways are controlled; (2) the rostral medulla, where multiple antinociceptive descending pathways originate; and (3) the spinal cord, where the nociceptive information enters the CNS.

The cells in the PAG are under the influence of activity originating in the hypothalamus. This is the main excitatory input to the PAG. The descending system can also be activated via collaterals of ascending axons (on the left-hand side of the figure) that contact cells at the three levels. In the PAG, the cells of the antinociceptive system can be driven by such collaterals via two inhibitory interneurons. The boutons of these interneurons are marked by *filled red triangles*. Activation of the first (enkephalinergic) neuron (*light red*) inhibits the inhibitory second cell, which probably uses GABA as a transmitter. The double inhibition leads to a disinhibition (activation) of the large cell at the origin of the antinociceptive system.

This PAG cell drives the neurons in the rostral medulla by releasing excitatory amino acids (*EAA*, e.g., glutamate or aspartate) or possibly neurotensin (*NT*). The final inhibition of the nociceptive cells at the spinal level is mediated mainly by norepinephrine (*NE*) or serotonin (5-hydroxytryptamine [5-HT]).

Note that at each level there are enkephalinergic neurons that inhibit postsynaptic cells, either directly (spinal level) or indirectly, by inhibiting an inhibitory cell and thus activating the antinociception (medulla and PAG). Therefore, systemic administration of morphine (which has an action similar to enkephalin) contributes to the alleviation of pain at these three levels. (Redrawn after Basbaum AI, Fields HL: Endogenous pain control system: brainstem spinal pathways and endorphin circuitry. *Ann Rev Neurosci* 7:309–338, 1984.)

the coordinated movements required in a life-endangering situation. It is conceivable that the antinociceptive system is particularly important for animals in herds that are often attacked and wounded by predators such as lions and tigers. For the wounded animal, the only way to save its life is to stay in contact with the herd and to flee.

The descending inhibitory system may have still another function that may be unrelated to nociception. The descending inhibitory activity may increase the signal-to-noise ratio in the CNS by suppressing the background activity of sensory neurons and thus improve the detection of a peripheral stimulus.[172]

Tonic Inhibition of Dorsal Horn Neurons Presumably Mediating Deep Somatic Pain. In animal experiments, cooling of the spinal cord between the medulla and the recording site in the spinal dorsal horn can be used to block neuronal activity in the descending antinociceptive tracts. In dorsal horn neurons driven by input from deep somatic tissues, spinal cord cooling induced an increase in resting activity, in response magnitude to noxious stimulation of muscle (Fig. 7-13), in convergence from different receptor types, and in the number of RFs per neuron.[92, 99] These data indicate that dorsal horn neurons that presumably mediate deep pain are subjected to a strong descending inhibition that is tonically active (otherwise, it could not be abolished by interruption of conduction in descending pathways).

Parts of the descending antinociceptive system appear to act specifically on the input from nociceptors in deep tissues. This statement is based on the finding that in dorsal horn neurons with convergent input from cutaneous and deep nociceptors, the responses to stimulation of deep tissues were strongly enhanced by the spinal cold block, whereas the effects of cutaneous stimulation on the same neuron were much less affected[209] (Fig. 7-14). A similar tonically active descending inhibition has been observed in neurons with input from joints.[30]

The tonic nature of the descending inhibition suggests that a transmitter substance is continuously released at the supraspinal origin of the antinociceptive tract(s). Injections of transmitter antagonists into the third cerebral ventricle in rats have demonstrated that the tonic inhibitory influence on dorsal horn neurons with input from deep nociceptors can be abolished by the opioid antagonist, naloxone (Fig. 7-15). Neither the α-adrenergic receptor blocker, phentolamine, nor the serotonergic blocker, methysergide, was effective in this regard.[211] Injections of dye solutions showed that the antagonists injected into the third ventricle reached the PAG and the medulla, but not the spinal cord. Therefore, the site of action of the antagonists was supraspinal.

In neurons with convergent input from nociceptors in both deep tissues and skin, the intracerebroventricular injection of naloxone enhanced the responses to deep stimulation more than threefold, with little effect on the responses to activation of cutaneous nociceptors. The data suggest that at the supraspinal level, the inhibitory pathways that act tonically on deep nociception use endogenous opioids as a transmitter substance.

A speculative interpretation of these data would be that a pathologic disturbance of that part of the descending antinociceptive system controlling nociception from muscle could result in a chronic disinhibition of the dorsal horn neurons that mediate muscle pain. In humans, this could lead to generalized spontaneous pain exclusively or predominantly in muscle and other deep somatic tissues. This symptom is a prominent characteristic of the fibromyalgia syndrome (FMS). The hypothesis that a dysfunction of the descending antinociceptive system may be involved in the pain of patients with FMS has been extensively discussed by Henriksson and Mense.[87]

Results from both human studies and animal experiments indicate that at least some of the effects of massage and acupuncture are mediated by the descending inhibition. The afferent limb of the pathway activating the antinociceptive system

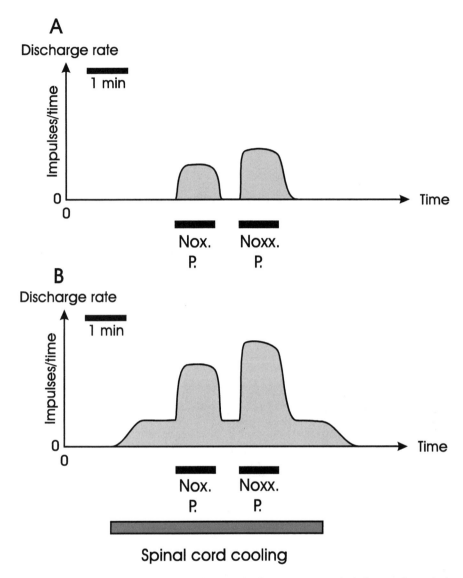

Figure 7-13. Disinhibition of a nociceptive dorsal horn neuron by a cold block of the descending antinociceptive system. In this animal experiment, the spinal cord between the medulla and the recording site at the lumbosacral level (i.e., cranial to the recording site) was cooled (*red bar*) so that conduction in the antinociceptive pathways was interrupted.

A. Responses of the neuron to noxious mechanical stimulation of the hindlimb. *Nox. P.*, noxious pressure stimulation; *Noxx. P.*, noxious pressure stimulation of higher intensity. **B.** The same stimuli as in **A** were repeated during cooling of the spinal cord. Note that directly after onset of the cooling, the neuron developed resting activity (which is likely to elicit spontaneous pain in an awake individual) and exhibited increased responses to the noxious stimuli (which means hyperalgesia in an awake organism).

That interruption of the descending system caused resting activity indicates that normally the system is tonically active and inhibits the occurrence of discharges in the absence of external stimuli.

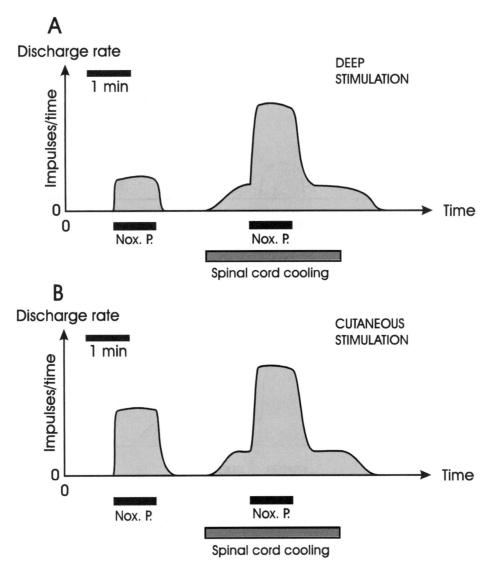

Figure 7-14. Differential action of the antinociceptive system on the responses of a single neuron to input from deep and cutaneous nociceptors. The nociceptive neuron studied had two high-threshold receptive fields (RFs), one in the skin of the hindlimb and the other in the deep tissues around the ankle joint.

A. Responses to noxious stimulation of the deep RF before and during interruption of the descending inhibition by spinal cord cooling. **B.** Responses of the same neuron to noxious stimulation of the cutaneous RF. Note that during cooling, both responses were increased, but the response to stimulation of the deep RF showed a larger increase than the response to stimulation of the cutaneous RF.

These data demonstrate that even in the same neuron, the activation by deep nociceptors is subjected to a stronger descending inhibitory influence than is the activation by cutaneous nociceptors. Therefore, a dysfunction of the descending inhibition is likely to cause spontaneous pain and hyperalgesia predominantly in deep tissues.

Discharge rate

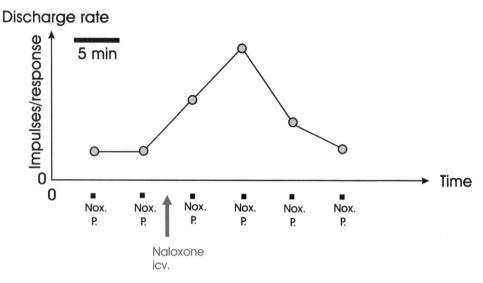

Figure 7-15. Naloxone-induced disinhibition of the responses of a dorsal horn neuron to nociceptive input from deep tissues. On the *ordinate*, the sum of impulses per stimulus fired by the neuron is shown. Noxious pressure stimulation (*Nox. P.*) of the neuron's receptive field was repeated every 5 to 6 minutes. After the second response, Naloxone (a morphine antagonist) was injected intracerebroventricularly (*icv.*) into the third cerebral ventricle. Naloxone led to a strong increase in the magnitude of response for approximately 15 minutes. This effect corresponds to a hyperalgesic state, i.e., the opposite of the effect of morphine.

The data show that the tonic activity of the descending antinociceptive system is maintained by continuous release of a substance (probably enkephalin or endorphin) acting on opioid receptors at the origin of the descending system (PAG or medulla). Because of the intracerebroventricular injection, an action of naloxone on the spinal cord could be excluded.

probably includes at least two types of afferent units:

1. The first of these consists of non-nociceptive receptors in deep tissues with slowly conducting afferent fibers (e.g., mechanosensitive and ergoreceptive group III muscle afferents), which are likely to be strongly excited by massage and muscular contractions. Long-lasting physical exercise is known to have an analgesic action that can lead to massive lesions of the skeletomotor system because overuse of muscles and joints is not perceived as painful. That the injury went unnoticed by the athlete may likewise be the result of strong activation of this part of the spectrum of muscle afferents (see references in Ref. 142). Experiments in rats have shown that running in a wheel increases the pain threshold. The same effect can be obtained by electrical stimulation of slowly conducting (group III and IV) muscle afferents.

2. An important input for acupuncture effects and also for the effects of strong massage stimuli (e.g., periosteal massage) presumably reaches the spinal cord via nociceptive thin myelinated afferents from deep somatic tissues, including muscle. The classical Chinese needle acupuncture requires deep penetration of subcutaneous tissues for proper treatment of functional disturbances (e.g., 4 cm deep in the stomach point 31).[4]

Descending Facilitation of Nociceptive Dorsal Horn Neurons. Nociceptive dorsal horn neurons are subjected to descending inhibitory and facilitating or excitatory influences.[124, 133] "Facilitating" means that the reaction of a (nociceptive) spinal neuron to a (noxious) stimulus is enhanced. The origin of some of the facilitating pathways are nuclei in the rostral ventral medulla, i.e., in the same area where antinociceptive cells are located.[131, 212] An important transmitter substance used by this system to facilitate spinal neurons is serotonin (5-HT) acting on $5-HT_1$ receptors.[212] This latter finding demonstrates that serotonin can inhibit (as in the descending antinociceptive system) or facilitate spinal neurons, depending on the receptor molecules that are present in the membrane of the spinal cell.

Some of the facilitating neurons have been shown to fire a short burst of action potentials just before a reaction to a painful stimulus takes place (e.g., the tail flick in animal experiments). These cells have been called "on-cells"; they are assumed to start the nociceptive tail flick reflex by facilitating the responses of spinal dorsal horn neurons to the noxious stimulus. In the rostral ventral medulla are "off-cells" that are tonically active and stop discharging just before the tail flick occurs. These neurons are assumed to have an inhibitory influence on nociceptive dorsal horn neurons.[59, 60] The neurons in the rostral medulla are known to have axonal arborizations that extend caudally to many spinal segments. Therefore, these cells are capable of influencing large populations of spinal neurons and changing the pain sensations in large regions of the body.[62]

Likewise, the wind-up behavior of dorsal horn neurons (i.e., increased responses to repeated stimuli) present in arthritic rats in response to A-fiber stimulation has been found to be dependent on a descending (facilitating) influence from supraspinal centers.[90] This A-fiber–induced wind-up is probably an indication of hyperexcitability, because normally the wind-up response requires C-fiber input. In humans, a wind-up response of nociceptive cells to A-fiber input likely leads to allodynia.

There is evidence indicating that under physiologic circumstances, activation of afferent fibers in the vagus nerve may facilitate the nociceptive tail flick via a relay in the medulla and forebrain.[69] This mechanism offers the possibility that mental or psychologic processes can increase pain sensations, because pain elicits stress and fear, which, in turn, enhance the pain. Another finding pointing in this direction is that a high level of attention improves the detection of a noxious stimulus.[19]

Collectively, the data show that the sensation of pain depends not only on the presence of a noxious stimulus but also on a large number of modulating factors. Among these factors are the activity in thick afferent fibers (leading to segmental pain inhibition) and the discharge frequency in descending antinociceptive and pain-facilitating pathways.

5. Supraspinal Mechanisms of Nociception From Muscle

Trigeminal Level. In comparison with limb muscles, much less information is available on the afferent fibers from masticatory and other head muscles. The data indicate that many of the slowly conducting muscle afferent units, including nociceptive ones, project to the subnucleus caudalis and interpolaris of the trigeminal spinal tract nucleus.[5, 155, 156, 179] In this area, second-order neurons can be found that behave similarly to those in the spinal dorsal horn[50]: Only a few cells receive exclusively nociceptive input from deep tissues, and many nociceptive neurons have convergent input from several sources, including masticatory muscles, temporomandibular joint, facial or intraoral skin, and cervical viscera (e.g., larynx). Neurons of this type are located predominantly in the superficial layers (laminae I and II) and in laminae V and VI of the subnucleus caudalis[1, 177] (Fig. 7-16), i.e., in areas that are equivalent to the superficial laminae and neck of the spinal dorsal horn.

The extensive convergence and large RF size of the nociceptive cells in the subnucleus caudalis have been considered as the neurophysiologic basis of the diffuse nature and referral that are typical features of craniofacial and temporomandibular joint pain. Signs of neuroplastic changes in convergent trigeminal neurons, following noxious stimulation of hypoglossal muscle afferents, have likewise been described.[177]

A

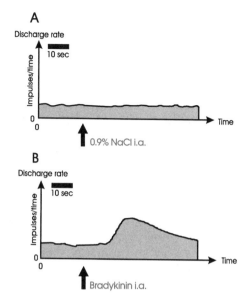

B

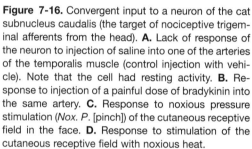

C

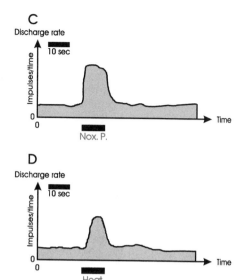

D

Figure 7-16. Convergent input to a neuron of the cat subnucleus caudalis (the target of nociceptive trigeminal afferents from the head). **A.** Lack of response of the neuron to injection of saline into one of the arteries of the temporalis muscle (control injection with vehicle). Note that the cell had resting activity. **B.** Response to injection of a painful dose of bradykinin into the same artery. **C.** Response to noxious pressure stimulation (*Nox. P.* [pinch]) of the cutaneous receptive field in the face. **D.** Response to stimulation of the cutaneous receptive field with noxious heat.

The results show that the neuron had convergent input from mechanonociceptors and heat nociceptors in the skin and chemonociceptors in muscle. In addition, it responded to innocuous pressure stimulation of the facial skin (not shown). (Redrawn after Amano N, Hu JW, Sessle BJ: Responses of neurons in feline trigeminal subnucleus caudalis (medullary dorsal horn) to cutaneous, intraoral, and muscle afferent stimuli. *J Neurophysiol* 55:227–243, 1986.)

An interesting finding that may be relevant for understanding temporomandibular disorders in patients is that noxious chemical stimulation of the temporomandibular joint in cats leads to reflex activation of masticatory muscles.[13] Such reflexes may induce transient increases in tension of craniofacial muscles for several minutes.

When considering motor reflexes at the trigeminal level, differences in organization between spinal and trigeminal reflex pathways should be kept in mind. Whereas input via muscle afferent fibers at the *spinal* level induces reciprocal motor effects ipsilaterally and contralaterally (e.g., inhibition of ipsilateral extensors and activation of contralateral extensors), muscle input at the *trigeminal* level has the same action on the ipsilateral and contralateral motoneurons of a given muscle.[154] As discussed with regard to muscle spasms in locomotor muscles in Chapter 5, however, the in-

crease in tension induced by noxious stimuli in masticatory muscles was over after several minutes; i.e., no long-lasting spasm was induced.

Thalamic Level. Little information is available concerning the processing of information from muscle nociceptors in the thalamus. In experiments employing electrical stimulation of muscle nerves and recording of the associated evoked potentials in the thalamus, Mallart[126] found an exclusive input from thin myelinated muscle afferents in the cat hindlimb to the ventrobasal complex and the medial thalamus. More recent data show that a small number of nociceptive neurons with musculotendinous input are present in the ventral and dorsolateral periphery of the ventral posterolateral nucleus and in the transitional zone between the ventral posterolateral and ventrolateral nucleus of the cat (the so-called "ventral periphery"[98, 118]), i.e., in one of the regions where spinothalamic tract cells are known to terminate in this species.[23, 72]

The location of nociceptive neurons in the periphery of the ventral posterolateral nucleus appears to be typical for the cat; in the rat, nociceptive cells with cutaneous and articular input have been found intermingled with tactile neurons within the ventrobasal complex proper.[77, 79, 85] Recent data suggest that the caudal ventromedial nucleus is a specific nucleus for deep pain in the rat.[63]

In primates, the spinothalamic tract with its nociceptive fibers has been shown to terminate mainly in the ventral posterolateral, ventroposterior inferior, and centralis lateralis nucleus.[72] There is indirect evidence that the nucleus ventroposterior inferior of the monkey may correspond to the "ventral periphery" or the ventral "shell region" of the ventral posterolateral and nucleus ventralis posteromedialis of the cat[208] and to the nucleus ventralis caudalis parvicellularis in humans, which has been discussed as being involved in pain sensations.[83]

The novel technique of positron emission tomography (PET) has yielded data in humans that indicate that the posterior thalamus is involved in pain processing.[101] Interestingly, with this method a reduction in regional blood flow (suggestive of a decrease in neuronal activity) of the thalamus was found in some pain patients. Evidence for a reduction of neuronal activity in the thalamus was also present in women with FMS.[152] The clinical significance of these findings is still obscure.

It is possible, however, that other nuclei of the thalamus (e.g., the posterior and medial nuclei) also process information from small-caliber deep afferents, at least from nociceptive ones. The posterior nuclei in the cat have been found to contain cells with nociceptive properties,[78] and some of the units in the medial thalamus were reported to respond to noxious stimulation of deep tissues in this species.[44] It is questionable, however, whether nociceptive cells in the medial and posterior thalamic nuclei are capable of mediating the sensory-discriminative component of pain. Recordings in awake monkeys have shown that these neurons have large, often

bilateral RFs and, therefore, are not capable of localizing a noxious stimulus with accuracy. (The sensory-discriminative pain component gives information on the nature, intensity, location, and time course of the stimulus.)

In contrast to the relatively unspecific neurons in the medial and posterior nuclei, the ventrobasal complex of the monkey contains neurons that respond differentially to innocuous and noxious stimuli and have small, contralateral RFs.[25] Whether muscle and joint pain are processed in different thalamic nuclei is unknown. Evidence indicates that at least the proprioceptive information from muscle and joint projects to separate areas near the nucleus ventralis intermedius.[82]

In polyarthritic rats, cells of the ventrobasal complex have unusual response characteristics with long afterdischarges and lowered mechanical thresholds.[68] Interestingly, cells of the nucleus centralis lateralis of arthritic rats acquire an input from the inflamed joints that is not present in normal animals. These data suggest that under pathologic conditions, nociceptive pathways to the thalamus may be opened that are silent or ineffective in the intact animal.[77] Such changes are probably associated with a (central) sensitization of thalamic neurons.[80]

The acquisition of a new input by a neuron requires that the information in afferent pathways deviates from its normal route. The underlying mechanism probably is a change in efficacy of synaptic connections that converge on the same neuron. Similar to neuroplastic processes in the spinal cord, such changes could be brought about in the thalamus by unmasking of ineffective (silent or latent) synapses. The processes at the thalamic level probably resemble those presented above as a possible explanation for spread and referral of muscle pain. Actually, no information is available as to where in the CNS the information from muscle nociceptors deviates from the normal pathway to elicit spread and referral of pain. The spinal cord is the first, but not the only, possible site for such a deviation.

Cortical Level.   The significance of the somatosensory cortex for the processing of nociceptive information is still hard to assess, and this is particularly true for nociception from muscle. At the beginning of this century, the predominant opinion was that the appreciation of pain is not or is only minimally represented in the cortex;[84, 187] this view has changed in recent years (for a discussion of the role of the cortex in pain perception, see Sweet[187]).

In some areas of the somatosensory cortex (Brodmann areas 3b and 1) in the monkey, neurons that receive input from cutaneous nociceptors have been shown to exist.[116] Many cells in the primate primary somatosensory cortex fulfill an important requirement of nociceptive neurons, in that they not only respond differentially to innocuous and noxious stimuli but also encode the intensity of a stimulus in the noxious range.[117] The somatosensory cortex of the rat likewise receives a remarkable nociceptive input, as has been shown in a study performed by Lamour et al.[119]: Of 292 neurons with peripheral RFs, 91 responded to noxious stimulation. Among these, 13 cells were driven from deep tissues. The proportion of cortical neurons driven by deep input has been reported to change if pathologic alterations occur in the body periphery. In arthritic rats, the main nociceptive input from joints shifts from cortical layer VI to layer V, and the pathologic input invades cortical laminae (such as layer IV) that do not normally respond to joint input[77, 120] (Fig. 7-17).

As to input from skeletal muscle, data from the cat and monkey show that activity in group I muscle afferents (which supply muscle spindles and Golgi tendon organs, respectively) influences mainly neurons in Brodmann areas 3a and 3b,[110, 181] whereas the input from group II and III muscle afferents projects to area 4 and the secondary somatosensory cortex.[81, 100, 201] The segregation between these two input sources is not distinct, however; and in the face region of the primary somatosensory cortex of the awake monkey (areas 3b, 1, and 2), few neurons were encountered that responded to deep input at all.[103]

Up to now, only a few reports have dealt specifically with the input from muscle nociceptors to cortical neurons. In one of theses studies,[109] noxious stimuli (strong local pressure and injections of algesic substances) were applied to the gastrocnemius-soleus muscle in cats during

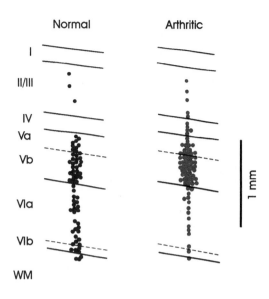

Figure 7-17. Shift in the input from joint nociceptors to cortical neurons induced by an experimental arthritis in rats. The figure shows the localization of neurons receiving nociceptive input from joint in the rat somatosensory cortex. In normal rats (*left panel*), the activated neurons were distributed over laminae V and VI, whereas in arthritic animals (*right panel*), the majority of active neurons were located in lamina Va and Vb. The data demonstrate the existence of strong neuroplastic changes at the cortical level following peripheral lesions. (Redrawn after Guilbaud G: Peripheral and central electrophysiological mechanisms of joint and muscle pain. *Proceedings of the 5th World Congress on Pain.* Edited by Dubner R, Gebhart GF, Bond MR. Elsevier, Amsterdam, 1988 (pp. 201–215).)

a systematic search for neurons in area 3a responding to these stimuli. The authors found that a small fraction (less than 10%) of the cells with deep input from the contralateral hindlimb were responsive to nociceptive input from muscle.

In humans, many of the available data stem from patients who suffered cortical wounds in World Wars I and II. Surprisingly, small lesions of the primary somatosensory cortex, particularly of the posterior wall of the central sulcus (Brodmann area 3), were found to be followed by more severe impairment of pain sensations than were larger lesions.[128, 171] In Marshall's study,[128] muscle pain also was tested by injecting hypertonic saline intramuscularly. Impairment of the pain sense was found to affect cutaneous and deep pain similarly.

Another cortical region that has been associated with pain perception is the secondary somatosensory cortex, which overlaps with the parietal operculum at the lower end of the postcentral gyrus and has fiber connections with the thalamic ventroposterior nuclei.[10, 34, 74] Surgical removal of large portions of the face area in the secondary somatosensory cortex, in the primary somatomotor cortex, and in the primary somatosensory cortex reportedly yield long-lasting relief of facial pain, whereas removal of parts of the primary somatosensory cortex only did not abolish the pain permanently.[122] Supporting data have been obtained in the monkey, wherein the secondary somatosensory cortex was demonstrated to receive its main afferent inflow from the thalamic nucleus ventroposterior inferior.[35, 45, 66]

Data obtained in awake humans with the use of PET and magnetic resonance imaging demonstrated that noxious stimulation of the skin leads to an increase in blood flow (indicative of neuronal activation) in the contralateral primary and secondary somatosensory cortex and in the anterior cingulate cortex. Such a pain-specific activation of the somatosensory cortices, however, has not been found in all of the studies.[26, 111, 166, 188]

The nociceptive region in the anterior cingulate cortex (Brodmann area 24) has strong connections with the limbic system and is assumed by some to mediate the aversive (affective-emotional) component of pain. More recent PET data indicate that other areas of the cingulate cortex also may be involved in pain processing. Possibly, the various parts of the cingulate gyrus mediate different aspects (reflexes, suffering, enhancement, inhibition) of pain sensations.[193] In patients with chronic neuropathic pain, additional and bilateral activation was found in the anterior insular cortex.[101] Comparable studies employing noxious stimulation of muscles in humans have not yet been reported.

6. Possible Mechanisms for the Development of Central Muscle Pain

Based on the experimental data on neuroplasticity, a theoretical mechanism for central muscle pain would be that in the course of a chronic muscle lesion, neurons of central nervous pathways mediating muscle pain are sensitized to such an extent that they become spontaneously active and elicit ongoing pain sensations in that area, which is normally supplied by the hyperactive neurons.

A relatively common cause of central pain (including muscle pain) is a stroke-induced lesion to the spinothalamic tract at supraspinal levels. In a study of 27 patients with central pain following a cerebrovascular lesion of the brainstem and thalamus, the pain was superficial in 8 patients, deep in 11 patients, and both superficial and deep in 8 patients.[121] No differences in the location of the lesion between patients having deep and cutaneous pain were reported. In these cases, a possible mechanism for the pain is that the lesion of the spinothalamocortical pathway led to a deafferentation (removal of normal input to a cell, which in this case is assumed to be largely inhibitory) that produced a disinhibition of nociceptive neurons. The interruption of LTM afferents in the spinothalamic tract (or between thalamus and cortex) does not appear to play an important role in the development of this type of central pain, in that many patients had normal cutaneous tactile sensibility.

Another form of muscle pain for which a central nervous pathogenetic component has been discussed is fibromyalgia. The syndrome is characterized by a combination of widespread pain with tenderness of at least 11 of 18 prescribed points on the body (according to the American College of Rheumatology[190]; see Chapter 9 for a detailed description). Although it is now recognized that fibromyalgia (or generalized tendomyopathy, as it is called in many European countries[153]) is primarily a disturbance of central pain processing, experimental evidence has suggested that peripheral sensitization could be a contributing factor. This issue is complicated because most, if not all, FMS patients also have some myofascial TrPs (MTrPs) that do cause sensitization of nociceptors in muscle and are associated with marked local hypoxia (see Fig. 8-21). Relative hypoxia associated with uneven capillary perfusion was detected by an in vivo electrode placed on the muscle surface over trapezius and brachioradialis TrPs in patients who had FMS.[86, 125] Chemical analysis of biopsies of 15 MTrPs in FMS patients for concentrations of high phosphates, compared with normal control biopsies,[8] showed that the patients had significantly decreased concentrations of adenine triphosphate and phosphoryl creatine but increased adenosine monophosphate, which corresponds to the changes characteristic of hypoxic muscle. Biopsies from tibialis anterior muscles free of MTrPs in the FMS patients did not show the adenine triphosphate and phosphoryl creatine changes indicative of hypoxia. It appears possible, but unlikely, that these findings account for peripheral sensitization that contributes to the pain in FMS patients because of the FMS but may relate more to sensitized nociceptors of concurrent MTrPs. In a biopsy study of trapezius muscle in FMS patients (in which the presence of MTrPs was not considered),[112] the moth-eaten appearance of some muscle fibers was assumed to be caused by local ischemia and spasm. In an earlier study of fibrositis (Weichteil-rheumatismus) in patients with symptoms more suggestive of MTrPs than FMS,[57] similar findings were interpreted in the same way.

The painful muscles of FMS patients exhibit neither increased tension nor raised activity by surface electromyography.[213] Although the surface oxygen tension of muscles over MTrPs of patients with FMS showed relative hypoxia,[125] polarographic needle probes in muscles of FMS patients[16] revealed an elevated mean tissue oxygen tension, which would not be expected to sensitize nociceptors. The reason for these conflicting results, other than the difference in the depth of the muscle tissue being measured, is not known. On the other hand, that same polarographic technique[16] revealed hypoxic levels of oxygen concentration at the core of the tender nodules of myogelosis (MTrPs).

The beneficial effect of a sympathetic block on the spontaneous pain and the pain arising from tender points has been interpreted as indicating that sympathetic efferent activity may be a pathogenetic factor in FMS.[7] Recent microneurographic data, however, have not supported the assumption that in FMS patients the sympathetic activity in muscle nerves is increased.[55] (In this kind of study, recordings of the activity of nerve fibers in humans were obtained by inserting metal microelectrodes through the intact skin into a nerve.) The analgesic effect of a sympathetic block therefore cannot be attributed to the reduction of an increased sympathetic activity but can be attributed to other reasons, e.g., removal of hypersensitivity of blood vessels or nociceptors to normal levels of sympathetic activity and neurotransmitters (see above).

Originally, the hypothesis that changes in the CNS may be relevant for the pathogenesis of FMS rested largely on the lack of pathologic findings in routine laboratory tests. More special tests showed that the cerebrospinal fluid level of SP is increased[170, 192] and the serum level of 5-HT is decreased in FMS patients.[148, 169] Interestingly, there was a correlation between the severity of the symptoms,[185] or number of tender points,[202] and the serum level of 5-HT (for a detailed report on these aspects, see Ref. 168 and Chapter 9).

As SP is considered to be a pain-promoting substance and 5-HT is known to be a transmitter in the descending antinociceptive system,[6] these findings may be indicative of an altered processing of the pain information in central nervous pathways (for a discussion of possible pathogenetic factors of fibromyalgia, see Refs. 86, 87, 167, 168).

B. DIAGNOSIS AND TREATMENT OF CENTRAL AND CENTRALLY MODIFIED PAIN

In recent years, the mechanisms by which the CNS can originate and augment pain have become much more widely recognized and the patients' complaints are more likely to be accepted at face value, despite there being no evidence for a peripheral source of the pain. The pain of FMS is an outstanding example of pain experienced in the musculoskeletal system that results from augmentation of pain sensation by central pathophysiologic mechanisms.

1. Spinal Cord Lesions Causing Pain of Central Origin

The incidence of central pain associated with spinal cord lesions is subject to many variables, including marked differences among individuals with similar lesions. The presence of central pain ranges from 80 to 94% among those with traumatic injuries.[189] For many patients with spinal cord lesions, the most distressing aspect of their misfortune is the severe intractable central pain. It can lead to chemical dependency, severe depression, and even suicide. Ironically for patients, the pain is often experienced in body regions that are anesthetic or have diminished or altered sensation as the result of injury.[176] Until recently, the pain has been essentially unexplained (for a review of the current hypotheses, see Yezierski[207]) and is still difficult to treat.

Traumatic lesions are among the most common causes of pain generated by the CNS, partly because these lesions are so common and partly because of the longevity of those patients. Central pain may also originate from neoplasms, external compression by herniated discs or spinal stenosis, internal pressure from syringomyelia, and postsurgical or postradiation pain of iatrogenic origin.[189]

The pain from a complete transection of the cord is often delayed in onset and nearly always diffusely burning below the level of the lesion, especially perineal pain. It is often a spontaneous cramp-like or aching pain in the abdomen and/or back that resembles visceral or musculoskeletal pain. At the level of the lesion, it is often a girdling hyperpathia that produces a distressing sensitivity to clothing. Incomplete lesions commonly (and predictably) produce hyperpathia in partially denervated parts and may also have intermittent lancinating pain, especially in the lower extremities.[189]

Pain is usually produced in an area of spinothalamic somatosensory loss, whether or not it is accompanied by loss in other modalities; but it may also occur with lesions that exhibit no clinically detectable loss. Incomplete spinal lesions are likely to cause allodynia and/or hyperpathia, corresponding to the symptoms at the level of complete lesions.[189] In addition, nerve or nerve root damage can cause peripheral neuropathic pain as in those with no spinal injury, and pain primarily of muscular origin (such as trigger points) can cause all of the symptoms characteristic of central pain, including pain referred to anesthetic regions of the spinal cord-injured patient.

Surgery and electrical stimulation therapy for relief of pain in spinal lesions have been disappointing. Usually, at best, peripheral nerve stimulation for medullary and thalamic lesions and posterior column stimulation or intracerebral stimulation for central pain have produced only temporary relief. Surgery can aggravate the pain problem, sometimes irreversibly.[159]

Unfortunately, drug therapy is generally ineffective. The best, but mixed, results have been reported with carbamazepine (Tegretol). In the presence of depression, amitriptyline and imipramine (helpful in chronic pain syndromes) can be tried. Administration of 5-hydroxytryptophan (5-HTP) has been more helpful in patients with deafferentation central pain than in those with central pain from spinal lesions. Prolonged dosage with tryptophan may be helpful,[159] but concerns about the development of eosinophilia myalgia syndrome[104] with supplemental oral tryptophan continue to limit its routine usage.

Recent studies report some progress in the understanding of the source of central pain. Comparison of painful and nonpainful denervated skin areas resulting from spinal cord injury in 16 patients by Eide et al.[54] indicated that their allodynia and wind-up–like pain (expressed as increasing response to serial pinpricks) depended on hyperexcitability in nociceptive spinothalamic tract neurons. Herman et al.[89] found in animal experiments that dysesthetic pain and pain related to spasm of central origin were mediated by different central mechanisms. Intrathecal baclofen suppressed spontaneous dysesthesia and evoked allodynia apparently by its effect on a dysfunctional $GABA_B$-receptor system. Clinically, the addition of clonidine to baclofen administered intrathecally to a patient with incomplete tetraplegia (anterior cord syndrome) relieved severe intractable anal spasm that followed a hemorrhoidectomy when intrathecal baclofen alone was ineffective.[147]

Xu et al.[206] reported that in rats with incomplete ischemic spinal cord injury, abnormal central sensory processing was under tonic opioidergic control as a result of upregulation of type B receptors for the endogenous neuropeptide, cholecystokinin.

Both animal[71] and human studies[53] indicate that the effectiveness of ketamine on spontaneous continuous intermittent pain and on evoked allodynia and wind-up–like pain depends on its control of the release of excitatory amino acids by its antagonistic effect on NMDA receptor function.

2. Post-traumatic Hyperirritability Syndromes

The term "post-traumatic hyperirritability syndrome" was introduced[108, 180] to identify a limited number of patients with myofascial pain who exhibit marked hyperirritability of the sensory nervous system and of existing trigger points (TrPs). One can think of this condition as a sensory counterpart to motor spasticity initiated by a specific traumatic event. A similar condition had been described by Margoles as the *stress neuromyelopathic syndrome*.[127]

The post-traumatic hyperirritability syndrome appears immediately following a major trauma, such as an automobile accident, a fall, or a severe blow to the body, that is apparently sufficient to injure the sensory modulation mechanisms of the CNS. These patients have constant pain that can be exacerbated by the vibration of a moving vehicle, the slamming of a door, a loud noise (a firecracker at close range), jarring (bumping into something or being jostled), mild thumps (a pat on the back), transient severe pain (a TrP injection), prolonged physical activity, and intense emotional stress (such as anger). Recovery from an episode of stimulation is slow. Even with mild exacerbations it may take the patient many minutes or hours to return to the baseline pain level. Severe exacerbation of pain may require days, weeks, or longer to return to the previous baseline pain level.

These patients characteristically give a history of having coped well in life prior to their injury, having paid no more attention to pain than did their friends and family. They were no more sensitive to sensory stimuli than other persons. From the moment of the initial trauma, however, pain suddenly became the focus of their life. They must pay close attention to the avoidance of strong sensory stimuli; they must ration physical activity, because even mild to moderate muscular stress or fatigue intensifies the pain. Any additional fall or motor vehicle accident that would ordinarily be considered minor can severely exacerbate the hyperirritability syndrome for months, possibly for years. Unfortunately, with successive traumas, the individual may become increasingly vulnerable to subsequent trauma. A frequent finding is a series of increasingly disabling motor vehicle accidents over a period of years. Efforts to increase exercise tolerance are self-defeating unless managed with great care. Similar phenomena were subsequently described as the *cumulative trauma disorder*[17] and the *jolt syndrome*.[56]

These patients suffer greatly, are poorly understood, and, through no fault of their own, are difficult to help. This condition may be a form of unusually severe FMS induced by an episode of physical trauma. The sensory nervous system behaves much as the motor system does when the spinal cord has lost supraspinal inhibition. A group of patients with traumatic brain injury has a similar chronic pain syndrome.[2]

In post-traumatic hyperirritability syndrome, a strong sensory input of almost any kind can activate nonspecific motor activity for an extended period of time in the same manner that it causes a generalized increase in the excitability of the nociceptive system. In addition, these patients may show lability of the autonomic nervous system with skin temperature changes and swelling that resolve with inactivation of regional TrPs. Because routine medical examination of these suffering patients fails to show any organic cause for their symptoms, they have often been identified as "crocks" or malingerers.

The post-traumatic hyperirritability syndrome is not the same as post-traumatic stress disorder, which commonly follows traumatic experiences in military service, especially if there is a history of abuse as a prisoner of war. Post-traumatic stress disorder can be confusingly similar to FMS, and the two are likely to coexist.[40]

3. Phantom Pain and Thalamic Pain

Phantom limbs and phantom pain are challenging phenomena that until recently, the medical profession could neither understand nor treat effectively. Because physicians (and others) did not take patients' mention of these symptoms seriously and respond with understanding, patients quickly learned not to talk about them.

Ronald Melzack has been a pioneer scientific investigator and informant[135] concerning these phenomena.

In 1978, Melzack and Loeser[137] presented case histories of five paraplegic patients in whom an entire section of spinal cord was removed (complete removal was confirmed visually) based on the assumption that their persistent severe pain must have been transmitted by a few remaining functioning fibers. In all five cases, their pain either persisted or returned postoperatively. In these and other cases, sympathetic blocks or sympathectomy usually failed to relieve the pain. Psychologic factors at times were a contributing factor to, but clearly were not the primary cause of, the pain. This pioneer paper concluded with the hypothesis that a central pattern-generating mechanism was located cranial to the lesion responsible for the pain.

In 1981, using intraneural microelectrodes, Nyström and Hagbarth[157] examined the nerve supplying the phantom area in two patients suffering phantom limb pain and found that tapping a distal neuroma augmented the recorded spontaneous activity and also the phantom pain. Blocking the neuroma with lidocaine blocked the tapping response. The block, however, had no effect on either the spontaneous neural activity or the phantom pain. This reinforced the realization that there must be a central origin of the pain.

Nearly a decade later, Katz and Melzack[113] summarized previous literature and a study of pain "memories" in the phantom phenomena of 68 amputees. These neural memories are predominantly replicas of distress experienced from the preamputation lesions or of the pain experienced in the amputated limb at or near the time of amputation. The phantom sensations had the same qualities as the preamputation pain. The patients report experiencing real pain, which they can describe in vivid detail, and insist that the experience is not merely a cognitive recollection of an earlier pain but is a reliving of the original experience.

Such reports were less common when there had been a pain-free interval between the pain and amputation. Conversely, the reports were not related to the duration of

preamputation pain, time since amputation, age, gender, use of prosthetic devices, level of amputation, number of limbs amputated, and whether amputation followed an accident or illness. Specific examples of these observations are most impressive.[135] The affect or emotional tone that accompanies these phantom pain experiences appears not to be a reactivation of stored memories but to be generated on a moment-by-moment basis. Katz and Melzack[113] emphasize the importance not only of minimizing the pain preceding amputation but also of blocking the pain **at the spinal level** during amputation.

A study of rat responses to sectioning of the sciatic and saphenous nerves, with or without preoperative painful experiences, confirmed the principles described above[114] and helped in the formulation of Melzack's neuromatrix theory.[134] This theory is based on the concept that the body we normally feel must be represented in some way in the brain by neural networks that can be activated by other than corresponding peripheral inputs. This means the body is perceived as a unity and identified as a "self" internally. This perception can be independent of external sensory input: "You don't need a body to feel a body." One of the most eloquent examples of this is the experience of a phantom limb in patients who were born without the limb and never had the limb. To some extent, there must be a "built-in" genetic substrate of a body self-image.

The current details of this theory[136] and the controversies it is generating[32] need not be covered in detail here. The important point is the implications of these undeniable principles to our understanding of muscle pain phenomena. It strongly reinforces the importance of taking with open-minded seriousness the descriptions of pain that patients experience. The fact that the descriptions do not fit our current understanding of pain mechanisms or what we would "expect" is most likely due to our state of ignorance than due to a problem with the patient's psyche.

Thalamic pain (as part of the so-called "thalamic syndrome"[41]) occurs most often as a sequel to a stroke or another lesion of the ventral posterolateral thalamus and associated tracts (see Fig. 7-1 for the location of the thalamus in the pain pathway). The patients complain of spontaneous pain combined with impairment of evoked pain and temperature sensation in the region supplied by the damaged region of the thalamus.[27, 165] In their original description of the thalamic syndrome, Dejerine and Roussy[41] emphasized that deep sensations are much more affected than cutaneous ones. Patients, however, describe the pain as mainly superficial. Often, the distal limbs are the sites of the most intense pain; sometimes, however, the entire contralateral body is involved. The pain is spontaneous, with bouts of severe pain superimposed; these bouts can be triggered by weak stimuli, such as noises and light. The pain is often combined with hyperalgesia of the skin and deep tissues in the affected body regions. Sometimes, the skin is hypoesthetic; in these cases, hyperalgesia of the deep structures can be demonstrated by local pressure stimulation.

Thalamic pain is often intractable; morphine and other strong analgesics do not help, as Dejerine and Roussy[41] noted in their original description. Today, the failure of morphine to abolish thalamic pain can be explained by data indicating that morphine exerts its action largely via activation of the descending antinociceptive system. Because thalamic pain originates in the thalamus and the descending antinociceptive system does not terminate in that region, morphine is not effective in alleviating thalamic pain. This is an important diagnostic distinction.

4. Modulation of Muscle Pain by Psychologic Factors

This section deals with pain that has a peripheral origin but has been modified by psychologic factors. The next section deals with pain that originates in dysfunctional CNS activity without a peripheral origin. This distinction can be hard to make reliably when both are present. Recent advances in visualization of regional brain activity should help to clarify much of this ambiguity.

An understanding of the relative importance of the affective feeling state and cortical sensation in the perception of pain has an interesting history.[38] To the ancient Greeks, pain was an affective feeling state rather than a sensation. With the rapid advances in basic medical knowledge in the 19th and 20th centuries, the sensory qualities of pain were emphasized, and the affective dimensions were relegated to secondary importance.

Recent studies imaging regions of brain activity have shown that both were partially right. Acute painful stimuli appear to be processed in the sensorimotor cortical areas (among others), in keeping with 19th and 20th century concepts. Hsieh et al.,[101] however, showed that in patients with chronic unilateral neuropathic pain, the pain activated *bilateral* anterior insula, posterior parietal, lateral inferior prefrontal, and posterior cingulate cortices, and Brodmann area 24, regardless of the side of pain. These are areas closely associated with emotional tone rather than sensation. This indicates that chronic pain can be the result of processes in regions of the CNS that differ from those mediating acute pain sensation and that chronic pain is likely to be perceived more as suffering than as a sensory experience. A number of schools of thought have developed conceptual models of the relationship between the psyche and the soma in chronic pain states.

Chapman[31] described four models that reflect diverse opinions, which need to be resolved for the sake of patients. The **stress** model takes a psychophysiologic approach, which is a variation of the classic medical model. This model postulates that stress caused by the environment, intrapsychic tensions, or both results in neurophysiologic processes that produce pain and other symptoms. Some stressed individuals can adapt and function well, however, while others engage in behavior disorders such as alcoholism, or escape reality by developing a thought disorder such as schizophrenic or paranoid thinking, or suffer an affective disorder of anxiety or depression. The **psychodynamic** model also conforms to the classic medical model of pain and sees the pain as the product of an underlying psychiatric disorder. As we learn more about the complexities of the psyche as related to pain, it becomes increasingly difficult to be sure what is normal and what is disordered psychic function. A few years ago, phantom limb pain was ascribed to disordered psychic function. Now it is recognized as a normal CNS response to the presence of strong nociceptive input, followed by an absence of normal nonpainful sensations. The **learned pain behavior** model assumes that a peripheral source of pain no longer exists, and all that remain are pain behaviors that signal pain to others, who respond sympathetically and reinforce the pain behavior. The **illness behavior** model views the patient's pain as the product of an interaction between intrapsychic tensions and the social network within which the patient operates. This model emphasizes the importance of beliefs and attitudes as forces that determine the patient's interaction with the health care system.

Psychophysiologic (Stress) Model. As well summarized by Sternbach,[184] individuals subjected to multiple life stresses may respond to the psychic stress by developing physical signs and symptoms, including pain. This process is commonly called "somatization," which can also operate in reverse. Peripheral injury and nociceptive input can influence CNS responses that aggravate pain. Somatization can involve autonomic and reflex responses. Strong affective reactions such as anxiety, resentment, dependent longing, and rage may be expressed physiologically as sweaty palms, tachycardia, gastric hyperactivity, and elevated diastolic blood pressure.[184]

When pain is involved, it is often ambiguous as to whether the pain caused reflex physiologic responses or whether the disturbed physiologic responses contributed to the pain. Anxiety can cause increased muscle tension (poor relaxation), but there is no acceptable evidence that the resulting muscle activity is responsible for the pain. Biofeedback to reduce muscle tension for treatment of pain has been unsatisfactory.[191] Similarly, individuals frequently experience these disturbed physiologic functions without any pain. We consider it much more likely that commonly overlooked peripheral sources of

pain, such as articular dysfunctions and TrPs, are responsible for much of the psychologic distress. Frequently, the primary somatic source of the pain has simply not been identified.

Part of the misinterpretation arises because the emotional and social situation can greatly influence and modify the perception of pain. In the couvade syndrome, the husband develops the complaints of aches and pains characteristic of his pregnant wife. Injured children may not become alarmed or display pain until they realize that their predicament has upset adults.[38] Anxiety most reliably relates to high levels of pain. Anxiety is increased by fear of the unknown, and a medical environment tends to reinforce fears of a life-threatening condition or painful experience. Anxiety of family members is often transferred directly to the patient and serves to reinforce or reactivate fears.[37] Conversely, seriously injured soldiers in battle often report little or no pain, presumably because it promises honorable relief from an intolerable, life-threatening situation. It is obscure at present whether this psychologic mechanism is an alternative explanation to the stress-induced activation of the descending antinociceptive system (see Section A4, "Organization of the Descending Antinociceptive System" and "Tonic Inhibition of Dorsal Horn Neurons Presumably Mediating Deep Somatic Pain") or whether the psychologic stress simply activates the descending system.

Psychodynamic Model. A pain complaint is much more common among patients with a diagnosis of neurosis than among those diagnosed as having a psychosis.[145] Among patients with neuroses, pain was most strongly associated with hysteria.[146] Merskey[145] reported that pain originating from psychologic illness is usually continuously present with irregular fluctuations but rarely, if ever, keeps the patient awake at night.

The degree to which pain is associated with depression depends strongly on the rigor of the criteria used to diagnose depression and can range from 10 to 80%.[145] Animal studies indicate that uncontrolled noxious stimulation results in a state of "learned helplessness" having the characteristics of depression. Depression helps to focus the patient's attention on the pain, rather than on how to cope with it. This can aggravate the suffering associated with the pain experience. In patients with chronic pain, therefore, it is important to treat the depression associated with it.[199] Sometimes, adequate treatment of the depression alone relieves the pain. In other cases, elimination of the pain eliminates the depression. Either can cause the other, and both states tend to aggravate each other.

When this psychophysiologic model is employed, relief of the pain and of the suffering associated with the pain is commonly approached through control of sympathetic arousal, psychologic intervention, manipulation of attention, social modeling, patient instruction, and use of selective cognitive interventions. These measures can be substantially helpful.[33]

Pain Behavior Model. Chapman and Turner[33] listed typical pain behaviors: grimacing (skin drawn tightly around closed eyes, horizontally stretched mouth, and deepening of the nasolabial furrow), posturing, bracing, rubbing, and grasping and moaning. These are all musculoskeletal activities. This is not surprising because recent imaging techniques show that both the sensory and motor cortex are activated in response to acute pain. This helps to explain why pain is so universally expressed as motor activity and may have something to do with the fact that it is so commonly felt in the muscles and related deep tissues.

When those who are a part of the patient's environment respond to these behaviors with sympathy and kindness that is not otherwise obtainable, the responses can reinforce the behaviors without the patient realizing what is happening. They are learning pain behavior, which persists only if it leads to reinforcing consequences. *If* the original source of the pain has resolved but only the behavior remains, this is appropriately treated as a behavior problem, not a medical one. Among those patients for whom this situation applies, the process is applied in reverse. The patient is placed on a time-contingent, not pain-contingent, activity program that reinforces achievement and not complaint. Those who come in close contact with the patient are taught how to avoid reinforcing pain behavior, and for appropriate patients, the results are remarkable.[64] This is a prime example of pain and suffering strongly modified by psychologic factors.

When there is an unrecognized and untreated but treatable source of pain, the results of an inappropriately applied behavior modification program are limited and can impose great injustice on the patient. This is commonly seen in patients suffering from unrecognized or poorly treated myofascial TrPs.

Illness Behavior Model. As described by the recognized leader of this concept, Pilowsky[161] defines abnormal illness behavior as a disagreement between the patient and the physician as to the nature of the sick role to which the patient is entitled. In other words, these patients have concerns about symptoms that their physician feels are not justified based on the physician's diagnosis. This approach assumes no error with regard to physician diagnostic acumen and serves to place all responsibility for the disagreement squarely on the patient.

In this context, sick role and illness have specific definitions. A **sick role** is granted to those whose condition is considered undesirable and who are not responsible for the condition, in the sense that they are unable to reverse or correct it voluntarily. When a sick role is granted, the patient is deserving of care and attention and is obliged to seek advice and assistance from a person regarded as competent to diagnose and treat the condition and to be cooperative.[161]

An **illness** is the property or attributes of an individual that entitles him or her to a sick role. This distinguishes illness from disease, which is the organismic state characterized by agreed objective patterns of clinical features that form the basis of an illness. Often, it is some time before a disease that has been identified by medical science becomes accepted as an illness by society.[161]

Pilowsky[161] then classifies the forms of **abnormal illness behavior** in terms of neurotic disorders, somatization disorders, conversion disorders, somatoform pain disorders, and hypochondriasis. He eloquently makes the critical point: "Obviously, this definition places a considerable and explicit responsibility on the physician to perform his or her role fastidiously, so that the patient's persistent abnormal pain behavior cannot be attributed to inadequacies on the physician's part."

Unfortunately, when it comes to musculoskeletal pain, a major part of the pain under consideration in this paradigm, the widespread lack of understanding of three of the most common sources of musculoskeletal pain—MTrPs, articular dysfunctions, and FMS—dooms many patients to unjustified psychiatric diagnoses and social stigma because of their physician's inadequate training or skills.

When the health care system fails to identify and address the source of the patient's pain, the patient and the health care delivery system are bound to react to the frustration of the situation, each in their own way. The behavioral models represent one response of the medical establishment to this predicament.

5. Psychogenic Muscle Pain

The distinction between pain that originates primarily in the peripheral nervous system but is augmented by psychologic factors and pain that originates primarily in the CNS presents a large gray area that often makes an unequivocal distinction difficult. Although the pain of a phantom limb that replicates the pain experienced immediately before loss of the limb is unquestionably of central origin, it is also characteristic of individuals who are completely normal psychologically; they simply lost a limb. Thus, just because pain is purely central in origin does not automatically stigmatize it as representing sick or abnormal psychologic function.

Pain is likely to be psychogenic, meaning that it originates as an abnormal functioning of the CNS when the pain seems to be dependent on an unambiguous psychiatric disease. Even then, one must be careful that the patient does not have two concurrent conditions: a pain-free psychosis and a peripheral source of pain. The distinction is critical because the treatment approach for dealing with the pain (and its effectiveness) can be different in each case. It is noteworthy, in this connection, how rarely pain is a complaint among psychotic patients and how common a pain complaint is among neurotic patients.[146] Based on the previous section, it is possible that the diagnosis of neurosis in some such patients is actually based on an unidentified peripheral source of pain. That hypothesis would provide at least one reason for the high degree of association between the two.

Two situations have been presented[38] as unequivocal examples of pain of psychogenic origin: pain during hallucinations, as in schizophrenia, and pain associated with conversion hysteria. It is noteworthy that one of the hallmarks of organic psychoses and schizophrenia is a diminished sensitivity to pain. This feature obscures the occurrence of normally painful conditions such as myocardial infarction, perforated peptic ulcer, acute appendicitis, and a fractured femur in these patients.[146] Merskey[146] called attention to the plight of psychiatric patients who develop a physical illness that is ignored or misdiagnosed because the patients' complaints are not accepted as valid. This is an aggravated version of the plight of people with normal psychologic function who have myogenic pain that is not properly recognized by their physician.

6. Medications

The following descriptions of representative medications cited in the text were abstracted from standard reference services.[70, 132, 158, 182] They provide useful data about the medications. For ease in finding a given agent, they are listed alphabetically by category and then by generic name. The standard classification may have little to do with the reason for including the agent in this chapter. Most of the uses suggested are not officially approved indications from the U. S. Food and Drug Administration (FDA). It is the responsibility of the health care provider to appropriately apply this information to a given patient or clinical situation. Most of the listed medications require careful monitoring for continued benefit and for adverse effects.

Anticonvulsants

Generic Name: *carbamazepine*
Brand Name: Tegretol, Epitol
   Dosage: For trigeminal neuralgia, begin with 100 mg PO bid and gradually increase to a maximum of 1.2 g/day in two to three divided doses. Maintenance dosage may range from 200 mg/day to 1.2 g/day but usually ranges from 400 to 800 mg/day.
   Action: Carbamazepine is structurally related to tricyclic antidepressants such as amitriptyline. Like phenytoin, carbamazepine reduces synaptic transmission within the trigeminal nucleus. It also exhibits sedative, antidepressant, and muscle relaxant actions. It is absorbed slowly from the gastrointestinal tract, with peak plasma levels from a single dose of 200 mg achieved in 2 to 8 hours. Steady-state plasma levels may not be reached for 2 to 4 days. Therapeutic levels range from 3 to 14 μg/mL. The plasma half-life ranges from 8 to 72 hours, with the major source of metabolism being the liver. Carbamazepine can induce liver microsomal enzymes to enhance its own metabolism and that of other drugs.
   Indication: The main indications are seizure disorders (generalized, partial complex), trigeminal neuralgia, neurogenic pain (especially lightning pains of tabes dorsalis), multiple sclerosis-related pain, acute idiopathic polyneuritis (Landry-Guillain-Barré syndrome), pain of post-traumatic paresthesia, and pain of diabetic neuropathy. It is sometimes helpful in muscle pain of central origin. This list does not include all of the disorders that may have been or have been observed to be responsive to this agent.
   Side Effects: Many potential adverse effects are associated with use of carbamazepine. They can include CNS effects (confusion, blurred vision, dizziness, insomnia, headache, hyperacusis, speech disturbances, visual hallucinations, oculomotor disturbances, aseptic meningitis, cataracts); cardiovascular system effects (tachycardia, arrhythmias, atrioventricular block, aggravation of hypertension, hypotension, syncope, edema, thrombophlebitis, congestive failure); gastrointestinal tract effects (nausea, vomiting, constipation, epigastric pain, dysphagia, weight loss, xerostomia, stomatitis); hepatic effects (toxic hepatitis, hepatocellular jaundice, cholestatic jaundice, acute intermittent porphyria); genitourinary system effects (urinary retention, oliguria, and frequency, elevated blood pressure, renal failure, impotence, proteinuria); skin effects (photosensitive reactions, urticaria, Stevens-Johnson syndrome, toxic epidermal necrolysis, drug-induced systemic lupus erythematosus); lymphatic system effects (localized or generalized lymphadenopathy, serum sickness); blood system effects (thrombocytopenia, leukopenia, granulocytopenia, pancytopenia, macrocytosis, megaloblastic anemia responsive to folic acid therapy); musculoskeletal system effects (myalgia, arthralgia, muscle cramps); and endocrine system effects (hyponatremia, inappropriate antidiuretic syndrome). A complete blood count, liver function tests, and renal function tests should be evaluated prior to initiating therapy and then periodically thereafter. Carbamazepine should be used with caution in combination with other anticonvulsants, calcium channel blocking agents, erythromycin, doxycycline, psychotherapeutic agents, and warfarin because of crossed effects on metabolism.
   Considerations: Carbamazepine is potentially helpful in a variety of neuropathies, but the risk of adverse events is also high. It is more likely than phenytoin to be helpful in those disorders.

Sedative Hypnotics

Generic Name: *amitriptyline hydrochloride*
Brand Name: Elavil
   Dosage: When used for insomnia or pain, the dosage is usually lower than is indicated for major depression. Although parenteral forms are available, oral therapy is typically used for treatment of pain. The dosage is usually 10 to 50 mg PO qhs.
   Action: The analgesic effect is apparently independent of its antidepressant effect. The plasma half-life is 10 to 50 hours.
   Side Effects: The most frequent adverse effects associated with short-term use relate to anticholinergic effects such as xerostomia, palpitations, constipation, and urinary retention. CNS effects can include somnolence, dizziness, psychosis, confusion, and even coma. Less common are hepatic, hematologic, and cutaneous effects.
   Considerations: Administration at night offers the benefit of improved sleep for patients with chronic pain. There may be synergy with other analgesic drugs. The relative benefit/risk ratio should be reassessed after 2 to 3 months of therapy because tachyphylaxis may occur.

Generic Name: *imipramine hydrochloride*
Brand Name: Tofranil, Janimine
   Dosage: When used for pain, the dosage is usually lower than is indicated for major depression. Although parenteral forms are available, oral therapy is usual for pain. Oral dosage is 10 to 75 mg qhs with fluid.
   Action: The analgesic effect is apparently independent of its antidepressant effect. The plasma half-life is 10 to 50 hours.
   Side Effects: As with amitriptyline, the most frequent adverse effects associated with short-term use relate to anticholinergic effects such as xerostomia, palpitations, constipation, and urinary

retention. CNS effects can include somnolence, dizziness, psychosis, confusion, and even coma. Less common are hepatic, hematologic, and cutaneous effects.

Considerations: Administration at night offers the benefit of improved sleep for patients with chronic pain. There may be synergy with other analgesic drugs. The relative benefit/risk ratio should be reassessed after 2 to 3 months of therapy because tachyphylaxis may occur at about that time.[22]

Nutritional/Metabolic

Generic Name: *5-hydroxytryptophan (5-HTP)*

Brand Name: Not established, but it has orphan drug status with the FDA

Dosage: The usual adult starting dose for postanoxic myoclonus is 25 mg PO four times daily; the dose may be increased by 100 mg/day every 3 to 5 days as tolerated. A reduction in postanoxic myoclonus is usually seen at doses of 600 to 1000 mg/day. For this indication, carbidopa should be started with L-5-HTP and discontinued only when the L-5-HTP has been stopped. For fibromyalgia, the recommended dosage is 100 mg three times per day.

Action: L-5-HTP is a natural aromatic amino acid that is the immediate precursor of the neurotransmitter, serotonin. It is metabolically beyond a committed enzyme reaction, which begins the conversion of tryptophan to serotonin. L-5-HTP is absorbed from the small intestine, with peak plasma concentrations occurring 1 to 2 hours after administration. Approximately 25% of the administered dose is eliminated by first-pass metabolism. The major metabolic pathway is decarboxylation by L-aromatic amino acid decarboxylase to serotonin. The average half-life of the parent compound is 4.3 hours.

Indication: An orphan indication is treatment of postanoxic intention myoclonus. It has been found in one study[24] to reduce the severity of FMS symptoms, but that application would be considered "off label" because it is not an officially approved indication.

Side Effects: The most frequently occurring adverse effects include anorexia, diarrhea, nausea, and vomiting. Gradual increases in dose may alleviate some of these effects.

Considerations: L-5-HTP is currently an investigational agent intended for use in the treatment protocol of patients with postanoxic myoclonus (cited 12/30/97). For more information about orphan product designations, contact the Office of Orphan Products Development, available on the World Wide Web at http://www.fda.gov/orphan.

Skeletal Muscle Relaxants

Generic Name: *baclofen*

Brand Name: Lioresal

Dosage: Oral dosage for muscle spasm must be individualized. Initially, dosage of 5 mg tid to qid can be increased every 3 to 5 days to a maximum of 80 mg/day. Discontinuation should not be abrupt, but dosage reduction can follow the same pattern as initiating dosage. A parenteral form by the same brand name is available for pump-driven intrathecal administration.

Action: The mechanism of baclofen is incompletely understood. It is a structural analog of GABA, coupled to a phenylethylamine moiety. It appears that the main mode of action is inhibition of afferent signal transmission in the spinal cord, because there is little penetration of the blood-brain barrier. There is evidence for both antinociceptive effects and inhibition of motor neuron-related muscle spasticity. Indications for use of oral baclofen include muscle spasticity of spinal cord origin, associated with multiple sclerosis and other cord injuries. Unapproved uses for baclofen include Huntington's choreiform movements, spasticity of cerebral lesions, stiff-man syndrome, and rheumatic diseases. Approved uses for intrathecal administration include severe spasticity in patients with multiple sclerosis, spinal cord injury, or cerebral palsy, for which the agent is listed as an orphan drug. The onset of action after oral administration is approximately 2 hours, and its plasma half-life is 2.5 to 4 hours.

Side Effects: The most common adverse effect is drowsiness; thus, patient operation of mechanical equipment may be hazardous. Other effects may involve the sensory organs or cause seizure exacerbations, mood disturbances, anticholinergic-like symptoms, dyspnea, alterations in blood pressure, rash, diaphoresis, hyperglycemia, and transaminitis. Caution should be exercised when treating patients with seizure disorders, equipment operators, peptic ulcer patients, and psychotic individuals. Withdrawal of this drug too rapidly can cause hallucinations, seizures, and recurrence of muscle spasms.

Considerations: Compared with 30 mg of diazepam daily, 60 mg of baclofen per day has been found to be equipotent in reducing painful spasticity but is less sedating. The dosage of baclofen should be reduced in patients with renal insufficiency.

Hypotensive Agent

Generic Name: *clonidine*

Brand Name: Catapres, available in oral and transdermal forms (a parenteral form has been studied)

Dosage: For management of hypertension, clonidine is begun with 0.05 to 0.1 mg bid and the daily dosage is increased by 0.1 to 0.2 mg every 3 days until the least effective dosage or a maximum of 2.4 mg/day in two to three divided doses is achieved. Transdermal dosage begins with a single patch applied every 7 days, which delivers 0.1 mg/day. Dosage for other applications is extrapolated from the antihypertensive therapy dosage. For sharp, shooting, chronic body pain, a 12-day trial of a patch may be effective in some patients.

Action: Clonidine appears to stimulate α_2-adrenergic receptors in the CNS (mainly in the medulla oblongata), causing inhibition, but not blockade, of sympathetic vasomotor centers, which results in a reduction in peripheral sympathetic nervous system activity and a decrease in the excretion of urinary catecholamines. Clonidine transiently stimulates the release of growth hormone, but chronic administration does not result in a persistent elevation of growth hormone levels. Clonidine reduces heart rate, blood pressure, intestinal motility in diarrhea states, and intraocular pressure in glaucoma. To the extent that some musculoskeletal pain disorders are sympathetically maintained, clonidine may represent a theoretical solution. It is somewhat sedating, so it may help people with insomnia if it is given only at bedtime. Its antihypertensive effects are: onset, 30 to 60 minutes after oral or intravenous dosing; peak, within 2 to 4 hours; and duration, 6 to 10 hours. Clonidine's oral bioavailability ranges from 65 to 96%, with an elimination half-life of 6 to 23 hours; approximately 20 to 40% of clonidine is bound to plasma proteins. Hepatic metabolism of clonidine to inactive metabolites is accompanied by renal and fecal excretion of unchanged compound (65 and 22%, respectively). Because the drug is excreted by the kidney, the dosage must be decreased in patients with severe renal insufficiency. The tricyclic antidepressant drugs and ibuprofen may reduce the antihypertensive effects of clonidine.

Indication: Currently, the main approved indication for use of clonidine is systemic hypertension. Other uses have included treatment of pheochromocytoma, vasodilation states such as migraine headache, dysmenorrhea, menopausal flushing, opiate withdrawal, and glaucoma. Other potential uses are listed under "Considerations."

Side Effects: The most common adverse effects include sedation (12%), xerostomia, and constipation. Clonidine can cause headache, dizziness, nausea, vomiting, fatigue, weakness, weight gain, gynecomastia, pruritus, and even alopecia. Approximately 20% of patients using the transdermal patch form develop hypersensitivity to clonidine. Impotence or loss of libido has occurred with the oral form at approximately 3% but is rarely problematic with the transdermal form. Muscle pain, muscle spasm, and joint pain have occurred in 3 to 6%.

Considerations: Clonidine can be therapeutic for pain. It has orphan drug status for use in the treatment of cancer pain. Potentially unapproved uses include profound analgesia that can result from injecting the parenteral form epidurally, but it should not be given by this route above the C4 dermatome. Clonidine has been used to treat Tourette's syndrome, wherein nearly 50% of patients report beneficial effects of the drug, but bothersome side effects reduce compliance when taken orally. Clonidine has been successful in the treatment of the restless leg syndrome. It is also effective in controlling postoperative shivering. Epidural or subarachnoid or transdermal clonidine can provide symptomatic pain relief from a variety of chronic pain states in which the onset of relief begins within 20 minutes and lasts up to 6 hours. Clonidine is probably helpful as adjunctive therapy in baclofen-refractory cases of spinal cord injury spasticity. Quadriplegics may be more responsive than paraplegics. There is some evidence for improved mortality in tetanus when clonidine is used to control autonomic dysfunction. The tricyclic antidepressant drugs and ibuprofen may reduce the antihypertensive effects of clonidine.

NMDA Antagonist

Generic Name: *ketamine*

Brand Name: Ketalar solution for injection (10, 50, and 100 mg/mL)

Dosage: For induction of dissociative anesthesia, recommended doses of ketamine are 1 to 4.5 mg/kg IV or 5 to 10 mg/kg IM; maintenance of anesthesia is achieved with an intravenous infusion of 0.1 to 0.5 mg/minute or one-half to the full induction dose intravenously or intramuscularly, repeated as required. For sedation and analgesia, intramuscular doses of 2 to 4 mg/kg or intravenous doses of 0.2 to 0.75 mg/kg have been employed; ketamine has also been given orally, rectally, and epidurally.

Action: Ketamine is a nonbarbiturate anesthetic/analgesic agent that should be viewed as another CNS depressant. Peak serum levels of ketamine occur 5 to 30 minutes after intramuscular injection and 30 minutes following oral doses; anesthesia is usually induced within 30 seconds and 4 minutes following intravenous and intramuscular induction doses, respectively. Similar to thiopental, ketamine is rapidly distributed to highly perfused tissues (e.g., brain, heart, lungs) following parenteral doses and then is redistributed to muscle, peripheral tissues, and fat. Ketamine is metabolized in the liver, and hepatic clearance is required for termination of clinical effects. A prolonged duration of action may occur in patients with cirrhosis or other type of liver impairment; thus, dose reductions should be considered in these patients. Norketamine is an active metabolite of ketamine; most of a dose of ketamine is excreted in the urine as hydroxylated and conjugated metabolites. Less than 4% appears in urine as unchanged drug or norketamine; the elimination half-life of ketamine is 2 to 3 hours. Its duration of action is not prolonged in the presence of decreased renal function; thus, dose adjustments do not appear warranted in renal insufficiency. Unlike inhalational agents and narcotics, which suppress the reticular activating system, ketamine induces a dissociative anesthesia, described as a functional and electrophysiologic dissociation between the thalamoneocortical and limbic systems. This prevents the higher centers from perceiving auditory, visual, or painful stimuli. With adequate anesthetic doses, a trance-like, cataleptic state with amnesia is produced with no impairment of laryngeal and pharyngeal reflexes or depression of respiration. The eyes remain open with a "disconnected" stare, and nystagmus is usually observed; the patient may appear to be awake but is dissociated from the environment, immobile, and unresponsive to pain.

Indication: Ketamine is useful as an anesthetic and analgesic/sedative in a variety of specialized procedures and clinical settings, particularly in children and in asthmatics, for relief of severe bronchospasm. Ketamine may be used in conjunction with anesthetic agents for the purpose of inducing and maintaining anesthesia, postoperative pain control, chronic pain control, radiologic and diagnostic procedures, and conscious sedation. Epidural ketamine has been useful in treating various types of pain, but it does not appear to offer much advantage over epidural morphine.

Side Effects: Adverse effects associated with ketamine include emergence phenomena (vivid dreams, hallucinations, delirium), cardiovascular stimulation (tachycardia, hypertension), hypersalivation, elevation of intracranial and intraocular pressures, nausea, vomiting, skeletal muscle hyperactivity, nystagmus, and skin rash; respiratory depression is usually not observed. Benzodiazepines or clonidine have been useful in attenuating cardiovascular effects and preventing emergence phenomena. Low-dose ketamine is safe for administration to obstetric patients. Ketamine is contraindicated in cases of hypersensitivity to the drug and where a significant elevation of blood pressure is hazardous (e.g., patients with poorly controlled hypertension, aneurysms, acute right- or left-sided heart failure, angina, cerebral trauma, recent myocardial infarction). Special caution must be exercised when administering ketamine to patients with hypertension, chronic congestive heart failure tachyarrhythmias, or myocardial ischemia. The same applies to patients with neurotic traits or psychiatric illness, alcohol intoxication or alcohol abuse, acute intermittent porphyria, seizure disorders, glaucoma, hyperthyroidism or receiving thyroid replacement (increased risk of hypertension, tachycardia, pulmonary or upper respiratory infection [ketamine sensitizes the gag reflex, potentially causing laryngospasm]), intracranial mass lesions, head injury, globe injuries, or hydrocephalus.

Considerations: Unapproved potential uses of ketamine include phantom limb pain, priapism, acute pain resulting from musculoskeletal trauma, and FMS.

Narcotics

Generic Name: *morphine sulfate*
Brand Name: Morphine Sulfate (oral tablets 15 mg, 30 mg; oral solution; rectal suppositories 5 mg, 10 mg, 20 mg, 30 mg; and parenteral injection)

Dosage: The usual adult dosage is 10 to 30 mg every 4 hours as needed for severe pain. The smallest effective dose should be used for the shortest period of time.

Action: (See codeine in Chapter 3, Section G7.)
Indication: Morphine sulfate is a strong analgesic to be used for relief of severe, acute pain or moderately severe, chronic, terminal pain (e.g., terminal cancer). It is also used to treat anxiety in congestive heart failure.

Side Effects: Similar but substantially more severe than with codeine (see codeine under Chapter 3, Section G7).

Considerations: Morphine sulfate is a potent analgesic available in a wide variety of administration forms. There will be few indications for this agent in the management of chronic pain conditions other than malignancy.

REFERENCES

1. Amano N, Hu JW, Sessle BJ: Responses of neurons in feline trigeminal subnucleus caudalis (medullary dorsal horn) to cutaneous, intraoral, and muscle afferent stimuli. *J Neurophysiol* 55:227–243, 1986.
2. Andary MT, Vincent F, Esselman PC: Chronic pain following head injury. *Phys Med Rehab Clin North Am* 4:141–150, 1993.
3. Angaut-Petit D: The dorsal column system: I. Existence of long ascending postsynaptic fibres in the cat's fasciculus gracilis. *Exp Brain Res* 22:457–470, 1975.
4. *An Outline of Chinese Acupuncture*. The Academy of Traditional Chinese Medicine. Foreign Language Press, Peking, 1975.
5. Arvidsson J, Raappana P: An HRP study of the central projections from primary sensory neurons innervating the rat masseter muscle. *Brain Res* 480:111–118, 1989.
6. Basbaum AI, Fields HL: Endogenous pain control system: brainstem spinal pathways and endorphin circuitry. *Ann Rev Neurosci* 7:309–338, 1984.
7. Bengtsson A, Bengtsson M: Regional sympathetic blockade in primary fibromyalgia. *Pain* 33:161–167, 1988.
8. Bengtsson A, Henriksson KG, Larsson I: Reduced high-energy phosphate levels in the painful muscles of patients with primary fibromyalgia. *Arthritis Rheum* 29:817–821, 1986.
9. Bennet GJ, Nishikawa N, Guo-Wei Lu, *et al.*: The morphology of dorsal column postsynaptic spinomedullary neurons in the cat. *J Comp Neurol* 224:568–578, 1984.
10. Biemond A: The conduction of pain above the level of the thalamus opticus. *AMA Arch Neurol Psychtr* 75:231–244, 1956.
11. Bliss TV, Collingridge GL: A synaptic model of memory: long-term potentiation in the hippocampus. *Nature* 361:31–39, 1993.
12. Bravo R: Growth factor inducible genes in fibroblasts. *Growth Factors, Differentiation Factors and*

Cytokines. Edited by Habenicht A. Springer, Berlin, 1990 (pp. 324–343).

13. Broton JG, Sessle BJ: Reflex excitation of masticatory muscles induced by algesic chemicals applied to the temporomandibular joint of the cat. *Arch Oral Biol* 33:741–747, 1988.

14. Brown AG: Ascending and long spinal pathways: Dorsal columns, spinocervical tract and spinothalamic tact. *Handbook of Sensory Physiology, Vol. 2, Somatosensory System*. Edited by Iggo A. Springer Verlag, Berlin, Heidelberg, New York, 1973 (pp. 315–338).

15. Brown AG: *Organization in Spinal Cord. The Anatomy and Physiology of Identified Neurones.* Springer Verlag, Berlin, 1981.

16. Brückle W, Suckfüll M, Fleckenstein W, *et al.*: Gewebe-pO$_2$-Messung in der verspannten Rückenmuskulatur (M. erector spinae). *Z Rheumatol* 49:208–216, 1990.

17. Burnette JT, Ayoub MA: Cumulative trauma disorders. Part I. The problem. *Pain Manage* 2:196–209, 1989.

18. Burstein R, Cliffer KD, Giesler GJ: Cells of origin of the spinohypothalamic tract in the rat. *J Comp Neurol* 291:329–344, 1990.

19. Bushnell MC, Duncan GH, Dubner R, *et al.*: Attentional influences on noxious and innocuous cutaneous heat detection in humans and monkeys. *J Neurosci* 5:1103–1110, 1985.

20. Calverley RKS, Jones DG: Contributions of dendritic spines and perforated synapses to synaptic plasticity. *Brain Res Rev* 15:215–249, 1990.

21. Calvino B, Villanueva L, le Bars D: Dorsal horn (convergent) neurons in the intact anaesthetized arthritic rat. I. Segmental excitatory influences. *Pain* 28:81–98, 1986.

22. Carette S, Bell MJ, Reynolds WJ, *et al.*: Comparison of amitriptyline, cyclobenzaprine, and placebo in the treatment of fibromyalgia: a randomized, double-blind clinical trial. *Arthritis Rheum* 37:32–40, 1994.

23. Carstens E, Trevino DL: Laminar origins of spinothalamic projections in the cat as determined by the retrograde transport of horseradish peroxidase. *J Comp Neurol* 182:151–166, 1978.

24. Caruso I, Sarzi Puttini P, Cazzola M, Azzolini V: Double-blind study of 5-hydroxytryptophan versus placebo in the treatment of primary fibromyalgia syndrome. *J Intern Med Res* 18:201–209, 1990.

25. Casey KL, Morrow TJ: Ventral posterior thalamic neurons differentially responsive to noxious stimulation of the awake monkey. *Science* 221:675–677, 1983.

26. Casey KL, Minoshima S, Morrow TJ, *et al.*: Comparison of human cerebral activation pattern during cutaneous warmth, heat pain, and deep cold pain. *J Neurophysiol* 76:571–581, 1996.

27. Cassinari V, Pagni CA: *Central Pain: A Neurosurgical Survey*. Harvard University Press, Cambridge, MA, 1969.

28. Cervero F: Somatic and visceral inputs to the thoracic spinal cord of the cat: effects of noxious stimulation of the biliary system. *J Physiol* 337:51–67, 1983.

29. Cervero F, Iggo A, Ogawa H: Nociceptor-driven dorsal horn neurones in the lumbar spinal cord of the cat. *Pain* 2:2–24, 1976.

30. Cervero F, Schaible H-G, Schmidt RF: Tonic descending inhibition of spinal cord neurones driven by joint afferents in normal cats and in cats with an inflamed knee joint. *Exp Brain Res* 83:675–678, 1991.

31. Chapman CR: Introduction, Section B. *The Management of Pain, Vol. 1*. Ed. 2. Edited by Bonica JJ. Lea & Febiger, Philadelphia, 1990 (pp. 284–286).

32. Chapman CR: Neuromatrix theory: do we need it? *Pain Forum* 5:139–142, 1996.

33. Chapman CR, Turner JA: Psychological and psychosocial aspects of acute pain, Chapter 5. *The Management of Pain, Vol. 1*. Ed. 2. Edited by Bonica JJ. Lea & Febiger, Philadelphia, 1990 (pp. 122–132).

34. Chatrian GE, Canfield RC, Knauss TA, *et al.*: Cerebral responses to electrical tooth pulp stimulation in man—an objective correlate of acute experimental pain. *Neurology* 25:745–757, 1975.

35. Chudler EH, Dong WK, Kawakami Y: Cortical nociceptive responses and behavioral correlates in the monkey. *Brain Res* 397:47–60, 1986.

36. Collingridge GL, Lester RAJ: Excitatory amino acid receptors in the vertebrate central nervous system. *Pharmacol Rev* 40:143–210, 1989.

37. Cousins M: Acute and postoperative pain, Chapter 18. *Textbook of Pain*. Ed. 2. Edited by Wall PD, Melzack R. Churchill Livingstone, New York, 1989 (pp. 284–305).

38. Craig KD: Emotional aspects of pain, Chapter 12. *Textbook of Pain*. Ed. 2. Edited by Wall PD, Melzack R. Churchill Livingstone, New York, 1989 (pp. 220–230).

39. Craig AD, Kniffki K-D: Spinothalamic lumbosacral lamina I cells responsive to skin and muscle stimulation in the cat. *J Physiol* 365:197–221, 1985.

40. Culclasure TF, Enzenauer RJ, West SG: Posttraumatic stress disorder presenting as fibromyalgia. *Am J Med* 94:548–549, 1993.

41. Dejerine J, Roussy G: Le syndrome thalamique. *Rev Neurol* 14:521–532, 1906.

42. Desimone R: The physiology of memory: recordings of things past. *Science* 258:245–246, 1992.

43. Dickenson AH, Sullivan AF: NMDA receptors and central hyperalgesic states. *Pain* 46:344–345, 1991.

44. Dong WK, Ryu H, Wagman IH: Nociceptive responses of neurons in medial thalamus and their relationship to spinothalamic pathways. *J Neurophysiol* 41:1592–1613, 1978.

45. Dong WK, Salonen LD, Kawakami Y, *et al.*: Nociceptive responses of trigeminal neurons in SII-7b cortex of awake monkeys. *Brain Res* 484: 314–324, 1989.

46. Dougherty PM, Willis WD: Enhancement of spinothalamic neuron responses to chemical and mechanical stimuli following combined microiontophoretic application of N-methyl-D-aspartic acid and substance P. *Pain* 47:85–93, 1991.

47. Dragunow M, Currie RW, Faull RLM, *et al.*: Immediate-early genes, kindling and long-term potentiation. *Neurosci Biobehav Rev* 13:301–313, 1989.

48. Draisci G, Iadarola MJ: Temporal analysis of increases in c-fos preprodynorphin and preproenkephalin mRNAs in rat spinal cord. *Mol Brain Res* 6:31–37, 1989.

49. Dubner R: Hyperalgesia and expanded receptive fields. *Pain* 48:3–4, 1992.

50. Dubner R, Bennett GJ: Spinal and trigeminal mechanisms of nociception. *Annu Rev Neurosci* 6:381–418, 1983.

51. Dubner R, Ruda MA: Activity-dependent neuronal plasticity following tissue injury and inflammation. *TINS* 15:96–103, 1992.

52. Dubner R, Kenshalo DR, Maixner W, *et al.*: The correlation of monkey medullary dorsal horn neuronal activity and the perceived intensity of noxious heat stimuli. *J Neurophysiol* 62:450–457, 1989.

53. Eide PK, Stubhaug A, Stenehjem AE: Central dysesthesia pain after traumatic spinal cord injury is dependent on *N*-methyl-D-aspartate receptor activation. *Neurosurgery* 37:1080–1087, 1995.

54. Eide PK, Jorum E, Stenehjem AE: Somatosensory findings in patients with spinal cord injury and central dysaesthesia pain. *J Neurol Neurosurg Psychiatry* 60:411–415, 1996.

55. Elam M, Johansson G, Wallin BG: Do patients with primary fibromyalgia have an altered muscle sympathetic nerve activity? *Pain* 48:371–375, 1992.

56. Elson LM: The jolt syndrome. Muscle dysfunction following low-velocity impact. *Pain Manage* 3: 317–326, 1990.

57. Fassbender HG, Wegner K: Morphologie und Pathogenese des Weichteilrheumatismus. *Z Rheumaforsch* 32:355–374, 1973.

58. Fields HL: *Pain*. McGraw-Hill, New York, 1987.

59. Fields HL: Is there a facilitating component to central pain modulation? *APS J* 1:139–141, 1992.

60. Fields HL, Heinricher MM: Anatomy and physiology of a nociceptive modulatory system. *Phil Trans R Soc Lond B* 308:361–374, 1985.

61. Fields HL, Clanton CH, Anderson SD: Somatosensory properties of spinoreticular neurons in the cat. *Brain Res* 120:49–66, 1977.

62. Fields HL, Malick A, Burstein R: Dorsal horn projection targets of ON and OFF cells in the rostral ventromedial medulla. *J Neurophysiol* 74:1742–1759, 1995.

63. Floyd NS, Keay KA, Bandler R: A calbindin immunoreactive "deep pain" recipient thalamic nucleus in the rat. *Neuro Rep* 7:622–626, 1996.

64. Fordyce WE: Learned pain: pain as behavior, Chapter 16. *The Management of Pain, Vol. 1*. Ed. 2. Edited by Bonica JJ. Lea & Febiger, Philadelphia, 1990 (pp. 291–299).

65. Foreman RD, Blair RW, Weber RN: Viscerosomatic convergence onto T2–T4 spinoreticular, spinoreticular-spinothalamic, and spinothalamic tract neurons in the cat. *Exp Neurol* 85:597–619, 1984.

66. Friedman DP, Murray EA: Thalamic connectivity of the second somatosensory area and neighboring somatosensory fields of the lateral sulcus of the macaque. *J Comp Neurol* 252:348–373, 1986.

67. Garthwaite J: Glutamate, nitric oxide and cell-cell signalling in the nervous system. *TINS* 14:60–67, 1991.

68. Gautron M, Guilbaud G: Somatic responses of ventrobasal thalamic neurones in polyarthritic rats. *Brain Res* 237:459–471, 1982.

69. Gebhart GF: Can endogenous systems produce pain? *APS J* 1:79–81, 1992.

70. Gelman CR, Rumack BH, Hess AJ (Eds.): *DRUGDEX System*. Micromedex, Englewood, CO (revised: June 1997).

71. Ghorpade A, Advokat C: Evidence of a role for *N*-methyl-D-aspartate (NMDA) receptors in the facilitation of tail withdrawal after spinal transection. *Pharmacol Biochem Behav* 48:175–181, 1994.

72. Gingold SI, Greenspan JD, Apkarian AV: Anatomic evidence of nociceptive inputs to primary somatosensory cortex: relationship between spinothalamic terminals and thalamocortical cells in squirrel monkeys. *J Comp Neurol* 308:467–490, 1991.

73. Graven-Nielsen T, Arendt-Nielsen L, Svensson P, Jensen TS: Experimental muscle pain: a quantitative study of local and referred pain in humans following injection of hypertonic saline. *J Musculoskeletal Pain* 5(2):49–69, 1997.

74. Greenspan JD, Winfield JA: Reversible pain and tactile deficits associated with cerebral tumor compressing the posterior insula and parietal operculum. *Pain* 50:29–39, 1992.

75. Gregor M, Zimmermann M: Characteristics of spinal neurones responding to cutaneous myelinated and unmyelinated fibres. *J Physiol* 221:555–576, 1972.

76. Guilbaud G: Peripheral and central electrophysiological mechanisms of joint and muscle pain. *Proceedings of the 5th World Congress on Pain*. edited by Dubner R, Gebhart GF, Bond MR. Elsevier, Amsterdam, 1988 (pp. 201–215).

77. Guilbaud G: Central neurophysiological processing of joint pain on the basis of studies performed in normal animals and in models of experimental arthritis. *Can J Physiol Pharmacol* 69:637–646, 1991.

78. Guilbaud G, Caille D, Besson JM, *et al.*: Single unit activities in ventral posterior and posterior group thalamic nuclei during nociceptive and non-nociceptive stimulations in the cat. *Arch Ital Biol* 115:38–56, 1977.

79. Guilbaud G, Peschanski M, Gautron M, *et al.*: Neurones responding to noxious stimulation in VB complex and caudal adjacent regions in the thalamus of the rat. *Pain* 8:303–318, 1980.

80. Guilbaud G, Benoist JM, Eschalier A, *et al.*: Evidence for central phenomena participating in the changes of responses of ventrobasal thalamic neurons in arthritic rats. *Brain Res* 484:383–388, 1989.

81. Hanson J: Hypoglossal high threshold afferents projecting to the secondary somatosensory area in the cat. *Arch Ital Biol* 123:63–68, 1985.

82. Hardy TL, Bertrand G, Thompson CJ: Position and organization of thalamic cellular activity during diencephalic recording. II. Joint- and muscle-evoked activity. *Appl Neurophysiol* 43:28–36, 1980.

83. Hassler R: Wechselwirkungen zwischen dem System der schnellen Schmerzempfindung und dem des langsamen, nachhaltigen Schmerzgefühles. *Langenbecks Arch Chir* 342:47–61, 1976.

84. Head H, Holmes G: Sensory disturbances from cerebral lesions. *Brain* 34:102–254, 1911.
85. Hellon RF, Mitchell D: Characteristics of neurones in the ventro-basal thalamus of the rat which respond to noxious stimulation of the tail. *J Physiol* 250:29–30, 1975.
86. Henriksson KG, Bengtsson A: Fibromyalgia—a clinical entity? *Can J Physiol Pharmacol* 69:672–677, 1991.
87. Henriksson KG, Mense S: Pain and nociception in fibromyalgia: clinical and neurobiological considerations on aetiology and pathogenesis. *Pain Rev* 1:245–260, 1994.
88. Henry JL: Effects of substance P on functionally identified units in cat spinal cord. *Brain Res* 114:439–451, 1976.
89. Herman RM, D'Luzansky SC, Ippolito R: Intrathecal baclofen suppresses central pain in patients with spinal lesions. A pilot study. *Clin J Pain* 8:338–345, 1992.
90. Herrero JF, Cervero F: Supraspinal influences on the facilitation of rat nociceptive reflexes induced by carrageenan monoarthritis. *Neurosci Lett* 209:21–24, 1996.
91. Hoheisel U, Mense S: Long-term changes in discharge behaviour of cat dorsal horn neurones following noxious stimulation of deep tissues. *Pain* 36:239–247, 1989.
92. Hoheisel U, Mense S: Response behaviour of cat dorsal horn neurones receiving input from skeletal muscle and other deep somatic tissues. *J Physiol* 426:265–280, 1990.
93. Hoheisel U, Lehmann-Willenbrock E, Mense S: Termination patterns of identified group II and III afferent fibres from deep tissues in the spinal cord of the cat. *Neuroscience* 28:495–507, 1989.
94. Hoheisel U, Mense S, Simons DG, et al.: Appearance of new receptive fields in rat dorsal horn neurones following noxious stimulation of skeletal muscle: a model for referral of muscle pain? *Neurosci Lett* 153:9–12, 1993.
95. Hoheisel U, Koch K, Mense S: Functional reorganization in the rat dorsal horn during an experimental myositis. *Pain* 59:11–118, 1994.
96. Hoheisel U, Mense S, Scherotzke R: Calcitonin gene-related peptide immunoreactivity in functionally identified primary afferent neurons in the rat. *Anat Embryol* 189:41–49, 1994.
97. Hoheisel U, Mense S, Ratkai M: Effects of spinal cord superfusion with substance P on the excitability of rat dorsal horn neurons processing input from deep tissues. *J Musculoskeletal Pain* 3:23–43, 1995.
98. Honda CN, Mense S, Perl ER: Neurons in ventrobasal region of cat thalamus selectively responsive to noxious mechanical stimulation. *J Neurophysiol* 49:662–673, 1983.
99. Hong SK, Kniffki K-D, Mense S, et al.: Descending influences on the responses of spinocervical tract neurones to chemical stimulation of fine muscle afferents. *J Physiol* 290:129–140, 1979.
100. Hore J, Preston JB, Durkovic RG, et al.: Responses of cortical neurons (area 3a and 4) to ramp stretch of hindlimb muscles in the baboon. *J Neurophysiol* 39:484–500, 1976.
101. Hsieh JC, Belfrage M, Stone-Elander S, et al.: Central representation of chronic ongoing neuropathic pain studied by positron emission tomography. *Pain* 63:225–236, 1995.
102. Hu JW, Sessle BJ, Raboisson P, et al.: Stimulation of craniofacial muscle afferents induces prolonged facilitatory effects in trigeminal nociceptive brainstem neurones. *Pain* 48:53–60, 1992.
103. Huang C-S, Hiraba H, Sessle BJ: Input-output relationships of the primary face motor cortex in the monkey (Macaca fascicularis). *J Neurophysiol* 61:350–362, 1989.
104. Hudson J, Pope H, Daniels S, Horwitz R, et al.: Fibromyalgia and eosinophilia-myalgia syndrome. *J Musculoskeletal Pain* 3(1):63–75, 1995.
105. Hunt SP, Pini A, Evan G: Induction of c-fos-like protein in spinal cord neurons following sensory stimulation. *Nature* 328:632–634, 1987.
106. Hylden JLK, Hayashi H, Dubner R, et al.: Physiology and morphology of the lamina I spinomesencephalic projection. *J Comp Neurol* 247:505–515, 1986.
107. Hylden JLK, Nahin RL, Traub RJ, et al.: Expansion of receptive fields of spinal lamina I projection neurons in rats with unilateral adjuvant-induced inflammation: the contribution of dorsal horn mechanisms. *Pain* 37:229–243, 1989.
108. Institute of Medicine: *Pain and Disability: Clinical Behavioral and Public Policy Perspectives.* National Academy Press, Washington, DC, 1987.
109. Iwamura Y, Kniffki K-D, Mizumura K, et al.: Responses of feline SI neurones to noxious stimulation of muscle and tendon. *Pain* 1:213, 1981.
110. Iwata K, Itoga H, Ikukawa A, et al.: Distribution and response characteristics of masseteric nerve-driven neurons in two separate cortical projection areas of cats. *Brain Res* 342:179–182, 1985.
111. Jones AKP, Brown WD, Friston KJ, et al.: Cortical and subcortical localization of response to pain in man using positron emission tomography. *Proc R Soc Lond B Biol Sci* 244:39–44, 1991.
112. Kalyan-Raman UP, Kalyan-Raman K, Yunus MB, et al.: Muscle pathology in primary fibromyalgia syndrome: a light microscopic, histochemical, and ultrastructural study. *J Rheumatol* 11:808–813, 1984.
113. Katz J, Melzack R: Pain 'memories' in phantom limbs: review and clinical observations. *Pain* 43:319–336, 1990.
114. Katz J, Vaccarino AL, Coderre TJ, et al.: Injury prior to neurectomy alters the pattern of autotomy in rats. *Anesthesiology* 75:876–883, 1991.
115. Keay KA, Bandler R: Deep and superficial noxious stimulation increases Fos-like immunoreactivity in different regions of the midbrain periaqueductal grey of the rat. *Neurosci Lett* 154:23–26, 1993.
116. Kenshalo DR, Isensee O: Responses of primate SI cortical neurons to noxious stimuli. *J Neurophysiol* 50:1479–1496, 1983.
117. Kenshalo DR, Chudler EH, Anton F, et al.: SI nociceptive neurons participate in the encoding process by which monkeys perceive the intensity of noxious thermal stimulation. *Brain Res* 454:378–382, 1988.

118. Kniffki K-D, Mizumura K: Responses of neurons in VPL and VPL–VL region of the cat to algesic stimulation of muscle and tendon. *J Neurophysiol* 49:649–661, 1983.

119. Lamour Y, Willer JC, Guilbaud G: Rat somatosensory (Sm I) cortex: I. Characteristics of neuronal responses to noxious stimulation and comparison with responses to non-noxious stimulation. *Exp Brain Res* 49:35–45, 1983.

120. Lamour Y, Guilbaud G, Willer JC: Rat somatosensory (Sm I) cortex. II. Laminar and columnar organization of noxious and non-noxious inputs. *Exp Brain Res* 49:46–54, 1983.

121. Leijon G, Boivie J, Johansson I: Central post-stroke pain—neurological symptoms and pain characteristics. *Pain* 36:13–25, 1989.

122. Lende RA, Kirsch WM, Druckman R: Relief of facial pain after combined removal of precentral and postcentral cortex. *J Neurosurg* 34:537–543, 1971.

123. Light AR, Trevino DL, Perl ER: Morphological features of functionally defined neurons in the marginal zone and substantia gelatinosa of the spinal dorsal horn. *J Comp Neurol* 186:151–171, 1979.

124. Light AR, Casale EJ, Menétrey DM: The effects of focal stimulation in nucleus raphe magnus and periaqueductal gray on intracellularly recorded neurons in spinal laminae I and II. *J Neurophysiol* 56:555–571, 1986.

124a. Lima D: Anatomical basis for the dynamic processing of nociceptive input. *Eur J Pain* 2:195–202, 1998.

125. Lund M, Bengtsson A, Thorborg P: Muscle tissue oxygen pressure in primary fibromyalgia. *Scand J Rheumatol* 15:165–173, 1986.

126. Mallart A: Thalamic projection of muscle nerve afferents in the cat. *J Physiol* 194:337–353, 1968.

127. Margoles MS: Stress neuromyelopathic pain syndrome (SNPS): report of 333 patients. *J Neurol Orthop Surg* 4:317–322, 1983.

128. Marshall J: Sensory disturbances in cortical wounds with special reference to pain. *J Neurol Neurosurg Psychiatry* 14:187–204, 1951.

129. Marx JL: The fos gene as a "master switch." *Science* 237:854–856, 1987.

130. Maunz RA, Pitts NG, Peterson BW: Cat spinoreticular neurons: locations, responses, and changes in responses during repetitive stimulation. *Brain Res* 148:365–379, 1978.

131. McCreery DB, Bloedel JR, Hames EG: Effects of stimulating in raphe nuclei and in reticular formation on response of spinothalamic neurons to mechanical stimuli. *J Neurophysiol* 42:166–182, 1979.

132. McEvoy GK (Ed.): *AHFS Drug Information.* American Society of Health-Systems Pharmacists, Bethesda, MD, 1996.

133. McMahon SB, Wall PD: Descending excitation and inhibition of spinal cord lamina I projection neurons. *J Neurophysiol* 59:1204–1219, 1988.

134. Melzack R: The gate control theory 25 years later: new perspectives on phantom limb pain, Chapter 2. *Proceedings of the 6th World Congress on Pain.* Edited by Bond MR, Charlton JE, Woolf CJ. Elsevier, Amsterdam, 1991 (pp. 9–21).

135. Melzack R: Phantom limbs. *Sci Am* 266:120–126, 1992.

136. Melzack R: Gate control theory: on the evolution of pain concepts. *Pain Forum* 5:128–138, 1996.

137. Melzack R, Loeser JD: Phantom body pain in paraplegics: evidence of a central "pattern generating mechanism" for pain. *Pain* 4:195–210, 1978.

138. Melzack R, Wall PD: Pain mechanisms: a new theory. *Science* 150:971–979, 1965.

139. Menétrey D, Chaouch A, Besson JM: Location and properties of dorsal horn neurons at origin of spinoreticular tract in lumbar enlargement of the rat. *J Neurophysiol* 44:862–877, 1980.

140. Mense S: Nervous outflow from skeletal muscle following chemical noxious stimulation. *J Physiol* 267:75–88, 1977.

141. Mense S: Structure-function relationships in identified afferent neurones. *Anat Embryol* 181:1–17, 1990.

142. Mense S: Nociception from skeletal muscle in relation to clinical muscle pain. *Pain* 54:241–289, 1993.

143. Mense S, Meyer H: Bradykinin-induced modulation of the response behaviour of different types of feline group III and IV muscle receptors. *J Physiol* 398:49–63, 1988.

144. Mense S, Light AR, Perl ER: Spinal terminations of subcutaneous high-threshold mechanoreceptors. *Spinal Cord Sensation.* Edited by Brown AG, Réthelyi M. Scottish Academic Press, Edinburgh, 1981 (pp. 79–86).

145. Merskey H: Pain and psychological medicine, Chapter 46. *Textbook of Pain.* Ed. 2. Edited by Wall PD, Melzack R. Churchill Livingstone, New York, 1989 (pp. 656–666).

146. Merskey H: Chronic pain and psychiatric illness, Chapter 19. *The Management of Pain, Vol. 1.* Ed. 2. Edited by Bonica JJ. Lea & Febiger, Philadelphia, 1990 (pp. 320–327).

147. Middleton JW, Siddall PJ, Walker S, *et al.*: Intrathecal clonidine and baclofen in the management of spasticity and neuropathic pain following spinal cord injury: a case study. *Arch Phys Med Rehabil* 77:824–826, 1996.

148. Moldofsky H: Rheumatic pain modulation syndromes: the interrelationships between sleep, central nervous system, serotonin and pain. *Adv Neurol* 33:51–57, 1982.

149. Moncada S, Palmer RMR, Higgs EA: Nitric oxide: physiology, pathophysiology and pharmacology. *Pharmacol Rev* 43:109–142, 1991.

150. Mooney R: Synaptic basis for developmental plasticity in a birdsong nucleus. *J Neurosci* 12:2464–2477, 1992.

151. Morgan IT, Curran T: Stimulus-transcription coupling in neurones: role of cellular immediate-early genes. *TINS* 12:459–462, 1989.

152. Mountz JM, Bradley LA, Modell JG, *et al.*: Fibromyalgia in women. Abnormalities of regional cerebral blood flow in the thalamus and the caudate nucleus are associated with low pain threshold levels. *Arthritis Rheum* 38:926–938, 1995.

153. Müller W (Ed.): *Generalisierte Tendomyopathie (Fibromyalgie).* Steinkopff, Darmstadt, 1991.

154. Nakamura Y, Nagashima H, Mori S: Bilateral effects of the afferent impulses from the masseteric muscle on the trigeminal motoneuron of the cat. *Brain Res* 57:15–27, 1973.

155. Nazruddin, Suemune S, Shirana Y, et al.: The cells of origin of the hypoglossal afferent nerves and central projections in the cat. *Brain Res* 400:219–235, 1989.

156. Nishimori T, Sera M, Suemune S, et al.: The distribution of muscle primary afferents from the masseter nerve to the trigeminal sensory nuclei. *Brain Res* 372:375–381, 1986.

157. Nyström B, Hagbarth KE: Microelectrode recording from transected nerves in amputees with phantom limb pain. *Neurosci Lett* 27:211–216, 1981.

158. Olin BR, Editor in Chief: *Facts and Comparisons.* Facts and Comparisons, St. Louis, 1992.

159. Pagni CA: Central pain due to spinal cord and brain stem damage, Chapter 49. *Textbook of Pain.* Ed. 2. Edited by Wall PD, Melzack R. Churchill Livingstone, New York, 1989 (pp. 634–655).

160. Perl ER: Afferent basis of nociception and pain: evidence from the characteristics of sensory receptors and their projections to the spinal dorsal horn. *Pain.* Edited by Bonica JJ. Raven Press, New York, 1980 (pp. 19–45).

161. Pilowsky I: Pain and chronic illness behavior, Chapter 17. *The Management of Pain, Vol. 1.* Ed. 2. Edited by Bonica JJ. Lea & Febiger, Philadelphia, 1990 (pp. 300–309).

162. Pomeranz B, Wall PD, Weber WV: Cord cells responding to fine myelinated afferents from viscera, muscle and skin. *J Physiol* 199:511–532, 1968.

163. Randic M, Miletic V: Effect of substance P in cat dorsal horn neurones activated by noxious stimuli. *Brain Res* 128:164–169, 1977.

164. Rexed B: The cytoarchitectonic organization of the spinal cord in the cat. *J Comp Neurol* 96:415–496, 1952.

165. Riddoch G: The clinical features of central pain. *Lancet* 1:1093–1209, 1939.

166. Roland P: Cortical representation of pain. *TINS* 15:3–5, 1992.

167. Russell IJ: Neurohormonal aspects of fibromyalgia syndrome. *Rheum Dis Clin North Am* 15:149–168, 1989.

168. Russell IJ: Neurochemical pathogenesis of fibromyalgia syndrome. *J Musculoskeletal Pain* 1(1&2):61–92, 1996.

169. Russell IJ, Michalek JE, Vipraio GA, et al.: Platelet 3H-imipramine uptake receptor density and serum serotonin levels in patients with fibromyalgia/fibrositis syndrome. *J Rheumatol* 19:104–109, 1992.

170. Russell IJ, Orr MD, Littman B, et al.: Elevated cerebrospinal levels of substance P in patients with fibromyalgia syndrome. *Arthritis Rheum* 37:1593–1601, 1994.

171. Russell WR: Transient disturbances following gunshot wounds of the head. *Brain* 68:6–97, 1945.

172. Sandkühler J: The organization and function of endogenous antinociceptive systems. *Progr Neurobiol* 50:49–81, 1996.

173. Satoh M, Kuraishi Y, Kawamura M: Effects of intrathecal antibodies to substance P, calcitonin gene-related peptide and galanin on repeated cold stress-induced hyperalgesia: comparison with carrageenan-induced hyperalgesia. *Pain* 49:273–278, 1992.

174. Schaible H-G, Schmidt RF, Willis WD: Enhancement of responses of ascending tract cells in the cat spinal cord by acute inflammation of the knee joint. *Exp Brain Res* 66:489–499, 1987.

175. Schmidt RF: Die Gate-Control—Theorie des Schmerzes: eine unwahrscheinliche Hypothese. *Schmerz.* Edited by Janzen R, Keidel WD, Herz A, Steichele C. Thieme, Stuttgart, 1972 (pp. 133–135).

176. Segatore M: Understanding chronic pain after spinal cord injury. *J Neurosci Nurs* 26:230–236, 1994.

177. Sessle JB, Hu JW: Mechanisms of pain arising from articular tissues. *Can J Physiol Pharmacol* 69:617–626, 1991.

178. Sher GD, Cartmell SM, Gelgor L, et al.: Role of N-methyl-D-aspartate and opiate receptors in nociception during and after ischaemia in rats. *Pain* 49:241–248, 1992.

179. Shigena Y, Sera M, Nishimori T, et al.: The central projection of masticatory afferent fibers to the trigeminal sensory nuclear complex and upper cervical spinal cord. *J Comp Neurol* 268:489–507, 1988.

180. Simons DG: Myofascial pain syndrome due to trigger points, Chapter 45. *Rehabilitation Medicine.* Edited by Goodgold J. CV Mosby, St. Louis, 1988 (pp. 686–723).

181. Sirisko MA, Sessle BJ: Corticobulbar projections and orofacial muscle afferent inputs to neurones in primate sensorimotor cerebral cortex. *Exp Neurol* 82:716–720, 1983.

182. Siston DW, Special Projects Editor: *Physicians' Desk Reference.* Medical Economics, Montvale, NJ, 1997.

183. Spitzer NC: A developmental handshake: neuronal control of ionic currents and their control of neuronal differentiation. *J Neurobiol* 22:659–673, 1991.

184. Sternbach RA: Psychophysiological pain syndromes, Chapter 15. *The Management of Pain, Vol. 1.* Ed. 2. Edited by Bonica JJ. Lea & Febiger, Philadelphia, 1990 (pp. 287–290).

185. Stratz T, Samborski W, Hrycai P, et al.: Serotonin concentration in serum of patients with generalized tendomyopathy (fibromyalgia) and chronic polyarthritis. [German.] *Med Klin* 88:458–462, 1993.

186. Sutula T, He X-X, Cavazos J, et al.: Synaptic reorganization in the hippocampus induced by abnormal functional activity. *Science* 239:1147–1150, 1988.

187. Sweet WH: Cerebral localization of pain. *New Perspectives in Cerebral Localization.* Edited by Thompson RA, Green JR. Raven Press, New York, 1982.

188. Talbot JD, Marrett S, Evans AC, et al.: Multiple representations of pain in human cerebral cortex. *Science* 251:1355–1358, 1991.

189. Tasker RR: Pain resulting from central nervous system pathology (central pain), Chapter 14. *The Management of Pain, Vol. 1.* Ed. 2. Edited by

Bonica JJ. Lea & Febiger, Philadelphia, 1990 (pp. 264–275).

190. The American College of Rheumatology: Criteria for the classification of fibromyalgia. Report of the multicenter criteria committee. *Arthritis Rheum* 33:160–172, 1990.

191. Turk DC, Meichenbaum DH, Berman WH: Application of biofeedback for the regulation of pain: a critical review. *Psychol Bull* 86:1322–1338, 1979.

192. Vaeroy H, Helle R, Forre O, *et al.*: Elevated CSF levels of substance P and high incidence of Raynaud's phenomenon in patients with fibromyalgia: new features of diagnosis. *Pain* 33:21–26, 1988.

193. Vogt BA, Derbyshire S, Jones AK: Pain processing in four regions of human cingulate cortex localized with co-registered PET and MR imaging. *Eur J Neurosci* 8:1461–1473, 1996.

194. Wall PD: The presence of ineffective synapses and circumstances which unmask them. *Phil Trans R Soc Lond B* 278:361–372, 1977.

195. Wall PD: The gate control theory of pain mechanisms. A re-examination and restatements. *Brain* 101:1–18, 1978.

196. Wall PD: The prevention of postoperative pain. [Editorial.] *Pain* 33:289–290, 1988.

197. Wall PD, Cronly-Dillon JR: Pain, itch and vibration. *Arch Neurol* 2:365–375, 1960.

198. Wall PD, Woolf CJ: Muscle but not cutaneous C-afferent input produces prolonged increases in the excitability of the flexion reflex in the rat. *J Physiol* 356:443–458, 1984.

199. Ward NG: Pain and depression, Chapter 18. *The Management of Pain, Vol. 1*. Ed. 2. Edited by Bonica JJ. Lea & Febiger, Philadelphia, 1990 (pp. 310–319).

200. Wiberg M, Blomqvist A: The spinomesencephalic tract in the cat: its cells of origin and termination pattern as demonstrated by the intra-axonal transport method. *Brain Res* 291:1–18, 1984.

201. Wiesendanger M: Input from muscle and cutaneous nerves of the hand and forearm to neurones of the precentral gyrus of baboons and monkeys. *J Physiol* 228:203–219, 1973.

202. Wolfe F, Russell IJ, Vipraio GA, *et al.*: Serotonin levels, pain threshold, and FM. *J Rheumatol* 24:555–559, 1997.

203. Woolf CJ, Thompson SWN: The induction and maintenance of central sensitization is dependent on N-methyl-D-aspartic acid receptor activation; implications for the treatment of post-injury pain hypersensitivity states. *Pain* 44:293–299, 1991.

204. Woolf CJ, Wall PD: Relative effectiveness of C primary afferent fibers of different origins in evoking a prolonged facilitation of the flexor reflex in the rat. *J Neurosci* 6:1433–1442, 1986.

205. Woolf CJ, Shortland P, Sivilotti LG: Sensitization of high mechanothreshold superficial dorsal horn and flexor motor neurons following chemosensitive primary afferent activation. *Pain* 58:141–155, 1994.

206. Xu XJ, Hao JX, Seiger A, *et al.*: Chronic pain-related behaviors in spinally injured rats: evidence for functional alterations of the endogenous cholecystokinin and opioid systems. *Pain* 56:271–277, 1994.

207. Yezierski RP: Pain following spinal cord injury: the clinical problem and experimental studies. *Pain* 68:185–194, 1996.

208. Yokota T, Nishikawa Y, Koyama N: Tooth pulp input to the shell region of nucleus ventralis posteromedialis of the cat thalamus. *J Neurophysiol* 56:80–98, 1986.

209. Yu X-M, Mense S: Response properties and descending control of rat dorsal horn neurons with deep receptive fields. *Neuroscience* 39:823–831, 1990.

210. Yu X-M, Mense S: Somatotopical arrangement of rat spinal dorsal horn cells processing input from deep tissues. *Neurosci Lett* 108:43–47, 1990.

211. Yu X-M, Hua M, Mense S: The effects of intracerebroventricular injection of naloxone, phentolamine and methysergide on the transmission of nociceptive signals in rat dorsal horn neurones with convergent cutaneous-deep input. *Neuroscience* 44:715–723, 1991.

212. Zhuo M, Gebhart GF: Spinal serotonin receptors mediate descending facilitation of a nociceptive reflex from the nuclei reticularis gigantocellularis and gigantocellularis pars alpha in the rat. *Brain Res* 550:35–48, 1991.

213. Zidar J, Bäckman E, Bengtsson A, *et al.*: Quantitative EMG and muscle tension in painful muscles in fibromyalgia. *Pain* 40:429–454, 1990.

214. Zieglgänsberger W, Tulloch IF: Effects of substance P on neurones in the dorsal horn of the spinal cord of the cat. *Brain Res* 166:273–282, 1979.

CHAPTER 8
Myofascial Pain Caused by Trigger Points

SUMMARY: The **myofascial pain syndrome,** in its strict sense, is a regional pain syndrome characterized by the presence of myofascial trigger points (TrPs). Many overlapping and some confusingly similar muscle pain syndromes must be distinguished from each other. The most distinctive **clinical characteristics of TrPs** include circumscribed spot tenderness in a nodule that is part of a palpably tense band of muscle fibers, patient recognition of the pain that is evoked by pressure on the tender spot as being familiar, pain referred in the pattern characteristic of TrPs in that muscle, a local twitch response, painful limitation of stretch range of motion, and some weakness of that muscle. Promising **testing methods** to demonstrate the presence of TrPs include a specific needle electromyographic (EMG) technique, ultrasound, surface electromyography, algometry, and thermography. Referred motor dysfunctions during activity can be tested using surface EMG techniques. Recommended **diagnostic criteria** of an active TrP for general clinical use are the presence of a circumscribed spot tenderness in a nodule of a palpable taut band and patient recognition of the pain evoked by pressure on the tender spot as being a source of spontaneous pain. The **differential diagnosis and confusions** section of this chapter lists many conditions mimicked by TrPs. It emphasizes the importance of examining for, and understanding the distinguishing characteristics of, fibromyalgia and articular dysfunctions as compared with myofascial TrPs. A **dysfunctional neuromuscular endplate** appears to be the central factor for the development of TrPs. The newly discovered **electrodiagnostic characteristics of TrPs** include spontaneous electrical activity and spikes at active loci that are closely associated with dysfunctional motor endplates. The newly identified **histogenesis of TrPs** recognizes contraction knots as the key feature, which apparently are closely related to active loci. This leads to an **integrated hypothesis of TrPs** that postulates a local energy crisis resulting from the dysfunctional endplates at active loci. The extensive research on the **local twitch response** is summarized. Appropriate **treatment** of patients with TrPs may involve many forms of stretch, several techniques to augment muscle release, injection of TrPs, management of perpetuating factors, and a home self-treatment program.

A. BACKGROUND

1. Prevalence

Myofascial trigger points (TrPs) are extremely common and become a painful part of nearly everyone's life at one time or another. *Latent* TrPs, which often cause motor dysfunction (stiffness and restricted range of motion) without pain, are more common than the painful *active* TrPs (see Section B1).

Among 200 unselected, asymptomatic young adults, Sola et al.[269] found focal tenderness representing latent TrPs in the shoulder girdle muscles of 54% of the female and 45% of the male subjects. Referred pain was demonstrated in 25% of these subjects. A recent study of 269 *unselected* female student nurses with or without pain symptoms[238] showed a similar high prevalence of TrPs in masticatory muscles. A TrP was identified by palpating a taut band for spot tenderness of sufficient sensitivity to cause a pain reaction. No effort was made to distinguish between active and latent TrPs, but a considerable number of TrPs were likely active because 28% of subjects were aware of pain in the temple area. In masticatory muscles, TrPs were found in 54% of right lateral pterygoid muscles, in 45% of right deep masseter muscles, in 43% of right anterior tempo-

ralis muscles, and in 40% of intraoral examinations of the right medial pterygoid muscle. Among the neck muscles, TrPs were identified in 35% of the right splenius capitis muscles and in 33% of the right upper trapezius muscles. The insertion of the right upper trapezius to the clavicle was also tender in 42% of those muscles with TrPs. Enthesopathy of this muscle was common.[238]

Fröhlich and Fröhlich[87] examined 100 asymptomatic control subjects for latent TrPs in lumbogluteal muscles. They found latent TrPs in the following muscles: quadratus lumborum (45% of patients), gluteus medius (41%), iliopsoas (24%), gluteus minimus (11%), and piriformis (5%).

Individual reports of the prevalence of myofascial TrPs in patient populations are available and, together, indicate a high prevalence of this condition among individuals with a regional pain complaint. The reports that follow are summarized in Table 8-1.

In an internal medicine group practice,[265] 54 of 172 patients presented with a pain complaint. Sixteen (30%) of the pain patients met the criteria for myofascial TrPs. Four of these sixteen patients had a pain duration of less than 1 month; three, a duration of 1 to 6 months;

Table 8-1 *Prevalence of Trigger Point Pain in Selected Patient Populations*

Region	Practice	Number Studied	% With Myofascial Pain	Source
General	Medical	172 (54)	30	Skootsky et al.[265]
General	Pain Medicine Center	96	93	Gerwin[94]
General	Comprehensive Pain Center	283	85	Fishbain et al.[83]
Craniofacial	Head & Neck Pain Clinic	164	55	Fricton et al.[86]
Lumbogluteal	Orthopaedic Clinic	97	21	Fröhlich and Fröhlich[87]

and nine, a pain duration of more than 6 months.

A neurologist examining 96 patients from a community pain medical center[94] found that myofascial TrPs caused at least part of the pain in 93% of the patients and were the primary cause of the pain in 74% of the patients.

Among 283 consecutive admissions to a comprehensive pain center, a primary organic diagnosis of myofascial syndrome was assigned in 85% of cases.[83] A neurosurgeon and a physiatrist made this diagnosis independently, based on physical examination as described by Simons and Travell.[256]

Of 164 patients referred to a dental clinic for chronic head and neck pain of at least 6 months duration, 55% had a primary diagnosis of myofascial pain syndrome (MPS) caused by active TrPs.[86]

Five lumbogluteal muscles in 97 patients complaining of pain in the locomotor system were examined in an orthopaedic clinic.[87] Forty-nine percent presented with latent TrPs, and 21% presented with active TrPs in the piriformis muscle.

The wide range in prevalence of myofascial pain caused by TrPs that is reported in different studies is, in part, the result of differences in the patient populations examined and in the degree of chronicity. Probably even more important are differences in the criteria used to make the diagnosis of myofascial TrPs and differences in the training and skill level of the examiners. Few of these studies gave a detailed description of the diagnostic examinations employed. This summary excludes papers that used the term "myofascial pain" categorically[251] instead of referring to the specific clinical disorder MPS that is caused by TrPs. To distinguish between these two diagnostic meanings unambiguously, the term *soft tissue pain* is recommended to identify a nonspecific, categoric cause of tender musculature for any reason, and the term *myofascial TrPs* is recommended to identify MPS caused specifically by TrPs. Active myofascial TrPs are clearly common and are a major source of musculoskeletal pain and dysfunction, but the poor agreement on appropriate diagnostic criteria imposes a serious handicap. One study critically tested interrater reliability for five manual examinations in five different muscles[98] and demonstrated good to excellent agreement for all muscles. The one examination component that lagged behind the other features was the local twitch response (LTR), which was only moderately reliable for some of the muscles tested.

In a population of hospitalized and ambulatory physical medicine and rehabilitation service patients diagnosed as having fibrositis (findings compatible with MPS caused by TrPs), most were between 31 and 50 years of age. These data agree with our clinical impression that individuals in their mature years of maximum activity are most likely to suffer from the pain syndromes of active myofascial TrPs. With the reduced activity of more advanced age, the stiffness and restricted range of motion of latent TrPs tends to become more prominent than the pain of active TrPs. This important clinical observation needs experimental verification.

2. Importance

Voluntary (skeletal) muscle is the largest single organ of the human body and accounts for 40% or more of body weight.[7, 38, 183] The number of muscles counted depends on the extent of muscle subdivision that is accepted taxonomically and on the number of variable muscles that are included. Not counting heads, bellies, and other parts of muscles, the *Nomina Anatomica,* reported by the International Anatomical Nomenclature Committee under the Berne Convention,[144] lists more than 200 paired muscles, for a total of more than 400 muscles. Any one of these muscles can develop myofascial TrPs that refer pain and motor dysfunction, often to another location.

The clinical importance of myofascial TrPs to practitioners has been described in the literature for acupuncturists,[117, 196] anesthesiologists,[21, 268] chronic pain managers,[231] dentists,[86, 105, 149, 279] family practitioners,[193, 213] gynecologists,[223] neurologists,[91] nurses,[23] orthopaedic surgeons,[4, 8, 43] pediatricians,[9, 69] physical therapists,[208, 209] physiatrists,[29, 147, 229, 230, 233] rheumatologists,[85, 93, 225] and veterinarians.[152] Yet, the muscles in general and TrPs in particular receive little attention as a major source of pain and dysfunction in modern medical school teaching and in medical textbooks. This chapter describes a neglected, major cause of pain and dysfunction in the largest organ of the body. The contractile muscle tissues are a primary target of the wear and tear of daily activities, but it is the bones, joints, bursae, and nerves on which physicians usually concentrate their attention.

Severity. The severity of symptoms caused by myofascial TrPs ranges from the agonizing, incapacitating pain caused by extremely active TrPs to the painless restriction of movement and distortion of posture caused by latent TrPs. The influence of latent TrPs on physical function is commonly overlooked. The potential severity of acute activation of a TrP is illustrated by one housewife who, while bending over cooking, activated a quadratus lumborum TrP that felled her to the floor and caused pain so severe that she was unable to reach up and turn the stove off to prevent a pot from burning through its bottom.

Patients who have had other kinds of severe pain, such as that caused by a heart attack, broken bones, or renal colic, say that the myofascial pain from TrPs can be just as severe. Despite their painfulness, myofascial TrPs are not directly life-threatening. Conversely, their painfulness can, and often does, impact drastically on the affected person's quality of life.

Cost. Unrecognized myofascial headache, shoulder pain, and low back pain that have become chronic are major causes of industrial lost work time and of compensation applications. Bonica[19] pointed out that disabling chronic pain costs the American people billions of dollars annually. Low back pain alone costs the people of California $200 million annually. Analgesics taken to relieve chronic pain are costly and can be an important cause of interstitial nephropathy.[101] A considerable portion of the chronic pain caused by myofascial TrPs likely could be prevented by prompt diagnosis with appropriate treatment.

How many more people not included in these studies carry on, yet bear the misery of nagging TrP pain that would improve if the correct diagnosis were made and the patient were treated appropriately? When the myofascial nature of pain is unrecognized, such as the pain caused by TrPs in the pectoral muscles that mimics cardiac pain, the TrP symptoms can lead to misdiagnoses, such as neurotic, psychogenic, or behavioral disorders. This adds frustration and self-doubt to the patient's misery and impedes appropriate diagnosis and treatment. Active myofascial TrPs are likely a major overlooked cause for that enigmatic scourge of mankind that is referred to categorically as soft tissue pain. The total cost is incalculable but enormous, and much of it is unnecessary.

3. Historical Review

The history of growth in our understanding of musculoskeletal pain is the history of the identification of specific sources and causes of the pain. Examples include neuropathic sources, articular dysfunction, muscular origins, and modulation of central nervous system (CNS) processing of pain. The history of muscle pain for much of the 20th century was reviewed,[226, 244, 245] and recently has been updated.[248]

This review identifies a number of historically noteworthy publications that provide a background to our present understanding of myofascial pain caused by TrPs. Progress has been slow and intermittent. Medical conditions with distinctly different causes can produce confusingly similar symptoms of muscle pain and tenderness. The medical community is just beginning to sort out this complex puzzle. To clinically clarify what TrPs are, it may help to define more clearly what they are not and how the various other diagnoses may be interrelated. Major progress has been made during the past decade with the recognition of a possible CNS involvement in the muscle pain and tenderness of fibromyalgia syndrome (FMS), distinguishing it from the regional muscular dysfunction of MPS. The relative contributions of articular (somatic) dysfunctions to TrP symptoms remain to be as clearly delineated. This review demonstrates how adherents to a given school of thought have single-mindedly concentrated on part of the total clinical picture of myofascial TrPs, introduced new names, and overlooked the more comprehensive picture.

Froriep (1843)[88] is an example of one of the pre-20th century authors who used several names to describe extremely tender, palpable hardenings in muscles for which effective treatment afforded the patient much pain relief. By the turn of the 20th century (1900) in America, Adler[2] associated the English language term "muscular rheumatism" with the concept of pain radiating from a tender spot in muscle. In England, Gowers,[104] Stockman,[272] and Llewellyn and Jones[182] promoted the term "fibrositis" for the same symptom complex. In Germany, Schmidt's publications used the German counterpart to muscular rheumatism, *Muskelrheumatismus.*[239] Other authors used the term *"Weichteilrheumatismus,"* literally meaning "soft-parts rheumatism," which is commonly translated into English as *nonarticular rheumatism.* The cause was enigmatic and/or controversial in every case.

In 1919, Schade[236] reported that the hardness of previously tender ropiness in muscles persisted during deep anesthesia and even after death until it was obscured by diffuse rigor mortis. These findings seem to exclude nerve-activated, muscular contraction as the cause of the palpable bands but are still consistent with an endogenous contracture of sarcomeres. Schade[237] later postulated a localized increase in the viscosity of muscle colloid and proposed the term "Myogelosen," literally translated as "muscle gellings" and identified in English as myogelosis. In the same year, two orthopaedic surgeons in Munich, F. Lange and G. Eversbusch,[172] coined the term "Muskelhärten" to describe tender points associated with regions of palpable hardness in skeletal muscles. This term is translated literally into English as "muscle hardenings" or "indurations." F. Lange's student, M. Lange, later equated these muscle hardenings to Schade's myogeloses. He used fingers, knuckles, or a blunt wood probe to apply forceful, ecchymosis-producing massage (Gelotripsie). His com-

prehensive clinical book[173] also presented the history and experimental basis of the concept of myogeloses (prior to the discovery of the actin-myosin contractile mechanism). This work essentially ignored the referred pain aspect of TrPs.

Before coming to the United States from Germany, Hans Kraus, an early pioneer in this field, first reported the therapeutic use of ethyl chloride spray for relief of *Muskelhärten* in 1937,[166] for relief of fibrositis in 1952,[167] and for relief of TrPs in 1959.[168] Until his death, he continued to promote the concept of exercise for recovering and maintaining full range of motion for good health and to emphasize the importance of TrPs.

In 1938, Kellgren,[159] working under the influence of Sir Thomas Lewis, published a major milestone paper. He established unequivocally for most major postural muscles of the body that each muscle and many fascial structures had a characteristic referred pain pattern when injected with a small amount of painful salt solution. (See also his later paper on deep pain.[160]) Shortly thereafter, three clinicians on three continents[102, 161, 287] concurrently and independently published a series of papers in English emphasizing four cardinal features: a palpable nodular or band-like hardness in the muscle, a highly localized spot of extreme tenderness in that band, reproduction of the patient's distant pain complaint by digital pressure on that spot, and relief of the pain by massage or injection of the tender spot. Each author reported pain syndromes of specific muscles throughout the body in large numbers of patients. All three had identified myofascial TrPs. However, each used different diagnostic terms and seemed to have been unaware of the others. The commonality of their observations was first noticed by M. Reynolds[225, 226] decades later.

One of the three, Michael Gutstein, who later published as Good,[102] used many diagnostic terms to describe the same condition: myalgia, idiopathic myalgia, rheumatic myalgia, and nonarticular rheumatism. He illustrated the referred pain patterns of many patients as case reports. He repeatedly held that the process responsible for the "myalgic spots" was a local constriction of blood vessels caused by overactivity of the sympathetic fibers supplying them.

Michael Kelly published nearly a dozen papers on fibrositis between 1941[161] and 1963.[162] He was impressed both by the palpable hardness of the "nodule" associated with the tender point in the muscle and by the distant referral of pain from the afflicted muscle. Kelly gradually evolved the concept that fibrositis was a functional, neurologic disturbance that originated at the myalgic lesion. He envisioned little or no local pathology, but a CNS reflex disturbance that caused the referred pain.

Janet Travell published more than 40 papers on myofascial TrPs between 1942[287] and 1990.[283] Her two volumes of *The Trigger Point Manual* were published with Simons in 1983 and in 1992. In 1952, she and Rinzler reported the pain patterns of TrPs in 32 skeletal muscles as "the myofascial genesis of pain,"[285] which quickly became the classical source for TrP pain patterns. It was her opinion that any fibroblastic proliferation was secondary to a functional disorder; pathologic changes occurred only after the condition continued for a long time. She maintained that the self-sustaining characteristic of TrPs depended on a feedback mechanism between the TrP and the CNS. Of those three pioneers, Gutstein (Good), Kelly, and Travell, only Travell's influence has withstood the test of time.

To date, there is no adequate histologic study of human myofascial TrPs. The few biopsy studies that did evaluate the tender nodule of myogelosis or of fibrositis must have included many myofascial TrPs. Among them, the study by Miehlke *et al.*[202] of the *Fibrositissyndrom* (fibrositis syndrome) was the most extensive and thorough. They reported minimal findings in mild cases and increasingly marked non-specific dystrophic findings in the progressively more symptomatic cases. Since the pathophysiology of TrPs seems to involve primarily a dysfunction in the immediate region of a motor endplate, there has been no reason to expect that ordinary histologic studies would clearly reveal the cause. A recent histologic study of the palpable nod-

ules associated with myogelosis at TrP sites, however, found evidence of local muscle fiber contracture.[224]

Throughout most of the 20th century, the term "fibrositis" described a condition that was compatible with myofascial TrPs, although ambiguously so. In 1977, Smythe and Moldofsky[266] introduced another and very different meaning that redefined the concept of fibrositis.[226] They described a condition of generalized pain marked by multiple tender points when tested by palpation. Four years later, Yunus *et al.*[306] proposed the term "fibromyalgia" as a more appropriate name for this condition. Since the diagnoses of MPS and FMS now account for nearly all of the patients previously diagnosed as having fibrositis, the latter term has became an outmoded diagnosis. Ten years ago it was unclear how closely the pathophysiology of FMS and MPS related to each other; the etiology of both was highly speculative.

In 1990, rheumatologists under the leadership of Wolfe[299] officially established diagnostic criteria for fibromyalgia. The criteria were simple and the examination was easily and quickly performed, which helped focus the attention of the medical community on this syndrome. Since then, remarkable progress has been made, and now the opinion prevails that a CNS dysfunction is responsible for the increased pain sensitivity of fibromyalgia.[234]

In the mid-1980s, Fischer[72, 75] introduced pressure algometry, which is a quantitative method for measuring the sensitivity of myofascial TrPs and of fibromyalgia tender points.

An important milestone of progress was reached by Hubbard and Berkoff in 1993 when they reported needle EMG activity characteristic of myofascial TrPs.[141] The following year, Hong and Torigoe[134] demonstrated that the rabbit was a suitable experimental model for studying the LTR that is characteristic of human TrPs. In 1995, Simons *et al.*[261] confirmed in rabbit experiments the electrical activity reported by Hubbard and Berkoff. Their rabbit study, and a concomitant human study,[260] strongly implicated a dysfunctional endplate region as the prime site of TrP pathophysiology.[252]

Progress was again made with the report by Gerwin *et al.*[98] of an interrater reliability study that identified appropriate criteria for recognizing myofascial TrPs in five muscles. The integrated hypothesis that is described in Section D of this chapter moves our understanding of TrPs another major step forward.[253]

4. Related Diagnostic Terms

The cause of muscle pain syndromes, or musculoskeletal pain, has perplexed the medical community for more than a century. The subject has been plagued by a multitude of terms that emphasized different aspects of basically the same phenomenon[244, 245] and that have been reported in different languages. A brief review of some of the more important diagnostic terms currently encountered will help to put the available literature into perspective.

Anatomically Oriented Terms. Many authors through the years have "discovered" a "new" muscle pain syndrome related to a specific part of the body and given it a name corresponding to that region. Characteristically, myofascial TrPs contribute significantly to the pain syndrome identified. Common examples are tension headache,[149, 280, 293] the scapulocostal syndrome,[201, 212, 213] and epicondylitis (tennis elbow).

Fibromyalgia. Fibromyalgia is fundamentally a different condition than MPS but often presents with confusingly similar symptoms.[243] It is characterized by an augmentation of nociception, which causes generalized deep-tissue tenderness that includes muscles. It has a different etiology than that of myofascial TrPs, but many of the tender points diagnostic of FMS are also common sites for TrPs, and many patients have both conditions. In the German literature, fibromyalgia is usually equated with *Generalisierte Tendomyopathie* (generalized tendomyopathy). Fibromyalgia is considered in detail in Chapter 9.

Fibrositis. The term "fibrositis" appeared in the English literature in 1904[104] and was soon adopted into German as the *Fibrositissyndrom* (in English, *fibrositis syndrome*[165]). For most of the 20th century, it was generally characterized by the presence of tender palpable "fibrositic" nodules. Many of these patients had TrPs. In time, fibrositis became an increasingly controversial diagnosis because of multiple definitions and no satisfactory histopathologic basis for the palpable nodules. The diagnosis was completely redefined in 1977,[266] and the new definition was officially established in 1990 as fibromyalgia.[299] According to the current definition of fibromyalgia, it is unrelated to the original concept of fibrositis. Fibrositis is currently an outmoded diagnosis.

Muskelhärten. By 1921, the term *"Muskelhärten"*[172] was a recognized part of and still appears occasionally in German literature, but it is rarely encountered in English literature. It literally means "muscle indurations" and refers to the palpable firmness of the tender nodule responsible for the patient's pain. Another German term, *Myogelosen*[173] (literally "muscle gellings"), refers to the same phenomena, and the two terms have frequently been used interchangeably. *Muskelhärten* has often been used to describe the physical findings, and *Myogelosen* has been used to identify the diagnosis.

Myofascial Pain Syndrome. This term has acquired both a general and a specific meaning, which need to be distinguished.[251] The general meaning includes a regional muscle pain syndrome of any soft tissue origin that is associated with muscle tenderness,[170, 304] and it is commonly used in this sense by dentists.[12] The other meaning is specifically a MPS caused by TrPs. This is a focal hyperirritability in muscle that can strongly modulate CNS functions and is the subject of this chapter.

Myofascitis. The term "myofascitis" is now rarely (and should not be) used as synonymous with myofascial TrPs.[212] Myofascitis is properly used to identify infected muscles. A somewhat similar term, "myositis," is used categorically to describe a group of disorders resulting from autoimmune and other inflammatory muscle injuries, as with dermatomyositis and polymyositis.

Myogelosis. The term "myogelosis" is the English form of a German term, *"Myo-*

gelosen," which is still occasionally used and is generally considered synonymous with *Muskelhärten* (see above). The name *myogelosis* was based on an outmoded hypothesis to account for muscle contraction that was proposed before the actin-myosin contractile mechanism was discovered. This term may be related to the English term "gelling," currently used to denote the stiffness that develops in the joints or muscles of arthritic individuals after sitting still for some time, usually more than 30 minutes.

Nonarticular Rheumatism.   Nonarticular rheumatism is a commonly used, but not clearly defined, categoric term for soft tissue pain syndromes to distinguish them from disorders primarily associated with joint dysfunction or joint disease (articular rheumatism). The nonarticular term is now not commonly used. It may have derived from the German term *"Weichteilrheumatismus,"* which was commonly used to describe a wide range of conditions that included myofascial pain caused by TrPs. Currently, Romano[228] employs "nonarticular" to identify papers dealing with soft tissue pain syndromes that are *not* fibromyalgia and are *not* attributed to myofascial TrPs. The literature reviews by Romano[228] provide information about localized soft tissue pain conditions such as adhesive capsulitis, periarticular arthritis, bursitis, epicondylitis, insertion tendinosis, and tennis elbow, which are frequently myofascial TrP syndromes masquerading as another diagnosis.

Osteochondrosis.   This term is an inclusive term used by Russian vertebroneurologists to cover the interaction of neural and muscular conditions, such as fibromyalgia, myofascial TrPs, and spinal nerve compromise.

Soft Tissue Rheumatism.   This term is usually used synonymously with nonarticular rheumatism described above.

Tendomyopathy.   Tendomyopathy, the English version of a German term, can be divided into general and local categories. General tendomyopathy is considered synonymous with fibromyalgia.[206] Regionalized tendomyopathy is comparable in many ways to myofascial TrPs but is not as clearly defined.

B. CLINICAL CHARACTERISTICS OF TRIGGER POINTS

The clinical characteristics of TrPs and an etiologic basis for each are introduced and presented in this section. Testing techniques that are useful for experimental purposes and some of which have potential routine clinical application are likewise dealt with in more detail here.

Diagnosis and treatment of acute single-muscle myofascial pain syndromes can be simple and easy. When an acute myofascial TrP syndrome is neglected and allowed to become chronic, it can become unnecessarily complicated, more painful, and increasingly time-consuming, frustrating, and expensive to treat.

1. Symptoms

Onset.   Active TrPs, unlike latent TrPs, cause a clinical pain complaint or other abnormal sensory symptoms. Latent TrPs may show all the other characteristics of active TrPs but usually to a lesser degree. Both active and latent TrPs can cause significant motor dysfunction. The same factors responsible for the development of an active TrP can, to a lesser degree, apparently cause a latent TrP.

The activation of a TrP is usually associated with some degree of mechanical abuse of the muscle in the form of *muscle overload*, which may be acute, sustained, and/or repetitive. Leaving the muscle in a *shortened position* can convert a latent TrP to an active TrP; this process is greatly accelerated if the muscle is contracted while in the shortened position. In paraspinal[36] and lower extremity[301] muscles, a degree of *nerve compression* that causes identifiable neuropathic EMG changes is associated with an increase in the numbers of active TrPs. In addition, a satellite TrP can develop from a key TrP in another muscle.

The patient is aware of the pain caused by an active TrP but may or may not be aware of the dysfunction it causes. Latent TrPs characteristically cause some degree of disturbed motor function, which often escapes the patient's attention or is simply tolerated. The patient becomes aware of pain originating from a latent TrP only when pressure is applied to it. Spontaneous referred pain appears with increased irritability of the TrP.[137]

The patient usually presents with complaints resulting from the most recently activated TrP. When this TrP has been successfully eliminated, the pain pattern may shift to that of an earlier, key TrP, which also must be inactivated. If the key TrP is inactivated first, the patient may recover without further treatment. The intensity and the extent of the referred pain pattern depend on the degree of irritability of the TrP, not on the size of the muscle. Myofascial TrPs in small, obscure, or variable muscles can be as troublesome to the patient as TrPs in large familiar muscles.

As illustrated in Figure 8-1, TrPs are activated directly by acute overload, overwork fatigue, radiculopathy, and gross trauma. TrPs are activated indirectly by other TrPs, visceral disease, arthritic joints, joint dysfunctions, and emotional distress. Satellite TrPs are prone to develop in muscles that lie within the pain reference zone of key myofascial TrPs or within the zone of pain referred from a diseased viscus, such as the pain of myocardial infarction, peptic ulcer, cholelithiasis, or renal colic. Any perpetuating factor can increase the likelihood of overload stress converting a TrP from a latent to an active one.

Clinically, it is often observed that with gentle, normal activity and in the absence of perpetuating factors, an *acute* active TrP may revert spontaneously to a latent state. Pain symptoms disappear, but occasional reactivation of the TrP by exceeding that muscle's stress tolerance can account for a

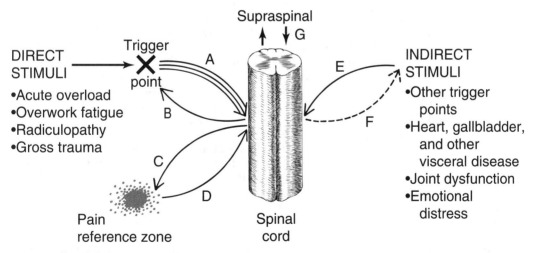

Figure 8-1. Schematic of central nervous system interactions with a TrP (*X*). *Triple arrow A,* running from the TrP to the spinal cord, represents sensory, autonomic, and motor effects. *Arrow B,* running from the spinal cord to the TrP, includes autonomic modulation of the intensity of TrP activation. *Arrow C,* running to the pain reference zone, represents the appearance of referred pain and tenderness at distant sites that may be several neurologic segments removed from the TrP. *Arrow D* indicates the influence of the vapocoolant spray in the region of the reference zone that facilitates release of the TrP. *Arrow E* signifies the activating effect of indirect stimuli on the TrP. *Dashed arrow F* denotes effects of TrPs on visceral function. *Vertical thick arrows G* identify TrP interactions at the supraspinal level. (Adapted from Travell J: Myofascial trigger points: clinical view. *Advances in Pain Research and Therapy, Volume 1.* Edited by Bonica JJ, Albe-Fessard D. Raven Press, New York, 1976 (pp. 919–926) (figure 10).)

history of recurrent episodes of the same pain over a period of years. This important clinical observation needs to be tested by critical research experiments.

Pain Complaint. Patients with active myofascial TrPs usually complain of aching pain characteristic of deep tissues, such as muscle and joints. They rarely complain of sharp, clearly localized cutaneous-type pain. The myofascial pain is often referred to a site some distance from the TrP in a pattern that is characteristic for each muscle. Sometimes, the patient is aware of numbness or paresthesia rather than pain.

Infants have been observed with point tenderness of the rectus abdominis muscle and colic. Both were relieved by sweeps of a stream of vapocoolant over the muscle, which helps to inactivate myofascial TrPs.

When children with musculoskeletal pain complaints were examined for myofascial TrPs, the TrPs were found to be a common source of their pain.[10] It is our impression that the likelihood of developing pain-producing *active* TrPs increases with age into the most active, middle years. As activity becomes less strenuous in later years, individuals are more likely to exhibit the stiffness and restricted range of motion of *latent* TrPs.

Sola[267] found that laborers who exercise their muscles heavily every day are less likely to develop active TrPs than are sedentary workers who are prone to intermittent bouts of vigorous physical activity. Our clinical experience has been similar.

Active TrPs are found commonly in postural muscles of the neck, shoulder, and pelvic girdles and in the masticatory muscles. In addition, the upper trapezius, scalene, sternocleidomastoid, levator scapulae, and quadratus lumborum muscles are commonly involved.

Dysfunctions. In addition to the clinical symptoms produced by the sensory disturbances of referred pain, dysesthesias, and hypesthesias, patients can experience clinically important disturbances of autonomic and motor functions.

Disturbances of **autonomic functions** that can be caused by TrPs include local cutaneous hyperthermia, referred cutaneous hypothermia, and persistent lacrimation (if the TrP is located in the head and neck region). Related proprioceptive disturbances caused by TrPs include imbalance, dizziness, tinnitus, and distorted weight perception of lifted objects.

Disturbances of **motor functions** caused by TrPs include weakness of the involved muscle function, loss of coordination by the involved muscle, and decreased work tolerance of the involved muscle. Weakness and the loss of work tolerance are often interpreted as an indication for increased exercise, but if this is attempted without inactivating the responsible TrPs, the exercise is likely to encourage and further ingrain substitution by other muscles, with further weakening and deconditioning of the involved muscle. The combination of weakness and loss of arm/hand muscle coordination makes hand grip unreliable; objects sometimes slip unexpectedly from the patient's grasp.

The patient is prone to intuitively substitute without realizing that, for instance, he or she is carrying the grocery bag in the nondominant but now-stronger arm. The weakness results from reflex motor inhibition (see Chapter 6, Section A) and characteristically occurs without atrophy of the affected muscle.

Sleep Disturbances. Sleep disturbance can be a problem for patients with a painful TrP syndrome. The influence of TrPs on sleep has not been studied systematically, but Moldofsky[205] has shown in a series of studies that other painful conditions, such as FMS and rheumatoid arthritis, can seriously disturb sleep. One study of MPS patients with active TrPs indicated that they commonly exhibited the same electroencephalographic changes during sleep. This sleep disturbance can, in turn, increase pain sensitivity the next day. Active myofascial TrPs become more painful when the muscle is held in the shortened position for long periods of time and if body weight is compressing the TrP. Thus, for patients with active TrPs, sleep positioning is critical to avoid unnecessary disturbance of sleep.

2. Physical Findings

A muscle harboring a TrP usually exhibits painful restriction of full range of motion and some losses of strength and/or endurance. Clinically, the TrP is identified as a localized spot of tenderness in a nodule or a palpable taut band of muscle fibers. Painfully restricted stretch range of motion and palpable increase in muscle tenseness (decreased compliance) are more severe in more active TrPs. An active TrP is identified when patients recognize the pain that is induced by applying pressure to the TrP as "their" pain. The taut band fibers usually respond with a LTR, when the taut band is accessible and is stimulated by properly applied snapping palpation. Taut bands respond consistently when the TrP is penetrated by a needle.

Taut Band. By gently rubbing across the direction of the muscle fibers of a superficial muscle, the examiner can feel a nodule at the TrP and a rope-like induration that extends from this nodule to the attachment at each end of the involved muscle fibers. The taut band can be snapped or rolled under the finger in accessible muscles. With effective inactivation of the TrP, this palpable sign becomes less tense and often (but not always) disappears, sometimes immediately.

Tender Nodule. Palpation along the taut band reveals a highly localized, exquisitely tender spot characteristic of a TrP that often feels nodular. Displacement of the pain threshold algometer by 2 cm along the band produced a statistically significant decrement in the algometer readings.[137, 222] Clinically, displacement of the induced pressure by 1 or 2 mm at a TrP can result in a markedly reduced pain response.

This critical clinical distribution of tenderness in the vicinity of a TrP corresponds to the sensitivity of the experimental LTR as demonstrated in rabbit experiments.[135] A 5-mm displacement to either side of the TrP (perpendicular to the taut band) resulted in almost total loss of response. The response faded out more slowly, however, when

stimulated over a range of several centimeters along the taut band (see "Local Twitch Response" in Section D of this chapter).

It now appears that sensitized nociceptors in the vicinity of dysfunctional motor endplates with contraction knots are most likely at the heart of these TrP phenomena. Experimental data indicate that there are many such active loci in any one TrP.[232, 235] From this it would follow that the more of these highly sensitive dysfunctional loci that are present, the larger and more sensitive would be the TrP.

Recognition. The application of digital pressure on either an active or a latent TrP can elicit a referred pain pattern characteristic of TrPs in that muscle. If the patient "recognizes" the elicited sensation as familiar clinically, however, this establishes the TrP as being active and is one of the most important diagnostic criteria available when the palpable findings are also present.[98, 252] Similar recognition is frequently observed when a needle penetrates the TrP and encounters an active locus.[129, 260]

Referred Sensory Signs. In addition to referring pain to the reference zone, TrPs characteristically refer tenderness and, sometimes, dysesthesias or hypoesthesia. The nature of this referred tenderness has been demonstrated experimentally by Vecchiet et al.[289]

Local Twitch Response. Snapping palpation of the TrP frequently evokes a transient twitch response of the taut band fibers. Its pathophysiologic nature is considered in Section D of this chapter. Twitch responses can be elicited from both active and latent TrPs. No difference in EMG response was noted in twitch responses, whether elicited by snapping palpation or by needle penetration.[257]

Limited Range of Motion. Muscles with active myofascial TrPs have a restricted stretch range of motion because of pain, as demonstrated by Macdonald.[187] An attempt to passively stretch the muscle beyond this limit produces increasingly severe pain, presumably because the muscle fibers of the taut band are already under substantially increased tension at rest length. The limitation of stretch resulting from pain is not quite as great with active as with passive lengthening of the muscle, at least partly as the result of reciprocal inhibition. When the TrP is inactivated and the taut band is released, the range of motion returns to normal. The degree of limitation produced by TrPs is much more marked in some muscles (e.g., subscapularis) than in others (e.g., latissimus dorsi).

Painful Contraction. When a muscle with an active TrP is strongly contracted against fixed resistance, the patient feels pain,[187] especially at attachment TrPs. This effect is most marked when an attempt is made to contract the muscle in a shortened position. This combination would maximize shortening of the sarcomeres in the contraction knot, aggravating the TrP mechanism to induce local cramping and, sometimes, referred pain.

Weakness. Although weakness is generally characteristic of a muscle with active myofascial TrPs, the magnitude is variable from muscle to muscle and from subject to subject. EMG studies indicate that in muscles with active TrPs, the muscle starts out fatigued, fatigues more rapidly, and becomes exhausted sooner than do normal muscles. This issue is presented in more detail under "Surface Electromyography" in Section C of this chapter.

3. Testing

No laboratory test or imaging technique has been generally established as diagnostic of TrPs. Three measurable phenomena, however, help greatly to substantiate objectively the presence of a TrP and are valuable as research tools. Two of them, electromyography and ultrasound, have much potential for clinical application in the diagnosis and treatment of TrPs. Magnetic resonance imaging and tissue impedance imaging of TrPs are unexplored possibilities.

Needle Electromyography. In 1993, Hubbard and Berkoff[141] reported finding EMG activity identified as specific to myofascial TrPs in a group of FMS patients. The utilization of FMS patients in this study would raise a concern about the generalizability of the findings to MPS patients without associated FMS. This same phe-

nomenon, however, had been noted in 1957 by Weeks and Travell.[294] Subsequent rabbit and human studies[259, 261, 262a] have confirmed the presence of spontaneous low-amplitude "noise" activity that is highly characteristic of myofascial TrPs but is not pathognomonic. The source of the high-amplitude spikes can be ambiguous. When the noise-like activity is also observed, it is a strongly confirmatory finding and an invaluable research tool. A detailed consideration of this phenomenon appears later in this chapter.

Ultrasound Imaging. Visualization of a LTR by use of ultrasound was first reported by Michael Margolis.[190] This observation was followed up with a study by Gerwin[95, 96] (Fig. 8-2) and applied clinically.[81] This imaging procedure provides a second means of substantiating and studying the LTR. In addition, it has potential for providing imaging that can be used to substantiate the clinical diagnosis of MPS caused by TrPs. This test would require the examiner to use the skill-demanding snapping palpation technique or to insert a needle into the TrP to elicit the twitch response.

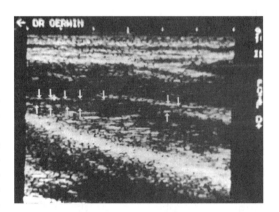

Figure 8-2. High-resolution ultrasound image of a LTR in the taut band fibers. The twitch was elicited by needle penetration of the TrP in a taut band of a right infraspinatus muscle. *White arrows* identify the band across the middle of the figure, seen to contract by ultrasound imaging. The transient contraction coincided with the patient's verbal report that he felt his typical pain and experienced a referred pain to his shoulder and arm. (Reproduced with permission from Gerwin RD, Shannon S, Hong C-Z, et al.: Interrater reliability in myofascial trigger point examination. *Pain* 69:65–73, 1997.)

Surface Electromyography. Surface EMG testing helps greatly to identify the source of increased resting muscle tension. The various causes of increased muscle tonus and the important role of EMG evaluation have recently been extensively reviewed.[258] (See also Chapter 5.) When the tension is caused entirely by the TrP-induced contracture of skeletal muscle (which occurs in the absence of action potentials), the EMG record is silent. When the tension results from muscle contraction originating neurogenically (through activation of the neuromuscular endplate), the EMG activity can locate the action potentials causing the tension.

TrPs cause distortion or disruption of normal muscle function. Functionally, the muscle with the TrP evidences a threefold problem: It exhibits *increased responsiveness*, *delayed relaxation*, and *increased fatigability*. Together, these dysfunctions cause overload and reduced work tolerance. In addition, the TrP can produce *referred spasm* and *referred inhibition* in other muscles. With the recent appearance of on-line computer analysis of EMG amplitude and mean power spectral frequency, a few pioneering investigators have reported the effects of TrPs on muscle activity. The reports indicate that TrPs can influence motor function of the muscle in which they occur *and* that their influence can be transmitted through the CNS to other muscles. To date, there has not been a sufficient number of well-controlled studies to establish the clinical reliability and application of these observations, but the few studies of TrP effects are promising.[121, 122]

The strong clinical effects of TrPs on sensation through referred pain have been mentioned in this chapter. It is well known that strong cutaneous stimuli (electric shocks) can cause reflex motor effects (flexion or flexor reflex).[119] If skin can modulate motor activity and TrPs can modulate sensory activity, it should be no surprise that TrPs can also strongly affect motor activity. In fact, the motor effects of TrPs may be the most important influence they exert, because the motor dysfunction they produce may result in overload of compensating muscles and spread the TrP problem from muscle to muscle. Accumu-

lating evidence now indicates that the muscles targeted for referred spasm from TrPs also usually have TrPs themselves.[121] These motor phenomena of TrPs deserve serious research investigation.

An **increased responsiveness** of the affected muscle is indicated by the abnormally high amplitude of EMG activity when the muscle is voluntarily contracted and loaded. Characteristically, the muscle with the TrP shows no motor unit activity at rest but tends to "overreact" with activity.[59] During flexion/extension movements of the head, the upper trapezius and/or sternocleidomastoid muscles with TrPs presented surface EMG amplitude more than 20% greater than asymptomatic muscles in 80% of cases. Headley[122] demonstrated a similar, marked augmentation of EMG activity in the upper trapezius with TrPs, compared with the uninvolved muscle on the contralateral side, when the patient attempted to shrug both shoulders equally.

Hagberg and Kvarnström[120] demonstrated **accelerated fatigability** electromyographically and in terms of work tolerance of the trapezius muscle, which had myofascial TrPs, compared with the contralateral muscle, which was pain-free. The EMG amplitude increased and median power frequency decreased significantly in the involved muscle compared with the uninvolved muscle. Both of these changes are characteristic of initial fatigue. Mannion and Dolan[188] showed a nearly linear relationship between the decline in median power frequency and the decline in strength of maximum voluntary contraction, tested intermittently, during fatiguing exercise. The increasing fatigue of the muscle was demonstrable as increasing weakness.

There is general acceptance of median power frequency as a valid criterion of muscle fatigue. Headley[123] studied **delayed recovery** following fatiguing exercise in 55 patients with muscle-related cumulative trauma disorder. Myofascial TrPs were common in the involved muscles in this group. Median power spectral analysis of surface EMG activity of bilateral lower trapezius muscles was monitored preexercise and postexercise and after a 7-minute rest. A statistically significant difference between preexercise and postexercise mean power spectral values and the postexercise values showed minimal recovery in 7 minutes, whereas normal muscles showed 70 to 90% recovery within 1 minute.

Delayed relaxation is commonly seen in muscle-overload work situations.[123] This failure to relax is a common surface EMG finding during repetitive exercises of muscles with myofascial TrPs. Headley[123] emphasized the importance of the brief surface EMG gaps observed in normal records of repetitive movements. Loss of these gaps can contribute significantly to muscle fatigue. Ivanichev[146] demonstrated delayed relaxation (loss of clean gaps with loss of muscle coordination) in a study of patients who had TrPs only in flexor or only in extensor forearm muscles. When doing rapid alternating movements of wrist flexion and extension, the muscles with TrPs showed the loss of coordination.

The presence of a sustained low-level EMG activity when the muscle could and should be relaxed is sometimes referred to as a static load. This persistent unnecessary activity also accelerates fatigue of the muscle.

Figure 8-3 illustrates schematically the EMG changes observed in exercised muscles with TrPs. The involved muscle shows a degree of fatigue at the beginning of a repetitive task, with accelerated fatigability and delayed recovery. These features apparently are hallmarks of the motor dysfunction of muscles containing myofascial TrPs.

The TrP can also induce motor activity (referred spasm) in other muscles, as already shown in Figure 6-7.[121] Pressure on a TrP in one (the infraspinatus) muscle induced a strong spasm response in another (the anterior deltoid) muscle. This response failed to occur following inactivation of the infraspinatus TrP. The muscle in which spasm is induced often also has TrPs, and this fits with the observation that muscles with TrPs are more readily activated and, therefore, are more likely to become target muscles for referred spasm than are muscles free of TrPs.

Certain muscles tend to be targets of referred spasm, so that TrPs in a number of distant muscles can accentuate EMG activity and irritability of a target muscle. The

upper trapezius, masseter, posterior cervicals, and lumbar paraspinal muscles appear to be common target muscles. These are also muscles that are prone to develop tightness, according to Janda.[151]

Carlson et al.[30] demonstrated the TrP-target muscle relationship for referred spasm between the upper trapezius and the ipsilateral masseter muscle. Following TrP injection of the trapezius muscle, there was a significant reduction in pain intensity ratings and EMG activity in the masseter muscle. Every one of these patients had localized TrP tenderness in the masseter TrP location, reinforcing the suspicion that target muscles characteristically have TrPs, but not necessarily active TrPs.

These examples are analogous to the activated segment concept described by Korr et al.[164] In their report, the spasm was demonstrated by paraspinal muscles acting as target muscles at the same level as nearby vertebrae, showing pressure sensitivity indicative of articular (somatic) dysfunction. The spasm response was most marked when pressure was applied to painfully pressure-sensitive vertebra.[54]

Spasm may be referred by TrPs independent of pain referral. Headley[121] noted that distant TrPs that referred spasm to the paraspinal muscles were not prone to refer pain and were rated as only mildly painful on application of pressure. She reported that inactivation of TrPs in these key spasm-inducing muscles resulted in marked reduction of low back pain.

The capacity of TrPs to refer **inhibition** can cause major disruption of normal muscle function. Headley[122] illustrated two clear examples of movement-specific inhibition in which the muscle worked well during isometric strength testing but did not contract at all during a movement for which it would normally serve as prime or assisting mover. A frequently seen example is an anterior deltoid muscle that is strongly inhibited during shoulder flexion but is recruited essentially normally during shoulder abduction. The normal functional pattern returned with inactivation of the TrP in the infraspinatus muscle.[123a]

Another example of referred inhibition[122] was an active TrP in the quadratus lumborum that inhibited gluteal muscles. Normal function of the gluteal

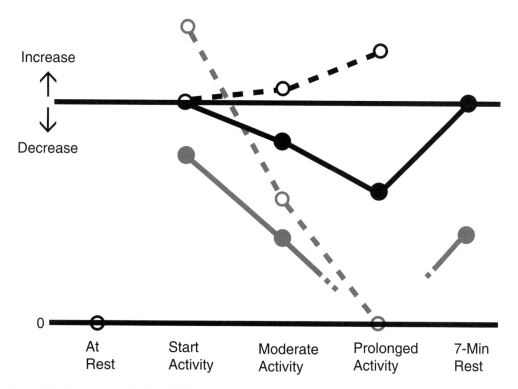

○··○ Amplitude, normal muscle

○··○ Amplitude, TrP muscle

●—● Median frequency, normal muscle

●—● Median frequency, TrP muscle

Increase

↑
↓

Decrease

0

| At Rest | Start Activity | Moderate Activity | Prolonged Activity | 7-Min Rest |

Figure 8-3. Comparison of surface EMG response to fatiguing exercise of normal muscle (*black lines*) and muscle with active TrPs (*red lines*). The averaged amplitude (*open circles*) and mean power frequency (*solid circles*) of the EMG record from the muscle with TrPs start out as if the muscle is already fatigued and show that the muscle with TrPs reaches exhaustion more quickly than does normal muscle. These changes are accompanied by accelerated fatigue and weakness of the muscle with TrPs. (Reproduced with permission from Simons DG, Travell JG, Simons LS: *Travell and Simons' Myofascial Pain and Dysfunction: The Trigger Point Manual, Volume 1. Upper Half of Body.* Ed. 2. Williams & Wilkins, Baltimore, 1999.)

muscles was restored when the TrP was inactivated. The immediate restoration of normal strength and normal median power spectral frequency during repetitive activity confirms that the recruited muscle was not lacking strength before the test but was neurologically inhibited by the quadratus lumborum TrP. With sufficient repetitions in a work situation, these ab-normal patterns become "well learned," and the muscle no longer returns immediately to a normal pattern with inactivation of the TrP. When that occurs, it is necessary to retrain the muscle to a normal pattern *after* inactivation of the responsible TrPs. Surface EMG biofeedback from the inhibited muscle(s) can facilitate retraining.

Algometry. Algometry (measurement of pain), in practice, is the measurement of tenderness in response to a force applied perpendicularly to the skin. Three endpoints are available: the onset of local pain (pressure pain threshold), the onset of referred pain (referred pain threshold), and intolerable pressure (pain tolerance). Most commonly, the pressure required to reach a pain threshold is measured directly from a spring scale calibrated in kilograms, Newtons, or pounds. Since the pressure is applied through a circular footplate, its diameter is a factor, and the actual measurement being made is stress (kg/cm^2) applied to skin. Since one of the most common algometers has a footplate area of $1\ cm^2$, the meter reading in kilograms is numerically the same as kg/cm^2; thus, no conversion is needed.

A convenient handheld spring algometer that is commercially available was described in 1986 and 1997,[73,79] and standard values were published in 1987.[74] Since then, it has been widely used in research papers. This device is useful for making a measurement of pain pressure threshold at a TrP site so that the initial tenderness can be compared with subsequent measurements following a therapeutic or experimental intervention. It is relatively objective, since the subject need not see the meter display, but the reading does depend on the subject's report of a subjective sensation. It is useful for research studies and helpful in many clinical situations, but the user must be aware of four kinds of limitations, listed below.

First, the measurement *per se* says absolutely nothing about the source or cause of the tenderness being measured. The tenderness may be caused by TrPs of myofascial pain, tender points of fibromyalgia, bursitis, severe spasm, etc. Therefore, by itself, the tenderness cannot serve as a diagnostic criterion. The cause of the tenderness must be established in combination with other diagnostic tests.

Second, the absolute value obtained at any one site can be strongly influenced by variations in the thickness and compliance of subcutaneous tissues from subject to subject and by inherent differences in the sensitivity of different muscles.[74]

Third, the relatively high degree of skill required to use this instrument effectively and the exquisite specificity of the location of the tender spot being measured are generally underrated. The precise location of maximum tenderness of that TrP must first be established by palpation or with the subject's cooperation. Since the tenderness of the *nodule* in a *taut band* is being measured, the footplate must be centered over the point of maximum tenderness in the nodule, and pressure must be aimed precisely in the direction of the nodule. The footplate *must remain* in this position throughout the measurement. If the footplate slips off the nodule and compresses the tissue adjacent to the nodule (which it is prone to do), an entirely different and erroneously high reading is obtained. For these reasons, errors are usually underestimations, not overestimations of the tenderness. By placing a finger on each side of the nodule or taut band and positioning the footplate between the fingers, the fingers can serve as a guide to maintain the footplate position over the point of maximum tenderness.

Fourth, the rate of application of pressure is important and is standardized at 1 kg/sec. If the rate is faster, FMS patients tend to report pain at less pressure. These difficulties would be at least partly ameliorated by averaging the lowest two of three readings if they are in reasonable agreement.

What constitutes appropriate interpretation of results from algometry of TrPs has recently been greatly clarified by Hong et al.[132, 137] Those authors, using algometry, examined three sites associated with latent and active TrPs of the extensor digitorum communis muscle of the middle finger. The three sites were on the TrP, the taut band 2 cm distal to the TrP, and, as a control (normal muscle) site, 1 cm further distal and 1 cm lateral to the taut band site. At each site, they measured three kinds of thresholds: onset of (local) pain, onset of referred pain, and intolerable pain. The authors[137] showed convincingly that eliciting referred pain in the expected pattern for that muscle is *not* a specific finding of TrPs. Instead, its presence is primarily dependent on the amount of pressure applied to the site. In all 25 examinations, referred pain was elicited from both the active TrP site and its taut band site (2 cm removed from the TrP). At the control site in these patients, referred pain was elicited in *half* of the examinations before reaching pain tolerance. In the subjects with latent TrPs, characteristic referred pain was elicited in *one fourth* of the examinations at the normal muscle site. These findings agree with those of Scudds *et al.*[242] that referred pain frequently can be elicited from normal muscle with the application of sufficient pressure in subjects with no pain complaint. The presence of local tenderness at these apparently normal muscle sites is even more common in patients suffering from TrP pain or fibromyalgia.

Hong *et al.*[137] found that referred pain could be elicited from every active TrP site but from only 47% of the latent TrP sites. Stated another way, it took less pressure to elicit referred pain from an active TrP than from a latent TrP. As would be expected, all three kinds of thresholds were significantly lower ($P < 0.01$) at active TrPs than at latent TrPs. The more irritable the TrP, the lower its pain threshold. Considerable overlap existed, however, between values obtained from active and latent TrPs; thus, threshold measurements alone in this muscle were not sufficient to distinguish active from latent TrPs. This study demonstrates that algometry can be a powerful research tool.

Another form of algometer is an electronic pressure-sensitive film that can be placed on the fingertip. Such a device was described as a palpometer.[14] All of the versions tried so far had a problem with adequate sensitivity and linearity of instrumental response at small pressure values, where resolution and accuracy are most important. When these technical problems have been solved, this device will have several advantages.

Thermography. Thermograms can be recorded by infrared radiometry or with films of liquid crystal. Recording infrared radiation (electronic thermography) with computer analysis provides a powerful tool for the accurate rapid visualization of skin temperature changes over large areas. This technique can demonstrate cutaneous reflex phenomena characteristic of myofascial TrPs. The less expensive contact sheets of liquid crystal have limitations that make reliable interpretation of the findings considerably more difficult.

Each of these thermographic techniques measures the skin surface temperature to a depth of only a few millimeters. The temperature changes correspond to changes in the circulation within but not beneath the skin. The endogenous cause of these temperature changes is usually sympathetic nervous system activity. Thermographic changes in skin temperature, therefore, are comparable in meaning to changes in skin resistance or changes in sweat production. Electronic infrared thermography is, however, superior to the other two measures in convenience and in spatial as well as temporal resolution.

The following research studies indicate that just finding a hot spot on the thermogram is *not* sufficient to identify a TrP beneath it. A similar temperature change can be expected from radiculopathy, an articular dysfunction, enthesopathy, or the result of a local subcutaneous inflammation. The thermographic hot spot of a TrP is described as a discoid region 5 to 10 cm in diameter, displaced slightly from directly over the TrP.[72] Five studies reported a region of hyperthermia over the TrP (a total of 170 TrPs)[56, 57, 75, 82, 171]; none reported a finding of hypothermia. No such agreement exists with regard to skin temperature changes in the region of referred pain. Available data suggest an interesting possibility, however. Undisturbed TrPs referring spontaneous autonomic cutaneous effects may tend to induce hyperthermia in a limited area of the skin overlying the TrP, whereas mechanical stimulation of the TrP that induces additional pain also induces a "reflex" hypothermia dependent on the stimulus. This latter phenomenon may be a far more discriminating criterion of a TrP. Research studies are needed, however, to investigate whether this reflex hypothermia is distinguishable from that which may occur when painful pressure is applied to a tender articular dysfunction, an area of bursitis, or an area of enthesopathy.

A thermographic hot spot was used by Kruse and Christiansen[171] as an initial identifier of the location of a TrP. Then, the presence of the TrP was confirmed by physical examination. This procedure eliminated TrPs that might not be thermographically active.

Swerdlow and Dieter[273] examined 165 patients who suffered whiplash injury and found that 139 of them had TrPs in the upper, middle, or lower trapezius muscles. Using Fischer's thermographic criteria, they found 40% false positives and 20% false negatives among these patients, which is unacceptable as a diagnostic criterion.

Scudds et al.[242] examined the backs of 49 fibromyalgia patients and 19 myofascial pain patients, using infrared thermography under resting conditions in conjunction with a dolorimeter study of referred pain. They found that the average skin temperature of the myofascial pain patients was 0.65°C warmer than that of the fibromyalgia patients. Apparently this study identified TrPs only by spot tenderness and referral of pain, which a subsequent study showed can also occur in normal subjects.[242] All TrPs caused referred pain, and half of the most tender spot in a fibromyalgia patient also referred pain. This result may mean that half of the fibromyalgia patients also had TrPs, which is consistent with the finding of another investigator who looked for that possibility,[92] or it may mean that some tender points that are not TrPs may also refer pain. These studies do suggest that patients selected primarily for myofascial TrPs are more likely to exhibit hyperthermia than are patients with fibromyalgia. The active loci responsible for TrPs not only can cause referred pain, but they also can refer local cutaneous hyperthermia.

Diakow[57] conducted a study to see if active TrPs exhibited a region of hyperthermia extending toward the pain reference zone beyond the usually hot spot, as compared with latent TrPs, which were assumed not to do so. In addition, he analyzed a subgroup who showed evidence of articular dysfunction in the location that would be likely to cause hyperthermia in the same region to which a TrP might refer hyperthermia. By eliminating this subgroup of 25 patients (leaving 104), the discrimination of active versus latent TrPs on the basis of Cohen's Kappa statistic improved from 0.44 to 0.55 (bad to poor) and specificity improved from 0.70 to 0.82 (fair to good). These results suggest that articular dysfunction can be an additional source of hot spots, which fits with Korr's studies of facilitated segments.[164]

Two studies indicated that when referred pain is produced by compressing the TrP, the reference zone becomes hypothermic. Travell described one patient who showed this very clearly.

Kruse and Christiansen[171] did a well-controlled study of temperature change in the reference zone of TrPs in response to pressure stimulation of middle trapezius TrPs. Infrared thermograms were obtained bilaterally from 5 prescribed upper extremity locations of 11 student volunteers with symptomatic TrPs in the middle trapezius muscle and in 11 asymptomatic controls. Initially, thermograms were used to locate thermally active TrPs that were confirmed as TrPs by palpation. The pressure thresholds of the TrP and of the corresponding control sites were determined by algometry. Pressure was then applied to the TrP until the subject felt referred pain, and it was maintained for 1 minute while thermograms were recorded every 15 seconds.

Initially, the region of the TrP site always showed increased temperature, as compared with its control site. The referred pain zone, initially, often showed a lesser increase.[171] With compression of the TrP, the areas of thermal response (in the direction of referred pain) showed a statistically significant reduction in temperature, whereas corresponding control sites showed a nonsignificant increase in temperature. The region of thermal response was remarkably more extensive than the region of referred pain. The pressure pain threshold values at TrP sites were significantly ($P < 0.001$) lower (more tender) than at control sites.

The literature, to date, fails to address a number of critical questions concerning thermographic changes associated with TrPs. Since many acupuncture practitioners use a skin-resistance point finder to locate the appropriate place to insert the needle for inactivating a TrP (or for treating a pain-type acupuncture point), it would be of considerable interest to explore the region of a hot spot for a point of low resistance to see how consistently this is found in a blinded study and to what extent a point of low resistance is located within the hot spot and how consistently the low-resistance point has a TrP (active or latent) nearby, beneath it. The presence of a TrP should be determined by adequate diagnostic criteria applied by examiners tested for good interrater reliability. Since it appears that this measurable characteristic of TrPs is modulated by sympathetic nervous system activity, research studies of the effects of TrPs on sympathetic control of skin perfusion should help to improve our understanding of the functional relationships between myofascial TrPs and the autonomic nervous system.

4. Diagnostic Criteria

The lack of general agreement as to appropriate diagnostic criteria for examining TrPs has been an increasingly serious impediment to more widespread recognition of myofascial TrPs and to comparable studies of the effectiveness of treatment.

Interrater Reliability. In a review of four recent studies on interrater reliability of TrP examinations, the first three reported unsatisfactory to marginal interrater reliability. The fourth study showed why. It demonstrated convincingly the need for all examiners to be both experienced and trained to perform reproducible examinations. This section summarizes these studies and the lessons learned.

Four well-designed studies have recently evaluated the reliability of various myofascial TrP examinations. Results are summarized in Table 8-2. In 1992, Wolfe et al.[300] reported a study part of which involved the

evaluation of eight muscles in eight patients by four physicians experienced in examining patients for TrPs. Each of the four examiners had many years of independent experience but had no chance to agree on a technique for examining the upper body TrPs prior to this study (i.e., were untrained, experienced examiners). The physicians examined each muscle for five findings characteristic of TrPs (Table 8-2). Since subsequent studies reported interrater reliability results in terms of the kappa statistic, two coauthors of this study (Simons and Skootsky) analyzed the original data for the kappa statistic, which corrects for chance agreement. They obtained poor interrater reliability.

Nice et al.[207] reported on the examination of three sites in the thoracolumbar paraspinal muscles of 50 patients with low back pain by 12 experienced full-time physical therapists who routinely treated patients with low back pain. "A practice session was held to allow the therapists to practice this method on each other until all physical therapists reported that they felt capable of using the method on patients,"[207] which is inadequate training when there was no evaluation of uniformity of technique. Again, these were inadequately trained, experienced examiners, and the study also resulted in poor interrater reliability.

Njoo and Van der Does[210] reported the examination of two muscles (quadratus lumborum and gluteus medius) in 61 patients with low back pain by two examiners picked from a pool of one general practitioner and four medical students. Each

Table 8-2   Interrater Reliability of Examinations for Trigger Point Characteristics, Kappa Values

Examination	Wolfe et al.[300]	Nice et al.[207]	Njoo et al.[210]	Gerwin et al.[97]	Mean
Spot tenderness	0.61		0.66	0.84	0.70
Jump sign			0.70		0.70
Pain recognition	0.30		0.58	0.88	0.59
Palpable band	0.29		0.49	0.85	0.54
Referred pain	0.40	0.38	0.41	0.69	0.47
Twitch response	0.16		0.09	0.44	0.23
Mean	0.35	0.38	0.49	0.74	

medical student was well-trained by the physician over a 3-month period but was inexperienced. Four of the five examiners were well-trained but inexperienced. Their interrater reliability was better, but not good.

Gerwin et al.[98] reported a double study in which four experienced physicians examined five muscles bilaterally in each of 10 subjects with myofascial TrPs. A preliminary study[97] and the first half of this study were conducted with the assumption that the four experienced examiners employed essentially the same examination technique. They achieved the same poor interrater reliability of other experienced, untrained examiners. In a second study by the same four physicians, but following a 3-hour training session, however, agreement among doctors was assessed statistically and found to be reliable before proceeding with the study. The study showed that examination of the extensor digitorum communis and latissimus dorsi muscles was most reliable. Examination of the sternocleidomastoid and upper trapezius muscles was less reliable; examination of the infraspinatus muscle was least reliable, suggesting that, of the five muscles tested, it is the most difficult to examine reliably.

A recent well-controlled study confirmed that extensive training of inexperienced examiners results in unskilled, unreliable examinations.[138a]

Clearly, to obtain reliable results, a clinical or experimental research study of human myofascial TrPs must employ both experienced and trained examiners who have been tested for interrater reliability *before* the study is conducted. The necessary skill can be learned. Fricton,[85] in a diagnostic study of masticatory myofascial pain, likewise found that experienced raters were more reliable than inexperienced raters; they also concluded that findings by palpation are technique-sensitive.

Diagnostic Value of Examinations. A second question must be considered: "What is the diagnostic value of the examination technique in terms of its specificity for identifying TrPs?"

An examination for **spot tenderness** or the **jump sign** is essentially the same test. The vigorousness of the jump sign is an indicator of the amount of pressure applied and the degree of spot tenderness. Either of these findings alone has limited diagnostic value because of ambiguity as to the cause of tenderness. The tenderness might be caused by myofascial TrPs, fibromyalgia, enthesopathy, bursitis, tendinitis, etc. The response observed is strongly dependent on the amount of pressure applied.[137] For reliable results, the pressure must be quantitatively standardized in some way. If a quantitative estimate of spot tenderness is desired, properly administered algometry[73, 74, 81] is superior to testing for the jump sign.

Pain recognition is a relatively reliable test as long as patients understand that the examiner is asking them for pain that they recognize as a familiar one that they have experienced recently and that they are not to identify a referred pain that is new to them. One source of confusion in this test is the presence of another referred pain coming from a diseased viscus or an articular dysfunction that is producing the *same* referred pain pattern.[142] In this case, inactivating the TrP will not eliminate the pain because the TrP is not the only source. *If* the patient recognizes the pain generated by pressure on a TrP, then that tender spot can be considered a source (trigger) that is contributing to at least part of the patient's pain.

The finding of a **palpable taut band**, by itself, may be ambiguous because it can sometimes be observed in pain-free subjects without other clinical evidence of TrP phenomena.[210, 300] The presence of a palpable nodule in the taut band has not been tested as a possible criterion of myofascial TrPs, but some clinicians observe the phenomenon routinely, and the nodule is to be expected, based on the integrated hypothesis (see Section D3). Normal structures, such as intramuscular septa, should not be tender. The value of examining for a taut band alone is further limited by the inaccessibility of many muscles to satisfactory manual palpation. Available data indicate that the presence of spot tenderness combined with a palpable band should prove highly reliable, if the examiner were sufficiently skillful and the muscle were sufficiently superficial. The addition of a palpable nodule at the tender spot as a criterion may enhance diagnostic sensitivity. Historically, focal tenderness or a tender nodule in a tense muscle has been one basis for diagnosing fibrositis, Myogelosen, Muskel-härten, and other closely related conditions. The combination of a tender nodule and a taut band is important because other conditions, such as lipomas, keratoacanthomas, subcutaneous calcification, thrombosed vessels, and the nodular panniculitis of Weber-Christian, usually exhibit only one of the features.

Recognized referred pain that reproduces the patient's pain complaint identifies an active TrP and adds greatly to the specificity of the diagnosis. A referred pain that corresponds to the known referral zones of the TrP being examined but is not recognized by the patient as a familiar pain is seriously nonspecific.[137] No study is known that has examined, under controlled conditions, specifically how commonly referred pain can be elicited from tender points of fibromyalgia when those tender points are not also TrPs. Tender points of fibromyalgia *per se* should *not* have the other palpable TrP characteristics, however.

The Trigger Point Manual[263] has pain patterns for individual muscles that are valuable for tracing backward to find the muscle or muscles that likely contain putative TrPs. Reproducing one of these pain patterns that is *not* recognized as a familiar pain by the patient is, however, likely to locate a latent rather than an active TrP.

Twitch responses are strongly associated with the presence of TrPs, and this finding is probably the most specific single clinical test of a TrP.[262a] The extent to which twitch responses can be elicited from other parts of the muscle, particularly in an area of enthesopathy, however, has not been critically evaluated. Enthesopathy, by definition, is found only in the region of attachment of the muscle structure to bone or a joint capsule, whereas TrPs are closely associated with endplates located near the middle of muscle fibers. Unfortunately, at this time, the clinical diagnostic usefulness of the LTR is limited to those muscles in which it can be relatively easily identified. The LTR is the most difficult of the diagnostic signs to reliably elicit manually.

Conversely, it does seem to be highly specific and is readily elicited by needle penetration of the TrP. The addition of ultrasound imaging may greatly increase the importance of this test and provide an objective indication of the relative skill of examiners.

The LTR demands the highest level of skill for reliable results, but with ultrasound imaging, it also has the potential for providing a specific, objective, recordable, clinically available imaging test for myofascial TrPs.

Painfully reduced **range of motion** appears to be a fundamental characteristic of TrPs that is easily performed but has not been subjected to testing for interrater reliability among examiners.

Recommendation. Clearly, no one diagnostic examination by itself is a satisfactory criterion for routine clinical identification of an active TrP. Based on information now available,[98] *spot tenderness in a palpable band and subject recognition of the pain are minimum acceptable criteria.* Additional supportive findings include eliciting the established pain pattern for that muscle, observing a twitch response, and finding painfully reduced stretch range of motion. *Most important,* at present, every author reporting a study of myofascial TrPs should identify, in the methods section, specifically which TrP examinations were used as diagnostic criteria and should describe *in detail* exactly how they were performed. Some muscles need different criteria than others. A consensus document that establishes official diagnostic criteria is urgently needed.

5. Differential Diagnosis and Confusions

When evaluating a patient for musculoskeletal pain, three possible sources of the pain are common and commonly overlooked: myofascial TrPs, fibromyalgia, and articular (somatic) dysfunction. These three conditions often interact with one another, require different diagnostic examination techniques, and need different treatment approaches.

One developing confusion is the use of the term *myofascial pain* for two different concepts.[251] Sometimes, myofascial pain is used in a nonspecific way that applies to almost any muscle syndrome of soft tissue origin.[113, 170, 203, 216, 304, 305] Historically, MPS has been used in the specific sense of the syndrome, which is caused by TrPs within a muscle belly (not scar, ligamentous, or periosteal TrPs).[92, 256, 263, 268, 285] Since the *nonspecific usage* includes many conditions that cause muscle pain without reference to and in absence of TrPs, the use of that terminology is ambiguous and confusing to those who think in terms of MPS with TrPs. Myofascial TrP is only one condition that is included in the nonspecific usage. For authors, one unambiguous approach is to specify *MPS caused by TrPs* or use *regional muscle pain syndrome or soft tissue pain* to identify the more general usage. The unmodified, unspecified use of the term "myofascial pain" is discouraged.

This section starts with a listing of common diagnoses that are often mistakenly made without considering the possibility of TrPs. Patients with one (and often more than one) of these diagnoses are frequently referred to myofascial TrP experts when the patient's pain problem was actually caused by undiagnosed or inadequately treated myofascial TrPs.

This section next emphasizes two common conditions that are closely related to myofascial TrPs and require different treatment approaches: the FMS and articular (somatic) dysfunctions. It also considers how TrPs relate to occupational myalgia, acupuncture points, nonmyofascial TrPs, and the post-traumatic hyperirritability syndrome.

Myofascial Trigger Points Mistakenly Diagnosed as Other Conditions. Those clinicians who have become skilled at diagnosing and effectively managing myofascial TrPs frequently evaluate patients who were referred to them as a last resort by fellow practitioners. These patients commonly arrive with a long list of diagnostic procedures and diagnoses, none of which satisfactorily explained the cause of, or relieved, the patient's pain. Table 8-3 lists examples of these diagnoses. Beside each diagnosis are listed likely TrP sources of that pain. This frustrating situation is understandable because

few medical schools or physical therapy schools teach myofascial TrPs as a regular part of their curriculum, so that most physicians and therapists now in practice have received *at most* a hit-or-miss exposure to myofascial TrPs. For most, any understanding of and competence achieved in diagnosing myofascial TrPs must have been accomplished through supplemental learning and practice following graduation.

This list reminds us that every skeletal muscle of the body can develop TrPs, and many of them commonly do. Since myofascial TrP pain is so common and because patients are most likely to experience the pain at sites other than the TrP location, the clinician is at risk of missing the diagnosis unless he or she considers the possibility of, and specifically searches for, the responsible displaced TrP culprit(s).

Fibromyalgia Syndrome. Two of the three most common muscle pain syndromes, fibromyalgia and myofascial TrPs, are now recognized as separate clinical[94, 135] and etiologic[234, 252] entities. Since both conditions are likely to cause severe muscle pain and frequently coexist but need a different treatment approach, it is of great importance for the patient's sake that any clinician dealing with patients who have muscle pain be able to clearly distinguish these two conditions. For those interested in understanding what fibromyalgia is, what it means to the patient, and how best to manage it, the reader is referred to an authoritative, comprehensive, readable summary written for patients.[84] For those interested in a comparable manual that similarly identifies the clinical nature of both fibromyalgia and chronic myofascial pain caused by TrPs, the reader should refer to the work by Starlanyl and Copeland.[271] A third authoritative patient manual focused on myofascial TrPs is also available, written by a physical therapist who is personally acquainted with the condition.[123] A comprehensive treatise on FMS for the health care provider and clinical investigator is provided in Chapter 9 of this book.

Table 8-3   *Common Referral Diagnoses Received When Overlooked Trigger Points Were Actually the Cause of Patients' Symptoms*

Initial Diagnosis	Some Likely Trigger Point Sources
Angina pectoris (atypical)	Pectoralis major
Appendicitis	Lower rectus abdominis
Atypical angina	Pectoralis major
Atypical facial neuralgia[282]	Masseter
	Temporalis
	Sternal division of sternocleidomastoid
	Upper trapezius
Atypical migraine	Sternocleidomastoid
	Temporalis
	Posterior cervical
Back pain, middle	Upper rectus abdominis
	Thoracic paraspinals
Back pain, low[256]	Lower rectus abdominis
	Thoracolumbar paraspinals
Bicipital tendinitis	Long head of biceps humerus
Chronic abdominal wall pain[110]	Abdominal muscles
Dysmenorrhea	Lower rectus abdominis
Earache (enigmatic)	Deep masseter
Epicondylitis	Wrist extensors
	Supinator
	Triceps brachii
Frozen shoulder	Subscapularis
Myofascial pain dysfunction	Masticatory muscles
Occipital headache[106]	Posterior cervicals
Postherpetic neuralgia	Serratus anterior
	Intercostals
Radiculopathy, C_6	Pectoralis minor
	Scalenes
Scapulocostal syndrome	Scalenes
	Middle trapezius
	Levator scapulae
Subacromial bursitis	Middle deltoid
Temporomandibular joint disorder	Masseter
	Lateral pterygoid
Tennis elbow	Finger extensors
	Supinator
Tension headache[149]	Sternocleidomastoid
	Masticatory muscles
	Posterior cervicals
	Suboccipital muscles
	Upper trapezius
Thoracic outlet syndrome[133]	Scalenes
	Subscapularis
	Pectoralis minor and major
	Latissimus dorsi
	Teres major
Tietze's syndrome	Pectoralis major enthesopathy
	Internal intercostals

At the beginning of this decade, the American College of Rheumatology (ACR) established official criteria for the classification of FMS. Anyone conducting clinical research on FMS or writing a paper that identifies subjects as having FMS should adhere closely to those criteria. When examining patients for the possibility of FMS, the situation is less clear. The ACR criteria were not directly intended as clinical diagnostic criteria for clinical care, even though it was recognized that they would be so used. One cannot be certain that a person with 9 or 10 tender points on the occasion of a given examination would not have exhibited 11 on a previous occasion. The provision of care for a person who seems clinically to have FMS despite failure to meet some criterion is not hard to justify. The certification of that same individual for disability or some form of compensation represents a much more difficult issue. Furthermore, the ACR criteria provide a clinical operational definition that makes no pretense at relating to an etiology. The tender sites that comprise the diagnostic criteria were selected because they contributed statistically to distinguishing patients with FMS from patients with other painful conditions. Importantly, they demonstrate that the patient exhibits widespread lowering of the pressure pain threshold (allodynia).

Fibromyalgia can be thought of as a set of core features and two types of ancillary features. The core features are generalized pain and tenderness over 11 of 18 prescribed anatomic sites. Characteristic ancillary features occur in more than three fourths of individuals: fatigue, nonrestorative sleep, and morning stiffness. Less common findings, in perhaps 25% of cases, include irritable bowel syndrome, Raynaud's phenomenon, headache, subjective swelling, nondermatomal paresthesia, psychologic stress, and marked functional disability. Patients with FMS experience at least as much pain as those with other painful disease states.[192]

The etiology of myofascial TrPs clearly includes a focal muscular dysfunction in the region of motor endplates, which can exert a strong influence on all major parts of the nervous system and lead to spinal level plasticity changes that help to convert an acute pain problem into a chronic one.

Conversely, even though FMS was at first thought to originate in skeletal muscles, careful histologic and ultrastructural study has shown no abnormality of skeletal muscles that was sufficiently common for that to be considered the cause of FMS.[16, 234]

There is strong research support for a systemic, metabolic/neurochemical pathogenesis of FMS. Fibromyalgia is considered an upward modulation of pain sensitivity throughout the body. Extensive research in recent years has led to the "serotonin deficiency hypothesis,"[234] which involves measurable disturbance in nociception, including serotonin regulation of the hypothalamic pituitary axis and the pituitary adrenal axis, and substance P. A close relationship between substance P and calcitonin gene-related peptide also appears to be involved.[234] Experimental evidence also indicates that NMDA receptors of the CNS are involved in the pain mechanisms of FMS.[270] A specific and hard-to-detect thyroid dysfunction may be a commonly overlooked, but treatable, factor in FMS.[186] Muscle nociceptive input may contribute to the pathogenesis or severity of FMS.[16]

Many studies show that a considerable number of FMS patients also have myofascial TrPs. In three studies, the percentage of FMS patients who also have TrPs were 100%,[71] 72%,[94] and 68%.[108] A study of 22 FMS patients[124] found that 40% needed TrP injections and that 89% of those reported relief. One early author incorrectly considered the presence of myofascial TrPs to be an essential feature of primary FMS.[42] Jayson[153] considered injection of TrPs an important part of treating FMS. Others[227, 240] emphasized the clinical importance of clearly distinguishing FMS and myofascial TrP pain.

Distinguishing myofascial TrPs and FMS is simple when the myofascial TrPs are acute, but it can be much more difficult when the myofascial TrPs have evolved into a chronic pain syndrome through neglect. Fibromyalgia, by definition, is a chronic pain syndrome. Table 8-4 lists a number of clinical features that distinguish myofascial pain caused by TrPs from the pain of FMS. The following comments relate to this table.

TrPs occur with nearly equal prevalence in male and female subjects,[269] whereas usually four to nine times as many females as males are observed to have

Table 8-4   *Clinical Features Distinguishing Myofascial Pain From Trigger Points (TrPs) and Fibromyalgia*

Myofascial Pain (TrPs)	Fibromyalgia
1 female:1 male	4–9 females:1 male
Regional pain	Widespread, general pain
Focal tenderness	Widespread tenderness
Muscle feels tense (taut bands)	Muscle feels soft and doughy
Restricted range of motion	Hypermobile
Examine for TrPs	Examine for tender points
Immediate response to injection of TrPs	Delayed and poorer response to injection of TrPs
20% also have fibromyalgia[a]	72% also have active TrPs[a]

[a]Taken from Gerwin RD: A study of 96 subjects examined both for fibromyalgia and myofascial pain. *J Musculoskeletal Pain* 3(Suppl. 1):121, 1995.

FMS,[191] depending on the population studied. Since FMS, by definition, is characterized by widespread, generalized pain and tenderness, this provides a basic distinction from a myofascial TrP, which causes a specific localized pain and tenderness pattern originating from a lesion in a muscle.

When examined, muscles harboring TrPs feel tense because of the contraction knots and taut bands, whereas muscles of a patient with FMS feel softer and more doughy, unless the FMS patient also has TrPs in the muscle being examined. Restricted range of motion is characteristic of muscles containing TrPs, whereas hypermobility is abnormally prevalent (approximately 40%) in children[90] and in adults[298] who have FMS.

Myofascial pain patients are examined for myofascial TrPs as described in this chapter, whereas FMS patients are examined for tender points. Myofascial TrPs and tender points are equally tender at the cutaneous, subcutaneous, and intramuscular level. The two conditions are sharply distinguished, however, by the fact that locations other than tender point sites in FMS patients are as tender at all three depths of tissue as are their tender point sites,[290] whereas non-TrP sites in myofascial pain patients have the same high pain thresholds as corresponding sites in normal subjects. FMS patients are abnormally tender almost everywhere. Myofascial pain patients are abnormally tender only at sharply circumscribed TrP sites and specific sites of referred tenderness.

A number of tender point sites in the FMS examination are designated as lying over tendinous attachments. In this case, because primary (central) TrPs are found in the midbelly portion of the muscle, the tenderness would not be the tenderness of a TrP itself. This attachment-tenderness can be enthesopathically produced secondarily, however, by central TrPs in that muscle.

Hong and Hsueh[135] found that TrPs injected in patients who also have FMS showed a delayed and poorer response than TrPs injected in patients who have MPS without FMS.

Articular Dysfunctions. Articular dysfunctions are one of the three major categories of musculoskeletal pain syndromes responsible for most muscle pain. Traditional medical physicians pioneered an understanding of TrPs, while osteopaths, chiropractors, and practitioners of orthopaedic medicine have developed and promoted manual medical techniques.[204] Until recently, the two have, for the most part, followed separate paths. Currently, at least one college of osteopathy emphasizes the importance of the close relation between TrPs and articular dysfunction. Rarely do medical schools teach mobilization of joints. Physical therapy schools are more likely to include articular dysfunctions than TrPs in their curriculum.

An outstanding osteopathic pioneer in the establishment of physiologic dysfunctions associated with articular dysfunction, Irvin Korr, explored and promoted the concept of the facilitated segment. In the segmental vicinity of an "osteopathic lesion" (vertebra with evidence of articular dysfunction), Korr and associates demonstrated decreased pain thresholds, increased sympathetic activity (decreased skin resistance), and facilitation of motor pathways.[164] With coworkers,[54] Korr demonstrated a muscular component to the facilitated segment. They reported a marked increase in paraspinal muscle activity associated with dysfunctional articular segments. They were, however, unaware of myofascial TrPs and how they related to the muscle tenderness that the authors associated closely with the articular dysfunction.

There is a remarkable analogy between this concept of a facilitated segment, which can strongly influence the three components of the nervous system—motor, sensory, and autonomic—and the nervous system effects produced by myofascial TrPs. The important relationship between the muscles and articular dysfunction is well recognized by many clinicians but has been badly neglected as a subject for serious research investigation.

Karl Lewit[177, 178] published his extensive experience as a neurologist practicing manual medicine and described the close relationship between articular dysfunction and myofascial TrPs. He emphasizes the importance of addressing therapeutically the muscle-dysfunction component and articular-dysfunction component when both are present.[179] The increased tension of TrP taut bands and facilitation of motor activity can maintain displacement stress on the joint while abnormal sensory input from the displaced joint can reflexly activate the TrP dysfunction.

Recently, the chiropractic profession has become increasingly interested in myofascial TrPs as such. One of their members has presented the only published report[185] of which we are aware that looked specifically at the relationship between articular dysfunction and TrPs. In this preliminary test, Lowe examined the relative amount of EMG activity that appeared in paraspinal muscles of normal, slightly involved, and severely involved segments in response to pressure on a distant TrP. He found that induction of additional pain by pressure on a distant active TrP markedly augmented the EMG activity of severely subluxed segments more than of normal segments. This indicates that articular dysfunction can effectively increase the responsiveness

of motor neurons of adjacent muscles to nociceptive input from distant TrPs.

Occupational Myalgias. The subject of occupational myalgias has attracted increasing interest in recent years. A MEDLINE search from 1990 through 1995 recovered 56 abstracted articles on the subject. The five most common of the eleven terms used by the authors were cumulative trauma disorder, repetitive strain injury, repetitive motion injury, repetitive motion study, and overuse syndrome. This is another example of many authors using different terms to identify essentially the same muscle pain syndrome. All authors had one root concern: Patients developed musculoskeletal pain symptoms as a result of work activity. Many authors expressed frustration at the lack of a satisfactory explanation for the cause of the pain itself.

A cardinal feature of myofascial TrPs is that they are activated either by an acute overload or by repeated overuse. The one common denominator in all 56 articles is the association of musculoskeletal pain with overload and/or overuse of the muscle. Placing a muscle in an awkward position that requires sustained contraction of specific muscles to maintain that posture is one of the most common examples of overuse. Headley[123] emphasized how commonly the symptoms in patients with cumulative trauma disorder are caused by myofascial TrPs. She demonstrated electromyographically abnormal function of muscles, caused by the TrPs in these patients.

Remarkably, *not one* of these 56 occupational myalgia abstracts indicated that the authors had considered the possibility that myofascial TrPs may be contributing to the worker's or patient's problem. Fortunately, most authors approached the problem by reducing the overload and/or overuse whenever possible. In this way, the mechanical perpetuating factors aggravating the TrPs were ameliorated or eliminated, allowing the muscle to partially or, occasionally, completely recover normal function.

If the TrP source of pain and dysfunction had been specifically related to TrPs in the muscle causing it, however, local TrP management of that muscle would expedite return to normal function. The employees or patients could be trained to recognize for themselves activities that abused the involved muscles and permit them to tailor routine activities and stretching exercises to maintain normal function of those muscles, which would greatly reduce the likelihood of reactivation. Rosen[229, 230] emphasizes the importance of the awareness of TrPs in the management of muscles that are used beyond their "critical load," especially among performing artists.

Trigger Points and Acupuncture. The distinction between TrPs and acupuncture points *for the relief of pain* is blurred for a number of understandable reasons. First, the mechanisms responsible for the pain relief associated with the two concepts have until recently been enigmatic or controversial. Second, as reported by Melzack et al.,[196] there is a high degree of correspondence (71%, based on their analysis) between published locations of TrPs and classical acupuncture points for the relief of pain. Third, a number of clinicians report just as good results when dry needling TrPs using acupuncture needles as when using hypodermic needles with injected solution.[116, 129, 150]

The evidence that TrP phenomena originate in the vicinity of dysfunctional endplates is presented later in this chapter. Classical acupuncture points are identified as prescribed points along meridians defined by ancient Chinese documents. As Melzack et al.[196] showed, the ancient Chinese clinicians were astute enough to recognize the importance of many common TrP locations and to include them in their charts of acupuncture points for pain.

Currently, a number of practitioners of acupuncture use a modified definition of acupuncture points, which selectively identifies TrP locations. As described by Belgrade,[11] "tender points are acupuncture points and can often be chosen for therapy." If one defines an acupuncture point for treatment of pain as a tender spot, one is using a cardinal definition of TrPs as a criterion for an acupuncture point, which would greatly increase the likelihood of treating a TrP and calling it an acupuncture point. Supporting this concept, Loh et al.[184] compared acupuncture and medical treatment for migraine and muscle tension headaches and found that benefit from acupuncture was more likely to occur when treated at local tender muscular points. Some classical acupuncture points for pain, such as those in the ear, cannot be myofascial TrPs because they occur only in muscle tissue.

Some authors assume that pain relief experienced from classical acupuncture points is associated with an endorphin response in the CNS.[11] The reduction of pain by inactivating a TrP is produced, however, by eliminating the nociceptive focus in a muscle that is responsible for the pain. That nociceptive input from the TrP can cause some central modulation of endorphins[70] tends to complicate the issue but does not change the primary muscular site of the TrP mechanism.

One student of acupuncture, Pomeranz,[217] emphasized the importance of the Deqi phenomenon for the identification of an acupuncture point. The Deqi phenomenon is described as a sensation of fullness, distension, and pins and needles when the inserted needle encounters the acupuncture point. Essentially the same sensory phenomenon is frequently observed, however, when injecting a TrP and the LTR is observed.[129] In a study of the analgesia obtained by electroacupuncture, the authors[219] concluded that the effect may be the result of intense stimulation of TrPs.

Ward[292] examined 12 acupuncture sites that were also common TrP sites in either a trapezius or infraspinatus muscle for the electrical activity characteristic of an active locus in a TrP (see Section D, "Nature of Trigger Points"). Characteristic spike activity was observed in every case.

In conclusion, frequently the acupuncture point selected for the treatment of pain is also a TrP, but sometimes it is not (for a more detailed discussion, see Baldry[6]). Because of the fundamental differences in mechanism, approach to management, and prognostic implications, it is important that clinicians identify TrPs as such so they can institute an appropriate home program and correct perpetuating factors, if present.

Nonmyofascial Trigger Points. TrPs that refer pain may also be observed in what appears to be normal skin,[264, 288] scar tissue,[20, 46] fascia and ligaments,[55, 103, 169, 175, 276, 277, 284] and the periosteum.[111, 174] The reason for sensitization of nociceptors at these sites needs to be clarified but must be different from the TrP mechanism that relates to dysfunctional motor endplates. These nonmyofascial TrPs are considered in detail elsewhere.[263]

Post-traumatic Hyperirritability Syndrome. The term "post-traumatic hyperirritability syndrome" was introduced[143, 247] to identify a limited number of patients with myofascial pain who exhibit marked hyperirritability of the sensory nervous system and of existing TrPs. A similar syndrome was described earlier by Margoles as the *stress neuromyelopathic syndrome.*[189] This syndrome has been addressed in Chapter 7, Section B2. The patients have constant pain, which may be exacerbated by weak stimuli of any kind. Similar phenomena were subsequently described as the *cumulative trauma disorder*[28] and the *jolt syndrome.*[63]

Patients with these symptoms are also identified as having a particularly severe form of FMS. Patients with whiplash injury are especially likely to develop FMS (22% within 18 months).[28a]

C. MUSCLE STRUCTURE AND FUNCTION IN RELATION TO TRIGGER POINT DEVELOPMENT

The basic features of muscle are dealt with in Chapter 2, Section A. To better understand the nature of myofascial TrPs, some special aspects are emphasized here.

1. Muscle Structure and Contractile Mechanism

A striated (skeletal) muscle is an assembly of fascicles, each of which is a bundle of muscle fibers on the order of 100 fibers. Each muscle fiber (a muscle cell) encloses approximately 2000 myofibrils in most skeletal muscles. A myofibril consists of a chain of sarcomeres connected end-to-end. The basic contractile unit of skeletal muscle is the sarcomere. Sarcomeres are connected to each other by their Z lines (or bands), like links in a chain. Each sarcomere contains an array of filaments that consist of actin and myosin molecules, which interact to produce the contractile force.

In the presence of both free calcium and adenosine triphosphate (ATP), the actin and myosin continue to interact, expending energy and exerting force to shorten the sarcomere. This interaction of actin and myosin, which produces tension and consumes energy, cannot happen if the sarcomeres are lengthened (the muscle stretched) until no overlap remains between the actin and the myosin heads. Each sarcomere of a muscle can generate maximum force only in the midrange of its length. The contractile force that any one sarcomere can exert on activation depends strongly on its length. The force approaches zero as the sarcomere reaches maximum or minimum length (fully stretched or fully shortened).

The calcium is normally sequestered in the tubular network of the sarcoplasmic reticulum that surrounds each myofibril. Calcium is released from the sarcoplasmic reticulum when a propagated action potential reaches it from the surface of the cell through T-tubules. Normally, after it has been released, the free calcium is quickly pumped back into the sarcoplasmic reticulum. The absence of free calcium terminates the contractile activity of the sarcomeres. In the absence of ATP, the myosin heads remain firmly attached (failure to "recock"), and the muscle becomes stiff, as in rigor mortis.

2. The Motor Unit

Motor units are the final common pathway through which the CNS controls voluntary muscular activity. Figure 8-4 schematically illustrates a motor unit, which consists of the cell body of an α-motor neuron in the anterior horn of the spinal cord; its axon, which passes through the spinal nerve and then through the motor nerve and enters the muscle where it branches to many muscle fibers (cells); and the multiple motor endplates, where each nerve branch terminates on one muscle fiber. The motor unit includes all of those muscle fibers that one neuron controls. In summary, a motor unit includes one α-motor neuron and all of the muscle fibers that it supplies. Any one muscle fiber normally receives its nerve supply from only one motor endplate and therefore only one motor neuron. The motor neuron determines the fiber type of all of the muscle fibers that it supplies. In postural and limb muscles, one motor unit controls between 300 and 1500 muscle fibers. The fewer fibers controlled by the motor neurons of a muscle (smaller

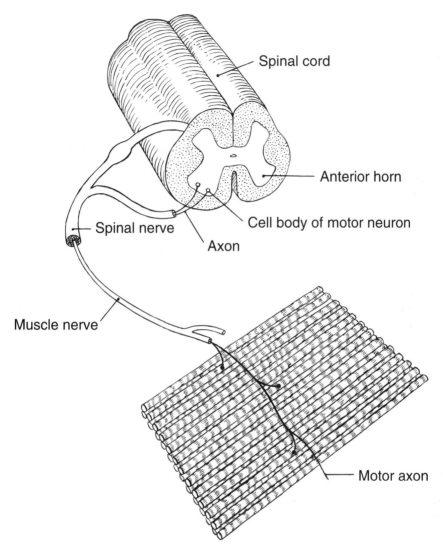

Figure 8-4. Schematic of a motor unit. The motor unit includes the cell body of a motor neuron, its axon, all its arborizations, and the muscle fibers that it supplies (usually approximately 500). In human skeletal muscle, each final arborization terminates at one motor endplate (*solid black circle*). Approximately 10 motor units interdigitate at any one location, so that one axon sends a branch to approximately every tenth muscle fiber. (Reproduced with permission from Travell JG, Simons DG: *Myofascial Pain and Dysfunction: The Trigger Point Manual, Volume 2.* Williams & Wilkins, Baltimore, 1992.)

motor units), the finer the motor control in that muscle.

One motor unit of a human limb muscle usually spans a territory 5 to 10 mm in diameter.[26] The diameter of one motor unit in the biceps brachii muscle can vary from 2 to 15 mm. This allows space for the intermingling of the fibers of approximately 15 to 30 motor units. Both EMG and glycogen-depletion studies show that the density of muscle fibers supplied by one neuron is greater in the center of the motor unit territory than toward its periphery.[26] Two recent studies of the diameter of masseter motor units reported mean values of 8.8 ± 3.4 mm[194] and 3.7 ± 2.3 mm, with the latter ranging between 0.4 and 13.1 mm.[275] Detailed three-dimensional analysis of the distribution of fibers in five motor units of cat tibialis anterior muscles showed some marked variations in diameter throughout the length of a motor unit.[232] Thus, if a taut band were produced by only one motor unit, its size could vary greatly, and it could have more or less sharply defined borders, depending on the uniformity of muscle fiber density within that motor unit. A similar variability could result from the involvement of selected muscle fibers of several interdigitating motor units.

3. The Motor Endplate Zone

The motor endplate is the structure that links a terminal nerve fiber of the motor neuron to a muscle fiber. It contains the synapse where the electrical signal of the nerve fiber is converted to a chemical messenger (acetylcholine), which in turn initiates another electrical signal in the cell membrane (sarcolemma) of the muscle fiber.

The endplate zone is the region where motor endplates innervate the muscle fibers of the muscle.[40, 241] This region is now known as the motor point.[163] The motor point is identified clinically as the area where a visible or palpable muscle twitch can be elicited in response to minimal surface electrical stimulation.

4. Location of Motor Endplates

Understanding the location of motor endplates is important for the clinical diagnosis and management of myofascial TrPs. Since the pathophysiology of TrPs is intimately associated with endplates, one expects to find TrPs only where there are motor endplates. Endplates in nearly all skeletal muscles are located near the middle of each fiber, midway between its attachments. This principle in human muscles was illustrated schematically (Fig. 8-5) by Coërs and Woolf.[41] Christensen[35] illustrated the midfiber distribution of endplates in stillborn infants in the opponens pollicis, brachioradialis, semitendinosus (two transverse bands of endplates), biceps brachii, gracilis (two distinct transverse bands), sartorius (scattered endplates), triceps brachii, gastrocnemius, tibialis anterior, opponens digiti quinti, rectus femoris, extensor digitorum brevis, cricothyroid, and deltoid muscles.

As the illustration shows, the principle applies regardless of the fiber arrangement of the muscle. For that reason, knowledge of the arrangement of fibers in a muscle is

essential to understanding the arrangement of the endplates within that muscle and, therefore, where one can expect to find TrPs. Fiber arrangements of muscles include parallel, parallel with tendinous insertions, fusiform, fusiform with two bellies, unipennate, bipennate, multipennate, and spiral (Fig. 8-6).

Among skeletal muscles, there are at least four kinds of exceptions to the general guideline that there is one endplate zone located in the midbelly region of the muscle:

1. Several human muscles, including the rectus abdominis, the semispinalis capitis, and the semitendinosus, have inscriptions dividing the muscle into serial segments, each of which has its own endplate zone.

2. The human sartorius muscle has endplates scattered throughout the muscle. The endplates supply parallel bundles of short fibers that interdigitate throughout the length of the muscle, with no well-defined endplate zone.[41] The human gracilis is described by one author[35] as having two transverse endplate zones like the semitendinosus but is described by others[41] as having multiple interdigitating fibers with a scattered endplate distribution like the sartorius. This interdigitating configuration is unusual in human skeletal muscles, and the endplate arrangement in these two muscles may be highly variable among individuals.

3. A review of compartmentalization seen within a muscle[64] emphasized that each compartment is isolated by a fascial plane. A separate motor nerve innervates the endplate zone of each compartment. Each compartment is also functionally distinct. Examples given are the proximal and distal partitions of the extensor carpi radialis longus and the distal partitions of the flexor carpi radialis muscle. The masseter muscle also shows evidence of motor unit compartmentalization.[194] Relatively few human muscles have been studied for this feature. It may be quite common.

4. The gastrocnemius muscle is an example of the arrangement of muscle fibers that increases strength by reducing

range of motion. The fibers are strongly angulated, so that one individual fiber is only a small percent of the total muscle length. Consequently, the endplate zone runs centrally down the length of each compartment of the muscle. An example of this arrangement is shown in Figure 8-5A.

Figure 8-7 schematically portrays two motor endplates and the small neurovascular bundles that cross the muscle fibers as

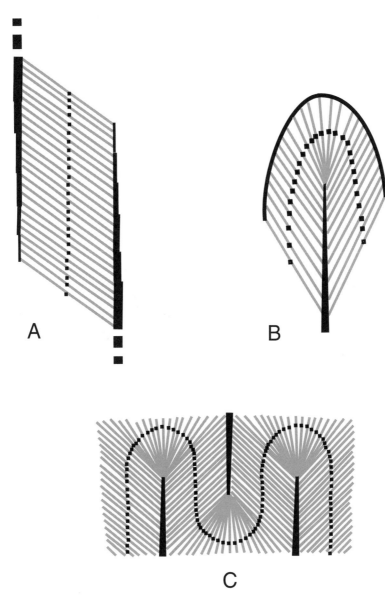

A

B

C

Figure 8-5. Location of endplates in human skeletal muscles of different structure. The *red lines* represent muscle fibers, the *black dots* represent motor endplates of those fibers, and the *black lines* represent aponeurotic attachments. Endplates are consistently found in the midregion of each muscle fiber. **A.** Simple oblique arrangement between two parallel aponeuroses, as seen in the gastrocnemius muscle. **B.** Circumpennate (feather-like) arrangement of endplates seen in the flexor carpi radialis and palmaris longus. **C.** Complex pennate arrangement of endplates found in the middle deltoid muscle. (Adapted from Coërs C: Contribution a l'étude de la jonction neuromusculaire. II. Topographie zonale de l'innervation motrice terminale dans les muscles striés. *Arch Biol Paris* 64:495–505, 1953.)

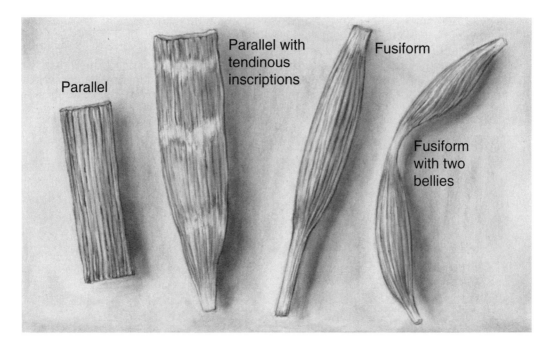

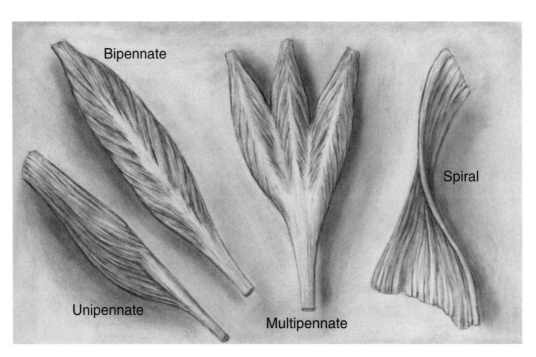

Figure 8-6. Parallel and fusiform fiber arrangements provide greater length change at the expense of force. Pennate arrangements provide more force at the expense of length change. Note that the attachments of muscle fibers in each muscle provide nearly equal length for all of its fibers. (Adapted from Clemente CD: *Gray's Anatomy of the Human Body.* American Ed. 30. Lea & Febiger, Philadelphia, 1985.)

the terminal axons supply motor end-plates.[62] The linear arrangement of endplates that follow the path of such a neurovascular bundle is oriented across the direction of the muscle fibers.[3, 41] The neurovascular bundle includes nociceptor sensory nerves and autonomic sympathetic nerves that are closely associated with these blood vessels. The close proximity of these structures to motor endplates is important for understanding the pathogenesis of TrPs, as well as the pain and autonomic phenomena associated with them.

5. Neuromuscular Junction

Different species have different topographic arrangements of the nerve terminal at an endplate. The frog has extended linear gutters. Rats and mice have a variation in which the gutters are curled and convoluted, as illustrated in Figure 8-7, but

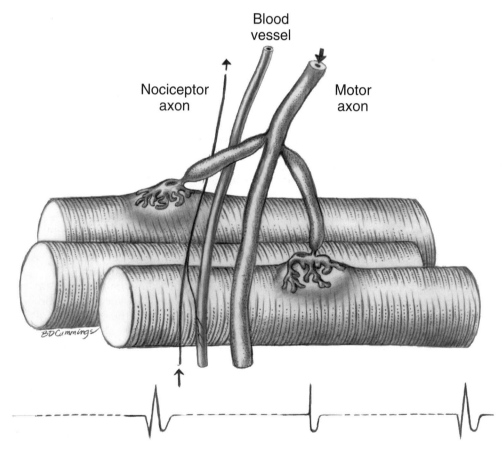

Figure 8-7. Sketch overview of two mammalian motor endplates and the neurovascular bundle associated with them. The nerve terminals of a motor axon are twisted into a compact neuromuscular junction that is imbedded into the slight elevation of the endplate region on the muscle fiber. The motor nerve fibers are accompanied by sensory nerve fibers and blood vessels. Autonomic nerves are found in close association with these small blood vessels in muscle tissue. As shown, muscle fiber action potentials recorded at the endplate region of a muscle fiber show an initially negative deflection. Beyond a very short distance to either side of the endplate, the action potentials of that fiber have a positive-first deflection. This is one way of localizing motor endplates electromyographically. (Adapted from Figure 5 of Salpeter MM: Vertebrate neuromuscular junctions: General morphology, molecular organization, and functional consequences, Chapter 1. *The Vertebrate Neuromuscular Junction.* Edited by Salpeter MM. Alan R. Liss, New York, 1987 [pp. 1–54].)

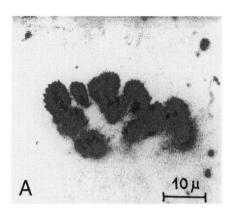

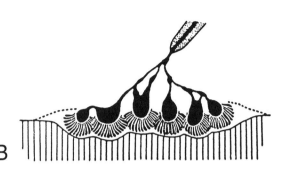

Figure 8-8. Structure of a motor endplate as seen on photomicrograph of the subneural apparatus and schematic cross section of the terminal arrangement in human muscle. **A.** Photomicrograph of human endplate region, stained by a modified Koelle's method to reveal cholinesterase, shows the multiple discrete groups of synaptic clefts of the subneural apparatus. This terminal motor nerve ending of one endplate shows 11 distinct round or oval couplets. This structural form is distinctly different than the tortuous and plexiform terminals in rats and mice. **B.** Schematic of cross section through the human motor endplate region. The unmyelinated terminal nerve ends in six terminal expansions (*black globules*). Each terminal expansion has its own synaptic gutter and system of postsynaptic folds. The *dotted lines* represent the Schwann cell extension that attaches to the sarcolemmal membrane of the cell and isolates the content of the synaptic cleft from the extracellular milieu. The *vertical parallel lines* represent the striations (Z lines) of the muscle fiber. (Reproduced with permission from Coërs C: Contribution a l'étude de la jonction neuromusculaire. Données nouvelles concernant la structure de l'arborisation terminale et de l'appareil sousneural chez l'homme. *Arch Biol Paris* 64:133–147, 1953.)

Figure 8-8 shows the usual human arrangement (see also Fig. 2-3). Cholinesterase stain of an endplate (Fig. 8-8*A*) clearly shows multiple, more or less separate synaptic clefts. With sufficient separation, this arrangement might effectively function as multiple small synapses, which could account for multiple sets of spikes originating in one active locus in one muscle fiber. Figure 8-8*B* is a schematic of this human endplate arrangement seen in cross section.

The neuromuscular junction is a synapse that, like many in the CNS, depends on acetylcholine (ACh) as the neurotransmitter.[39] The basic structure and function of a neuromuscular junction are shown in Figure 2-3. The nerve terminal produces packets of ACh. This process consumes energy that is largely supplied by mitochondria located in the nerve terminal.

The nerve terminal responds to the arrival of an action potential from the α-motor neuron by the opening of voltage-gated calcium channels. These channels allow ionized calcium to move from the synaptic cleft into the nerve terminal. The channels are located on either side of the specialized portion of the nerve membrane that normally releases packets of ACh in response to ionized calcium.

The simultaneous release of many packets of ACh quickly overwhelms the barrier of cholinesterase in the synaptic cleft. Most of the ACh then crosses the synaptic cleft to reach the crests of the folds of the postjunctional membrane of the muscle fiber, where the ACh receptors are located. The cholinesterase soon decomposes the remaining ACh, limiting its time of action. The synapse can now respond promptly to another action potential of the α-motor neuron.

The normal random release of individual packets of ACh from a nerve terminal produces well-separated individual miniature endplate potentials (MEPPs). The mass release of ACh from numerous vesicles in response to an action potential arriving at the nerve terminal depolarizes the postjunctional membrane enough to reach its threshold for excitation. This event initiates an action potential that is propagated by the surface membrane (sarcolemma) throughout the muscle fiber. Individual MEPPs, however, are not propagated and die out quickly.

6. Muscle Pain

The current understanding of the neurophysiology of muscle pain was summarized in 1993,[197, 198] and updated in 1994 and 1997.[199, 200, 250]

The anatomic and physiologic basis of muscle function is described in Chapters 1 through 6. Some important aspects regarding TrPs are repeated or added here: Endogenous substances such as bradykinin, E-type prostaglandins, and 5-hydroxytryptamine are known to sensitize muscle nociceptors. Peripheral sensitization of nociceptors is probably responsible for the local tenderness of TrPs to pressure. Several phenomena occurring at the spinal cord level can be related to referred pain. Injection of a pain-inducing substance into the muscular receptive field of a nociceptive neuron can result in the appearance of additional receptive fields in that limb.[127] This phenomenon is attributed to the "awakening" of "sleeping" nociceptive connections in the spinal cord. When action potentials from nociceptors in a given muscle use the "awakened" connection, they reach and excite neurons that process information from a region outside the muscle. Therefore, the pain is felt (mislocalized) in that region; i.e., the pain is referred to that region. The neuroanatomic basis for referral is a combination of divergence (the action potentials from one source reach more than one central neuron) and input convergence (one central neuron receives input from more than one source).

Inputs from several tissues to one sensory lumbar spinal neuron are common. In a study of cats, most of the 188 units studied (77%) were convergent and responded to nociceptive input from two or more deep tissues: facet joints, periosteum, ligaments, intervertebral disc, spinal dura, low back/hip/proximal leg muscles, and tendons.[99] Most of these units also had a cutaneous nociceptive site.[126] This corresponds to the clinical experience that low back pain and referred leg pain are neither well-localized nor attributable to a specific tissue without additional information.

The overwhelming majority of dorsal horn cells that have visceral input also have a somatic input that is nociceptive.[31] As one becomes more aware of the ubiquitousness of referred pain, both neurophysiologically and clinically, it becomes apparent that a patient's pain complaint is as likely or even more likely to be referred from another site as to originate at the site of pain complaint.

An awareness of neuroplastic changes in the CNS is a relatively new and fundamental development with profound clinical implications. An acute nociceptive input can induce prolonged changes, both structural and functional, in the processing of nociceptive signals in the CNS. Neurophysiologic evidence of this changed neuronal activity has recently been summarized by Yaksh and Abram.[302] More prolonged nociceptive input can induce more long-lasting changes that may *not* be reversible with time alone.

Much of the suffering from chronic pain is preventable if the acute pain is controlled promptly and effectively. Clinical examples of the importance of this principle are increasing rapidly. Specifically with regard to myofascial TrPs, Hong and Simons[133] demonstrated that the length of treatment required for patients who had developed a pectoralis myofascial TrP syndrome as the result of whiplash injury was directly related to the length of time between the accident and the beginning of TrP therapy. With longer initial delay, more treatments were required, and the likelihood of complete symptom relief was decreased.

The use of local analgesia at the time of surgery to prevent nociceptive signals from reaching the spinal cord is helpful[302] but is more effective if combined with meticulous postsurgical pain control. The concept of preventive analgesia was applied successfully by blocking pain from the TrP with preinjection blocks *prior to* a TrP injection.[77, 80] Katz et al.[158] showed that preventing acute surgical pain, in turn, prevents progression to chronic pain and that there is a direct relation between the severity of acute postoperative pain and the severity of subsequent chronic postoperative pain.

At the cortical level, recent investigations show that the brain activates different structures in response to experimentally induced acute pain compared with chronic neuropathic pain.[138] Via positron emission tomography, the latter shows a striking preferential activation of the right anterior cingulate cortex (Brodmann area 24), regardless of the side of the painful mononeuropathy. Activation of this region of the brain is associated with emotional distress (suffering). Acute pain activates both motor and sensory portions of the cortex, producing more of a cognitive and motor behavioral response than an emotional experience. This result emphasizes the importance of the affective-motivational dimension in chronic ongoing neuropathic pain that is not involved in acute pain. Chronic pain causes suffering that is processed differently in the brain than the way that an acute pain experience is processed. These neurophysiologic facts emphasize the importance to the patient and to the health care delivery system of *preventing* chronic pain and properly interpreting patients' descriptions and behavior. Newly activated myofascial TrPs that are poorly identified and poorly managed can become a major unnecessary cause of expensive, miserable chronic pain.

D. NATURE OF TRIGGER POINTS

TrPs have been so difficult to understand because there has been no method of studying them electrophysiologically, and those investigating pathology were looking for characteristic histologic changes distributed uniformly throughout the TrP or palpable nodule. Adding to the difficulty, differences in terminology often made it difficult to know whether different investigators were examining patients with basically the same medical condition that was identified by different names emphasizing different aspects of that condition.

Our current understanding of TrPs results from the convergence of two independent lines of investigation, one electrodiagnostic and the other histopathologic. Fitting together the lessons from each leads to an integrated hypothesis that can explain the nature of TrPs. It is now becoming clear that the region we are accustomed to calling a TrP or a tender nodule is a cluster of numerous microscopic loci of intense abnormality that are scattered throughout the TrP or nodule. The critical TrP abnormality now appears to be a neuromuscular dysfunction at the motor endplate of an extrafusal skeletal muscle fiber. This would make myofascial pain caused by TrPs a true neuromuscular disease. The following section and a previous publication[263] review the research data that provides the basis for this concept.

1. Electrodiagnostic Characteristics

The basis for the electrodiagnostic approach to the study of TrPs was anticipated by Weeks and Travell in 1957,[294] when they reported and illustrated that TrPs in the resting trapezius muscle exhibited a series of high-frequency spike-shaped discharges while adjacent sites in this muscle were electrically silent. Unfortunately, this observation was not effectively pursued. In 1993, Hubbard and Berkoff[141] reported similar electrical activity as being characteristic of myofascial TrPs. Their paper, as in the previous 1957 report, emphasized only the high-amplitude (>100 µV) spike potentials. Hubbard and Berkoff hypothesized that the source of the electrical activity was abnormal muscle spindles and dismissed the possibility that the potentials might be coming from motor endplates.

When Simons, Hong, and Simons started to investigate the electrical activity in TrPs as described by Hubbard and Berkoff,[141] they employed a 5-fold higher amplification and a 10-fold increase in sweep speed for their records. It was immediately apparent that there were two significant components to the electrical activity. In addition to the intermittent and variable high-amplitude spike potentials, there was a consistently present, lower-amplitude (maximum of approximately 60 µV) noise-like component that seemed to be every bit as important as, if not more important than, the high-amplitude component. Figure 8-9A shows the electrical activity recorded at the same slow speed that Hubbard and Berkoff reported. Only spikes are distinguishable in this record, and the polarity of their onset is not identifiable. Figure 8-9B presents similar electrical activity recorded at the same amplification but with a 10-fold increase in sweep speed. In this record, the

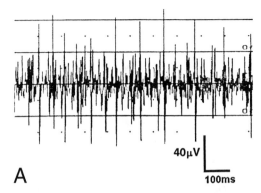

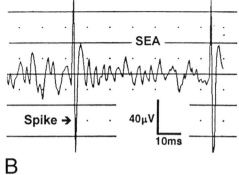

A

B

Figure 8-9. Typical recording of the spontaneous electrical activity (SEA) and spikes recorded from an active locus of a TrP at two different sweep speeds. **A.** Recording at the same slow sweep speed of 100 ms/division used by Hubbard and Berkoff[141] to report this electrical activity. Only spikes of unknown initial polarity are identifiable. **B.** A similar amplification but at a 10-times higher sweep speed of 10 ms/division, used in subsequent studies by others who also have observed the low-amplitude noise component as well as the polarity of initial deflection of the spikes from active loci. This additional information is of critical importance for understanding the source and nature of these potentials. (Reproduced with permission from Simons DG, Travell JG, Simons LS: *Travell and Simons' Myofascial Pain and Dysfunction: The Trigger Point Manual, Volume 1. Upper Half of Body.* Ed. 2. Williams & Wilkins, Baltimore, 1999.)

noise-like low-amplitude potentials are clearly apparent and distinguishable from the spike activity, and the polarity of the initial deflection of each spike potential is clearly evident.

To deal with the potential terminology confusion inherent in this situation, the three investigators[259] adopted the noncommittal term **spontaneous electrical activity** (SEA) to identify this noise-like component. Since spikes only, SEA only, or both might appear from one of these minute needle sites, the neutral term **active locus** was adopted to identify such a site. These three authors[259] used the same kind of needle and slow insertion technique reported by Hubbard and Berkoff.

In time, it became increasingly apparent to them that the potentials found at the active loci of TrPs corresponded completely to the potentials that are recognized by electromyographers as **normal** motor endplate potentials (EPPs). Electromyographers identify the low-amplitude component (SEA of TrPs) as endplate noise and the high-amplitude spike component as endplate spikes.[163] The similarity can be seen by comparing Figures 8-9*B* and 8-10*B*. The EPPs in Figure 8-10 are considered normal, as published in a current electrodiagnostic textbook,[163] based on the study by Wiederholt.[297] At this point it became necessary

for the three investigators to resolve what appeared to be the incompatible "facts" that the SEA and spikes characteristic of active loci in symptom-producing TrPs represented normal endplate activity.

Spontaneous Electrical Activity. To clearly resolve and reliably identify SEA electromyographically, it is necessary to use a relatively high amplification (20 μV/division) and high sweep speed (10 ms/division). If the needle examination is conducted by using the usual thrust technique, one is likely to pass an active locus without recognizing it or to elicit a LTR instead of finding SEA. A slow, gentle technique is required that includes back-and-forth rotation of the needle between the thumb and finger as it is advanced. On these higher-amplification records, the peak amplitudes of spikes are often off scale, but their presence is unmistakable, and their take-off polarity is observable in detail.

The SEA presented here was recorded with the commonly used, disposable, Teflon-coated, monopolar EMG needle. The exposed tip of this needle is relatively enormous compared with the diameter of a muscle fiber or of the endplate region of a muscle fiber. Figure 8-11 shows the relative size of the needle and muscle fibers. The

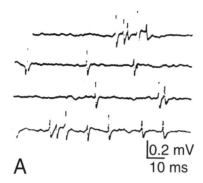

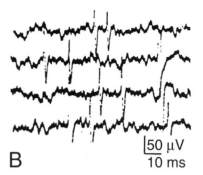

A   0.2 mV
     10 ms

B   50 µV
     10 ms

Figure 8-10. EMG recordings of electrical potentials identified as normal endplate activity of the tibialis anterior muscle, published in a current textbook of electrodiagnosis.[163] Recordings are at the higher sweep speed of 10 ms/division. **A.** Endplate spikes recorded at low amplification; the relatively low amplitude noise-like component is barely apparent. **B.** Recording at four-times higher amplification of endplate activity, showing both the continuous endplate noise and occasional spikes. (Reproduced with permission from Kimura J: *Electrodiagnosis in Diseases of Nerve and Muscle, Volume 2.* FA Davis, Philadelphia, 1989.)

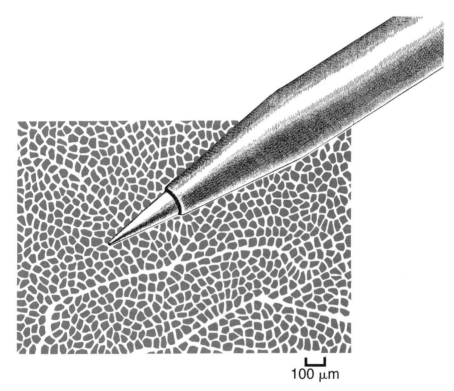

100 µm

Figure 8-11. Schematic that shows the relative size of the exposed tip of a standard Teflon-coated EMG needle in comparison with normal muscle fibers. Muscle fibers are generally approximately 50 µm in diameter. The exposed needle tip (without the Teflon coating) can extend approximately 450 µm and, therefore, could be in contact with approximately 18 muscle fibers, counting both sides of the needle. (Reproduced with permission from Simons DG, Travell JG, Simons LS: *Travell and Simons' Myofascial Pain and Dysfunction: The Trigger Point Manual, Volume 1. Upper Half of Body.* Ed. 2. Williams & Wilkins, Baltimore, 1999.)

exposed tip of a needle was approximately 0.45 mm (450 µm) long. The mean diameter of normal muscle fibers varies with fiber type, ranging from 41 to 59 µm.[60] Therefore, the exposed tip would contact approximately nine muscle fibers of 50 µm diameter on either side of it. A giant fiber (contraction knot) seen in TrPs can be 100 µm or more in diameter.[224] Such a large needle of this configuration would not be expected to detect individual MEPPs, which were difficult to detect extracellularly by using a microelectrode,[68] because their potentials are propagated such a short distance along the outer surface of the postjunctional membrane. The larger amplitude and much wider distribution of SEA over the endplate region should help to make it detectable with the monopolar needle. The smaller exposed electrode surface of a coaxial needle and its more directional receptive field may increase the chances of observing the normal MEPPs reported by physiologists.

Evidence indicates that the SEA may be present spontaneously regardless of the presence of the EMG needle. Since the needle is carefully advanced so slowly and smoothly, it usually evokes few or no insertion potentials. As the needle slowly advances through the TrP region in this electrically quiet background, the examiner occasionally hears a distant rumble of noise that swells to full SEA dimensions as the needle advances. This "acquisition" of SEA at an active locus in a TrP is illustrated in Figure 8-12A and presents a record of the needle approaching the immediate vicinity of the SEA. The transition represents a fraction of a millimeter of needle displacement. Sometimes, the SEA can be increased or decreased by simply applying gentle side pressure to the hub of the EMG needle. To what extent the presence of the needle causes increased ACh release has not been resolved.

Early in the study of the electrical activity found at active loci,[259] the investigators needed to test whether active loci were located at motor endplates. Figure 8-12B illustrates one strong indication that SEA originated at a motor endplate. As Buchthal et al.[27] showed, an initial negative deflection of a motor unit action potential indicates that the recording needle is close to (within 1 mm of) the origin of the action potential (a motor endplate). The lowest trace in Figure 8-12B shows the regular firing pattern of one motor unit. The upper trace presents in detail the action potential between the + marks. It has the initial negative deflection, followed by a rapid rise to peak negative voltage and the biphasic waveform characteristic of a motor unit action potential recorded at its origin, the motor endplate.[27] This potential was recorded at the site of an active locus. The middle trace is recorded from an adjacent control site approximately 1 cm away. Its waveform shows that the recording needle was not located at the origin of that electrical activity. It is, however, a simultaneous recording from the same motor unit. The potential in the upper trace that was recorded from the site of an active locus also originated from a site that was within a millimeter or so of a motor endplate of that same motor unit. This was a consistent finding. Frequently, when subjects initiated a gentle voluntary contraction, they initially recruited only, or very nearly only, the same motor unit that included the muscle fiber that was exhibiting SEA. This needs to be studied quantitatively in a controlled study. The result would indicate the degree to which the involved motor neurons are more excitable than others.

The issue of whether the EPPs now recognized by electromyographers as endplate noise arise from normal or abnormal endplates is critical and questions conventional belief. Figure 8-13 illustrates the difference between normal MEPPs (Fig. 8-13, A and C) and abnormal endplate noise (Fig. 8-13, B and D), which corresponds to the SEA of active loci in TrPs.

Since the paper by Wiederholt in 1970,[297] electromyographers have accepted his conclusion that the SEA represented normal MEPPs and often identified them as endplate (seashell) noise.[163] Wiederholt was correct in concluding that the low-amplitude potentials arose from endplates and illustrated a few discrete monophasic potentials having the configuration of normal MEPPs. The continuous noise-like EPPs that he also illustrated and that we

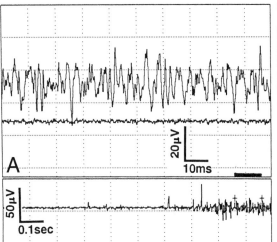

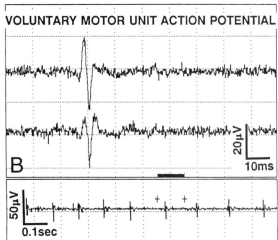

Figure 8-12. Two examples of electrical activity recorded at active loci in TrPs. **A.** The 1-second recording in the *lower panel* obtained as the needle approached the active locus shows the quiet baseline becoming increasingly active as a result of endplate noise (spontaneous electrical activity) as the investigators heard a corresponding development of a noise-like (seashell) sound. The last 0.1 second of that record from the search needle is displayed at increased amplification and 10 times the sweep speed in the upper trace of the *upper panel*. It shows SEA of approximately 20 μV amplitude. The lower trace of the *upper panel* displays the quiet baseline present throughout this record that was recorded from a control needle at a site near to, but outside of, the TrP.
B. The 1-second recording in the *lower panel* displays repetitive discharges of a motor unit recorded from an endplate location found by the appearance of SEA. The motor unit activity is in response to a minimal voluntary contraction of the muscle. The upper trace in the *upper panel* displays the sixth

action potential in detail. The abrupt, initially negative diphasic spike indicates that the recorded potential originated within 1 mm of the search needle, which means it had to be that close to the motor endplate. The lower trace of the *upper panel* was recorded from an adjacent site in the endplate zone but out of the TrP and shows a markedly triphasic, rounded, initially negative deflection of longer duration from the same motor unit. That both potentials came from the same motor unit was confirmed by a constant time relationship in all nine repetitions of them throughout the 1-second record. This illustrates how one can establish independently the presence of an endplate in the absence or presence of SEA. This substantiates the concept that the SEA observed in an active locus arises in the immediate vicinity of or at a motor endplate. (Reproduced with permission from Simons DG, Travell JG, Simons LS: *Travell and Simons' Myofascial Pain and Dysfunction: The Trigger Point Manual, Volume 1. Upper Half of Body.* Ed. 2. Williams & Wilkins, Baltimore, 1999.)

observe from active loci have, however, an entirely different noise-like configuration and an abnormal origin.

Three studies by physiologists (literature generally not familiar to electromyographers) indicate that the SEA (endplate noise) arises from a functionally disturbed endplate. In 1956, Liley[181] observed that even relatively minor mechanical disturbance applied to the endplate region could greatly increase the frequency of the postjunctional membrane potentials, from a normal maximum of 118/second to as high as 1000/second (an increase of one order of

magnitude). Minor mechanical stimuli (minor traumas), including pulling gently on the motor nerve, vibrating the endplate region, and visibly dimpling the surface of the muscle fiber by touching it with an electrode, induced this abnormal pattern (Fig. 8-13B). Once converted to abnormal, the pattern remained abnormal.[181]

Two decades later, studies by Miledi and coworkers identified excessive release of ACh packets as the cause of the increased electrical activity. These studies were published several years after Wiederholt's seminal paper.[297] In 1971, Heuser and

Miledi[125] demonstrated that exposure of the endplate region to lanthanum ions produced a 10,000-fold (four orders of magnitude) increase in the release of ACh, resulting in so many MEPPs that individual potentials were no longer discernible. In a subsequent study,[145] exposure of the endplate region to a foreign serum produced a similar result, as illustrated in Figure 8-13D. If the dysfunctional nerve terminal extends the length of the contraction knot (see Section D of this chapter), then the postjunctional membrane surrounding the entire nerve terminal could be expected to evidence the endplate noise.

Recently, Ertekin et al.[65] reported a marked increase in the number of MEPPs during an attack of hypokalemic periodic paralysis. This indicates that under resting conditions, low serum potassium can also lead to abnormally increased (but much less severe and also reversible) release of ACh.

This "acetylcholine noise," as Miledi and associates called it in their papers, looks remarkably like the potentials produced by Liley,[181] the endplate noise of electromyographers, and the SEA found in TrPs. This strongly suggests that the SEA that identifies active loci in TrPs is produced by grossly increased release of ACh resulting from a serious disturbance of normal endplate function and that the endplate noise identified by electromyographers is the signature of a dysfunctional endplate.

Based on his clinical experience and early studies of SEA, Hong[128] proposed that the clinically identified TrP consists of multiple discrete sensitive spots. It is now apparent that those sensitive spots are abnormal endplates evidencing SEA and

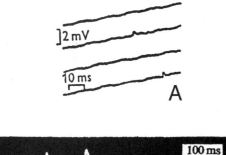

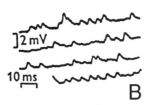

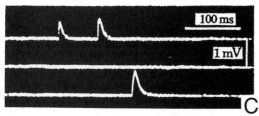

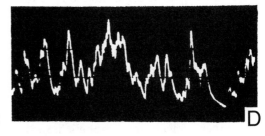

Figure 8-13. Physiologic studies of the EPPs characteristic of normal (**A** and **C**) and dysfunctional (**B** and **D**) endplates. **A** and **B** are early intracellular recordings published in 1956.[181] **A.** Two *normal* (isolated, monophasic, low-amplitude) MEPPs. **B.** A continuous series of overlapping, superimposed, noise-like, higher-amplitude **abnormal** potentials produced by almost any mechanical disturbance of the endplate region. (**A** and **B** are reproduced with permission from Liley AW: An investigation of spontaneous activity at the neuromuscular junction of the rat. *J Physiol* 132:650–666, 1956.)

C and **D** are slower recordings made in 1974 with greater amplification.[145] **C.** Normal, infrequent, individual, monophasic MEPPs. **D.** Response to exposure of the endplate region to incompatible blood serum. The continuous noise-like discharge corresponds to the endplate noise component of motor EPPs and to the spontaneous electrical activity observed in TrPs. This noise-like electrical discharge was caused by a 1000-fold increase in the rate of release of ACh from the nerve terminal. (**C** and **D** are reproduced with permission from Ito Y, Miledi R, Vincent A: Transmitter release induced by a 'factor' in rabbit serum. *Proc R Soc Lond B* 187:235–241, 1974.)

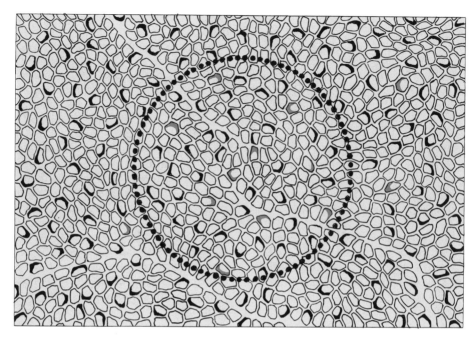

Figure 8-14. Schematic drawing of a cross-sectional view through a TrP (*dotted circle*). This schematic gives an indication of the relative frequency and distribution of active loci. It identifies muscle fibers without endplates in this section (*clear forms*), fibers with normal endplates (*forms with black crescents*), and fibers with active loci (*forms with red crescents*). The locations and frequency of normal endplates were identified by the presence of initially negative motor unit potentials that were produced by a minimal voluntary contraction. See text for more explanation. (Drawing is based on published data.[252, 259, 260])

are scattered among uninvolved normal endplates. This configuration is illustrated schematically as a cross section of the muscle fibers of a TrP in Figure 8-14.

Subsequent reports[18, 36, 259, 260, 261] concluded that the electrical activity characteristically found in TrPs is the same as the motor EPPs recognized as normal by electromyographers.[163, 297]

Spikes. Electromyographers now recognize that spikes originating in the endplate region are action potentials of the one skeletal muscle fiber supplied by that endplate.[163] To confirm this concept and to eliminate the possibility that SEA originates in intrafusal fibers of a dysfunctional muscle spindle, the taut band was monitored as far as 2.6 cm from the endplate for the same action potentials that originated at the endplate as spikes. The same potentials were observed at both locations.[262] These potentials were observed and must have been propagated by extrafusal rather than

intrafusal fibers, since that distance was more than twice the total length of an intrafusal muscle fiber.[140]

Contrary to experience with SEA while exploring TrPs, spikes were not recognized at a distance but appeared suddenly, often simultaneously with SEA. Spikes are often 10 times the voltage of SEA. In that case, they should be equally apparent when the needle is more than 3 times (square root of 10) as far from the source of the voltage. Repeatedly, very light side pressure on the hub of the EMG needle would terminate the spike potentials while release of pressure in one direction or added pressure in the other direction would restore them. These observations left the impression that the presence or absence of spikes depends significantly on the mechanical disturbance (stimulus) provided by the needle.[262]

When numerous spikes were present, it was not uncommon to see three or four different trains of spikes, each of which had its own waveform characteristics and repetition rate. This suggested three or four different sites of origin within one endplate or individual sites of origin from a cluster of involved endplates. If multiple trains of spikes originate from one muscle fiber, the multiple groups of synaptic clefts illustrated in Figures 8-8, *A* and *B*, could account for this phenomenon, provided that a train of spike potentials originated independently in one group of clefts of the myoneural junction. In case the spikes originate in a cluster of endplates, each source would be propagated in a different but nearby muscle fiber. Determination of which mechanism is operating would be an important issue to resolve experimentally.

Available data indicate that spikes occur when a sufficient number of ACh packets are released to depolarize the postjunctional membrane sufficiently to initiate a propagated action potential in that muscle fiber. The mechanical pressure exerted by the needle or related mechanical disturbances may facilitate ACh release sufficiently to produce spikes. More severely dysfunctional endplates of more active TrPs may produce spikes spontaneously without stimulation.

One must be aware of the danger of assuming that spikes observed in a TrP originate at an active locus when no SEA is identified. It can be difficult to distinguish spikes originating at a dysfunctional endplate from motor unit action potentials recorded from a normal endplate.

Distribution of Active Loci in a Muscle. A recent study[260] examined the location of active loci in different parts of a muscle with a TrP. The TrP was always found to be located within the endplate zone, the boundaries of which had been determined independently. This study examined three sites (Fig. 8-15) for active loci: in the TrP, in the endplate zone outside of a TrP, and in the taut band associated with that TrP but outside of the endplate zone (in the absence of a TrP). A fourth, control, location was monitored in the same muscle, but outside each of the three sites. Each of these sites was explored systematically (Fig. 8-16) by inserting the needle in three divergent tracks, stopping eight times in each track whenever SEA alone, spikes alone, SEA with spikes, or a LTR was observed and whenever the needle had advanced approximately 1.5 mm and no activity had been

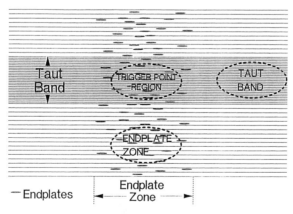

Figure 8-15. Schematic showing the three locations that were explored for active loci. One was the TrP region that was selected as a clinically identified TrP in a taut band. Another was an endplate zone site that was in the independently and electrically identified endplate zone but was outside of any clinically identifiable TrPs. The third was a taut band site that was beyond the endplate zone and not at a TrP. All of the TrPs were found to be located in the endplate zone. The distribution of endplates (*thin ovals*) determines the extent of the endplate zone. The taut band was identified by palpation. (Reproduced with permission from Simons DG, Travell JG, Simons LS: *Travell and Simons' Myofascial Pain and Dysfunction: The Trigger Point Manual, Volume 1. Upper Half of Body.* Ed. 2. Williams & Wilkins, Baltimore, 1999.)

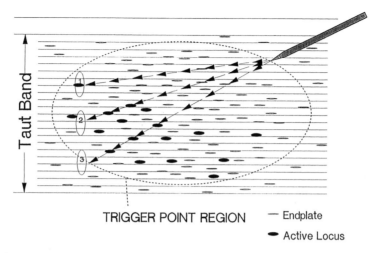

TRIGGER POINT REGION — Endplate

● Active Locus

Figure 8-16. Schematic of search pattern at each experimental site. The large *dotted oval* represents the region of the clinically identified TrP. The *filled ovals* represent normal active loci. The *thin open ovals* represent normal endplate locations that show no spontaneous electrical activity. The EMG needle is very slowly advanced eight times in each of three diverging tracks (labeled *1*, *2*, and *3*). Each needle advance is approximately 1.5 millimeters. (Reproduced with permission from Simons DG, Travell JG, Simons LS: *Travell and Simons' Myofascial Pain and Dysfunction: The Trigger Point Manual, Volume 1. Upper Half of Body.* Ed. 2. Williams & Wilkins, Baltimore, 1999.)

located. After each advance, gentle side pressure was applied to the hub of the Teflon monopolar EMG needle to see if activity appeared or changed. Needle advancement was slow, with gentle rotation of the needle back and forth to facilitate its smooth entry through the muscle tissue.

Using the presence of SEA with or without spikes as the criterion of an active locus, examination of 11 muscles (a total of 264 needle advances) showed active loci to be four times more common in TrPs than in the endplate zone outside of a TrP (35:9).[260] None were observed in the taut band outside of the endplate zone. Clearly, the SEA (noise) type of endplate electrical activity is significantly related to myofascial TrPs. This same SEA was significantly related to trigger spots of rabbits (similar to human TrPs), compared with adjacent non-taut band sites.[259] It is also clear, however, that the isolated observation of SEA alone does not ensure that the needle is located in a clinically identifiable TrP. It may represent a site of mechanical stress on the synaptic connection or an immune system reaction. It may also be a site of TrP activity that is too small to be clinically detectable.

In the human study,[260] the appearance of spikes in the absence of SEA was unrelated to TrPs. Of 15 appearances of spikes, only 1 occurred within a TrP, 12 occurred inside the endplate zone but outside of the TrP, and the other 2 appeared in the taut band. This result could easily have been due to the investigators' failure to distinguish the spike component of endplate electrical activity from motor unit action potentials that were present because of incomplete relaxation and that were being recorded from the search needle but not from the control needle in nearby muscle.

The question arose, "If the SEA and spike potentials that we are observing arise from dysfunctional endplates, then why don't we also see the normal configuration of individual MEPPs observed by physiologists and occasionally by electromyographers?"[25, 65, 297] Those normal potentials that were observed were recorded by using coaxial needle electrodes, which characteristically have a smaller exposed surface (0.03 mm^2),[25] compared with the tip of a monopolar needle (0.08 mm^2). The coaxial configuration also makes them more directional in sensitivity. Both of these factors could be important because of the minute area of extracellular endplate membrane from which a normal EPP can be recorded.[68] The first two reports illustrated both the endplate noise pattern and the lower-amplitude individual MEPP pattern, which is what would be expected if some recordings came from active loci and others from normal endplates.

In studies of active loci,[260, 261] it became important to confirm the presence of normal endplates in addition to the abnormal ones that were generating SEA. One can confirm the presence of a functional motor endplate by the presence of diphasic motor unit action potentials that have a sharp initial negative spike. In accordance with the volume conduction theory[61] and as observed by Buchthal *et al.*,[27] this waveform occurs when the potentials originate in the region of the needle tip. Figure 8-12*B* illustrates the differences in waveform when action potentials of the same motor unit are recorded at the origin of propagation at the endplate and elsewhere along the length of the fiber.

Using the technique described above to locate SEA, we examined several TrPs for the presence of SEA and for normal (SEA-free) motor endplate locations by sampling eight locations in each of two tracks in a TrP. The subject was asked to make a minimal voluntary contraction at each location. Of the 16 locations tested in the TrP (which was in the endplate zone), three locations were active loci (SEA appeared and each was at an endplate), nine were at an endplate (negative voluntary spikes without SEA), and four were at neither an endplate nor an active locus (no evidence of electrical activity beyond background). This is consistent with the concept that a dysfunctional motor endplate is at the heart of the TrP mechanism and that the dysfunctional endplates are a minority among many normal endplates.

If spikes originate at an active locus and are propagated action potentials in just that one muscle fiber, and if the taut band represents taut muscle fibers passing through the TrP, then it should be possible to record a train of spikes simultaneously from the active locus and from the taut band some distance from the TrP. This was observed in several human subjects and in several rabbits.[262] In one human subject, the distance between the TrP and the recording needle in the taut band was 2.6 cm, fully twice the total length of an intrafusal muscle fiber.

2. Histopathology of Trigger Points and Tender Palpable Nodules

Contraction knots, a characteristic histopathologic finding in TrPs and in tender palpable nodules, have been repeatedly noted, but their significance has not been appreciated. In 1951, Glogowski and Wallraff[100] reported finding numerous "*knotenförmig gequollene Muskelfasern*" (club-like swollen muscle fibers) in biopsies of *Muskelhärten (Myogelosen)* (muscle indurations or myogeloses). In 1960, Miehlke *et al.*[202] reported "*bauchige Anschwellungen*" (bulging swellings) of muscle fibers in longitudinal sections and also much variable width and staining intensity in cross sections of muscle fibers in biopsies taken from regions of *Muskelhärten* (muscle indurations) in patients with *Fibrositis syndrom* (fibrositis). And in 1976, Simons and Stolov,[254] using TrP criteria, examined canine muscles for a tender spot in a palpable taut band comparable with that observed in human patients. Under anesthesia, the same location in the muscle was identified by palpation and widely biopsied. Some isolated and some groups of darkly staining, enlarged, round muscle fibers appeared in cross sections (Fig. 8-17). In longitudinal sections, the corresponding feature was a number of contraction knots. Individual knots appeared as a segment of muscle fiber with extremely contracted sarcomeres. This contractured segment showed a corresponding increase in diameter of the muscle fiber, as illustrated in Figure 8-18.

The structural features of contraction knots, one of which is illustrated in Figure 8-18, are portrayed schematically in the lower half of Figure 8-19. This figure presents a likely explanation for the palpable nodules and the taut bands associated with TrPs. The *inset* below in Figure 8-19 shows three single contraction knots scattered among normal muscle fibers. Figures 8-18 and 8-19 illustrate that beyond the

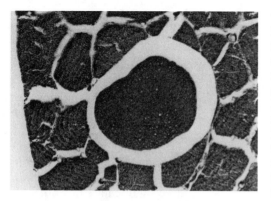

Figure 8-17. The giant round muscle fiber in the center of the figure is surrounded by normal-sized cells and an open space that may contain substances that could sensitize adjacent nociceptive nerve fibers. (Reproduced with permission from Simons DG, Stolov WC: Microscopic features and transient contraction of palpable bands in canine muscle. *Am J Phys Med* 55:65–88, 1976.)

thickened segment of contractured muscle fiber at the contraction knot, the muscle fiber becomes markedly thinned and consists of stretched sarcomeres to compensate for the contractured ones in the knot segment. In addition, a pair of contraction knots separated by empty sarcolemma are illustrated in the upper right of the *inset* of Figure 8-19. This previously reported feature[100, 254] may represent one of the first irreversible complications that result from the continued presence of the contraction knot.

The muscle fibers containing contraction knots are clearly under increased tension both at the contraction knot and beyond. The upper (total muscle schematic) part of Figure 8-19 illustrates that this sustained tension could produce local mechanical overload of the connective tissue attachment structures in the vicinity where the taut band fibers attach. This sustained

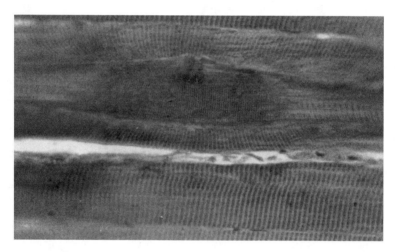

Figure 8-18. Longitudinal section of an example of the contraction knots seen in biopsies of canine muscles, in this case the gracilis. The biopsy site was an exquisitely tender spot in a taut band of the muscle. These are two essential TrP criteria. The striations (corresponding to sarcomere length) indicate severe contracture of the approximately 100 sarcomeres in the knot portion of the muscle fiber. The fiber diameter is markedly increased in the region of the oval contraction knot (center of figure) and abnormally decreased on either side of it. The sarcomeres on either side of the knot show compensatory elongation, compared with the normally spaced sarcomeres in the muscle fibers running across the bottom of the figure. The irregularity of the sarcolemma along the upper border of the sarcolemma in the center of the contraction knot may represent an endplate, which would be expected if this were also an active locus electromyographically. The distortion of the sarcomere alignment in adjacent muscle fibers represents sheer stresses in those fibers that may, in time, play a part in the propagation of this dysfunction to neighboring muscle fibers. (Reproduced with permission from Simons DG, Stolov WC: Microscopic features and transient contraction of palpable bands in canine muscle. *Am J Phys Med* 55: 65–88, 1976.)

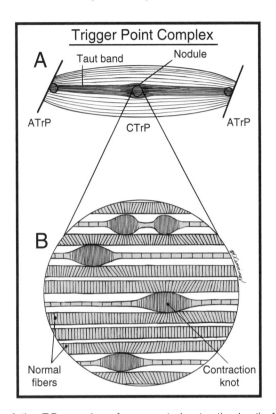

Figure 8-19. Schematic of the TrP complex of a muscle in longitudinal section. The upper drawing identifies three regions that can exhibit abnormal tenderness (*red*). The *enlarged circle* illustrates the microscopic contraction knots that can account for why the TrP feels nodular and the taut band feels tense. The contraction knots mark sites of electrically active loci. **A.** The **central trigger point** (*CTrP*) is found in the endplate zone and contains numerous electrically active loci and numerous contraction knots. The local tenderness of the CTrP is identified by a *red oval*. A taut band of muscle fibers extends from the TrP to the attachment at each end of the involved fiber. When sustained tension of the taut band induces a localized enthesopathy, that site is identified as an **attachment trigger point** (*ATrP*). The local tenderness of the enthesopathy at the ATrP is identified by a *red circle with a black border*.

B. This enlarged view of a microscopic part of the CTrP shows the distribution of five contraction knots and is based on Figure 8-17. The *vertical lines* in each muscle fiber identify the relative spacing of its striations. The space between two striations corresponds to the length of one sarcomere. Each contraction knot identifies a segment of muscle fiber experiencing strong contracture of its sarcomeres. The sarcomeres within one of these enlarged seg-

ments (contraction knot) of a muscle fiber are markedly shorter and wider than the sarcomeres of the neighboring normal muscle fibers, which are free of contraction knots. In fibers with these contraction knots (note the lower three individual knots), the sarcomeres in the part of the muscle fiber that extends beyond both ends of the contraction knot are elongated and narrow, compared with normal sarcomeres.

At the top of this enlarged view is a pair of contraction knots separated by an interval of empty sarcolemma between them that is devoid of contractile elements. This configuration suggests that the sustained maximal tension of the contractile elements in an individual contraction knot caused mechanical failure of the contractile elements in the middle of the knot. If that happened, the two halves would retract, leaving an interval of empty sarcolemma between them.

In patients, the CTrP would feel nodular, compared with the adjacent muscle tissue, because it contains numerous swollen contraction knots that take up additional space and are much more firm and tense than are uninvolved muscle fibers. (Reproduced with permission from Simons DG, Travell JG, Simons LS: *Travell and Simons' Myofascial Pain and Dysfunction: The Trigger Point Manual, Volume 1. Upper Half of Body.* Ed. 2. Williams & Wilkins, Baltimore, 1999.)

tissue distress could be expected to induce the release of sensitizing agents that would sensitize local nociceptors, producing an attachment TrP.

In 1996, Reitinger et al.[224] biopsied, from fresh cadavers, the still-palpable nodules of myogelosis that were located in the gluteus medius muscle where TrP 1 and TrP 2 are found, as described by Travell and Simons.[286] Cross sections showed the previously described, large, rounded, darkly staining muscle fibers and a statistically significant increase in the average diameter of muscle fibers in the myogelosis biopsies compared with nonmyogelotic control biopsies from the same muscle. Electromicroscopic cross sections showed an excess of the A-band and lack of the I-band configuration. Exclusive presence of A-band in the absence of I-band occurs only in fully contracted sarcomeres.[13]

It is highly likely that this fully contracted electromicroscopic pattern seen in cross sections corresponds to the fully contractured contraction knots seen in longitudinal sections under light microscopy.

Two features of Figure 8-18 suggest that the SEA does originate at a contraction knot and that the contraction knot may be caused by a dysfunctional endplate. First, this figure illustrates a longitudinal section of a contraction knot, which, in this case, is a segment of muscle fiber that includes approximately 100 maximally contractured sarcomeres. Normally, sarcomeres range in length from approximately 0.6 μm, when fully shortened to approximately 1.3 μm, when fully extended, which is a full 1:2 length ratio.[13] Based on a minimum sarcomere length of 0.6 μm, the 100 sarcomeres of the contraction knot would extend 60 μm. This is within the 20 to 80 μm range in the length of normal motor endplates, depending on the muscle.[235] Second, although one cannot be sure of this in the absence of acetylcholinesterase stain, the irregularity of the upper border in the middle of the contraction knot in Figure 8-18 fits exactly the shape one might expect if the motor endplate for that muscle fiber were centered over and

extended the length of the contraction knot.

3. Integrated Trigger Point Hypothesis

This section includes several diagnostic categories that have German names, which are explained in the historical review part of Section A of this chapter. The clinical symptoms characteristic of TrPs are related here to the integrated hypothesis. This single etiology seems to hold up remarkably well despite the variety of diagnostic criteria that have been used, the diversity of names given, the various medical disciplines involved, and the complexity resulting from moving across languages.

Energy Crisis Hypothesis. This hypothesis evolved from an effort to identify a pathophysiologic process that could account for (1) the lack of motor unit action potentials in the palpable taut band of the TrP when the muscle was at rest; (2) the fact that TrPs are often activated by muscle overload; (3) the release of substances that sensitize nociceptors in the TrP; and (4) the effectiveness of almost any therapeutic technique that restores the muscle's full-stretch length. This hypothesis was introduced in 1981[255] and recently updated.[199, 249] It fits nicely into the integrated hypothesis that follows.

Figure 8-20 shows the basic concept of the energy crisis hypothesis. It postulates that an initial insult, such as mechanical rupture of either the sarcoplasmic reticulum[249] or the muscle cell membrane (sarcolemma),[15] would release calcium that would maximally activate actin and myosin contractile activity. If the damage were repairable, however, the abnormality would be temporary. It is now apparent that a more likely mechanism is abnormal depolarization of the postjunctional membrane, which could persist indefinitely, based on excessive ACh release from the dysfunctional nerve terminal. In this way, maximum contracture of the muscle fibers in the vicinity of the motor endplate could be sustained indefinitely without motor unit action potentials.

The sustained contractile activity of the sarcomeres would markedly increase meta-

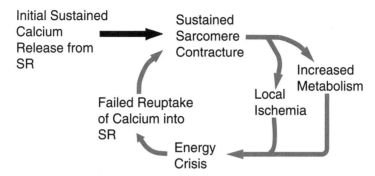

Figure 8-20. Schematic of the energy crisis hypothesis that postulates a vicious cycle (*red arrows*) of events that appears to contribute significantly to TrPs. The function of the sarcoplasmic reticulum (*SR*) is to store and release ionized calcium that induces activity of the contractile elements, which causes sarcomere shortening. An initiating event (*black arrow*), such as trauma or a marked increase in the endplate release of acetylcholine, can result in excessive release of calcium from the SR. This calcium produces maximal contracture of a segment of muscle, which creates a maximal energy demand and chokes off local circulation. The ischemia interrupts energy supply, which causes failure of the calcium pump of the sarcoplasmic reticulum, completing the cycle. (Reproduced with permission from Simons DG, Travell JG, Simons LS: *Travell and Simons' Myofascial Pain and Dysfunction: The Trigger Point Manual, Volume 1. Upper Half of Body.* Ed. 2. Williams & Wilkins, Baltimore, 1999.)

bolic demands and would squeeze shut the rich network of capillaries that supply the nutritional and oxygen needs of that region. Circulation in muscles fails during a sustained contraction that is more than 30 to 50% of maximum effort (depending on the involved muscle). This combination of increased metabolic demand and impaired metabolic supply could produce a severe, albeit local, energy crisis. The Ca^{++} pump that returns the calcium into the sarcoplasmic reticulum is dependent on an adequate supply of ATP and appears to be more sensitive to low ATP levels than is the contractile mechanism itself. Thus, when the pump fails, the contractile mechanism persists, assuring continued failure of the pump. When the ATP supply of the contractile mechanism is exhausted, a sustained contracture develops, as in McArdle's disease. This completes a vicious cycle. In addition, the severe local hypoxia and tissue energy crisis could be expected to stimulate production of neurovasoreactive substances that sensitize local nociceptors.

Thus, the hypothesis accounts for (1) the lack of motor unit action potentials because of the endogenous **contracture** rather than a nerve-initiated **contraction** of the muscle fibers; (2) the frequency with which muscle overload activates TrPs, most likely reflecting the mechanical vulnerability of the synaptic cleft region of an endplate; (3) the release of substances that could sensitize nociceptors in the region of the dysfunctional endplate as a result of tissue distress caused by the energy crisis; and (4) the effectiveness of essentially any technique that elongates the muscle out to its *full* stretch length, reducing energy demand.

This fourth point can be explained by the fact that the continued activity of the actin-myosin interaction depends on physical contact between the actin and myosin molecules, which occurs fully when the sarcomere is approximately midlength or less. The molecules lose overlap contact at full length. With cessation of contractile activity because of actin-myosin separation, both the energy consumption and compression of capillaries would be relieved. This opportunity to restore energy reserves could help to block two critical steps in the energy crisis cycle.

Based on this hypothesis, the TrP region should (1) be higher in temperature than surrounding muscle tissue because of increased energy expenditure with impaired circulation to remove heat; (2) be a region of significant hypoxia because of ischemia;

and (3) have shortened sarcomeres. In addition, the tendinous attachment of many of the muscles with taut bands would likely develop enthesitis because of the abnormally increased, sustained tension exerted by the double source of increased tension in each involved muscle fiber.

1. Only two studies have specifically addressed the temperature question: an informal report by Travell in 1954[278] and another described briefly in Russian in 1976 by Popelianskii et al.[218] Both recorded a focal increase in temperature in the region of the TrP. It would be relatively easy to repeat this experiment using modern instrumentation and patients who meet the current diagnostic criteria for TrPs.

2. One elegantly instrumented and validated study reported in German[24] examined affected muscle for focal hypoxia and encountered remarkably positive results. The study reported the findings in tender, tense indurations (Muskelhärten) in the back muscles of three patients diagnosed as having *Myogelosen* (myogelosis). Figure 8-21 presents the graphic results. The first 5 to 8 mm of sensor advancement show the normal random variation of tissue oxygen tension, with successive 0.7-mm steps of advancement outside of the TrP. As the probe approached the palpable border of the tender induration (TrP), the tissue oxygen tension increased as if there were a compensatory hyperemia surrounding the region of hypoxia. After reaching a peak, the tissue oxygen tension fell abruptly to nearly (but not quite) zero, indicating profound hypoxia in the central region of the induration. It is noteworthy that the volume of the region of increased oxygen tension surrounding the central region of oxygen deficit was calculated to be at least as large as the volume of hypoxic tissue.

3. The contraction knots and electromicroscopic findings described above confirm the presence of contractured sarcomeres. Although no experimental investigation of the development of enthesitis at the attachments of muscles with taut bands has been reported to date, its frequent clinical occurrence is illustrated repeatedly throughout this volume and confirmed by clinicians who look for it.

Integrated Concept of Trigger Point Formation. When combined, the two lines of experimental evidence, electrophysiologic and histologic, indicate that

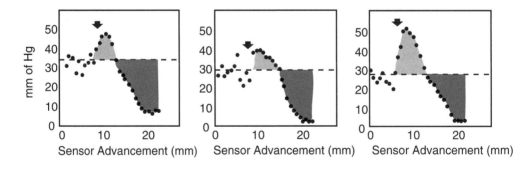

● Palpable border of the induration   – – – Normal mean pO$_2$

Figure 8-21. Tissue oxygen pressure values recorded by an oxygen probe that progressed in 0.7-mm steps through normal muscle and then into a tender, tense induration (Muskelhärte, another name for a TrP) in three patients with myogelosis. *Arrows* mark the palpable border of the induration. The *dashed line* indicates the mean oxygen pressure of adjacent normal muscle. The area *marked in red* identifies the severe oxygen deficiency recorded as the probe approached the center of the induration. Note the comparable region of increased oxygen pressure (*gray*) surrounding the central region of hypoxia. (Data are reproduced with permission from Brückle W, Suckfüll M, Fleckenstein W, *et al.*: Gewebe-pO$_2$-Messung in der verspannten Rückenmuskulatur (m. erector spinae). *Z Rheumatol* 49:208–216, 1990.)

Dysfunctional Endplate Region

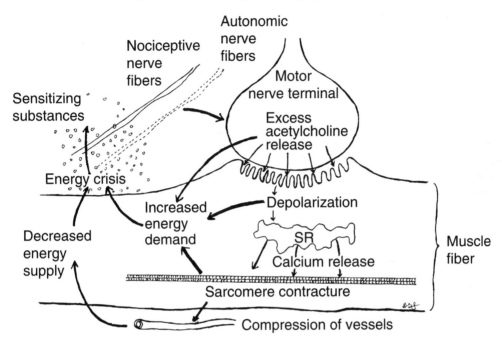

Figure 8-22. Integrated hypothesis. The primary dysfunction hypothesized here is an abnormal increase (by several orders of magnitude) in the **production and release of acetylcholine** packets from the motor nerve terminal under resting conditions. The greatly increased number of MEPPs produces endplate noise and **sustained depolarization of the postjunctional membrane** of the muscle fiber. This sustained depolarization could cause a **continuous release and inadequate uptake of calcium ions from local sarcoplasmic reticulum** (*SR*) and produce **sustained shortening (contracture) of sarcomeres**. Each of these four highlighted changes would increase energy demand. The sustained muscle fiber shortening compresses local blood vessels, thereby reducing the nutrient and oxygen supplies that normally meet the energy demands of this region. The increased energy demand in the face of an impaired energy supply would produce a local energy crisis, which leads to release of sensitizing substances that could interact with autonomic and sensory (some nociceptive) nerves traversing that region. Subsequent release of neuroactive substances could, in turn, contribute to excessive acetylcholine release from the nerve terminal, completing what then becomes a self-sustaining vicious cycle. (Reproduced with permission from Simons DG, Travell JG, Simons LS: *Travell and Simons' Myofascial Pain and Dysfunction: The Trigger Point Manual, Volume 1. Upper Half of Body.* Ed. 2. Williams & Wilkins, Baltimore, 1999.)

the spontaneous electrical activity and spikes observed at active loci within TrPs are the EPPs that are currently recognized by electromyographers as "normal" EPPs. Physiologic experiments, however, have shown that these potentials are not normal but are the result of a grossly abnormal increase in ACh release by the nerve terminal. An endplate exhibiting this SEA is identified as an active locus. Since it appears likely that the contraction knot is located at an endplate and is caused by this endplate dysfunction, the two are likely

intimately related. The following hypothesis proposes what that relationship may be. The hypothesis provides a model that can be used to design critical experiments with which to verify, refine, or refute the hypothesis.

Figure 8-22 presents the hypothesis schematically. The core of the hypothesis is the continuous excess ACh release from the motor nerve terminal into the synaptic cleft. There the ACh activates ACh receptors in the postjunctional membrane to produce greatly increased numbers of

MEPPs. These potentials are so numerous that they superimpose in order to produce endplate noise or SEA and a sustained partial depolarization of the postjunctional membrane. The excessive demand for production of ACh packets in the motor nerve terminal would increase its energy demand (evidenced by abnormal mitochondria in the nerve terminal). The increased activity of the postjunctional membrane and sustained depolarization would impose an additional energy demand. Increased numbers of subsarcolemmal mitochondria and abnormal mitochondria have been noted repeatedly in past studies and have led to use of the term "tagged red fibers" for the affected muscle cells. The above mechanism may be responsible for the presence of many ragged red fibers.

The calcium channels that trigger release of calcium from the sarcoplasmic reticulum are voltage-gated by depolarization of the T-tubule at the triad where the T-tubule communicates with the sarcoplasmic reticulum (see Fig. 2-2). The T-tubule is part of the same sarcolemmal membrane that forms the postjunctional membrane. This depolarization is one mechanism that might account for a tonic increase in the release of calcium from the sarcoplasmic reticulum to produce the local sarcomere contracture that is the most likely explanation for contraction knots. These knots could also explain why clinicians often describe palpating a nodule at the TrP in addition to a taut band. This contracture process appears to be much more intense in the immediate vicinity of the affected endplate. Sustained release of calcium from the sarcoplasmic reticulum would increase the energy demand of the calcium pumps in the sarcoplasmic membrane that return the calcium into the sarcoplasmic reticulum.

This sustained contracture of sarcomeres in the muscle fiber supplied by the affected endplate fits in nicely with the previously proposed energy crisis hypothesis reviewed in detail above. This energy crisis in the vicinity of the endplate can be expected to release neuroactive substances that sensitize and modify the function of sensory and autonomic nerves in that region. As noted above (Section C), small blood vessels, sensory nerves, and autonomic nerves normally are part of the same neurovascular bundle or complex that includes the motor nerve.

Sensitization of local nociceptors could readily account for the exquisite tenderness of the TrP, the referred pain originating at the TrP, and the origin of the LTR. Several lines of experimental evidence suggest that autonomic (probably sympathetic) nervous system activity can strongly modulate the abnormal release of ACh from the nerve terminal.

The clinical effectiveness of botulinum A toxin (BTx) injection for the treatment of myofascial TrPs[1, 33, 303] helps to substantiate dysfunctional endplates as an essential part of the pathophysiology of TrPs. This toxin specifically acts *only* on the neuromuscular junction, effectively denervating that muscle cell.

Several studies by Gevirtz and associates support the possibility that the autonomic nervous system can modulate spike activity (and, therefore, the rate of release of ACh packets) at a motor endplate. Trigger point EMG activity was increased by psychologic stressors both in normal subjects[195] and in patients with tension-type headache.[176] These two reports did not specify whether the TrP EMG activity being measured was SEA or spikes or some combination of both.

More recently, Hubbard[140] published additional experimental data indicating that the amount of electrical activity is strongly influenced by the autonomic nervous system. All intramuscular injections employed EMG guidance to place the injected solution close to the source of the TrP EMG potentials. Four patients were injected with phentolamine intramuscularly, and two patients were injected intravenously. In all six studies, the TrP EMG activity subsided for the duration of the phentolamine effect. Phentolamine is a competitive α-adrenergic blocker.[140] In a series of uncontrolled studies, a total of 108 patients received EMG-guided injections of phenoxybenzamine, which is a long-lasting, adrenergic, noncompetitive α-receptor blocking agent that can produce a chemical sympathectomy with no effect on the parasympathetic system. It has an intravenous half-life of 24 hours. Between one half and two thirds of the patients experienced at least 25% pain relief within 1 month of treatment, and relief lasted for 4 months. Apparently, few subjects realized complete relief. The phentolamine study is more convincing than the phenoxybenzamine study. In a subsequent rabbit study by Chen et al.,[32] intravenous injection of phentolamine caused as much as a 68% decrease in the integrated measure of SEA and spikes in 80 seconds. Activity then stabilized at this level. Apparently, approximately two thirds of the ACh release was dependent on local sympathetic nervous system effects.

In conjunction with a human study of active TrP loci,[260] the investigators confirmed a previous observation[139] that spike activity associated with SEA in the upper trapezius muscle in some subjects was increased by normal resting inhalation and was inhibited by exhalation. Exaggerated respiratory efforts exaggerated the response. They also noted an increase in the amplitude of SEA during inhalation.

Clinical Correlations. If multiple active loci are part of the same pathophysiologic process as multiple contraction knots and if this relationship applies equally to TrPs and to tender nodules, it would represent a major step forward in our understanding of myogenic pain. Based on the integrated hypothesis just described, many of the clinical features of this clinical condition can now be explained.

Two aspects of Figure 8-18 suggest that the SEA does originate at a contraction knot and that the contraction knot may be caused by a dysfunctional endplate. If we assume that this pathophysiologic interpretation is correct, it explains nicely a number of clinical features that apply to both TrPs and tender nodules, although some features have often been overlooked.

The *taut band* of TrPs would be caused by the increased tension of involved muscle fibers because of both the tension induced by the maximally shortened sarcomeres in the contraction knot and the increased (elastic) tension produced by all the remaining elongated (and abnormally thin) sarcomeres. Ordinarily, a muscle fiber runs from its musculotendinous attach-

ment at one end of a muscle to its musculotendinous attachment at the other end. In fusiform muscles (Fig. 8-6), each fiber runs the full length of the muscle.

Figure 8-18 shows clearly the abnormally shortened and abnormally lengthened sarcomeres of the muscle fiber that contains the contraction knot (which is in the center of the figure). These abnormal lengths contrast to the normal resting length of sarcomeres in the muscle fibers running across the lower part of the figure. With the involvement of a sufficient number of muscle fibers in each of several fascicles, the increased tension of the involved muscle fibers should be palpable as a taut band running the length of the muscle. This applies if the muscle fibers run nearly the full length of the muscle and the muscle has no inscriptions, which is the case in most muscles.

The *palpable nodule* of TrP-related diagnoses such as myogelosis can be explained by the presence of many contraction knots (Fig. 8-19). Since a sarcomere must maintain a nearly constant volume, it becomes broader as it shortens. The sarcomeres in a contraction knot appear to be at least twice the diameter of the distant sarcomeres in the same fiber. This difference corresponds to the giant round fibers that are 100 μ in diameter, compared with normal 50-μ-diameter fibers. The nodule feels larger and firmer than surrounding tissue because of the greater volume occupied by the contraction knots and the highly condensed state of their contractile elements. The region of contraction knots feels larger than the rest of the taut band because the normal fibers and the very stretched fibers in the taut band extend into the nodule unchanged. The contraction knots occupy additional volume (Fig. 8-19).

The *spot tenderness* of both TrPs and nodules would be the result of sensitized nociceptors. The nociceptors are most likely sensitized by substances released as a result of the local energy crisis and tissue distress, which apparently are associated with these histopathologic changes and endplate dysfunction. As reported in Chapter 2, bradykinin is an effective sensitizing agent that is released in hypoxic or ischemic tissue.

The *enthesopathy* (tenderness at the muscle attachment) is explained by the inability of the muscle attachment structures to withstand the unrelieved sustained tension produced by the taut band. In response, these tissues develop degenerative changes that are likely to produce substances that could sensitize local nociceptors. Fassbender and Wegner[67] presented impressive histologic evidence for the kind of degenerative changes to be expected in regions of TrP-induced enthesopathy.

The *myoglobin response to massage* of fibrositic nodules can be explained on the basis of the observed histopathologic changes in nodules. Repeated deep massage of the fibrositic nodules (TrPs) produced transient episodes of myoglobinuria that were not produced by similar massage of normal muscle.[44, 45] The intensity of myoglobin response, degree of tenderness, and firmness of the nodule progressively faded out with repeated treatments. The distended sarcoplasm of these contraction knots could well be more vulnerable to rupture by mechanical trauma than normal fibers. The pressure applied by the therapist and the resulting cell rupture could spill myoglobin and destroy the involved neuromuscular junction as a functional structure, thus effectively terminating the contracture and associated energy crisis. As more and more contraction knots were destroyed within the nodule, the patient was further relieved of symptoms.

The development of *histopathologic complications* that could contribute to chronicity and make treatment more difficult is suggested by two observations. First, Figure 8-18 clearly illustrates marked distortion of the striations (sarcomere arrangement) in adjacent muscle fibers for some distance beyond the contraction knot. This would produce unnatural shear forces between fibers that could seriously (and chronically) stress the sarcolemma of the adjacent muscle fibers. If the membrane were stressed to the point that it became pervious to the relatively high concentration of calcium in the extracellular space, the result could be massive contracture that would compound the shear forces. Bennett[15] described this mechanism clearly and how it could lead to severe local

contracture of the muscle contractile elements. This mechanism might account for the "keulenförmige gequollene Muskelfasern" (club-shaped swollen muscle fibers) described by Glogowski and Wallraff,[100] which look like elongated versions of a contraction knot. If this happens, it might occur anywhere along a muscle fiber where it has been affected by an adjacent contracture. This could explain the tendency for clumping of giant fibers mixed with unusually small fibers (segments of stretched sarcomeres) that can be observed in cross sections. This tendency for clumping was illustrated by Simons and Stolov[254] in their Figure 9 and by Reitinger et al.[224] in their *Abb.* 3c.

Second, the occasional finding of a segment of empty sarcolemmal tube between two contraction knots (Fig. 8-19) may represent an additional irreversible complication of a contraction knot. Miehlke et al.[202] described "Entleerung einzelner Sarkolemmschläuche" (evacuation of individual sarcolemmal tubes). Reitinger et al.[224] described "Muskelfasern mit optisch leerem, zystischem Innenraum (Myofibrillenverlust?)" (muscle fibers with an optically empty, cystic interior [loss of myofibrils?]). Simons and Stolov,[254] in their Figure 13, illustrated and described the complete emptying of the sarcolemmal tube between two contraction knots. This configuration appears as if the sustained maximal tension of the contractile elements in a contraction knot caused mechanical failure of the contractile elements in the middle of the knot. This allowed the two halves to retract, leaving an interval of empty sarcolemma between them. Electromicroscopic illustrations by Fassbender[66, 67] show disintegration of the actin filaments where they attach to the Z-line, suggesting that this is the location in the contractured sarcomeres where the mechanical failure may begin.

These additional histopathologic complications could contribute to chronicity and may relate to the transition from latent to active TrPs.

Confirmation. One relatively simple study could help greatly to definitively confirm or reject the integrated hypothesis.

The investigators would need to identify myofascial TrPs or tender nodules that are responsible for the patient's pain complaint; electrodiagnostically locate the SEA of an active locus in each;[252] mark that location electrolytically with iron from the EMG needle;[137, 297] biopsy the site; fix the biopsy by liquid nitrogen; and prepare *longitudinal* sections that are stained for iron,[137, 297] acetylcholinesterase,[297] and a base stain, such as one of the trichromes.[224] If the iron-stained regions include contraction knots with motor endplates attached to them, it would greatly advance the understanding and acceptance of the diagnoses of TrPs and conditions characterized by tender nodules.

4. Other Hypotheses

Pain-Spasm-Pain Cycle. The old concept of a pain-spasm-pain cycle does not stand up to experimental verification either from a physiologic point of view or from a clinical[109] point of view (see Chapter 7).

Physiologic studies show that muscle pain tends to inhibit, not facilitate, reflex contractile activity of the same muscle. Walsh[291] explained clearly how this misconception has been strongly reinforced by a misunderstanding of human motor reflexes, based on spinalized cat experiments, and has persisted throughout the 20th century.

In 1989, Ernest Johnson,[155] editor of the *American Journal of Physical Medicine*, summarized overwhelming evidence that the common perception of muscle pain being closely related to muscle spasm is a myth and that the myth has been strongly encouraged by commercial interests.[155] The term "tension headache" is a good example of this myth in action. The term originated with the assumption that muscle spasm (involuntary contraction) was responsible for the headache and that relaxing the pericranial muscles would relieve it. In 1991, an editorial in the journal *Pain*[211] reviewed this issue and emphasized that it was unambiguously clear that increased EMG activity did not account for the muscle tenderness and pain of tension-type headache (see also Jensen[154]). The editors had no satisfactory alternative solution and did not consider the role of

myofascial TrPs. A current variation of this pain-spasm-pain concept, the stress-hyperactivity-stress theory,[37] seems equally invalid for the same reasons.

Muscle Spindle Hypothesis. Hubbard and Berkoff in their initial communication[141] and Hubbard in his most recent report[140] concluded that the source of TrP EMG activity was a dysfunctional muscle spindle. The three reasons they[141] gave for dismissing the possibility that these potentials might arise from motor endplates were that the activity (1) is not localized enough to be generated in the endplate, (2) does not have the expected location, and (3) does not have the expected waveform morphology.

Existing literature and our experimental findings contradict these assertions. The degree of localization that is described in Section D1 under "Distribution of Active Loci in a Muscle" and "Spikes" corresponds closely to that previously described in the classical paper on the source of motor EPPs.[297] A recent study[262a] explicitly examined the distribution within the muscle of the electrically active loci and found that they were not found outside of the endplate zone. Muscle spindles are distributed more uniformly throughout a muscle, as shown for the cat by Chin *et al.*[34] and for humans by Radziemski *et al.*[221] (Fig. 8-23). Muscle spindles clearly are not concentrated just in the midmuscle endplate zone where TrPs are found. The studies associated with Figures 8-12 and 8-16 demonstrate that active loci occur at extrafusal motor endplates.

Readers can judge for themselves the similarity of waveforms by comparing the spikes and SEA in our recordings from an active locus (Fig. 8-9B) with the "normal" motor EPPs illustrated in an electromyography text (Fig. 8-10).

Other authors agree that these spikes and spontaneous electrical activity that are found in TrPs arise from motor endplates.[18, 36] Brown and Varkey[22] also attributed the spontaneous electrical activity to potentials of the endplate zone and the spikes to postsynaptic muscle-fiber action potentials that were presynaptically activated by mechanical irritation, which can

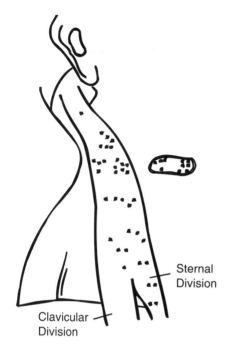

Sternal
Division

Clavicular
Division

Figure 8-23. An example of the distribution of muscle spindles in the sternocleidomastoid muscle of a 14-week-old human fetus. The spindles are distributed rather uniformly throughout the muscle and not clustered in the midbelly region in the manner of motor endplates. (Reproduced with permission from Radziemski A, Kudzia A, Jakubowicz M: Number and localization of the muscle spindles in the human fetal sternocleidomastoid muscle. *Folia Morphol* 50(1/2): 65–70, 1991.)

happen. In addition, the clinical effectiveness of botulinum A toxin (BTx) injection for the treatment of myofascial TrPs[1, 33, 303] supports the endplate hypothesis.

If muscle spindles were the location of TrPs, it would not help to explain the close relation between TrPs and taut bands, since propagated action potentials originating from motor neurons are not responsible for the tension of the band. It is true that a muscle spindle is an attractive source for the afferent limb of the LTR, but it is not necessary to postulate a dysfunctional muscle spindle. Some LTRs may originate in normal muscle spindles that preferentially excite motor neurons, which supply dysfunctional endplates characteristic of active loci.

Two issues need clarification. The recent report by Hubbard[140] of finding one muscle spindle in one biopsy needs to be put in

perspective. The first histologic study using iron deposition as an accurate marker,[156] in 1955, reported that in all 28 sites of electrical activity in rat muscles, "no other structures of muscle, including muscle spindles, had any consistent relationship to the area containing the iron deposits." They did not use a cholinesterase stain and so were unable to identify motor endplates. Wiederholt[297] used both iron stain and cholinesterase stain when he strongly associated the source of the electrical activity with endplates. He made no mention of muscle spindles, although it would be no surprise if a muscle spindle appeared in a few of his sections, since they are widely distributed in the muscle, including the endplate region.

The report[140] that in two subjects, EMG-guided intramuscular TrP injections of curare had no effect on either the amplitude or the frequency of the TrP-EMG activity would seem to be convincing evidence that the EMG activity did not come from motor endplate activity. In several pilot tests using intravenous injection of curare in the rabbit (Hong, Simons, Simons, unpublished data), however, they learned that unless one establishes by some independent means, such as motor nerve stimulation, that the motor endplates are effectively blocked by the curare, one cannot draw any conclusions with confidence concerning its effect on the electrical activity of active loci. This confirmation was lacking in the Hubbard study. This experiment needs to be repeated with proper controls.

Another study[214] suggested that spikes arise from intrafusal muscle fibers. Those authors discussed why spikes are not ectopic discharges of motor axons but did not consider the possibility that spikes are the result of mechanically induced release of abnormal amounts of ACh at the neuromuscular junction of an extrafusal fiber. All of their data were consistent with this latter possibility. Muscle spindles may, at times, contribute to TrP phenomena, but it seems extremely unlikely that muscle spindles are the primary site of the TrP mechanism.

Neuropathic Hypothesis. Back in 1980, Gunn[115] proposed that the cause of TrP hypersensitivity is neuropathy of the nerve serving the affected muscle. Recently, Chu[36] has presented extensive EMG evidence that neuropathic changes can be related to the presence of TrPs in the paraspinal musculature. There is much clinical evidence that compression of motor nerves can, at times, activate and perpetuate the primary TrP dysfunction at the motor endplate. Conversely, TrPs are commonly activated by an acute muscle overload that is unrelated to a compressive neuropathic process. Neuropathy can be, but is not always, a major activating factor.

Fibrotic Scar Tissue Hypothesis. The concept that the palpable firmness of the tissues at the TrP represents *fibrotic (scar) tissue* is based on the assumption that damaged muscle tissue has healed by scar formation.[76] This concept derives from histologic findings in a few most severely involved subjects in studies of Muskelhärten, Myogelosen, Fibrositis, and Weichteilrheumatismus reported in the German literature through the mid-20th century. Patients with myofascial TrPs would have been included under the diagnostic criteria used for these studies but so would almost any other muscular affliction with tender indurations. Unfortunately, to date, there has been a dearth of well-designed histologic studies of TrPs using discriminating TrP diagnostic criteria. The recently discovered endplate dysfunction described in this chapter and the taut bands caused by sarcomere contraction account for the clinical findings in patients with myofascial TrPs without invoking fibrosis as part of the process. The rapid resolution of the palpable taut band with specific TrP treatment argues against that explanation. A review by Simons of all biopsies of tender nodules reported in the 20th century consistently found few reports of scar tissue, and when scar tissue was reported, it was observed only in a relatively few cases.

If the endplate dysfunction is allowed to persist for an extended period of time, it may eventually lead to chronic fibrotic changes. The question of how quickly and under what circumstances this can occur must be resolved with appropriate experimental studies. The increasing refractoriness to local TrP therapy, with longer periods before effective treatment is started,[134] can just as well be attributed to

plastic changes of the CNS when subjected to prolonged nociceptive input. This central mechanism is now well-documented experimentally (see Chapter 7, Section A2).

5. Local Twitch Response

The LTR is a brisk transient contraction of the palpable taut band of muscle fibers elicited by mechanical stimulation of the TrP in that taut band. Mechanical stimulation may be produced by needle penetration of the TrP,[254] by mechanical impact applied directly to the muscle[134] (or to the skin over the TrP), or by snapping palpation of the TrP.[246]

Clinically, the response is most valuable as a confirmatory sign. When injecting a TrP, a LTR signals that the needle has reached a part of the TrP that will be therapeutically effective.[129] It is often not practical as a primary diagnostic criterion of a TrP because it can be prohibitively painful to the patient when it is elicited, it is often inaccessible to manual palpation because of overlying fat and/or muscle, and it requires a particularly high degree of manual skill for reliable examination.[98] When it does occur in the course of examination of a tender nodule or taut band, however, that is strong evidence for the presence of a TrP. The rabbit localized twitch response has proven to be a valuable research tool for investigating the nature of twitch responses.[134, 136]

Topographic Extent of the Local Twitch Response. To date, most experimental investigations of the LTR were conducted on rabbits. The pioneering study by Hong and Torigoe in 1994[134] identified a trigger spot (comparable to a human TrP) in the rabbit biceps femoris muscle by locating a taut band, using pincer palpation and testing along its length for a maximum twitch response to snapping palpation. This was designated the trigger spot. Mechanical stimulation was standardized by using a solenoid-driven rod to impact the surface of the muscle at selected locations. The response was recorded electromyographically with a monopolar Teflon-coated EMG needle placed in the taut band several centimeters distal to the trigger spot.

Figure 8-24A from this study compares the vigor of the twitch response with taps

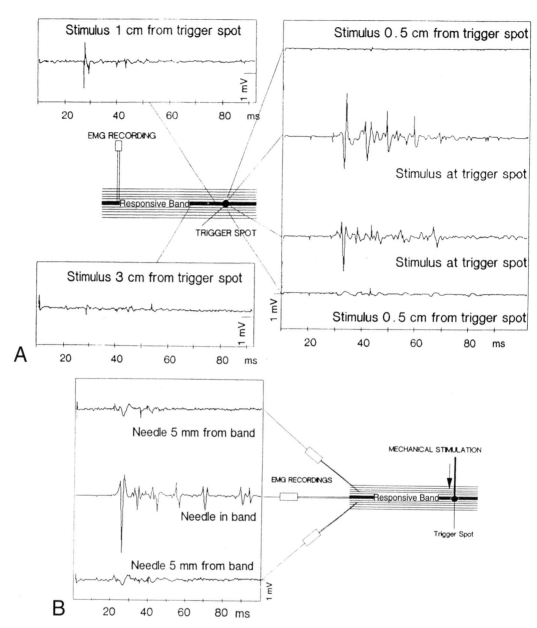

Figure 8-24. EMG recordings demonstrating the spacial specificity of the rabbit localized twitch response with regard to the region of the trigger spot that was stimulated mechanically to elicit the response and to the region of the taut band from which the response was recorded. The *solid black line* represents the taut band (marked *responsive band*) that was selected for testing by manual palpation.

A. Specificity of the point of stimulation in the region of the trigger spot and along the taut band. EMG recordings of twitch responses were obtained from a needle inserted in the taut band distant from the trigger spot. Stimuli were delivered directly on the trigger spot, to either side of it, and along the taut band toward the recording needle, as indicated by labels on the recordings and location of the label lines. The most vigorous response was observed at

the trigger spot, almost none to either side, and progressively less as the point of stimulation was farther from the trigger spot.

B. The *arrow* indicates mechanical stimulation of the TrP by a tap delivered with a solenoid-driven thin rod. The three EMG tracings were obtained in the taut band and 5 mm to either side of it. The recordings near but not in the taut band show only distant waveforms.

These observations substantiate the clinical impression that the LTR is specific to mechanical stimulation of the trigger spot (point) region and is ordinarily propagated only by the taut band fibers passing through the trigger spot. (Reproduced with permission from Hong C-Z, Hsueh T-C: Difference in pain relief after trigger point injections in myofascial pain patients with and without fibromyalgia. *Arch Phys Med Rehabil* 77(11):1161–1166, 1996.)

on the trigger spot and taps applied short distances away from it. Responses were unobtainable 5 mm to either side of the trigger spot, were greatly attenuated when applied in the taut band 1 cm from the trigger spot toward the recording needle, and were vestigial in the taut band 3 cm from the trigger spot. The vigor of the twitch response was extremely sensitive to small displacements of only a few *millimeters* when the stimulus was applied to muscle fibers adjacent to the trigger spot and was similarly attenuated by displacement a few *centimeters* along the same fibers that pass through the trigger spot. These findings correspond to the location of tenderness near TrPs in human patients. The increased responsiveness to snapping palpation at the nodule or the TrP is correspondingly greater, compared with responsiveness at a distance from it along the taut band. The findings also correspond to the meticulous accuracy with which one must stimulate the most sensitive location in the taut band by snapping palpation, and not at adjacent tissue, to evoke a LTR.

Figure 8-24*B* examines the effect of tapping the trigger spot and recording the twitch response with a needle in the taut band and with it placed 5 mm to either side of the taut band. The latter positions showed vestigial twitch responses. The action potentials of the twitch response were propagated in just those fibers passing through the trigger spot and did not involve adjacent muscle fibers. The LTR was highly localized to the trigger spot and to the taut band passing through it.

Origin and Propagation of the Local Twitch Response. No studies to determine the specific structures responsible for the origin of the LTR are known to date.

Clinically, the strong relation between the appearance of LTRs during successful needling of a TrP[129] and the severe pain frequently experienced by the subject when a twitch response occurs suggests that it can originate from stimulation of sensitized nociceptors in the region of the TrP.

The α-motor neurons with endplates suffering from excessive ACh release appear to be preferentially responsive to the strong sensory spinal input from these sensitized nociceptors. This possibility is reinforced by the observation that occasionally the snapping palpation of one TrP repeatedly resulted in simultaneous LTRs in the taut band of that TrP and in the taut band of another TrP in a nearby muscle. If this is true, then comparably strong nociceptive input from related muscle structures may also be able to initiate this reflex. That may include any nidus of sensitization in the muscle, including bursitis and enthesopathy in the region where the muscle attaches. Although LTRs were significantly more likely to occur at a TrP site than out of a TrP in one study,[259] the fact that responses did occur as the result of needling two other sites supports the possibility of less specific sites of origin for this response than just active loci at motor endplates.

Propagation of the LTR has been the subject of several studies by Hong and coworkers. His initial study of the rabbit twitch response with Torigoe,[134] part of which is described above, also reported that either anesthetizing the muscle nerve supplying the muscle or severing it with scissors terminated previously vigorous twitch responses to mechanical stimulation with a solenoid device. A subsequent study[136] in which the same technique was used in five rabbits examined the effect on the twitch response by first transecting the spinal cord at the T_4, T_5, or T_6 level and later cutting the sciatic nerve, as illustrated in Figure 8-25*A*. Figure 8-25*B* presents the duration of LTRs recorded before and repeatedly after each procedure. Immediately following spinal cord transection rostral to segments supplying the biceps femoris muscle, no twitch response was obtainable. As the spinal cord recovered from spinal shock caused by the spinal surgery, the duration of twitch responses recovered to their presurgical level. Following sectioning of the sciatic nerve, the duration of twitch responses again fell to zero and remained there until the end of the experiment an hour later. These results indicate that the rabbit localized twitch response is propagated essentially as a local spinal reflex that is not dependent on supraspinal influences.

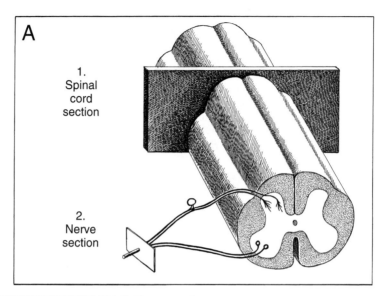

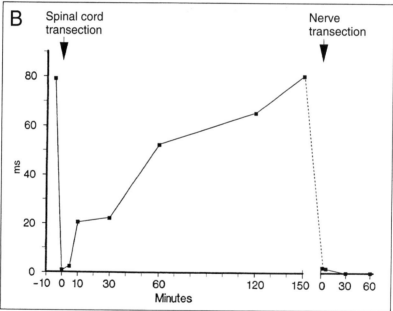

Figure 8-25. Evidence that the LTR is a spinal reflex not dependent on higher centers. **A.** Schematic of a procedure for a LTR experiment.[136] First, the spinal cord of the fully anesthetized rabbit was completely severed. Later, the motor nerve was severed. **B.** Results of the LTR experiment. *Abscissa,* time elapsed in minutes. *Ordinate,* mean duration of LTRs in milliseconds. As soon as the spinal cord was severed, the LTR disappeared as a result of spinal shock. As the animal recovered from spinal shock, the LTR slowly returned. After the motor nerve was severed, however, LTRs became unobtainable and remained that way. (Based on data reported in Hong C-Z, Torigoe Y, Yu J: The localized twitch responses in responsive taut bands of rabbit skeletal muscle fibers are related to the reflexes at spinal cord level. *J Musculoskeletal Pain* 3(1):15–34, 1995.)

A human study[130] followed changes in the LTR during the recovery phase after a brachial plexus injury marked by complete loss of nerve conduction. The EMG activity of twitch responses recovered in parallel with the recovery of nerve conduction. This result is consistent with the other evidence that the twitch response is largely, if not completely, a spinal reflex.

In a study[274] of the motor innervation of the cat gastrocnemius muscle, the authors described and illustrated what portion of the muscle contracted in response to electrical stimulation of one fascicle of the motor nerve. It fit nicely the appearance of twitch responses in rabbit muscle.[134] This is compatible with the other evidence suggesting that a LTR is the contraction of at least one or sometimes several interdigitating motor units.

6. Taut Band

In muscles accessible to palpation, a myofascial TrP is consistently found within a palpable taut band. Clinically, the taut band is a basic diagnostic criterion of a TrP.[98] By itself, however, it is an ambiguous finding. Taut bands are found in asymptomatic subjects with no evidence of tender nodules or TrPs.[300] Other muscle structures, such as intermuscular and intramuscular septa, can feel deceptively similar.

The source of increased tension palpable in the taut band is identified by the mechanism illustrated in Figure 8-19. Other explanations fail to explain how the tension can be relieved within seconds or minutes after inactivation of the TrP.

From a research point of view, the taut band remains one of the more neglected phenomena that are associated with musculoskeletal pain. It is difficult to measure with accuracy, specificity, and reliability. Several studies indicate that palpable taut bands can be present in normal muscles without any other indication of abnormality, such as tenderness or pain.[215, 300] This observation suggests that the symptoms of a clinical TrP represent additional spread and propagation of TrP pathology beyond a few simple contraction knots to much more extensive involvement of the muscle fibers. Club-like swellings, double knots with empty sarcoplasm between them, and areas

of degenerating fibers may be some of those additional complications. The newly proposed pathogenesis of taut bands opens up the possibility of histopathologic study of the endplate changes associated with taut bands that are in the early stages of development.

E. TREATMENT OF MYOFASCIAL PAIN CAUSED BY TRIGGER POINTS

This section considers various methods of treatment and the neurophysiologic basis for their effectiveness: muscle stretch, local tissue stretch, TrP injection, therapeutic ultrasound, and post-treatment procedures, which include use of drugs and biofeedback relaxation. These treatment issues are discussed in much greater detail in the two volumes of *The Trigger Point Manual*.[263, 286]

1. Muscle Stretch

A newly activated, single-muscle myofascial TrP is usually remarkably responsive to simple stretch therapy. This is especially true if the cause of activation was just a moderate overload. Stretching the entire muscle to increase its pain-free range of motion by almost any means is beneficial, and several augmentation techniques are remarkably effective. It is essential that the stretching be done slowly and only to the onset of discomfort. Rapid stretch and "bouncing" stretch tend to irritate TrPs, not release them.

The basis for the effectiveness of almost any kind of stretch has not been firmly established by experimental investigations, but there is one likely possibility. The energy crisis hypothesis includes contracture of sarcomeres in the region of the TrP as a key link in this chain of events. By lengthening the sarcomeres and reducing the overlap between actin and myosin molecules, the energy being consumed is reduced, and at full stretch length, it practically ceases. This would break an essential link needed to maintain the vicious cycle of the energy crisis.

Augmentation of Muscle Stretch. At least five ways can be used to augment simple muscle stretch: intermittent cold, postisometric relaxation, reciprocal inhibition, slow exhalation, and eye movement. These topics are discussed in detail (Chapter 3 of Simons *et al.*[263]).

Intermittent Cold.   The introduction of intermittent cold in the form of vapocoolant spray was a major advance in the augmentation of stretch to release muscles with active myofascial TrPs. The vapocoolant spray as used to treat TrPs exerts marked CNS as well as local effects. A strong centrally mediated effect is demonstrated by two observations. The release of muscle tension that it provides is the result of purely cutaneous stimulation that avoids cooling of the muscle itself. Also, application of the vapocoolant to the painful area can provide relief from referred pain that is of visceral origin.[268, 275a]

The vapocoolant spray also has a strong local anti-inflammatory action, as shown by its relief of the pain and inflammatory reaction from a ligamentous strain and the total abolition of the pain of a first- or second-degree burn, including the prevention of blister formation, when it is applied immediately. The pathway or pathways by which its CNS effects are mediated have not been established experimentally, to date, but are probably mediated at least partly by the autonomic nervous system because of its influence on the level of activity of an active locus.

Postisometric Relaxation Technique. The postisometric relaxation technique introduced by Lewit and Simons[180] essentially employs the contract-relax technique used by physical therapists, with the addition of very gentle stretch and release. It is often effectively augmented with coordinated slow exhalation and eye movement.

The exact mechanism responsible for the effectiveness of this relaxation technique is conjectural, but there is no question that relaxation and stretch of the muscle is facilitated following a gentle voluntary contraction. One possible mechanism would be that contraction activates Golgi tendon organs, which inhibit the homonymous motor neurons. One can demonstrate this technique on oneself by sequentially contracting major muscle groups to relax them for sleep at night. Similarly, patients having difficulty relaxing a muscle for an EMG examination can often achieve complete relaxation immediately following a gentle contraction of that muscle. Such relaxation would certainly be helpful when stretching a muscle, which requires that the muscle be as relaxed as possible.

Reciprocal Inhibition.   Reciprocal inhibition not only is a spinal level reflex but also is effective when contraction of the antagonist is initiated at the cortical level. When one muscle is contracted, its antagonist is inhibited. Thus, when one attempts to actively stretch a muscle by contracting its antagonist, one is reciprocally inhibiting the muscle to be stretched. This effect is so powerful that release of TrP tightness by passive stretching of a muscle can be augmented by simply having the patient imagine assisting the movement as if contracting the antagonist muscle group without executing the effort. Reciprocal inhibition can be used alone to augment a simple stretch, or it can be combined with postisometric relaxation.

The power of this reflex is illustrated by a subject in whom the electrical activity of the hamstring and rectus femoris muscles was monitored by surface EMG recordings, and motion of the knee was recorded simultaneously by using electrogoniometry. When he attempted to further flex the already-flexed knee, the subject developed a severe painful cramp of the hamstrings, which showed strong EMG activity. He was instructed to attempt to straighten his knee to control the cramping. *Before* the quadriceps femoris muscle evidenced any EMG activity and before there was any change in the knee angle, the hamstring EMG activity (and cramp) abruptly subsided. Just willing movement in the antagonist was sufficient to suppress the cramping, even before the motor result of the effort became evident.[78]

Slow Exhalation.   As one slowly exhales, muscles throughout the body generally tend to relax. With inhalation, their activity is facilitated.[179] One exception is the relaxing effect that deep inhalation (a yawn) has on jaw-closing muscles. Part of this reverse effect may be reciprocal inhibition of jaw-closing muscles by activation of their antagonists, the jaw-opening muscles. To be effective, respiration must be sufficiently slow and deep.[179]

The following experimental evidence suggests a significant relation between respiration and TrP activity. While conducting a human study of active loci in TrPs,[260] the authors made observations that confirmed previous observations.[139] In many subjects, spike activity associated with SEA in the upper trapezius muscle was turned on by normal resting inhalation and was turned off by exhalation. The authors also noted a corresponding waxing and waning in the amplitude of SEA during inhalation and exhalation.

Eye Movement. In general, eye movement facilitates movement of the head and trunk in the direction of gaze. This applies to lifting the head and torso as well as for torso flexion and rotation. The direction of gaze (eye movement) does not facilitate trunk movement to either side, but looking up does facilitate straightening up from the side-bent position. Eye movement should not be exaggerated because maximum-effort movement of the eyes may have a contrary effect.[179]

Local Tissue Stretch. Two forms are commonly practiced, and either can be effective: TrP pressure release and deep-stroking massage.

Trigger Point Pressure Release. The new term "trigger point pressure release" replaces the previous term "ischemic compression"[263] for two reasons. No experimental evidence substantiates ischemia as the primary mechanism for the effectiveness of this technique, and clinicians have been prone to apply unnecessarily excessive force, which can be counterproductive and painful to the patient. The technique now recommended conforms to the concept of barrier release. The operator applies gentle, gradually increasing pressure on the TrP until a definite increase in resistance is encountered (the barrier) and, at the same time, the patient begins to feel a degree of discomfort. By simply maintaining this degree of pressure, the palpable tension (barrier) releases and the finger advances slightly, taking advantage of the release that has occurred. This approach is tailored to the needs of that patient's individual muscles, which is more "user friendly" and more effective. Equally important, the patient learns what

optimal pressure feels like for subsequent self-treatment.

Deep-Stroking Massage. The technique of deep-stroking massage was historically the first widely accepted technique for treating fibrositis (many descriptions of which fit myofascial TrPs). It was widely practiced at the beginning of the 20th century[244, 245] and is still commonly used. Its effectiveness may be accounted for by the massage-producing elongation of contractured sarcomeres in contraction knots to interrupt an essential link in the chain of events postulated by the dysfunctional endplate hypothesis. Enough pressure to mechanically disrupt the endplate can totally inactivate that endplate and eliminate the cycle. Two experimental studies showed that vigorous massage of tender "fibrositis" nodules did disrupt muscle fibers sufficiently to release intracellular myoglobin. Comparable massage of normal muscle caused no such elevation of serum myoglobin. As the tenderness and tension of the "nodule" subsided with repeated treatments, the post-treatment increase of serum myoglobin became successively less and finally failed to appear when symptoms had abated.[44, 45] This finding strongly supports the concept that dysfunctional endplates may be more susceptible to mechanical trauma than are normal endplates and that properly placed local tissue stretch can inactivate them.

The effectiveness of pressure release and deep-stroking massage is enhanced by placing the muscles in a comfortably stretched position during the procedure. The full benefit of the treatment may not be realized until the next day. This treatment can then be repeated in another day or two if release was incomplete.

These forms of local tissue manipulation apparently produce a localized stretch effect that lengthens sarcomeres in the immediate vicinity of the applied pressure. The pressure itself may also help by physically dispersing the sensitizing substances released because of the hypoxic ischemia and by mechanical disruption of the dysfunctional endplate.

2. Trigger Point Injection

Several studies[129, 150] indicate that in terms of immediate inactivation of the TrP, dry needling may be as effective as injecting a local anesthetic such as procaine. Injection of an analgesic markedly reduces postinjection soreness, however.[129] Dry needling most likely is effective because it mechanically disrupts the integrity of dysfunctional endplates, which also explains why dry needling requires such precise localization and, when effective, elicits a LTR. Injection of any solution may be helpful by temporarily diluting and dissipating sensitizing substances in the region of the energy crisis.

One author[116] recommends identifying TrPs by spot tenderness in a palpable taut band and then using acupuncture techniques. He first identifies the TrP as a spot of localized tenderness in a taut band and then identifies the precise skin location through which to insert the acupuncture needle by using a dermometer (point finder or skin resistance detector). He then inserts the needle through this spot of low skin resistance into the TrP, where he feels a "grabbing" sensation at the needle tip as the needle enters the taut band, which is often associated with aching pain. A LTR is often observed. This is a good example of the confusing overlap that has developed between myofascial TrPs and acupuncture techniques. The critical goal is inactivation of the active loci and endplate dysfunction associated with the TrP. The particular technique used to do so is less important than the degree of skill that the clinician has developed in the use of that technique.

The recommended injection technique was presented in detail by Hong.[131] That paper describes the preferred way of holding the syringe for injection. The operator grasps the syringe between the thumb and last two fingers and uses the index finger to depress the plunger while *resting the wrist on the patient's body,* as indicated in Figure 8-26. This gives the operator much better control of the needle in case the patient jumps, sneezes, or moves unexpectedly. The operator's hand is well-anchored on the body, moves with the body, and brings with it the syringe and needle without further needle penetration. This technique is particularly important when injecting in the neighborhood of the chest, where guarding against unexpected additional depth of penetration may be of

critical importance to avoid producing a pneumothorax.

Another paper by Hong[129] lends new emphasis to the importance of noting LTRs while injecting a TrP. The effectiveness of injection therapy appears to be much greater if a LTR is elicited in the process.

Several authors have reported the successful use of botulinum A toxin (BTx) for the treatment of myofascial pain caused by TrPs,[1, 33, 303] including a recent review.[33a] In a small, double-blind, placebo-controlled study, four patients experienced 30% reduction of pain following BTx injection but not following saline injection.[33] The effectiveness of BTx injection is of great theoretic interest but can be easily abused in its therapeutic applications.

In therapeutic doses, BTx paralyzes muscles by blocking release of ACh from motor nerve terminals at the neuromuscular junction.[114] This eventually causes degeneration of that neuromuscular junction. The denervated muscle fiber normally becomes reinnervated in approximately 3 to 6 months. That BTx quickly inactivates myofascial TrPs is a strong indicator that the myofascial TrP mechanism is intimately associated with the neuromuscular junction.

Because of its destructiveness, however, BTx should be used with due precautions. It should be used only after more conservative, noninvasive measures, such as augmented stretch techniques, have been tried. Generally, the basic reason why noninvasive therapy or even dry needling provides only temporary relief is because perpetuating factors have not been adequately addressed.[263]

If the decision is made to inject botulinum A toxin (BTx), it is important that dosage be minimized. This requires precise localization of the TrP and injecting minimal quantities to avoid destroying motor endplates unnecessarily. An active TrP should be confirmed by patient recognition of his or her clinical pain complaint when the sensitive spot is compressed. Also, an active locus of a TrP should be confirmed by eliciting a LTR by snapping palpation or with the needle *before* injection. For those with the necessary equipment and skills, an even more specific and precise criterion is the identification of an active locus electro-

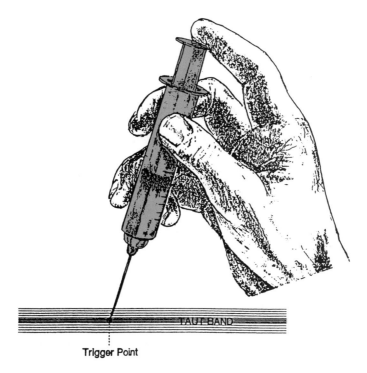

Trigger Point

Figure 8-26. Recommended way to hold the syringe for TrP injection to avoid overpenetration caused by unexpected movement. The wrist should rest solidly against the patient. (Reproduced with permission from Hong C-Z: Considerations and recommendations regarding myofascial trigger point injection. *J Musculoskeletal Pain* 2(1):29–59, 1994.)

myographically by its spontaneous electrical activity (commonly recognized as EPPs), as described by Simons *et al.*[259, 260] and by Hubbard and Berkoff.[141]

The one clear indication for the injection of botulinum A toxin (BTx) is the presence of an untreatable perpetuating factor, such as spasticity caused by CNS damage. Pain caused by TrPs also needs to be controlled.

3. Therapeutic Ultrasound

Many therapists find the application of ultrasound an effective way of inactivating TrPs. Ultrasound is particularly valuable for treating TrPs of deeper muscles that are hard to reach by manual therapeutic techniques. One can apply the ultrasound head to the spot tenderness in the muscle where digital pressure reproduces the patient's pain complaint.

The mechanism by which ultrasound could effectively inactivate TrPs is unknown. If sufficient pressure were applied with the head, it would be one way of applying a form of TrP pressure release and/or

massage. The ultrasound heats the tissues, which, if continued long enough at sufficient intensity, might terminate the local energy crisis. The increased heat and molecular excitation might augment the energy crisis pathophysiology to the point of self-destruction. Controlled research studies on the effect of ultrasound on well-diagnosed active TrPs are urgently needed.

4. Post-Treatment Procedures

Whatever technique is used to inactivate the TrPs, a number of post-treatment procedures provide a vital role to expedite return of normal function of the muscles and to help the patient learn how to avoid recurrence.

Post-Treatment Range of Motion. Following treatment, whether by some form of stretch or by injection, the patient should move the treated muscle through three cycles of *full* range of motion that include the *fully* shortened position and the *fully* lengthened position. This helps to restore normal muscle contractile activity throughout the muscle's full range. The muscle usually feels stiff to the patient toward the end of its full-stretch range of motion on the first cycle and less stiff on the second, and it returns to normal on about the third cycle. It is important that the muscle be moved slowly and that each cycle also include the fully shortened position of the muscle. This procedure can be thought of as helping to correct the inequality of sarcomere lengths between the middle and the ends of the muscle fibers that caused the hypertonus of the taut band. It could also help to reprogram motor control pathways to fully utilize the newly restored full-range capability of the muscle. Muscles learn.

Post-Treatment Surface Heat. Application of moist heat following either stretch-and-spray or injection serves several purposes. Following stretch-and-spray, it rewarms the skin. Following either procedure, it convinces patients that the operator is sincerely concerned for their comfort, an important part of the art of medicine. The sense of warmth and comfort helps the patient to fully relax, which is important for an effective therapeutic result. It also gives the patient's autonomic nervous system an opportunity to recover its equanimity if the injection was a painful experience. The TrPs in many muscles powerfully modulate autonomic nervous system activity.

Post-Treatment Electrical Stimulation. The use of electrical stimulation is common practice among many therapists as a supplementary modality in the treatment of TrPs. It sometimes is used as preliminary treatment but more commonly is applied following stretch and/or injections.[220] Clinical experience suggests that the most effective technique is to increase the electrical stimulus to the point of gentle muscular contraction in a cyclic mode. This is effectively a passive form of contract-relax. This technique, when done actively by the patient, is very effective but requires concentration and effort. This passive, electrical method may permit more accurately controlled dosage and for longer periods of time. Rachlin[220] recommends electrical stimulation routinely following TrP injec-

tion and needling. He describes using an intermittent current (that may be sinusoidal, surged, or ramped) for 15 minutes. If spasm is present, he recommends preceding this intermittent current with 10 minutes of tetanizing current to fatigue the muscle. The muscle achieves more complete relaxation following this fatiguing stimulation. If the patient rejects the use of electrical stimulation (because of discomfort), moist heat is substituted. A fuller description of the parameters of the electrical stimulation and of the rationale for its use is presented in the book by Kahn[157] under the heading "Electrical Stimulation."

Drug Therapy. The nonsteroidal antiinflammatory drugs are generally of little help for relief of pain caused by myofascial TrPs. These drugs are very helpful, however, for the postinjection soreness that is likely to peak a day or two after injection, especially if dry needling without a local analgesic was used. This suggests that the tissue injury of needling induces an inflammatory reaction that is not characteristic of the pathophysiology of TrPs. This is consistent with our new concept of the nature of myofascial TrPs. When injected in higher concentrations at the TrP, however, a prostaglandin-suppressing action seems to help relieve pain from TrPs.[89] Prostaglandins are a likely candidate as one of the more important agents involved in the sensitization of nociceptors in a TrP (see Chapter 2, Section A7). Hubbard[140] recommends the injection of phenoxybenzamine under needle EMG guidance. This noncompetitive α blocker should suppress, if not eliminate, that component of sympathetic nervous system influence at the TrP.

Ingestion of aspirin prior to injection is contraindicated because it enhances bleeding tendencies. If a patient bruises easily (because of increased capillary fragility), a course of 500 mg of ascorbic acid (vitamin C) three times daily for at least 2 days prior to injection is highly recommended.

In the past, use of muscle relaxants has been based primarily on the erroneous concept that muscle pain is the result of spasm and that spasm causes muscle pain; therefore, relieving the spasm should relieve the pain. Since this mechanism is not valid, we do not recommend the use of muscle relaxants.

The demonstrated effectiveness of botulinum A toxin (BTx) when injected in the region of TrPs helps to substantiate the concept that endplate dysfunction is at the heart of the TrP dysfunction. This toxin totally destroys endplate function, effectively denervating that muscle fiber. Use of this toxin is discussed in more detail above under the heading "Injection."

Biofeedback. The original idea of using biofeedback to break up what has turned out to be a nonexistent pain-spasm-pain cycle is no longer valid. Biofeedback is useful, however, to train tense patients with myofascial TrPs how to recognize their muscular tension and how to relax their overactive muscles. Unnecessary sustained muscle contraction that produces a minimum baseline level of EMG activity unnecessarily aggravates TrPs.

Another particularly valuable and rapidly developing use of biofeedback is to retrain muscles that have been inhibited by TrPs and must relearn normal functional activity. Muscles learn and remember the dysfunctional patterns imposed on them by TrPs. Retraining can progress much faster if patients can *see* what level of muscle activity they are achieving.

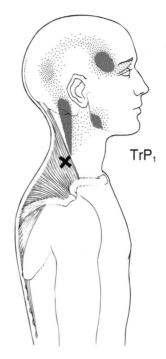

Figure 8-27. Referred pain pattern and location (X) of TrP 1 in the upper trapezius muscle. *Solid red* shows the essential referred pain zone; *stippling* maps the spillover zone. (Reproduced with permission from Simons DG, Travell JG, Simons LS: *Travell and Simons' Myofascial Pain and Dysfunction: The Trigger Point Manual, Volume 1. Upper Half of Body.* Ed. 2. Williams & Wilkins, Baltimore, 1999.)

F. MYOFASCIAL PAIN BY BODY REGION

The clinical characteristics of TrPs for individual muscles have been fully described.[263, 286] This section approaches the clinical characteristics of TrPs in terms of five regions of the body.

1. Head and Neck Region

The upper trapezius muscle is an example of one of the muscles most commonly afflicted with TrPs, especially among office workers. Any position or task that requires the shoulder to carry the weight of an upper extremity repeatedly or for prolonged periods of time overloads the upper trapezius muscle and strongly encourages the development of TrPs. As an example of muscles in this region, Figure 8-27 shows the pattern of referred pain characteristic of it, and Figure 8-28 illustrates the spray-and-stretch technique, using this muscle as an example. Fluori-Methane is the preferred

vapocoolant, but it is a fluorocarbon that compromises the ozone layer. It is being replaced by the environmentally friendly *Gebauer Spray and Stretch*. Ethyl chloride can be used if it is dispensed as a stream and not as a spray and if the operator realizes that it is flammable and a potent anesthetic that absolutely requires adequate ventilation to avoid inhaling concentrated fumes. It is colder than Fluori-Methane, so the nozzle should be held closer to the skin and the stream of spray advanced more rapidly. The details of this technique are described in Chapter 3 of a companion volume.[263]

The TrPs of one muscle can interact in many ways with other muscles. One such example is the key-muscle effect. A key muscle is one that induces a satellite TrP in another muscle. When the key TrP is inactivated, the satellite TrP be-

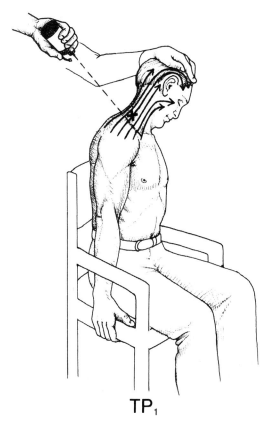

TP₁

Figure 8-28. Trapezius stretch position and spray pattern (*arrows*) for TrP 1 (*X*) in the upper trapezius muscle. (Reproduced with permission from Simons DG, Travell JG, Simons LS: *Travell and Simons' Myofascial Pain and Dysfunction: The Trigger Point Manual, Volume 1. Upper Half of Body.* Ed. 2. Williams & Wilkins, Baltimore, 1999.)

comes inactive without further treatment. For example, a key TrP in the sternocleidomastoid muscle can induce a satellite TrP in the temporalis, masseter, or digastric muscles.[131]

Myofascial TrPs are a frequent cause of common headaches. Dejung *et al.*[53] examined a series of 25 patients with headache for myofascial TrPs as a possible cause. All of them had ropy tension in various muscles that exhibited a zone of enhanced tenderness by local finger pressure. A majority of the patients had TrPs that were responsible for their headache, based on recognition of their head pain when it was reproduced by pressure on the tender spot in the muscle. The muscles most com-

monly responsible for headache were the sternocleidomastoid, upper trapezius, scalene, and deep cervical paraspinal (rotatores and multifidi) muscles.

Several kinds of headache are caused by myofascial TrPs. Tension-type headache is defined in a way that could include TrP pain as its cause. Jaeger, a dentist familiar with head and neck pain of TrP origin, illustrated how, in her experience, the combination of several head and neck active TrPs combine pain patterns to account for common tension-type headache descriptions.[149] She also showed that cervicogenic headaches were a combination of TrPs and cervical spine dysfunction.[148] Patients diagnosed as having occipital neuralgia turned out to be suffering primarily from TrPs.[106] Successful management of patients suffering from chronic head and neck pain continued to improve for a year following a treatment program that emphasized patient training and correction of perpetuating factors.[107] The relationship between the various official kinds of headache and myofascial TrPs is reviewed thoroughly in Chapter 5 of a companion volume.[263]

Articular dysfunctions of the cervical spine can be closely related to myofascial TrPs of cervical and head muscles. Referred pain patterns produced by cervical zygapophyseal joints can mimic closely referred pain patterns of cervical muscles.[17] The muscle shortening and the increased tension caused by TrPs in suboccipital and deep paraspinal muscles can seriously aggravate articular dysfunctions and maintain abnormal joint tension and compression in the joint(s) crossed by those muscles. Conversely, clinical evidence strongly indicates that the distressed joint can reflexly induce TrPs in functionally related muscles.[179] The diagnosis and treatment of both conditions are often required for relief of the patient's symptoms.

2. Shoulder and Upper Extremity Region

In this region of the body, the subscapularis muscle is an example of a critically important muscle because it is a frequently overlooked cause of the "frozen shoulder" syndrome.[263] In this syndrome, the patient has severely restricted abduction and external rotation at the shoulder joint, and the restriction can be so severe that the patient is unable to move the arm more than a few centimeters from the body. The characteristic pain pattern of this muscle and the usual location of its TrPs are shown in Figure 8-29. The restricted range of motion caused by the taut-band shortening and intolerance to stretch of the subscapularis fibers helps to induce active TrPs in the remaining shoulder girdle musculature. Attention to those more accessible TrPs alone fails to solve the problem until the subscapularis TrPs are also released. The technique for injecting its TrPs is shown in Figure 8-30. It is essential that the operator direct the needle *away* from the ribs to avoid a pneumothorax when injecting this muscle.

Many patients diagnosed as having thoracic outlet syndrome have symptoms caused by active TrPs. The manner in which the anterior scalene muscle does this is well described (Chapter 20 of Simons et al.[263]). In addition, a pseudothoracic outlet syndrome is produced by the combination of active TrPs in most or all of four internal rotators of the arm at the shoulder joint. These muscles include the pectoral group, subscapularis, teres major, and latissimus dorsi muscles. These same internal rotators also commonly develop TrPs in

stroke patients. These TrPs cause much pain and disability, which can be greatly improved by inactivating the TrPs. They ordinarily require repeated therapy (usually injection) because the spasticity perpetuates the TrPs. The TrPs also aggravate the spasticity. This is an example of a situation in which the use of *precise* EMG-guided injection of the TrPs with botulinum toxin is indicated.

A common complaint in this region of the body is interscapular pain. Dejung[49] describes the common origin of this complaint from TrPs in the serratus anterior muscle and explains how to diagnose and treat them.

Baker[5] examined 100 consecutive patients suffering an initial whiplash injury from an automobile accident and found common patterns of muscles that developed active TrPs, depending on the direction of impact. TrPs are a common cause of pain and disability following this kind of injury. The pectoralis minor muscle is a particularly important cause of TrP-generated radiculopathy symptoms in these patients. The longer the interval between the accident and institution of myofascial TrP therapy, the greater the number of treatments required and a de-

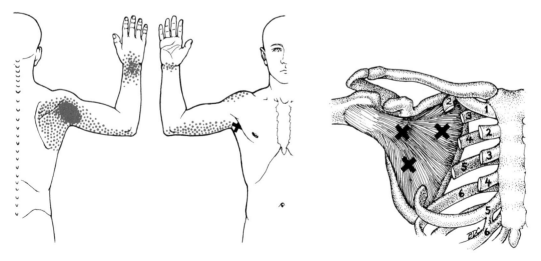

Figure 8-29. Referred pain pattern projected from TrPs (*Xs*) in the right subscapularis muscle. The essential referred pain zone is *solid red*; the spillover zone is *stippled red*. In the *right panel*, portions of the second through the fifth ribs have been removed for clarity. (Reproduced with permission from Simons DG, Travell JG, Simons LS: *Travell and Simons' Myofascial Pain and Dysfunction: The Trigger Point Manual, Volume 1. Upper Half of Body.* Ed. 2. Williams & Wilkins, Baltimore, 1999.)

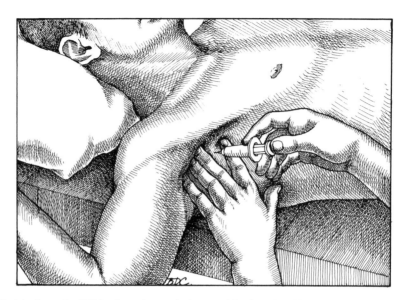

Figure 8-30. Injection of a TrP in the subscapularis muscle along the axillary border of the scapula. (Reproduced with permission from Simons DG, Travell JG, Simons LS: *Travell and Simons' Myofascial Pain and Dysfunction: The Trigger Point Manual, Volume 1. Upper Half of Body.* Ed. 2. Williams & Wilkins, Baltimore, 1999.)

creasing likelihood of complete resolution of symptoms.[134]

Pain and tenderness in the region of the lateral epicondyle are often diagnosed as epicondylitis, when, in fact, the cause is myofascial TrPs[51] of the brachialis, biceps brachii, pronator teres, supinator, and/or flexor group of muscles in the forearm.

3. Torso Region

Low back pain is currently an unresolved scourge of modern society, with no consensus as to its cause and appropriate management. There are a number of interacting and often overlooked causes that could help to explain the present level of medical and patient frustration. These include active TrPs, articular dysfunctions, interarticular ligamentous strain, and small tears in the annulus of an intervertebral disc.[58] The subject of low back pain is reviewed in Chapter 41 of a companion volume.[263]

The diagnosis and treatment of the 15 torso and pelvic muscles whose active TrPs cause low back pain have been summarized[256] and described in more detail.[263, 286] The quadratus lumborum and iliopsoas muscles are so often overlooked because special examination procedures are required to find their TrPs. They both are commonly involved, especially the quadratus lumborum. The paraspinal muscles appear to be special targets for referred reflex activation. Painful stimulation of lower-body TrPs is likely to selectively induce reflex motor unit activity in lumbar paraspinal muscles. Painful pressure applied to a TrP in the soleus muscle or tensor fasciae latae muscle induced a marked degree of muscle spasm in the lumbar paraspinal muscles that was reduced or eliminated by inactivating the TrPs.[121, 249] This helps to explain why, to resolve chronic back pain caused by TrPs, it is so important to resolve all active TrPs in the lower half of the body, including all paraspinal muscle TrPs.

When dealing with patients who have low back (sacroiliac) pain, Dejung[47] emphasized the importance of examining both the quadratus lumborum muscle for TrPs and the sacroiliac joint for blockage and of treating both if present, since each tends to aggravate the other. More recently, Dejung[50] described the identification, and illustrated the treatment, of TrPs in muscles commonly contributing to low back pain, including the longissimus dorsi, gluteus medius, iliacus, psoas, and abdominal muscles. Dejung[48] emphasized the importance of TrPs in the iliacus muscle as a commonly overlooked cause of lumbosacral (low back) pain and, in 1991, described in detail conservative management of TrPs in the iliacus and psoas muscles. Dejung and Ernst-Sandel[52] described how TrPs in the gluteus medius muscle are frequently responsible for patient complaints of lumbosacral pain and/or sciatica. Two other commonly involved muscles are the quadratus lumborum and the piriformis.

Practitioners of manual medicine applied to joints identify what is sometimes the primary cause of the backache and often a major contributing factor (in conjunction with active deep paraspinal TrPs). Figure 8-31 illustrates this anatomy and shows how shortening of short or long rotatores muscles on one side would tend to compress the zygapophyseal (facet) joint and neural foramen on the same side and put intervertebral ligaments under sustained stress on the other side, probably including the interspinous ligament. These structures do not well tolerate such unrelieved stress. Denslow et al.[54] reported that addition of stress to an existing articular dysfunction caused reflex spasm most markedly in the adjacent paraspinal muscles. This fits an increasing body of clinical evidence showing that articular dysfunctions can induce TrP activity and that TrP activity can aggravate corresponding articular dysfunctions. This helps to explain why it can be critically important to resolve therapeutically both the TrPs and the associated joint displacement. Some muscle energy techniques are well-suited for release of rotatores TrPs. They also can be inactivated by dry needling or injection, as shown in Figure 8-32.

4. Pelvic Region

Intrapelvic TrPs are probably the most consistently overlooked and neglected of any one group. Routine pelvic examinations do not include palpation of the musculature for TrPs, and those well acquainted with myofascial TrPs rarely do this special-purpose pelvic examination.[286] The levator ani is one of the most commonly involved intrapelvic muscles. Figure 8-33 presents its characteristic referred pain pattern and frequently seen TrP locations in that muscle. Coccygodynia is strongly associated with levator ani TrPs. Normally, one can slip the tip of the external examining finger beneath the tip of the coccyx and apply gentle pressure to the underside of it without any particular discomfort. It becomes intolerably painful as the finger applies lifting pressure to the coccyx, which stretches the levator ani and applies pressure on the attachment region of that muscle. The posterior gluteus maximus fibers are direct antagonists to the levator ani in the region of the coccyx and can be used to apply what is usually effective active stretch and reciprocal inhibition of the levator ani. Internally identified levator ani TrPs can be released with the digital pressure-release technique, with internal application of ultrasound, or with cyclic minimal contractions of the muscle by means of electrical stimulation.

The intrapelvic examination of these and of additional muscles for TrPs is fully described in Chapter 6 of Travell and Simons.[286] As gynecologists adopt this procedure, they discover that the endometriosis pain in many of their patients is fully accounted for by TrPs that respond well to TrP therapy. Similarly, urologists are discovering that the pain of many of their prostatitis patients is accounted for by intrapelvic (levator ani) TrPs. Fortunately, intrapelvic TrPs respond well to appropriate therapy in the hands of skilled practitioners.

5. Lower Extremity Region

Lower extremity TrPs are critically important because distortion of normal muscle function at this level frequently causes a chain-like reaction of compensatory dysfunctions at higher levels.[286] Thus, torso, head, and neck TrPs often respond poorly to treatment until the lower extremity dysfunctions are corrected. A common example is uncorrected pronation of the foot.

TrPs in the anterior portion of the gluteus minimus muscle refer pain down the lateral thigh and leg (Fig. 8-34A), and those in the posterior portion of this deep muscle refer pain in the distribution typical

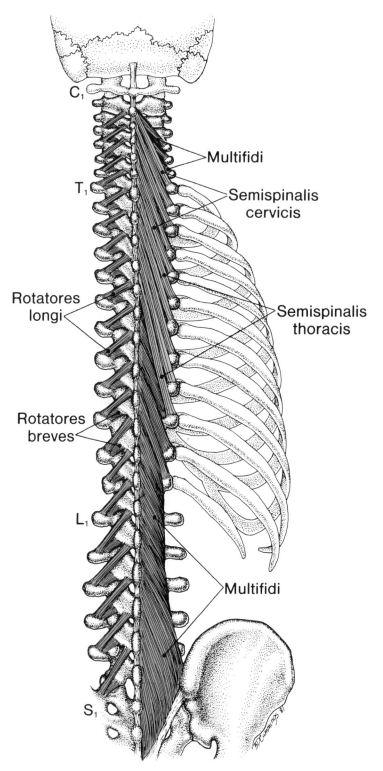

Figure 8-31. Attachment of the deep group of paraspinal muscles. **Right.** The more superficial of this group are the semispinalis thoracis at the thoracic level (*light red*), which overlies the multifidi, and the multifidi at the thoracic, lumbar, and sacral levels (*dark red*). **Left.** The rotatores form the deepest layer at both the thoracic and lumbar levels. (Reproduced with permission from Simons DG, Travell JG, Simons LS: *Travell and Simons' Myofascial Pain and Dysfunction: The Trigger Point Manual, Volume 1. Upper Half of Body.* Ed. 2. Williams & Wilkins, Baltimore, 1999.)

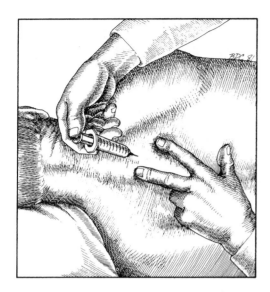

Figure 8-32. Injection of the right multifidus and rotatores muscles at the upper thoracic level. The needle is aimed slightly caudad to avoid penetrating between the vertebral laminae. (Reproduced with permission from Simons DG, Travell JG, Simons LS: *Travell and Simons' Myofascial Pain and Dysfunction: The Trigger Point Manual, Volume 1. Upper Half of Body.* Ed. 2. Williams & Wilkins, Baltimore, 1999.)

of sciatica (Fig. 8-34*B*). Although these TrPs are common, they are often overlooked because of the depth of the muscle and lack of familiarity with this pain pattern originating in muscle. The self-stretch technique that patients can learn to do at home is shown in Figure 8-35. This emphasizes the importance of teaching patients a home stretching exercise tailored to the muscles responsible for their pain. This figure shows how the patient employs contract-relax to augment stretch and notes the possible addition of assistive contraction of the antagonists to add the additional effect of reciprocal inhibition to help release muscle tension.

The knee joint is particularly vulnerable to muscle imbalance, which can induce painful abnormal stresses in the joint.[295] TrPs in the distal portion of the vastus lateralis or in the distal angulated fibers of the vastus medialis, which are sometimes distinguished as the vastus medialis oblique muscle because of their unique stabilizing function, are particularly likely to induce troublesome inhibition. TrPs in the vastus lateralis and/or vastus medialis

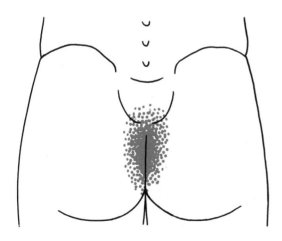

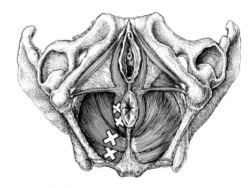

Sphincter ani, levator ani, and coccygeus (view from below)

Figure 8-33. Referred pain patterns (*solid red and red stippling*) generated by TrPs (*Xs*) in the right sphincter ani, levator ani, and coccygeus muscles. (Reproduced with permission from Travell JG, Simons DG: *Myofascial Pain and Dysfunction: The Trigger Point Manual, Volume 2.* Williams & Wilkins, Baltimore, 1992.)

can cause reflex inhibition of the adjacent rectus femoris muscle, causing a dangerous buckling knee syndrome (Chapter 14 of Travell and Simons[286]).

Muscles that are functionally weak because of inhibition by TrPs respond poorly to a simple strengthening program. The patient substitutes other muscles, and the strengthening exercise simply reinforces the abnormal contraction pattern. By inactivating the TrPs causing the inhibition, a normal functional pattern may be restored immediately. If the abnormal pattern has persisted too long, however, it may be necessary to retrain the inhibited muscle. This relearning process can be greatly accelerated with the use of EMG biofeedback.

Grossjean and Dejung[112] describe in detail their experience with 35 patients seen for a painful Achilles tendon, in whom they found TrPs in the soleus or, more commonly, in the medial or lateral gastrocnemius muscles. The tendon pain responded to treatment (massage or injection) of the TrPs (see also Hackett[118]).

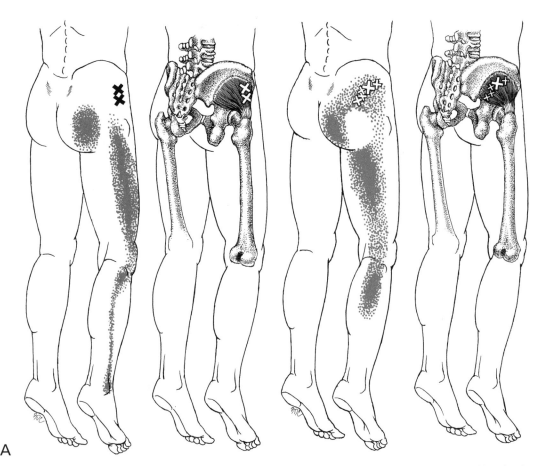

A

B

Figure 8-34. A. Pattern of referred pain from TrPs (*Xs*) in the anterior portion of the right gluteus minimus muscle (*light red*). The essential pain pattern is *solid red,* and the spillover extension observed when the muscle is more severely involved is *stippled*. **B.** Pain pattern (*dark red*) referred from TrPs (*Xs*) in the posterior part of the right gluteus minimus muscle (*light red*). The essential pain pattern is *solid red,* and the spillover pattern is *stippled*. The *large X* marks the most common location of TrPs in the posterior part of this muscle. The most anterior *small X* lies at the junction of the anterior and posterior portions of this muscle. (Reproduced with permission from Travell JG, Simons DG: *Myofascial Pain and Dysfunction: The Trigger Point Manual, Volume 2.* Williams & Wilkins, Baltimore, 1992.)

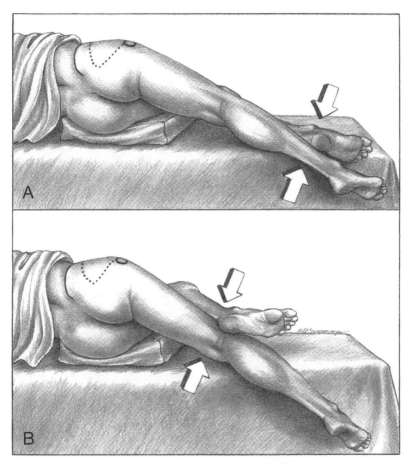

Figure 8-35. Self-stretch of the anterior fibers of the right gluteus minimus muscle. The *dotted line* identifies the posterior and the superior borders of the gluteus minimus muscle; these borders are closely related to the greater trochanter (*open circle*) and the crest of the ilium (*solid line*). **A.** Starting position. The individual contracts the muscle *gently* to press the right leg upward against resistance provided by the left heel. After 5 seconds of balanced pressure (*large arrows*) or after simply holding the weight of the thigh against the pull of gravity, the person relaxes and allows the right leg to drop downward over the edge of the table. This movement into adduction takes up the slack and lengthens the anterior part of the muscle.

B. Final stretch position after several cycles of the procedure described in **A**. Release of gluteus minimus muscle tension is enhanced when the patient tries to add stretch to the muscle (within comfort tolerance) by voluntarily contracting antagonists (in this case, adductor muscles). This effort adds the benefit of reciprocal inhibition. (Reproduced with permission from Travell JG, Simons DG: *Myofascial Pain and Dysfunction: The Trigger Point Manual, Volume 2.* Williams & Wilkins, Baltimore, 1992.)

G. COMMON MISCONCEPTIONS ABOUT THE TREATMENT OF TRIGGER POINTS

Effective treatment of MPS caused by TrPs usually involves more than simply applying a procedure to the TrPs. It is often necessary to consider and deal with what activated the TrPs, to identify and correct any perpetuating factors (which often are different than what activated the TrPs), and to help the patient restore and maintain normal muscle function.

There are a number of common misconceptions about the treatment of TrPs.

1. *Simply treating the TrP should be sufficient.* Occasionally, this may be true *if* the stress that activated the TrP is not

recurrent and *if* there are no perpetuating factors present. Otherwise, the TrP is likely to be reactivated again by the same stress. Ignoring perpetuating factors invites chronicity. After the TrPs have persisted for some time, failure to retrain the muscle to normal function or failure to reestablish its full-stretch range of motion results in a degree of persistent dysfunction.

2. *Since the pain has no demonstrable cause, it cannot be as severe as the patient indicates and must be largely psychogenic or behavioral.* The patients are trying to communicate their suffering. Believe them. It is severe. For instance, an appreciable amount of the pain reported by many patients with FMS comes from their TrPs. The pain of FMS patients rates fully as severe as the pain of rheumatoid arthritis. It is severe enough to cause CNS plasticity changes characteristic of chronic pain (see Chapter 1, Section D). Because of their chronic TrP and FMS pain, these patients often develop pain behavior that tends to reinforce dysfunction and suffering. Many patients have suffered grievously and needlessly because a series of physicians unacquainted with myofascial TrPs erroneously applied the psychogenic label to them covertly, if not overtly.

3. *Myofascial pain syndromes are self-limiting and will cure themselves.* It is possible for an acute uncomplicated TrP activated by an unusual activity or muscle overload to resolve spontaneously within a week or two *if* the muscle is not overstressed (used within tolerance, which may be limited) and *if* there are no perpetuating factors. Otherwise, if the acute syndrome is not properly managed, it evolves needlessly into a chronic MPS.

4. *Relief of pain by treatment of skeletal muscles for myofascial TrPs rules out serious visceral disease.* Because of the referred pain nature of visceral pain, application of vapocoolant spray or infiltration of a local anesthetic into the somatic reference zone can temporarily relieve the pain of myocardial infarction, angina, and acute abdominal disease.[296]

REFERENCES

1. Acquadro MA, Borodic GE: Treatment of myofascial pain with botulinum A toxin. [Letter]. *Anesthesiology* 80(3):705–706, 1994.
2. Adler I: Muscular rheumatism. *Med Rec* 57:529–535, 1900.
3. Aquilonius S-M, Askmark H, Gillberg P-G, et al.: Topographical localization of motor endplates in cryosections of whole human muscles. *Muscle Nerve* 7:287–293, 1984.
4. Arat A: *Neck Sprains As Muscle Injury, Tension Headache and Related Conditions.* Ed. 2. Guynes Printing Company, El Paso, TX, 1973 (pp. 134, 136).
5. Baker BA: The muscle trigger: evidence of overload injury. *J Neurol Orthop Med Surg* 7:35–44, 1986.
6. Baldry P: *Acupuncture, Trigger Points, and Musculoskeletal Pain.* Churchill Livingstone, New York, 1989.
7. Bardeen CR: The musculature, Sect. 5. *Morris's Human Anatomy.* Ed. 6. Edited by Jackson CM. Blakiston's Son & Co, Philadelphia, 1921 (p. 355).
8. Bateman JE: *The Shoulder and Neck.* WB Saunders, Philadelphia, 1972 (p. 182).
9. Bates T: Myofascial pain, Chapter 14. *Ambulatory Pediatrics II.* Edited by Green M, Haggerty RJ. WB Saunders, Philadelphia, 1977 (pp. 147, 148).
10. Bates T, Grunwaldt E: Myofascial pain in childhood. *J Pediatr* 53:198–209, 1958.
11. Belgrade M: Two decades after ping-pong diplomacy: is there a role for acupuncture in American pain medicine? *APS J* 3(2):73–83, 1994.
12. Bell WE: *Temporomandibular Disorders: Classification, Diagnosis, Management.* Year Book Medical Publishers, Chicago, 1990.
13. Bendall JR: *Muscles, Molecules, and Movement: An Essay in the Contraction of Muscles.* American Elsevier, New York, 1969.
14. Bendtsen L, Jensen R, Jensen NK, et al.: Muscle palpation with controlled finger pressure: new equipment for the study of tender myofascial tissues. *Pain* 59:235–239, 1994.
15. Bennett RM: Myofascial pain syndromes and the fibromyalgia syndrome: a comparative analysis, Chapter 2. *Myofascial Pain and FMS, Volume 17, Advances in Pain Research and Therapy.* Edited by Fricton JR, Awad EA. Raven Press, New York, 1990 (pp. 43–65).
16. Bennett RM: The contribution of muscle to the generation of fibromyalgia symptomatology. *J Musculoskeletal Pain* 4(1/2):35–59, 1996.
17. Bogduk N, Simons DG. Neck pain: joint pain or trigger points? Chapter 20. *Progress in Fibromyalgia and Myofascial Pain, Volume 6, Pain Research and Clinical Management.* Edited by Vaerøy H, Mersky H. Elsevier, Amsterdam, 1993 (pp. 267–273).
18. Bohr TW: Fibromyalgia syndrome and myofascial pain syndrome: do they exist? *Neurol Clin* 13(2):365–384, 1995.
19. Bonica JJ: Preface. *Advances in Neurology, Volume 4.* Edited by Bonica JJ. Raven Press, New York, 1974 (p. vii).

20. Bourne IHJ: Treatment of painful conditions of the abdominal wall with local injection. *Practitioner* 224:921–925, 1980.

21. Brown BR: Diagnosis and therapy of common myofascial syndromes. *JAMA* 239:646–648, 1978.

22. Brown WF, Varkey GP: The origin of spontaneous electrical activity at the end-plate zone. *Ann Neurol* 10:557–560, 1981.

23. Bruce E: Myofascial pain syndrome: early recognition and comprehensive management. *AAOHN J* 43(9):469–474, 1995.

24. Brückle W, Suckfüll M, Fleckenstein W, *et al.*: Gewebe-pO₂-Messung in der verspannten Rücken-muskulatur (m. erector spinae). *Z Rheumatol* 49:208–216, 1990.

25. Buchthal F, Rosenfalck P: Spontaneous electrical activity of human muscle. *Electroenceph Clin Neurophysiol* 20:321–336, 1966.

26. Buchthal F, Schmalbruch H: Motor unit of mammalian muscle. *Physiol Rev* 60:90–142, 1980.

27. Buchthal F, Guld C, Rosenfalck P: Innervation zone and propagation velocity in human muscle. *Acta Physiol Scand* 35:175–190, 1955.

28. Burnette JT, Ayoub MA: Cumulative trauma disorders. Part I. The problem. *Pain Manage* 2:196–209, 1989.

28a. Buskila D, Neumann L, Vaisberg G, *et al.* Increased rates of fibromyalgia following cervical spine injury: a controlled study of 161 cases of traumatic injury. *Arthritis Rheum* 40:446–452, 1997.

29. Cailliet R: *Low Back Pain Syndrome.* Ed. 3. FA Davis, Philadelphia, 1981 (pp. 86–87).

30. Carlson CR, Okeson JP, Falace DA, *et al.*: Reduction of pain and EMG activity in the masseter region by trapezius trigger point injection. *Pain* 55:397–400, 1993.

31. Cervero F: Visceral nociception: peripheral and central aspects of visceral nociceptive systems. *Philos Trans R Soc Lond B Biol Sci* 308:325–337, 1985.

32. Chen J-T, Chen S-M, Kuan T-S, *et al.*: Phentolamine effect on spontaneous electrical activity of active loci in a myofascial trigger spot of rabbit skeletal muscle. *Arch Phys Med Rehabil* 79(7):790–794, 1998.

33. Cheshire WP, Abashian SW, Mann JD: Botulinum toxin in the treatment of myofascial pain syndrome. *Pain* 59:65–69, 1994.

33a. Childers MK, Simons DG: Botulinum toxin use in myofascial pain syndromes, Chapter 21. *Pain Procedures in Clinical Practice.* Ed. 2. Edited by Lennard TA. Hanley & Belfus, Philadelphia, 2000 (pp. 191–202).

34. Chin NK, Cope M, Pang M: Number and distribution of spindle capsules in seven hindlimb muscles of the cat. *Symposium On Muscle Receptors.* Edited by Barker D. Hong Kong University Press, 1962 (pp. 241–248).

35. Christensen E: Topography of terminal motor innervation in striated muscles from stillborn infants. *The Innervation of Muscle.* Edited by Bouman HD, Woolf AL. Williams & Wilkins, Baltimore, 1960 (pp. 17–26).

36. Chu J: Dry needling (intramuscular stimulation) in myofascial pain related to lumbosacral radiculopathy. *Eur J Phys Med Rehabil* 5(4):106–121, 1995.

37. Clark GT: A critique of the stress-hyperactivity-pain theory of myogenic pain. *Pain Forum* 5(1):70–73, 1996.

38. Clemente CD: *Gray's Anatomy of the Human Body.* American Ed. 30. Lea & Febiger, Philadelphia, 1985.

39. Coërs C: Contribution a l'étude de la jonction neuromusculaire. Données nouvelles concernant la structure de l'arborisation terminale et de l'appareil sousneural chez l'homme. *Arch Biol Paris* 64:133–147, 1953.

40. Coërs C: Contribution a l'étude de la joncion neuromusculaire. II. Topographie zonale de l'innervation motrice terminale dans les muscles striés. *Arch Biol Paris* 64:495–505, 1953.

41. Coërs C, Woolf AL: *The Innervation of Muscle, A Biopsy Study.* Blackwell Scientific Publications, Oxford, 1959 (figs. 9–15).

42. Coulehan JL: Primary fibromyalgia. *Am Fam Phys* 32(3):170–177, 1985.

43. D'ambrosia RH: *Musculoskeletal Disorders: Regional Examination and Differential Diagnosis.* JB Lippincott, Philadelphia, 1977 (p. 332).

44. Danneskiold-Samsøe B, Christiansen E, Andersen RB: Regional muscle tension and pain ("Fibrositis"). *Scand J Rehabil Med* 15:17–20, 1983.

45. Danneskiold-Samsøe B, Christiansen E, Andersen RB: Myofascial pain and the role of myoglobin. *Scand J Rheumatol* 15:174–178, 1986.

46. Defalque RJ: Painful trigger points in surgical scars. *Anesth Analgesia* 61:518–520, 1982.

47. Dejung B: Iliosacralgelenksblockierungen—eine Verlaufsstudie. *Manuelle Medizin* 23:109–115, 1985.

48. Dejung B: Die Verspannung des M. iliacus als Ursache lumbosacraler Schmerzen. *Manuelle Medizin* 25:73–81, 1987.

49. Dejung B: Verspannungen des M. serratus anterior als Ursache interscapulärer Schmerzen. *Manuelle Medizin* 25:97–102, 1987.

50. Dejung B: Manuelle Triggerpunktbehandlung bei chronischer Lumbosakralgie. *Schweiz Med Wochenschr* 124(Suppl. 62):82–87, 1994.

51. Dejung B, Strub M: Die Behandlung der lateralen Epicondylodynie. *Physiotherapeut* 30(2):4–7, 1994.

52. Dejung B, Ernst-Sandel B: Triggerpunkte im M. glutaeus medius—eine häufige Ursache von Lumbosakralgie und ischialgiformem Schmerz. *Manuelle Medizin* 33:74–78, 1995.

53. Dejung B, Angerer B, Orasch J: Chronische Kopfschmerzen. *Physiotherapeut* 28(12):20–27, 1992.

54. Denslow JS, Korr IM, Krems AD: Quantitative studies of chronic facilitation in human motoneuron pools. *Am J Physiol* 105:229–238, 1947.

55. de Valera E, Raftery H: Lower abdominal and pelvic pain in women. *Advances in Pain Research and Therapy, Volume 1.* Edited by Bonica JJ, Albe-Fessard D. Raven Press, New York, 1976 (pp. 935–936).

56. Diakow PRP: Thermographic imaging of myofascial trigger points. *J Manipulative Physiol Ther* 11:114–117, 1988.

57. Diakow PRP: Differentiation of active and latent trigger points by thermography. *J Manipulative Physiol Ther* 15(7):439–441,1992.

58. Dittrich RJ: Low back pain-referred pain from the deep somatic structure of the back. *Lancet* 73:63–68, 1963.

59. Donaldson CCS, Skubick DL, Clasby RG, et al.: The evaluation of trigger-point activity using dynamic EMG techniques. *Am J Pain Manage* 4:118–122, 1994.

60. Dubowitz V, Brooke MH: *Muscle Biopsy: A Modern Approach.* WB Saunders, Philadelphia, 1973 (pp. 76, 77).

61. Dumitru D, DeLisa JA: AAEM mini monograph #10: volume conduction. *Muscle Nerve* 14:606–624, 1991.

62. Dutta CR, Basmajian JV: Gross and histological structure of the pharyngeal constrictors in the rabbit. *Anat Rec* 137:127–134, 1960.

63. Elson LM: The jolt syndrome. Muscle dysfunction following low-velocity impact. *Pain Manage* 3:317–326, 1990.

64. English AW, Wolf SL, Segal RL: Compartmentalization of muscles and their motor nuclei: the partitioning hypothesis. *Phys Ther* 73(12):857–867, 1993.

65. Ertekin C, Araç N, Uluda B, et al.: Enhancement of "end-plate monophasic waves" during an attack of hypokalemic periodic paralysis. [Letter]. *Muscle Nerve* 19(6):680–681, 1996.

66. Fassbender HG: Nonarticular rheumatism, Chapter 13. *Pathology of Rheumatic Disease.* Springer-Verlag, New York, 1975 (pp. 303–314).

67. Fassbender HG, Wegner K: Morphologie und Pathogenese des Weichteilrheumatismus. *Z Rheumaforsch* 32:355–374, 1973.

68. Fatt P, Katz B: Spontaneous subthreshold activity at motor nerve endings. *J Physiol* 117:109–128, 1952.

69. Fine PG: Myofascial trigger point pain in children. *J Pediatr* 111:547–548, 1987.

70. Fine PG, Milano R, Hare BD: The effects of myofascial trigger point injections are naloxone reversible. *Pain* 32:15–20, 1988.

71. Finestone DH, Willingham SGJ, Koffman GE, et al.: Physical and psychiatric impairment in patients with myofascial pain syndrome compared to patients with fibromyalgia. *J Musculoskeletal Pain* 3(Suppl. 1):86, 1995.

72. Fischer AA: Diagnosis and management of chronic pain in physical medicine and rehabilitation, Chapter 8. *Current Therapy in Physiatry.* Edited by Ruskin AP. WB Saunders, Philadelphia, 1984 (pp. 123–154).

73. Fischer AA: Pressure threshold meter: its use for quantification of tender spots. *Arch Phys Med Rehabil* 67:836–838, 1986.

74. Fischer AA: Pressure algometry over normal muscles. Standard values, validity and reproducibility of pressure threshold. *Pain* 30:115–126, 1987.

75. Fischer AA: Documentation of myofascial trigger points. *Arch Phys Med Rehabil* 69:286–291, 1988.

76. Fischer AA: Trigger point injection. *Physiatric Procedures in Clinical Practice.* Edited by Lennard TA. Hanley & Belfus, Philadelphia, 1995 (pp. 28–35).

77. Fischer AA: Trigger point injections can be performed pain-free using preinjection block (PIB). *J Musculoskeletal Pain* 3(Suppl. 1):140, 1995.

78. Fischer AA: Personal communication, 1996.

79. Fischer AA: New developments in diagnosis of myofascial pain and fibromyalgia. *Phys Med Rehabil Clin North Am* 8(1):1–21, 1997.

80. Fischer AA: New approaches in treatment of myofascial pain. *Phys Med Rehabil Clin North Am* 8(1):153–169, 1997.

81. Fischer AA: Algometry in diagnosis of musculoskeletal pain and evaluation of treatment outcome: an update. *J Musculoskeletal Pain* 6(1):5–32, 1998.

82. Fischer AA, Chang CH: Temperature and pressure threshold measurements in trigger points. *Thermology* 1:212–215, 1986.

83. Fishbain DA, Goldberg M, Meagher BR, et al.: Male and female chronic pain patients categorized by DSM-III psychiatric diagnostic criteria. *Pain* 26:181–197, 1986.

84. Fransen J, Russell IJ: *The Fibromyalgia Help Book.* Smith House Press, St. Paul, 1996.

85. Fricton JR: Myofascial Pain, Chapter 9. *Baillière's Clinical Rheumatology: Fibromyalgia and Myofascial Pain Syndromes, Volume 8, No. 4.* Edited by Masi AT. Baillière Tindall (Saunders), Philadelphia, 1994 (pp. 857–880).

86. Fricton JR, Kroening R, Haley D, et al.: Myofascial pain syndrome of the head and neck: a review of clinical characteristics of 164 patients. *Oral Surg* 60:615–623, 1985.

87. Fröhlich D, Fröhlich R: Das Piriformissyndrom: eine häufige Differentialdiagnose des lumboglutäalen Schmerzes (Piriformis syndrome: a frequent item in the differential diagnosis of lumbogluteal pain). *Man Med* 33:7–10, 1995.

88. Froriep: *Ein Beitrag zur Pathologie und Therapie des Rheumatismus.* Weimar, 1843.

89. Frost A: Diclofenac versus lidocaine as injection therapy in myofascial pain. *Scand J Rheumatol* 15:153–156, 1986.

90. Gedalia A, Press J, Klein M, et al.: Joint hypermobility and fibromyalgia in schoolchildren. *Ann Rheum Dis* 52(7):494–496, 1993.

91. Gerwin RD: Myofascial pain. The future of pain management: the perspective of a specialist in myofascial pain. *Am J Pain Manage* 1(1):9–10, 1991.

92. Gerwin RD: The management of myofascial pain syndromes. *J Musculoskeletal Pain* 1(3/4):83–94, 1993.

93. Gerwin RD: Neurobiology of the myofascial trigger point, Chapter 3. *Baillère's Clinical Rheumatology: Fibromyalgia and Myofascial Pain Syndromes, Volume 8, No. 4.* Edited by Masi AT. Baillière Tindall, London, 1994 (pp. 747–762).

94. Gerwin RD: A study of 96 subjects examined both for fibromyalgia and myofascial pain. *J Musculoskeletal Pain* 3(Suppl. 1):121, 1995.

95. Gerwin RD: Personal communication, 1996.

96. Gerwin RD, Duranleau D: Ultrasound identification of the myofascial trigger point. [Letter]. *Muscle Nerve* 20:767–768, 1997.

97. Gerwin RD, Shannon S, Hong C-Z, et al.: Identification of myofascial trigger points: inter-rater agreement and effect of training. *J Musculoskeletal Pain* 3(Suppl. 1):55, 1995.

98. Gerwin RD, Shannon S, Hong C-Z, *et al.*: Interrater reliability in myofascial trigger point examination. *Pain* 69:65–73, 1997.

99. Gillette RG, Kramis RC, Roberts WJ: Characterization of spinal somatosensory neurons having receptive fields in lumbar tissues of cats. *Pain* 54:85–98, 1993.

100. Glogowski G, Wallraff J: Ein Beitrag zur Klinik und Histologie der Muskelhärten (Myogelosen). *Z Orthop* 80:237–268, 1951.

101. Goldberg M, Murray TG: Analgesic-associated nephropathy. *N Engl J Med* 299:716–717, 1978.

102. Good M: Five hundred cases of myalgia in the British army. *Ann Rheum Dis* 3:118–138, 1942.

103. Gorrell RL: Troublesome ankle disorders and what to do about them. *Consultant* 16:64–69, 1976.

104. Gowers WR: Lumbago: its lesions and analogues. *Br Med J* 1:117–121, 1904.

105. Graff-Radford SB: Myofascial trigger points: their importance and diagnosis in the dental office. *J Dent Assoc S Afr* 39:237–240, 1984.

106. Graff-Radford SB, Jaeger B, Reeves JL: Myofascial pain may present clinically as occipital neuralgia. *Neurosurgery* 19(4):610–613, 1986.

107. Graff-Radford SB, Reeves JL, Jaeger B: Management of chronic headache and neck pain: the effectiveness of altering factors perpetuating myofascial pain. *Headache* 27:186–190, 1987.

108. Granges G, Littlejohn G: Prevalence of myofascial pain syndrome in fibromyalgia syndrome and regional pain syndrome: a comparative study. *J Musculoskeletal Pain* 1(2):19–35, 1993.

109. Graven-Nielsen T, Svensson P, Arendt-Nielsen L: Effects of experimental muscle pain on muscle activity and coordination during static and dynamic motor function. *Electroenceph Clin Neurophysiol* 105(2):156–164, 1997.

110. Greenbaum DS, Greenbaum RB, Joseph JG, *et al.*: Chronic abdominal wall pain: diagnostic validity and costs. *Dig Dis Sci* 39(9):1935–1941, 1994.

111. Gross D: *Therapeutische Lokalanästhesie.* Hippokrates Verlag, Stuttgart, 1972 (p. 142).

112. Grossjean B, Dejung B: Achillodynie—ein unlösbares Problem? *Schweiz Z Sportmed* 38:17–24, 1990.

113. Grzesiak RC: Psychological considerations in myofascial pain, fibromyalgia, and related musculoskeletal pain, Chapter 4. *Myofascial Pain and Fibromyalgia.* Edited by Rachlin ES. Mosby, St. Louis, 1994 (pp. 61–90).

114. Gundersen CB: The effects of botulinum toxin on the synthesis, storage and release of acetylcholine. *Prog Neurobiol* 14:99, 1980.

115. Gunn CC: Prespondylosis and some pain syndromes following denervation supersensitivity. *Spine* 5(2):185, 1980.

116. Gunn CC: *Treating Myofascial Pain: Intramuscular Stimulation (IMS) for Myofascial Pain Syndromes of Neuropathic Origin.* Multidisciplinary Pain Center, University of Washington Medical School, Seattle, 1989.

117. Gunn CC, Milbrandt WE: Utilizing trigger points. *Osteopathic Phys* 44:29–52, 1977.

118. Hackett GS: *Ligament and Tendon Relaxation Treated by Prolotherapy.* Ed. 3. Charles C Thomas, Springfield, IL, 1958 (pp. 27–36).

119. Hagbarth KE, Finer B: The plasticity of human withdrawal reflexes to noxious skin stimuli in lower limbs. *Prog Brain Res (Amsterdam)* 1:65–78, 1963.

120. Hagberg H, Kvarnström S: Muscular endurance and electromyographic fatigue in myofascial shoulder pain. *Arch Phys Med Rehabil* 65:522–525, 1984.

121. Headley BJ: Evaluation and treatment of myofascial pain syndrome utilizing biofeedback. *Clinical EMG for Surface Recordings, Volume 2.* Edited by Cram JR. Clinical Resources, Nevada City, CA, 1990 (pp. 235–254).

122. Headley BJ: The use of biofeedback in pain management. *Phys Ther Pract* 2(2):29–40, 1993.

123. Headley BJ: Physiologic risk factors. *Management of Cumulative Trauma Disorders.* Edited by Sanders M. Butterworth-Heineman, London, 1997 (pp. 107–127).

123a. Headley BJ: Personal communication, 1999.

124. Hess MJ, Borg-Stein J, Goldenberg DL: Role of rehabilitation in the management of fibromyalgia. *Arch Phys Med Rehabil* 76:1049, 1995.

125. Heuser J, Miledi R: Effect of lanthanum ions on function and structure of frog neuromuscular junctions. *Proc R Soc Lond B* 179:247–260, 1971.

126. Hoheisel U, Mense S: Response behaviour of cat dorsal horn neurones receiving input from skeletal muscle and other deep somatic tissues. *J Physiol* 426:265–280, 1990.

127. Hoheisel U, Mense S, Simons DG, *et al.*: Appearance of new receptive fields in rat dorsal horn neurons following noxious stimulation of skeletal muscle: a model for referred muscle pain? *Neurosci Lett* 153:9–12, 1993.

128. Hong C-Z: Myofascial trigger point injection. *Crit Rev Phys Med Rehabil* 5:203–217, 1993.

129. Hong C-Z: Lidocaine injection versus dry needling to myofascial trigger point: the importance of the local twitch response. *Am J Phys Med Rehabil* 73:256–263, 1994.

130. Hong C-Z: Persistence of local twitch response with loss of conduction to and from the spinal cord. *Arch Phys Med Rehabil* 75:12–16, 1994.

131. Hong C-Z: Considerations and recommendations regarding myofascial trigger point injection. *J Musculoskeletal Pain* 2(1):29–59, 1994.

132. Hong C-Z: Algometry in evaluation of trigger points and referred pain. *J Musculoskeletal Pain* 6(1):47–59, 1998.

133. Hong C-Z, Simons DG: Response to treatment for pectoralis minor myofascial pain syndrome after whiplash. *J Musculoskeletal Pain* 1(1):89–131, 1993.

134. Hong C-Z, Torigoe Y: Electrophysiological characteristics of localized twitch responses in responsive taut bands of rabbit skeletal muscle. *J Musculoskeletal Pain* 2(2):17–43, 1994.

135. Hong C-Z, Hsueh T-C: Difference in pain relief after trigger point injections in myofascial pain patients with and without fibromyalgia. *Arch Phys Med Rehabil* 77(11):1161–1166, 1996.

136. Hong C-Z, Torigoe Y, Yu J: The localized twitch responses in responsive taut bands of rabbit skeletal muscle fibers are related to the reflexes at

spinal cord level. *J Musculoskeletal Pain* 3(1):15–34, 1995.

137. Hong C-Z, Chen Y-N, Twehous DA, *et al.*: Pressure threshold for referred pain by compression on the trigger point and adjacent areas. *J Musculoskeletal Pain* 4(3):61–79, 1996.

137a. Hsieh C-Y, Hong C-Z, Adams AH, *et al.*: Interexaminer reliability of the palpation of trigger points in the trunk and lower limb muscles. *Arch Phys Med Rehabil* 81:258–264, 2000.

138. Hsieh JC, Belfrage M, Stone-Elander S, *et al.*: Central representation of chronic ongoing neuropathic pain studied by positron emission tomography. *Pain* 63:225–236, 1995.

139. Hubbard DR: Personal communication, 1994.

140. Hubbard DR: Chronic and recurrent muscle pain: pathophysiology and treatment, and review of pharmacologic studies. *J Musculoskeletal Pain* 4(1/2):124–143, 1996.

141. Hubbard DR, Berkoff GM: Myofascial trigger points show spontaneous needle EMG activity. *Spine* 18:1803–1807, 1993.

142. Inman VT, Saunders JB de CM: Referred pain from skeletal structures. *J Nerv Ment Dis* 99:660–667, 1944.

143. Institute of Medicine: *Pain and Disability: Clinical Behavioral and Public Policy Perspectives.* National Academy Press, Washington, DC, 1987.

144. International Anatomical Nomenclature Committee: *Nomina Anatomica.* Excerpta Medical Foundation, Amsterdam, 1966 (pp. 38–43).

145. Ito Y, Miledi R, Vincent A: Transmitter release induced by a 'factor' in rabbit serum. *Proc R Soc Lond B* 187:235–241, 1974.

146. Ivanichev GA: [*Painful Muscle Hypertonus*]. Russian. Kazan University Press, Kazan, 1990.

147. Jacob AT: Myofascial pain. *Physical Medicine and Rehabilitation: State of the Art Reviews, Volume 5/Number 3.* Edited by Schwab CD. Hanley & Belfus, Philadelphia, 1991 (pp. 573–583).

148. Jaeger B: Are "cervicogenic" headaches due to myofascial trigger point and cervical spine dysfunction? *Cephalalgia* 9(3):157–164, 1989.

149. Jaeger B: Differential diagnosis and management of craniofacial pain, Chapter 11. *Endodontics.* Ed. 4. Edited by Ingle JI, Bakland LK. Williams & Wilkins, Baltimore, 1994 (pp. 550–607).

150. Jaeger B, Skootsky SA: Double blind, controlled study of different myofascial trigger point injection techniques. *Pain* 4(Suppl.):S292, 1987.

151. Janda V: Evaluation of muscular imbalance, Chapter 6. *Rehabilitation of the Spine: A Practitioner's Manual.* Edited by Liebenson C. Williams & Wilkins, Baltimore, 1996 (pp. 97–112).

152. Janssens LA: Trigger points in 48 dogs with myofascial pain syndromes. *Vet Surg* 20:274–278, 1991.

153. Jayson MI: Fibromyalgia and trigger point injections. *Bull Hosp Jt Dis* 55(4):176–177, 1996.

154. Jensen R: Mechanisms of spontaneous tension-type headaches: an analysis of tenderness, pain thresholds and EMG. *Pain* 64:251–256, 1995.

155. Johnson EW: The myth of skeletal muscle spasm. [Editorial]. *Am J Phys Med* 68(1):1, 1989.

156. Jones RV Jr, Lambert EH, Sayre GP: Source of a type of "insertion activity" in electromyography

with evaluation of a histologic method of localization. *Arch Phys Med Rehabil* 36:301–310, 1955.

157. Kahn J: Electrical modalities in the treatment of myofascial conditions, Chapter 15. *Myofascial Pain and Fibromyalgia.* Edited by Rachlin ES. Mosby, St. Louis, 1994 (pp. 473–485).

158. Katz J, Jackson M, Kavanagh BP, *et al.*: Acute pain after thoracic surgery predicts long-term post-thoracotomy pain. *Clin J Pain* 12:50–55, 1996.

159. Kellgren JH: Observations on referred pain arising from muscle. *Clin Sci* 3:175–190, 1938.

160. Kellgren JH: Deep pain sensibility. *Lancet* 1:943–949, 1949.

161. Kelly M: The treatment of fibrositis and allied disorders by local anesthesia. *Med J Aust* 1:294–298, 1941.

162. Kelly M: The relief of facial pain by procaine (Novocain) injections. *J Am Geriatr Soc* 11:586–596, 1963.

163. Kimura J: *Electrodiagnosis in Diseases of Nerve and Muscle, Volume 2.* FA Davis, Philadelphia, 1989.

164. Korr IM, Thomas PE, Wright HM: Clinical significance of the facilitated state. *J Am Osteopath Assoc* 54:277–282, 1955.

165. Kraft GH, Johnson EW, LaBan MM: The fibrositis syndrome. *Arch Phys Med Rehabil* 49:155–162, 1968.

166. Kraus H: Behandlung akuter Muskelhärten. *Wien Klin Wochenschr* 50:1356–1357, 1937.

167. Kraus H: Diagnosis and treatment of low back pain. *GP* 5(4):55–60, 1952.

168. Kraus H: Evaluation and treatment of muscle function in athletic injury. *Am J Surg* 98:353–361, 1959.

169. Kraus H: *Clinical Treatment of Back and Neck Pain.* McGraw-Hill, New York, 1970 (pp. 95, 107).

170. Kraus H, Fischer AA: Diagnosis and treatment of myofascial pain. *Mt Sinai J Med* 58:235–249, 1991.

171. Kruse RA Jr, Christiansen JA: Thermographic imaging of myofascial trigger points: a follow-up study. *Arch Phys Med Rehabil* 73:819–823, 1992.

172. Lange F, Eversbusch G: Die Bedeutung der Muskelhärten für die allgemeine Praxis. *Münch Med Wochenschr* 68:418–420, 1921.

173. Lange M: *Die Muskelhärten (Myogelosen).* München, JF Lehmann's Verlag, 1931.

174. Lawrence RM: *Osteopuncture: Theory and Practice.* Presented at the annual meeting of the North American Academy of Manipulative Medicine, 1977.

175. Leriche R: Des effets de l'anesthésie à la novocaine des ligaments et des insertions tendineuses periarticulaires dans certaines maladies articulaires et dans vices de position fonctionnels des articulations. *Gazette Hopitaux* 103:1294, 1930.

176. Lewis C, Gevirtz R, Hubbard D, *et al.*: Needle trigger point and surface frontal EMG measurements of psychophysiological responses in tension-type headache patients. *Biofeedback Self Reg* 19(3):274–275, 1994.

177. Lewit K: *Manipulative Therapy in Rehabilitation of the Motor System.* Butterworths, London, 1985.

178. Lewit K: Chain reactions in disturbed function of the motor system. *Man Med* 3:27–29, 1987.

179. Lewit K: *Manipulative Therapy in Rehabilitation of the Locomotor System.* Ed. 2. Butterworth Heinemann, Oxford, 1991.

180. Lewit K, Simons DG: Myofascial pain: relief by post-isometric relaxation. *Arch Phys Med Rehabil* 65:452–456, 1984.

181. Liley AW: An investigation of spontaneous activity at the neuromuscular junction of the rat. *J Physiol* 132:650–666, 1956.

182. Llewellyn LJ, Jones AB: *Fibrositis.* London, Heinemann, 1915.

183. Lockhart RD, Hamilton GF, Fyfe FW: *Anatomy of the Human Body.* Ed. 2. JB Lippincott, Philadelphia, 1969 (p. 144).

184. Loh L, Nathan PW, Schott GD, *et al.*: Acupuncture versus medical treatment for migraine and muscle tension headaches. *J Neurol Neurosurg Psychiatry* 47:333–337, 1984.

185. Lowe JC: The subluxation and the trigger point: measuring how they interact. *Chiropractic J* 8(10): 32, 35, 1993.

186. Lowe JC: *The Metabolic Treatment of Fibromyalgia.* McDowell Publishing, Boulder, CO, 2000.

187. Macdonald AJR: Abnormally tender muscle regions and associated painful movements. *Pain* 8:197–205, 1980.

188. Mannion AF, Dolan P: Relationship between mechanical and electromyographic manifestations of fatigue in the quadriceps femoris muscle of humans. *Muscle Nerve* 4(Suppl.):S46, 1996.

189. Margoles MS: Stress neuromyelopathic pain syndrome (SNPS). *J Neurol Orthop Surg* 4:317–322, 1983.

190. Margolis M: Personal communication, 1996.

191. Masi AT: Review of the epidemiology and criteria of fibromyalgia and myofascial pain syndromes: concepts of illness in populations as applied to dysfunctional syndromes. *J Musculoskeletal Pain* 1(3/4):113–157, 1993.

192. McCain GA: A clinical overview of the fibromyalgia syndrome. *J Musculoskeletal Pain* 4(1/2):9–34, 1996.

193. McClaflin RR: Myofascial pain syndrome. Primary care strategies for early intervention. *Postgrad Med* 96(2):56–59, 63–66, 69–70, 1994.

194. McMillan AS, Hannam AG: Motor-unit territory in the human masseter muscle. *Arch Oral Biol* 36(6):435–441, 1991.

195. McNulty WH, Gevirtz RN, Hubbard DR, *et al.*: Needle electromyographic evaluation of trigger point response to a psychological stressor. *Psychophysiology* 31(3):313–316, 1994.

196. Melzack R, Stillwell DM, Fox EJ: Trigger points and acupuncture points for pain: correlations and implications. *Pain* 3:3–23, 1977.

197. Mense S: Nociception from skeletal muscle in relation to clinical muscle pain. *Pain* 54:241–289, 1993.

198. Mense S: Peripheral mechanisms of muscle nociception and local muscle pain. *J Musculoskeletal Pain* 1(1):133–170, 1993.

199. Mense S: Referral of muscle pain: new aspects. *Am Pain Soc J* 3:1–9, 1994.

200. Mense S: Pathophysiological basis of muscle pain syndromes. An update. *Phys Med Rehabil Clin North Am* 8:23–53, 1997.

201. Michele AA, Davies JJ, Krueger FJ, *et al.*: Scapulocostal syndrome (fatigue-postural paradox). *NY State J Med* 50:1353–1356, 1950.

202. Miehlke K, Schulze G, Eger W: Klinische und experimentelle Untersuchungen zum Fibrositissyndrom. *Z Rheumaforsch* 19:310–330, 1960.

203. Miller B: Manual therapy treatment of myofascial pain and dysfunction, Chapter 13. *Myofascial Pain and Fibromyalgia.* Edited by Rachlin ES. Mosby, St. Louis, 1994 (pp. 415–454).

204. Mitchell FL Jr, Moran PF, Pruzzo NA: *An Evaluation and Treatment Manual of Osteopathic Muscle Energy Procedures.* Mitchell, Moran and Pruzzo Associates, Valley Park, MO, 1979.

205. Moldofsky H: The contribution of sleep-wake physiology to fibromyalgia, Chapter 13. *Advances in Pain Research and Therapy, Volume 17: Myofascial Pain and Fibromyalgia.* Edited by Fricton JR, Awad EA. Raven Press, New York, 1990 (pp. 227–240).

206. Müller W: *Generalisierte Tendomyopathie (Fibromyalgie).* Steinkopf Verlag, Darmstadt, 1991.

207. Nice DA, Riddle DL, Lamb RL, *et al.*: Intertester reliability of judgments of the presence of trigger points in patients. *Arch Phys Med Rehabil* 73:893–898, 1992.

208. Nielsen AJ: Spray and stretch for myofascial pain. *Phys Ther* 58:567–569, 1978.

209. Nielsen AJ: Case study: myofascial pain of the posterior shoulder relieved by spray and stretch. *J Orthop Sports Phys Ther* 3:21–26, 1981.

210. Njoo KH, van der Does E: The occurrence and inter-rater reliability of myofascial trigger points in the quadratus lumborum and gluteus medius: a prospective study in non-specific low back pain patients and controls in general practice. *Pain* 58:317–323, 1994.

211. Olesen J, Jensen R: Getting away from simple muscle contraction as a mechanism of tension-type headache. [Editorial]. *Pain* 46:123–124, 1991.

212. Ormandy L: Scapulocostal syndrome. *Va Med Q* 121(2)(Spring):105–108, 1994.

213. Pace JB: Commonly overlooked pain syndromes responsive to simple therapy. *Postgrad Med* 58: 107–113, 1975.

214. Partanen JV, Nousiainen U: End-plate spikes in electromyography are fusimotor unit potentials. *Neurology* 33:1039–1043, 1983.

215. Pellegrino MJ, Waylonis GW, Sommer A: Familial occurrence of primary fibromyalgia. *Arch Phys Med Rehabil* 70:61–63, 1989.

216. Perry F, Heller PH, Kamiya J, *et al.*: Altered autonomic function in patients with arthritis or with chronic myofascial pain. *Pain* 39:77–84, 1989.

217. Pomeranz BH: Acupuncture in America: a commentary. *Am Pain Soc J* (2):96–100, 1994.

218. Popelianskii IA-IU, Zaslavskii ES, Veselovskii VP: [Medicosocial significance, etiology, pathogenesis, and diagnosis of nonarticular disease of soft tissues of the limbs and back.] Russian. *Vopr Revm* 3:38–43, 1976.

219. Price DD, Rafii A, Watkins LR, *et al.*: A psychophysical analysis of acupuncture analgesia. *Pain* 19:27–42, 1984.

220. Rachlin ES: Trigger point management, Chapter 9. *Myofascial Pain and Fibromyalgia.* Edited by Rachlin ES. Mosby, St. Louis, 1994 (pp. 173–195).
221. Radziemski A, Kudzia A, Jakubowicz M: Number and localization of the muscle spindles in the human fetal sternocleidomastoid muscle. *Folia Morphol* 50(1/2):65–70, 1991.
222. Reeves JL, Jaeger B, Graff-Radford S: Reliability of the pressure algometer as a measure of myofascial trigger point sensitivity. *Pain* 24:313–321, 1986.
223. Reiter RC, Gambone JC: Nongynecologic somatic pathology in women with chronic pelvic pain and negative laparoscopy. *J Reprod Med* 36(4):253–259, 1991.
224. Reitinger A, Radner H, Tilscher H, *et al.*: Morphologische Untersuchung an Triggerpunkten [Morphologic study of trigger points]. *Man Med* 34:256–262, 1996.
225. Reynolds MD: Myofascial trigger point syndromes in the practice of rheumatology. *Arch Phys Med Rehabil* 62:111–114, 1981 (table 2).
226. Reynolds MD: The development of the concept of fibrositis. *J Hist Med Allied Sci* 38:5–35, 1983.
227. Rogers EJ, Rogers R: Fibromyalgia and myofascial pain: either, neither, or both? *Orthop Rev* 18(11):1217–1224, 1989.
228. Romano TJ: Non-articular rheumatism. *J Musculoskeletal Pain* 1(2):133–143, 1993.
229. Rosen NB: Myofascial pain: the great mimicker and potentiator of other diseases in the performing artist. *Md Med J* 42(3):261–266, 1993.
230. Rosen NB: The myofascial pain syndromes. *Phys Med Rehabil Clin North Am* 4(Feb):41–63, 1993.
231. Rosomoff HL, Fishbain DA, Goldberg M, *et al.*: Physical findings in patients with chronic intractable benign pain of the neck and/or back. *Pain* 37:279–287, 1989.
232. Roy RR, Garfinkel A, Ounjian M, *et al.*: Three-dimensional structure of cat tibialis anterior motor units. *Muscle Nerve* 18:1187–1195, 1995.
233. Rubin D: Myofascial trigger point syndromes: an approach to management. *Arch Phys Med Rehabil* 62:107–110, 1981.
234. Russell IJ: Neurochemical pathogenesis of fibromyalgia syndrome. *J Musculoskeletal Pain* 4(1/2):61–92, 1996.
235. Salpeter MM: Vertebrate neuromuscular junctions: General morphology, molecular organization, and functional consequences, Chapter 1. *The Vertebrate Neuromuscular Junction.* Edited by Salpeter MM. Alan R. Liss, New York, 1987 (pp. 1–54).
236. Schade H: Beiträge zur Umgrenzung und Klärung einer Lehre von der Erkältung. *Z Ges Exp Med* 7:275–374, 1919.
237. Schade H: Untersuchungen in der Erkältungsfrage: III. Über den Rheumatismus, insbesondere den Muskelrheumatismus (Myogelose). *Münch Med Wochenschr* 68:95–99, 1921.
238. Schiffman EL, Fricton JR, Haley DP, *et al.*: The prevalence and treatment needs of subjects with temporomandibular disorders. *J Am Dent Assoc* 120:295–303, 1990.
239. Schmidt A: Zur Pathologie und Therapie des Muskelrheumatismus (Myalgie). *Münch Med Wochenschr* 63:593–595, 1916.

240. Schneider MJ: Tender points/fibromyalgia vs. trigger points/myofascial pain syndrome: a need for clarity in terminology and differential diagnosis. *J Manipulative Physiol Ther* 18(6):398–406, 1996.
241. Schwarzacher VHG: Zur Lage der motorischen Endplatten in den Skelettmuskeln. *Acta Anat* 30:758–774, 1957.
242. Scudds RA, Landry M, Birmingham T, *et al.*: The frequency of referred signs from muscle pressure in normal healthy subjects. *J Musculoskeletal Pain* 3(Suppl. 1):99, 1995.
243. Simms RW, Goldenberg DL, Felson DT, *et al.*: Tenderness in 75 anatomic sites distinguishing fibromyalgia patients from controls. *Arthritis Rheum* 31:183–187, 1988.
244. Simons DG: Muscle pain syndromes, Part I. *Am J Phys Med* 54:289–311, 1975.
245. Simons DG: Muscle pain syndromes, Part II. *Am J Phys Med* 55:15–42, 1976.
246. Simons DG: Electrogenic nature of palpable bands and "jump sign" associated with myofascial trigger points. *Advances in Pain Research and Therapy, Volume 1.* Edited by Bonica JJ, Albe-Fessard D. Raven Press, New York, 1976 (pp. 913–918).
247. Simons DG: Myofascial pain syndrome due to trigger points, Chapter 45. *Rehabilitation Medicine.* Edited by Goodgold J. CV Mosby Co, St. Louis, 1988 (pp. 686–723).
248. Simons DG: Muscular pain syndromes, Chapter 1. *Myofascial Pain and Fibromyalgia, Advances in Pain Research and Therapy, Volume 17.* Edited by Fricton JR, Awad EA. Raven Press, New York, 1990 (pp. 1–41).
249. Simons DG: Referred phenomena of myofascial trigger points, Chapter 28. *Pain Research and Clinical Management: New Trends in Referred Pain and Hyperalgesia, Volume 27.* Edited by Vecchiet L, Albe-Fessard D, Lindblom U, Giamberardino MA. Elsevier, Amsterdam, 1993 (pp. 341–357).
250. Simons DG: Neurophysiological basis of pain caused by trigger points. *Am Pain Soc J* 3:17–19, 1994.
251. Simons DG: Myofascial pain syndrome: one term but two concepts: a new understanding.[Editorial]. *J Musculoskeletal Pain* 3(1):7–13, 1995.
252. Simons DG: Clinical and etiological update of myofascial pain from trigger points. *J Musculoskeletal Pain* 4(1/2):97–125, 1996.
253. Simons DG: Myofascial trigger points: the critical experiment. *J Musculoskeletal Pain* 5(4):113–118, 1997.
254. Simons DG, Stolov WC: Microscopic features and transient contraction of palpable bands in canine muscle. *Am J Phys Med* 55:65–88, 1976.
255. Simons DG, Travell JG: Myofascial trigger points, a possible explanation. *Pain* 10:106–109, 1981.
256. Simons DG, Travell JG: Myofascial origins of low back pain. Parts 1, 2, 3. *Postgrad Med* 73:66–108, 1983.
257. Simons DG, Dexter JR: Comparison of local twitch responses elicited by palpation and needling of myofascial trigger points. *J Musculoskeletal Pain* 3(1):49–61, 1995.
258. Simons DG, Mense S: Understanding and measurement of muscle tone related to clinical muscle pain. *Pain* 75:1–17, 1998.

259. Simons DG, Hong C-Z, Simons LS: Prevalence of spontaneous electrical activity at trigger spots and control sites in rabbit muscle. *J Musculoskeletal Pain* 3(1):35–48, 1995.

260. Simons DG, Hong C-Z, Simons LS: Nature of myofascial trigger points, active loci. *J Musculoskeletal Pain* 3(Suppl. 1):62, 1995.

261. Simons DG, Hong C-Z, Simons LS: Spontaneous electrical activity of trigger points. *J Musculoskeletal Pain* 3(Suppl. 1):124, 1995.

262. Simons DG, Hong C-Z, Simons LS: Spike activity in trigger points. *J Musculoskeletal Pain* 3(Suppl. 1):125, 1995d.

262a. Simons DG, Hong C-Z, Simons LS: Presence of electrically active loci in human trigger points, end-plate zones, and taut bands. [Submitted for publication].

263. Simons DG, Travell JG, Simons LS: *Travell and Simons' Myofascial Pain and Dysfunction: The Trigger Point Manual, Volume 1. Upper Half of Body.* Ed. 2. Williams & Wilkins, Baltimore, 1999.

264. Sinclair DC: The remote reference of pain aroused in the skin. *Brain* 72:364–372, 1949.

265. Skootsky SA, Jaeger B, Oye RK: Prevalence of myofascial pain in general internal medicine practice. *West J Med* 151:157–160, 1989.

266. Smythe HA, Moldofsky H: Two contributions to understanding the "fibrositis syndrome." *Bull Rheum Dis* 28:928–931, 1977.

267. Sola AE: Personal communication, 1981.

268. Sola AE, Bonica JJ: Myofascial pain syndromes, Chapter 21. *The Management of Pain.* Ed. 2. Edited by Bonica JJ, Loeser JD, Chapman CR, Fordyce WE. Lea & Febiger, Philadelphia, 1990 (pp. 352–367).

269. Sola AE, Rodenberger ML, Gettys BB: Incidence of hypersensitive areas in posterior shoulder muscles. *Am J Phys Med* 34:585–590, 1955.

270. Sørensen J, Bengtsson A, Backman E, *et al.*: Pain analysis in patients with fibromyalgia. Effects of intravenous morphine, lidocaine, and ketamine. *Scand J Rheumatol* 24(6):360–365, 1995.

271. Starlanyl D, Copeland ME: *Fibromyalgia & Chronic Myofascial Pain Syndrome: A Survival Guide.* New Harbinger, Oakland, CA, 1996.

272. Stockman R: Chronic rheumatism, chronic muscular rheumatism, fibrositis, Chapter 2. *Rheumatism and Arthritis.* Edited by Stockman RW. Green & Son, Edinburgh, 1920 (pp. 41–56).

273. Swerdlow B, Dieter JNI: An evaluation of the sensitivity and specificity of medical thermography for the documentation of myofascial trigger points. *Pain* 48:205–213, 1992.

274. Swett JE, Eldred E, Buchwald JS: Somatotopic cord-to-muscle relations in efferent innervation of cat gastrocnemius. *Am J Physiol* 219(No 3):762–766, 1970.

275a. Theobald GW: The relief and prevention of referred pain. *J Obstet Gynaecol Br Commonw* 56:447–460, 1949.

275. Tonndorf ML, Hannam AL: Motor unit territory in relation to tendons in the human masseter muscle. *Muscle Nerve* 17:436–443, 1994.

276. Travell J: Basis for the multiple uses of local block of somatic trigger areas (procaine infiltration and ethyl chloride spray). *Miss Valley Med J* 71:13–22, 1949.

277. Travell J: Pain mechanisms in connective tissue. *Connective Tissues, Transactions of the Second Conference, 1951.* Edited by Ragan C. Josiah Macy Jr. Foundation, New York, 1952 (pp. 96–102, 105–109, 111).

278. Travell J: Introductory comments. *Connective Tissues, Transactions of the Fifth Conference, 1954.* Edited by Ragan C. Josiah Macy Jr. Foundation, New York, 1954 (pp. 12–22).

279. Travell J: Temporomandibular joint pain referred from muscles of the head and neck. *J Prosthet Dent* 10:745–763, 1960.

280. Travell J: Mechanical headache. *Headache* 7:23–29, 1967.

281. Travell J: Myofascial trigger points: clinical view. *Advances in Pain Research and Therapy, Volume 1.* Edited by Bonica JJ, Albe-Fessard D. Raven Press, New York, 1976 (pp. 919–926) (figure 10).

282. Travell J: Identification of myofascial trigger point syndromes: a case of atypical facial neuralgia. *Arch Phys Med Rehabil* 62:100–106, 1981.

283. Travell J: Chronic myofascial pain syndromes. Mysteries of the history, Chapter 6. *Advances in Pain Research and Therapy: Myofascial Pain and Fibromyalgia, Volume 17.* Edited by Fricton JR, Awad EA. Raven Press, New York, 1990 (pp. 129–137).

284. Travell J, Bobb AL: Mechanism of relief of pain in sprains by local injection techniques. *Fed Proc* 6:378, 1947.

285. Travell J, Rinzler SH: The myofascial genesis of pain. *Postgrad Med* 11:425–434, 1952.

286. Travell JG, Simons DG: *Myofascial Pain and Dysfunction: The Trigger Point Manual, Volume 2.* Williams & Wilkins, Baltimore, 1992.

287. Travell J, Rinzler S, Herman M: Pain and disability of the shoulder and arm: treatment by intramuscular infiltration with procaine hydrochloride. *JAMA* 120:417–422, 1942.

288. Trommer PR, Gellman MB: Trigger point syndrome. *Rheumatism* 8:67–72, 1952.

289. Vecchiet L, Galletti R, Giamberardino MA, *et al.*: Modifications of cutaneous, subcutaneous, and muscular sensory and pain thresholds after the induction of an experimental algogenic focus in the skeletal muscle. *Clin J Pain* 4:55–59, 1988.

290. Vecchiet L, Giamberardino MA, de Bigontina P, *et al.*: Comparative sensory evaluation of parietal tissues in painful and nonpainful areas in fibromyalgia and myofascial pain syndrome, Chapter 13. *Proceedings of the 7th World Congress on Pain: Progress in Pain Research and Management, Volume 2.* Edited by Gebhart GF, Hammond DL, Jensen TS. IASP Press, Seattle, 1994 (pp. 177–249).

291. Walsh EG: *Muscles, Masses and Motion. The Physiology of Normality, Hypotonicity, Spasticity and Rigidity.* Mac Keith Press, distributed by Cambridge University Press, New York, 1992.

292. Ward AA: Spontaneous electrical activity at combined acupuncture and myofascial trigger point sites. *Acupuncture Med* 14(2):75–79, 1996.

293. Webber TD: Diagnosis and modification of headache and shoulder-arm-hand syndrome. *J Am Osteopath Assoc* 72:697–710, 1973.

294. Weeks VD, Travell J: How to give painless injections. *AMA Scientific Exhibits 1957*, Grune & Stratton, New York, 1957 (pp. 318–322).

295. Weiser HI: Semimembranosus insertion syndrome: a treatable and frequent cause of persistent knee pain. *Arch Phys Med Rehabil* 60:317–319, 1979.

296. Weiss S, Davis D: The significance of the afferent impulses from the skin in the mechanism of visceral pain, skin infiltration as a useful therapeutic measure. *Am J Med Sci* 176:517–536, 1928.

297. Wiederholt WC: "End-plate noise" in electromyography. *Neurology* 20:214–224, 1970.

298. Wilkins JC, Meerschaert JR: Hypermobility syndrome: prevalence and manifestations. *Arch Phys Med Rehabil* 76:1047, 1995.

299. Wolfe F, Smythe HA, Yunus MB, *et al.*: The American College of Rheumatology 1990 Criteria for the Classification of Fibromyalgia: Report of the Multicenter Criteria Committee. *Arthritis Rheum* 33:160–172, 1990.

300. Wolfe F, Simons DG, Fricton JR, *et al.*: The fibromyalgia and myofascial pain syndromes: a preliminary study of tender points and trigger points in persons with fibromyalgia, myofascial pain syndrome and no disease. *J Rheumatol* 19:944–951, 1992.

301. Wu C-M, Chen H-H, Hong C-Z: Inactivation of myofascial trigger points associated with lumbar radiculopathy: surgery versus physical therapy. *Arch Phys Med Rehabil* 78:1040–1041, 1997.

302. Yaksh TL, Abram SE: Focus article: preemptive analgesia: a popular misnomer, but a clinically relevant truth? *Am Pain Soc J* 2:116–121, 1993.

303. Yue SK: Initial experience in the use of botulinum A toxin for the treatment of myofascial related muscle dysfunctions. *J Musculoskeletal Pain* 3(Suppl. 1):22, 1995.

304. Yunus MB: Research in fibromyalgia and myofascial pain syndrome: current status, problems and future decision. *J Musculoskeletal Pain* 1(1):23–41, 1993.

305. Yunus MB: Understanding myofascial pain syndromes: a reply. *J Musculoskeletal Pain* 2(1):147–149, 1994.

306. Yunus MB, Masi AT, Calabro JJ, *et al.*: Primary fibromyalgia (fibrositis): clinical study of 50 patients with matched normal controls. *Semin Arthritis Rheum* 11:151–171, 1981.

CHAPTER 9
Fibromyalgia Syndrome

I. Jon Russell

SUMMARY: Fibromyalgia syndrome (FMS) is a common medical condition characterized by widespread pain and tenderness to palpation at multiple anatomically defined soft tissue body sites. While much of this pain and many of these test sites are located in muscle, the allodynia is now believed to come primarily from central nervous system neurosensory amplification of nociception in general and not specifically from muscle pathology. While its gender distribution is about equal in childhood, it overwhelmingly affects adult females more than adult males. The symptoms pervade many aspects of daily life, with comorbidities such as depression, anxiety, insomnia, endocrinopathies, irritable bowel syndrome, and dysfunction of the autonomic nervous system. It can accompany and complicate a variety of medical conditions, such as rheumatoid arthritis, systemic lupus erythematosus, and hypothyroidism. Once considered to be a figment of the patient's imagination, FMS is now recognized as the human model for widespread allodynia. Laboratory tests were negative in the past because the proper tests were not being done. Appropriate tests show low platelet serotonin levels, elevated levels of spinal fluid substance P and nerve growth factor, abnormal cortisol and growth hormone regulation, and lower-than-normal regional blood flow in the brain. There is a growing awareness that clinical FMS may be etiologically heterogeneous, including a subset with compressive brainstem or cervical myelopathy. The challenge now is to better understand the pathogenesis of the documented abnormalities and how best to correct them. In those arenas, too, there has been encouraging progress. Multimodal therapies, including effective new medications, offer hope for reduced pain and functional improvement.

A. OVERVIEW

Fibromyalgia syndrome (FMS) is a common clinical condition in which the patient perceives widespread pain and exhibits reproducible tenderness to palpation at a variety of anatomically defined soft tissue areas of the body. It affects adult females much more commonly than it does males. Some clinicians suspect that it is increasing in frequency, but the most likely reason for such an impression is an increasing awareness of this syndrome among the medical community and in the public press. Generally accepted classification criteria for FMS now facilitate epidemiologic and pathogenic studies to further characterize the disorder.

Fibromyalgia probably is not a new malady, but because it leaves no permanent marks on bones or joints, there is no reason to expect that archeologic evidence would support its historical existence. Conversely, FMS is currently making its mark in today's legal and political arenas. That is because the level of physical dysfunction it causes can be moderately severe, compared with that of rheumatoid arthritis (RA), and it is more than twice as common as RA in the general population. As a result, the cost of this condition to affected individuals, families, employers, insurers, and governments is so high that it cannot be ignored.

The cause of FMS is unknown, but growing evidence indicates that its pathogenesis involves aberrant neurochemical processing of sensory signals in the central nervous system (CNS) (see Chapter 7). The symptomatic result is lowering of the pain thresholds and an amplification of normal sensory signals until the patient experiences nearly constant pain.

Unfortunately, a cure for FMS is not yet in sight. Multimodal therapy can reduce the severity of symptoms in most patients, but few can say that any combination of interventions has fully relieved their symptoms. The hope for cure of this disorder is through an active and multifaceted research program.

The discussions that follow offer insights into each of these aspects of FMS. We attempt to integrate clinical and lab-oratory features of FMS into a series of potentially testable hypotheses that are likely to usher in a new era for FMS in which the condition will be better understood and more effectively managed.

B. HISTORY

There is no way of knowing whether FMS was one of those ancient disorders that lured people of ages past to the relaxing warmth of natural hot pool spas in Europe, dating back to Roman times. Arthritic disorders have, through the years, been successively carved out of the old term "rheumatism" into many different disorders. In a similar manner, what was once nonarticular rheumatism is now divided into more than 100 different conditions classified under the contemporary heading of soft tissue pain disorders.

Early in the twentieth century, the term "fibrositis" was coined by Sir Edward Gowers,[50] who was attempting to further characterize lumbago. A dramatic milestone in modern thinking about fibrositis was the insight provided by Smythe and Moldofsky,[133] who apparently were the first to recognize that there was a group of patients whose widespread pain was accompanied by remarkably consistent tenderness to palpation at soft tissue body sites referred to as "tender points" (TPs). From the work of Moldofsky, a psychiatrist with training in sleep physiology, the concept of disrupted slow-wave sleep became associated with the fibrositis pattern of widespread pain and TPs.[83]

The diagnostic criteria developed by Smythe and Moldofsky were later modified by Yunus and colleagues[162] to require fewer TPs but to include a variety of constitutional manifestations. Among them was the prolonged morning stiffness that had prompted earlier authors to believe that fibrositis must have an inflammatory component like that of RA, but the erythrocyte sedimentation rate was usually normal in fibrositis, and no other objective inflammatory features were found. For that reason, it was argued that the disorder was poorly named (the suffix -itis inferring inflammation).

The name was changed to FMS; unfortunately, that name is similarly troublesome. It is not clear, for example, that either fibrous tissue (fibro . . .) or muscle (. . . my . . .) is pathologically involved in this disorder. Despite this, it seems wise to delay any further change in terminology until more information is known about the real pathogenesis of this disorder. When a change in terminology can properly be made, it also may be the right time to make the transition from syndrome to disease.

In his review on the concept of syndromology, Cohen[34] distinguished a "disease" as a homogeneous disorder with a known genesis, from a "syndrome," which lacks such stability. By his definition, a syndrome may be an assortment of signs and symptoms for which the pathogenesis is either poorly understood or may just represent the common manifestations of several distinct initiating etiologies. Conversely, the pattern of the signs and symptoms presented by affected individuals is sufficiently typical that they can be combined into a single group classification.

In FMS, the clinical symptoms of widespread body pain, multiple TPs, long-duration morning stiffness, and inefficient sleep are so characteristically patterned that statistical analysis against healthy normal controls (HNCs) typically results in P values of at least 10^{-3}. The larger problem may not be sensitivity but specificity. The overlap with a variety of comorbidities (discussed in more detail below), such as chronic fatigue syndrome, residua from physical or emotional trauma, affective disorders, and irritable bowel syndrome, makes it increasingly important that laboratory measures be developed to help with specificity assessments.

In affected individuals, there is usually no doubt that something is wrong. Despite this background in the clinical similarities of individuals with FMS, it is still possible or even likely that FMS is the ultimate manifestation of several distinct physiologic processes. These may involve one or more genetic predispositions, achievement of a susceptible age, chronic insomnia, neurochemical dysfunctions, endocrinopathies, CNS dysfunction, spinal stenosis, and perhaps even physical trauma. If so, it is possible that new revelations from biochemical measures or genetic markers will eventually allow identification of clinical or etiologic subsets of fibromyalgia that should be viewed or managed differently. Perhaps some forms of FMS can even be prospectively anticipated and prevented.

Before 1990, there was a proliferation of different criteria for the diagnosis of FMS, but none had been universally accepted. The criteria supported by the American College of Rheumatology (ACR)[153] had a slightly different purpose. They were called "classification criteria" to clearly distinguish them from "diagnostic criteria" and to indicate that they were intended to represent the minimal standard for entry of subjects into a research study investigating the clinical, biologic, epidemiologic, and management features of a narrowly identified group of people with pain. That clinicians all over the world now use these criteria as a guide for clinical diagnosis is a testimony to the great need for such criteria, to the influence of the ACR, and to the care with which the study was carried out.

Considering the wide-reaching effects of this study, a brief description of how it was conducted is warranted. Investigators from approximately 20 clinical centers in the United States and Canada first agreed on a potentially useful protocol and then carefully followed it to systematically evaluate the symptoms and signs found in people with a clinical diagnosis of FMS. A key feature of the protocol was that a respected FMS clinician at each study site identified persons with a qualified entry condition and referred them to a diagnosis-blinded colleague to conduct the study-related assessments without reference to a specific diagnosis. Groups of 20 FMS, 20 HNCs, and 20 disease controls with early RA, systemic lupus erythematosus, and other painful conditions were assessed identically.

Statistical analysis of the resultant data at a central location led to a classification based on two criteria, which was then endorsed by the ACR. The combination of a typical finding from history of chronic (>3 months) widespread pain and tenderness to palpation at 18 anatomically defined TPs exhibited a moderately high sensitivity (88.4%) and specificity (81.1%) for FMS and established the clinical distinction between FMS and other painful conditions.

The criteria have been criticized because they are largely subjective, but they continue to be used worldwide.

Viewed from the standpoint of research investigations conducted on FMS, a noteworthy change was made at about the same time. From the early 1970s until approximately 1990, the number of publications about FMS (including those using the term "fibrositis") was between 10 and 20 annually. After 1990, the number increased dramatically, to more than 100 annually (Fig. 9-1). The topic distribution during the years since 1970 is shown in Figure 9-2. MEDLINE-referenced publication has focused heavily on diagnosis, physiopathology, psychology, complications, and ethnology, with 200 to 400 articles in each area, but there are more than 100 articles each on epidemiology and diet therapy. The most likely explanation for the dramatic increase in the number of articles published seems to be the general acceptance of the ACR classification criteria.

Thus, in the wake of successful classification criteria, a surge of investigative energy in the early 1990s led to a number of important new observations. Fibromyalgia was found to be universally common. It was present in approximately 2% of the adult general population in the United States[155] and exhibited a similar distribution in most other countries where valid epidemiologic studies had been conducted. Adult women were affected five to seven times more commonly than were men. In children, the gender distribution was about equal for boys and girls.[20]

A debate over central versus peripheral pathogenesis developed in an attempt to better understand the etiology of FMS. Failing to find convincing histologic support for peripheral histopathology, the focus shifted heavily toward involvement of the CNS. As a result, findings in the neurochemical mechanisms of nociception and in the neuroendocrine system took the stage. Abnormal levels of biochemicals, such as tryptophan, serotonin, substance P,[107] and growth hormone, and the abnormal diurnal regulation of cortisol production were reported.[35] Anatomic and func-

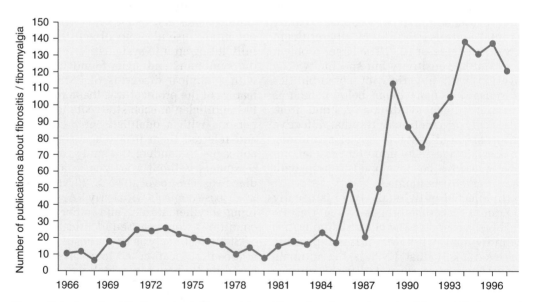

Figure 9-1. Annual publications about fibromyalgia. According to MEDLINE, the markers indicate the number of publications with a main topic of fibrositis or fibromyalgia syndrome (FMS). The total number of articles consistently ranged only slightly above or below 20 until approximately 1990, when classification criteria were endorsed by the ACR. Thereafter, the number of articles rapidly increased more than fivefold. The seven most common general topics by order of frequency were diagnosis, physiopathology, psychology, complications, ethnology, epidemiology, and diet therapy. (Source: MEDLINE [database on-line], National Library of Medicine, Bethesda, MD, 1999.)

Fibromyalgia Publications from 1966 to Present

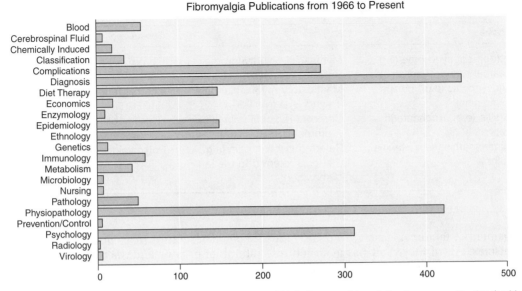

Figure 9-2. Topic frequency in publications about fibromyalgia from 1966 to 1998. There are two prominent topics (diagnosis, physiopathology) with more than 400 listings each, one (psychology) with 300 listings, and two (ethnology, complications) with more than 200 listings each. (Source: MEDLINE (database on-line), National Library of Medicine, Bethesda, MD, 1999.)

tional imaging of the brain and spinal cord will probably be the sources of important new revelations in the coming decade.[86]

Controversy still rages over whether FMS should be considered a disabling condition on par with painful conditions such as low back pain, RA, and osteoarthritis and be compared with neurologic conditions such as multiple sclerosis, myasthenia gravis, or diabetic neuropathy. The real controversy hinges over whether patients with FMS should receive financial compensation for the limitations they experience in routine daily activities and in their overall quality of life and on what basis such a decision should be made for a given individual. This issue will be important to affected individuals, to the families of patients, to insurance companies, and even to governments because the potential cost (currently more than $16 billion annually in the United States) is high.[157, 158]

C. DIAGNOSIS

1. Classification

Fibromyalgia is not a form of arthritis, as some patients suspect. The ranges of joint motion usually remain normal throughout the course of FMS, although some limitation of active range of motion may be present as a result of the considerable discomfort experienced. Joint swelling, inflammation, effusions, or increased temperature are not expected components of FMS. Occasionally, FMS may antedate or follow the onset of a rheumatic disease, but in the majority of cases, FMS is not simply the early stage of another medical condition. Fibromyalgia is properly classified as one of a large group of soft tissue pain syndromes. Some authors and many clinicians have improperly referred to this category of disorders generically as "myofascial pain disorders," but that confuses the issue of the distinct disorder called myofascial pain syndrome (MPS) (see Chapter 8). The latter disorder is complicated enough and does not benefit from confusion in taxonomy.

The large group of soft tissue pain syndromes is characterized by pain emanating from periarticular structures located outside of the joint capsule and periosteum. These syndromes differ from arthritic disorders, in that the synovial joints are not directly involved. The anatomic structures that appear to be symptomatic can include

Table 9-1   *Soft Tissue Pain Disorders*

Localized	Regional	Generalized
Entrapment syndrome (e.g., carpal tunnel syndrome)	Myofascial pain syndrome (MPS)	Fibromyalgia syndrome (FMS)
Tenosynovitis (e.g., biceps tendinitis)	Masticatory myofascial pain syndrome (MMPS)	Chronic fatigue syndrome (CFS)
Bursitis (e.g., trochanteric bursitis)	Complex regional pain syndrome (CRPS)	Hypermobility syndrome (HMS)
Enthesopathies (e.g., tennis elbow)	Referred visceral pain (e.g., angina referred to the left shoulder)	Polymyalgia rheumatica (PMR)

ligaments, tendons, fascia, bursae, and muscles. All of these soft tissue structures are known to facilitate mechanical functions of the diarthrodial joints. Any of these structures can become painful and dysfunctional alone or in association with distinct inflammatory, autoimmune, arthritic, or endocrine disorders. The resultant physical dysfunction and compromise in quality of life can be as severe as that associated with any of the arthritic diseases; thus, these soft tissue pain syndromes are not benign.

Table 9-1 shows a contemporary classification of soft tissue pain syndromes.[106] The main subheadings divide the syndromes into localized, regionalized, and generalized categories. Most of the "localized" conditions are believed to result from repetitive mechanical injury to inadequately conditioned tissues. They are often named anatomically and are disclosed by a typical history plus the exquisite tenderness elicited by digital palpation of the affected structures.

The syndromes with a regional distribution tend to result from "overuse." Even though they may involve more than one type of body structure, they are still limited in anatomic scope to a region or body quadrant. MPS[128] is characterized by trigger points (TrPs), in contrast to the TPs of FMS, and has traditionally been managed by physiatrists. Masticatory MPS involves the temporomandibular joint and/or TrPs in the muscles of mastication and is typically treated by dentists.[31] Several types of visceral pain can be referred to a musculo-

skeletal structure (e.g., angina felt in the shoulder or jaw), and the recently renamed complex regional pain syndrome (CRPS) (formerly reflex sympathetic dystrophy)[87] is classified in this category.

The "generalized" category implies a systemic process that affects the musculoskeletal system in a more global manner. Chronic fatigue syndrome is characterized by persistent idiopathic fatigue and a number of other constitutional symptoms.[59] It initially presented in epidemics, but more recent applications of that diagnosis have emphasized sporadic cases,[124] and current criteria no longer exclude FMS.[45] An overlap between FMS and chronic fatigue syndrome[49] has led to speculation that they are identical, but important historical and clinical differences suggest that they are separate family members of an overlapping soft tissue pain spectrum. People with FMS report chronic widespread pain and are characterized by tenderness to palpation at many of the same anatomic sites involved in some of the localized pain syndromes.[56]

2. Presentation of Fibromyalgia

The typical patient with FMS is a middle-aged woman who may say to her physician, "Doctor, I hurt all over." She may look fatigued, a little bewildered, or even agitated but usually does not appear chronically ill. Most patients with FMS present classically, with a history of widespread pain that has been symptomatic for 3 months or longer. The pain is most pronounced in the regions of soft tissues such as the muscles, ligaments, bursae, and tendons, near the diarthrodial joints but not in them. Two rather graphic but real descriptions of the pain associated with FMS are as follows: "I feel as if I fell out of a car traveling at 30 miles per hour"; or "I feel just like the time I played volleyball in the hot sun all day at the beach. I had a terrible sunburn and every muscle was sore. No position was comfortable and I couldn't sleep it off."

The pain has been described as a persistent, diffuse, deep, aching, throbbing, sometimes stabbing pain associated with distal extremity dysesthesias. The McGill Pain Questionnaire[79] is based on quantifying pain by the words that are chosen to describe the sensation of the pain. For example, terms like "lancinating," "burning," or "stabbing" would describe a pain of greater severity than the pain described by words such as "bothersome" or "uncomfortable." The more potent words would contribute more to the score of the administered questionnaire. Patients with FMS typically exhibit high scores on that kind of assessment because they choose dramatic words to describe their symptoms. Not uncommonly, the veracity of the FMS patient's claims has been questioned, if for no other reason than the dramatic verbal and facial portrayal of the pain. Recall that we have no way to objectively confirm or deny that the pain the patient describes is what is actually felt.

When patients were asked to document, on a body diagram, the locations of their pains, they usually indicated bilateral body sites involving the upper and lower extremities, the neck posteriorly, the anterior chest, and the low back (Fig. 9-3). Evidence now suggests that monitoring a patient's course with serial quantitative (percent shaded) pain diagrams may provide a reliable method for research outcome studies. A fairly easy method for quantifying the extent of involvement on a given drawing by the patient is Wallace's "rule of nines."[149] Over the next several years, it can be predicted that this methodology will be tested repeatedly against the most effective analgesic modalities that the pharmaceutical industry can develop.

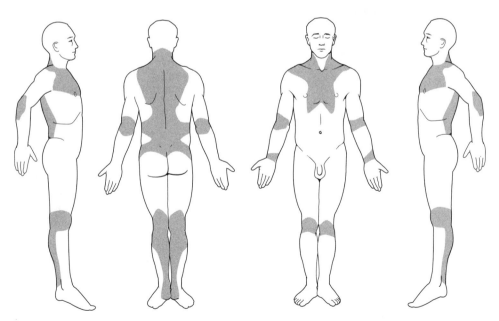

Figure 9-3. Fibromyalgia pain diagrams. The *shaded areas* on the set of four diagrams were marked by a patient with fibromyalgia to indicate the locations of her painful symptoms on the occasion of her entry into a clinical research study. The pattern of widespread pain is typical of pain diagrams by other fibromyalgia patients. Using the "rule of nines," numeric values can be derived to indicate the proportion of the entire figure affected. That number provides an estimate of the pain severity.

Although most patients with FMS present with widespread pain, some have presented quite differently. The incident complaint can mimic some other well-known medical conditions, such as the substernal chest pain of angina pectoris, the throbbing occipital head pain of recurrent muscle contraction headache, the mechanical lumbar area pain of a degenerative disc syndrome, or even the radiating lower extremity pain of sciatica (Table 9-2). When a patient presents in one of these ways, it is critical that the physician examine for tenderness at all 18 typical TPs (see "Tender Points" below) because often all will be extremely tender, even to the patient's surprise.

Other common presenting symptoms can include chronic insomnia, depression, anxiety, lightheadedness, prolonged morning stiffness, a tiredness resembling physical fatigue, crampy abdominal pains with loose stools and left upper quadrant abdominal tenderness resembling irritable bowel syndrome, and interstitial cystitis with frequency, urgency, and dysuria despite sterile urine and bladder area tenderness to deep palpation.

Despite these variations in presentation, the clinical identification of persons who have FMS is simple once the investigator or clinician has considered this diagnosis and become familiar with the characteristic features to be sought (Table 9-3).

3. Tender Points

On examination, the characteristic physical finding can be identified by pressing on each of 18 anatomically defined soft tissues TP sites.[153] The patient's physical response to palpation of a TP can be viewed as a semiobjective clinical sign, such as a deep tendon reflex. The anatomic sites do not appear to represent a single type of anatomic structure but rather can include skeletal muscles, ligaments, and bursae. At least 11 of the 18 TPs must exhibit painful sensitivity to 4 kg of palpation pressure.

Testing for FMS TPs is not difficult, but it helps to learn the method from an experienced examiner and then practice with a patient known to have FMS. The procedure can be accomplished in approximately 30 seconds on a clinic patient.

Rapid, sequential application of 4 kg of pressure on each of the TPs of a FMS patient will often induce an involuntary writhing withdrawal on the patient's part or even an unintended outburst of tears. This should not be viewed as an hysterical response, any more than would involuntary guarding to deep palpation of an acute abdomen. After a patient has been examined at each of 18 TPs, there will often be a residual deep ache that may be described as bone pain. The aching sensation may persist several days after such an examination, and a bruise may appear at some TP sites.

The pattern of the TP distribution in a given FMS individual is not known to have any pathogenic significance. Approximately one third of FMS patients will exhibit a preponderance of painful TP sites

---

Table 9-2   Clinical Symptoms Associated With Fibromyalgia Syndrome[a]

- Depression, anxiety
- Cognitive deficits, short-term memory loss
- Throbbing occipital pain of muscle contraction headache
- Lightheadedness, dizziness, syncope
- Chronic insomnia, nocturnal myoclonus, nocturnal bruxism
- Daytime tiredness resembling physical fatigue
- Prolonged morning stiffness, as from rheumatoid arthritis
- Chest wall pain mimicking angina pectoris, breast area pain
- Mechanical low back pain or sciatica-like radiation of pain
- Bursitis, tendinitis, myalgias, arthralgias, piriformis syndrome
- Numbness, tingling, dysesthesias in hands and feet
- Irritable bowel, abdominal pain, diarrhea, constipation
- Interstitial cystitis, frequency, urgency, sterile dysuria

Adapted from Russell IJ: Fibromyalgia syndrome: approaches to management. *Bull Rheum Dis* 45(3): 1–4, 1996.

[a]These symptoms may mix or match at different times in a given patient, but none of them is required for classifying a patient as having fibromyalgia syndrome.

Table 9-3   *The 1990 ACR Criteria for the Classification of Fibromyalgia Syndrome*

From History—Widespread Musculoskeletal Pain
Definition: For the past 3 months, pain has been experienced in four quadrants; the locations are counted as follows: both sides of the body, above and below the waist, in the trunk (e.g., cervical spine, anterior chest, thoracic spine, low back areas). Shoulder and buttock involvement count for both sides of the body. "Low back" counts as lower segment.

From Examination—Pain Induced by Palpation of Tender Points
Definition: Pain must be inducible at 11 or more of the following 18 (9 bilateral) tender point sites:
Anatomic Location of Tender Point Sites:
1, 2. Occiput: at the suboccipital muscle insertion
3, 4. Low cervical: at the anterior aspects of the intertransverse spaces at C5–C7
5, 6. Trapezius: at the midpoint of the upper muscle border
7, 8. Supraspinatus: near the origins, above the spine of the scapula
9, 10. Second rib: upper surface just lateral to the second costochondral junction
11, 12. Lateral epicondyle: extensor muscle, 2 cm distal to the epicondyle
13, 14. Gluteal: in upper outer quadrants of buttocks in anterior fold of muscle
15, 16. Greater trochanter: posterior to the trochanteric prominence
17, 18. Knees: at the medial fat pad proximal to the joint line and condyle

Adapted from Wolfe F, Smythe HA, Yunus MB, *et al:* The American College of Rheumatology 1990 criteria for the classification of fibromyalgia. *Arthritis Rheum* 33:160–172, 1990.

on one side of the body. Some patients seem to be more symptomatically affected in the upper half of the body than in the lower half or on one side of the body more than on the other side.

Three variables known to influence the reliability of this examination are the amount of digital palpation pressure applied, the rate at which it is applied, and whether it is applied singly or as a series of brief pulses of pressure.

Pressure gauges are available for standardization of the applied digital pressure and for research study. The most accurate means of standardizing the amount of pressure that should be applied by the examining finger is to press it against a calibrated dolorimeter or perhaps a pediatric scale (4 kg equals 1.6 lb). The standard method for use of a dolorimeter in measuring the pressure pain threshold is a steady increase in vertically applied pressure at a fixed rate of 1 kg/sec. A wafer-thin pressure transducer is available, which can be worn on the distal phalanx of the examiner to display the highest amount of pressure exerted.

A reasonably accurate clinical estimate of the correct amount of pressure can be achieved by pressing the palmar pad of the examining thumb or finger against a soft tissue resistance, such as the anterior thigh, until the distal portion of the nail blanches.

The tenderness at these TP sites in FMS is apparently located in the deep soft tissues, as topical anesthesia of the skin has no effect on the severity of pain induced by deep pressure stimuli.[69] Despite this apparently unique sensitivity of the TPs to palpation pressure, there is no convincing evidence that the tissues that hurt are histologically or functionally abnormal.[163]

4. Control Points

As investigators explored the application of the TP examination to people with FMS,[127] they observed body sites at which people with FMS exhibited little tenderness to deep palpation pressure. These so-called control points (CPs) were at first expected to provide a resource for checking the specificity of tenderness at the TPs. According to the original theory, if a patient reported pain after deep palpation pressure at a CP, there must have been some supratentorial (read emotive or psychologic) augmentation of the symptoms at the true TPs for the purpose of secondary gain.

Some investigators believed that tenderness to pressure at the CPs would invalidate the diagnosis of FMS.

This concept was later discounted when it was recognized that the consistently lower severity of tenderness at the CPs actually correlated closely with the severity of tenderness at the TPs.[100, 116] For example, the correlation between severity of tenderness at the TPs and the CPs was R = 0.52 for tender point index (TPI) and R = 0.80 for algometry.[116] It is now accepted that the pain thresholds at the control sites are diffusely but less severely lowered than the TPs in FMS. In addition, the concept of the affected CPs has provided substantial support for the hypothesis of a CNS rather than a peripheral muscle tissue pathogenesis of FMS.[107]

5. Trigger Points

A TP is defined differently than a TrP, and thus the two should not be used synonymously. A TP that is not also a myofascial TrP (MTrP) hurts locally, when pressed, but usually does not refer pain. In FMS there are multiple, symmetric TPs. By contrast, a TrP is a regional phenomenon that may be tender, like a TP, but that also refers pain to a symptomatic zone of reference that is usually more distal. A complex of symptoms and signs characterizes MPS (see Chapter 8).[137] Evidence suggests that some FMS patients can occasionally exhibit one or more TrPs in addition to a full complement of 18 TPs.[51] At least one TrP was found in 68% of FMS patients and in 20% of the normal controls.

If a typical TrP is present in a FMS patient, a concomitant diagnosis of MPS should be made. The two conditions should be treated separately, with the knowledge that TrPs in the setting of FMS are more resistant to treatment than when they present alone.[60] There is no convincing evidence to suggest that "widespread MPS" is a naturally occurring disorder or that progressive spreading of regional MPS can eventually become FMS. In fact, it seems likely that what has been referred to as widespread MPS was actually FMS. The distinction is important to diagnostic classification, understanding of pathogenesis, clinical management, and outcome assessment. Only MPS can often be cured with appropriate therapy and can be controlled even in a FMS patient with modified TrP therapy; there is no documented cure for FMS. The pain of MPS is probably amplified when it occurs in the setting of FMS.

6. Pain Thresholds

Healthy normal individuals generally do not perceive a 4-kg digital pressure stimulus as painful. Therefore, this finding in FMS seems to represent a lower-than-normal pain threshold and meets the clinical definition of a neurophysiologic phenomenon called allodynia (see also "Allodynia" in Section E).[16] For that reason, it was proposed that FMS could be viewed mechanistically as "chronic, widespread allodynia."[107] Allodynia is defined as a lower-than-normal pain threshold or a situation in which pain is perceived from a stimulus that is not normally painful. It is distinguished from hyperalgesia, which refers to an overly aggressive response by a person subjected to a stimulus that would be expected to be painful for a normal individual.[16]

There are at least two implications from such a view. First, FMS appears to represent a unique opportunity to better understand the process of disordered nociception. Second, neurochemicals, which had earlier been shown to induce or influence allodynia in animals, should be studied in FMS. To act on these concepts, effective clinical tools, including valid measures of pain severity, must be developed.

7. Assessment of Pain Severity

The clinical recognition of FMS by use of the ACR criteria is not adequate to document the syndrome's severity in a given patient. Many approaches have been taken to establish severity, including the use of self-report questionnaires and quantitative examination. Questionnaire formats used in the past have included the visual analog scale (VAS) for pain,[116] the McGill pain score,[52] and quantitative pain diagrams.[149]

Examination methods have included reporting the number of points,[153] calculating the TPI,[114] or calculating an average dolorimetry score,[127] which we now call the average pressure pain threshold (APT).

The TPI (a similar entity is called myalgic score by other authors) is easily determined and provides an objective measure to follow. As shown in Table 9-4, a tenderness scale is applied to the tenderness at each site examined (nontender = 0, tender without physical response = 1, tender plus wince or withdrawal = 2, exaggerated withdrawal = 3, too painful to touch = 4). The sum of the tenderness severities at all 18 sites is the TPI.

Deriving the APT requires the availability of a dolorimeter (algometer). One convenient device is shown in Figure 9-4. The

---

Table 9-4   *Clinical Determination of Tenderness Severity*

Calculating the Tender Point Index
A. Apply 4 kg of digital pressure to each tender point
B. Observe body language, especially the face, for response
C. Use the following scale to quantify each response:
    Not painful = 0
    Felt painful, no physical response = 1+
    Felt painful, wince or withdrawal = 2+
    Felt painful, exaggerated withdrawal = 3+
    Area too painful to allow pressure = 4+
D. Add the tenderness severities for all 18 sites
E. The sum is the tender point index (TPI)
F. The expected range for normal controls = 0–5
G. The expected range for fibromyalgia = 11–72

FMS research
H. Typical FMS research study TPI (mean ± SD) = 25.7 ± 9.7

Adapted from Russell IJ, Fletcher EM, Michalek JE, *et al:* Treatment of primary fibrositis/fibromyalgia syndrome with ibuprofen and alprazolam. A double-blind, placebo-controlled study. *Arthritis Rheum* 34:552–560, 1991.

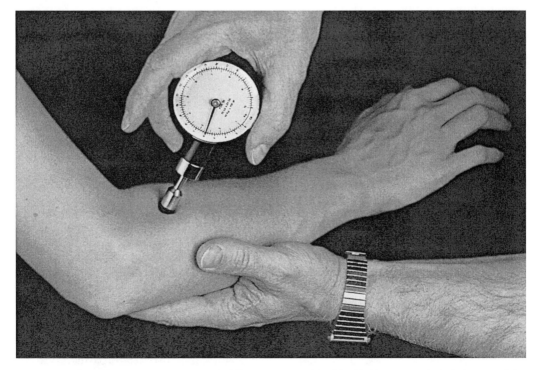

Figure 9-4. A Fischer dolorimeter in use at TP on lateral epicondyle. Notice the vertical placement of the instrument over the skin.

procedure should be illustrated for the subject on a control (fairly nontender) area, such as the midanterior thigh, with the subject in the seated position. The foot pad of the instrument is placed vertically on the skin of the area to be tested and advanced consistently at a rate of 1 kg/s. The subject is advised to say "now" when the pressure makes the expected transition from pressure to pain. Immediately, the examiner will withdraw the instrument and read from the gauge the maximum amount of pressure achieved. Between tests, the needle of the instrument is returned to 0 by pressing a button. This test can be repeated on the opposite thigh to check for reproducibility. Each of the anatomic TPs should then be examined in some defined order, perhaps interrupted periodically with examination of a CP. The sum of the values obtained from the 18 ACR criteria-designated TPs is divided by 18 to obtain the APT. Notice that this value will be inversely proportional to the TPI.

The TPI and the APT exhibit good interrater reliability, test-retest reliability, and intercorrelation ($R = -0.649$ for TPI versus APT) between measures.[105] A recent examination of these measures[110] has shown, however, that the APT exhibits a slightly higher reliability (Fig. 9-5). The TPI bears some correlation to the patient's level of anxiety and/or depression, which is not exhibited by the APT.

Actually, a Catch-22 has existed with regard to determining the ideal outcome variable. The best system for checking the performance of an outcome variable is to check it against effective therapy, but fully effective therapy for FMS has been elusive. Most outcome studies have utilized both self-report and examination measures in the hope that something would document the anticipated benefit. Recently, that problem has been partially remedied by a treatment study using tramadol.[122] Clinical benefit was clearly associated with administration of the drug. Both the TPI and APT exhibited significant improvement with treatment, providing direct evidence for their validity as outcome measures in FMS (Russell et al., unpublished data).

8. Comorbidities

The clinical manifestations of FMS are usually more complex than body pain

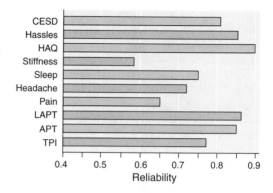

Figure 9-5. Reliability of outcome measures in fibromyalgia. Intraclass correlation coefficients of reliability for 90 subjects with paired measures 2 weeks apart. The Stanford Health Assessment Questionnaire (*HAQ*) (physical function), Hassles (anxiety), and Center for Epidemiology Studies Depression (*CESD*) (depression) scales were highly reliable in fibromyalgia. Close behind in reliability were the algometer-based measures of the average pressure pain threshold (*APT*) and limited APT (*LAPT*), which performed better than the tender point index (*TPI*) or the visual analog scale (*VAS*) for subjective perception of pain (*Pain*) or morning stiffness (*Stiffness*). Morning *Stiffness* was assessed by VAS; *Sleep* difficulty was assessed by VAS; *Headache* severity was assessed by VAS; *Pain* severity was assessed by VAS; *LAPT* was assessed by a limited APT involving algometry at only six sites; *APT* was assessed by algometry at 18 tender point sites; *TPI*, a unitless measure of tenderness severity, was assessed by graded palpation examination. (Adapted from Russell IJ, Michalek JE: Comparative reliability of digital palpation and algometry-based pain measures in patients with FMS. *J Rheumatol* [Submitted for publication].)

alone. For example, patients experience great frustration with their inability to achieve normal restorative sleep. They awaken feeling unrefreshed and are stiff for an extended period of time (usually several hours, as in RA) each morning. During the day, they are tired but have difficulty napping. They have chronic muscle contraction-type headaches, with pain in the occipital region extending over the scalp and leaving it sensitive to touch. Temporary relief can sometimes be achieved by taking a hot bath, massaging the neck, and then sleeping for at least 30 minutes with the neck supported by a small pillow.

The frequency of depression is increased in patients with FMS (30 to 40%) compared with normal controls (approximately 10%) or with people hospitalized for another medical condition (approximately 20%), but it does not differ significantly from the frequency of depression in patients with RA.[2] As with RA, it is reasonable to predict that the depression of FMS results from the pain and dysfunction, rather than being their cause.

If one considers the sleep loss and chronic headache associated with FMS, it is not surprising that patients complain bitterly of changes in cognitive functions. They have difficulty remembering events, patterns of behavior, task-related protocols, and numbers that had been second nature to them prior to the onset of FMS. This is an inadequately studied aspect of FMS, so it is not known whether it results from loss of sleep, from the distraction of head and body pain, or even from the numerous medications taken in hope of achieving relief. It is also unclear how reversible this deficit will be when effective treatment for the underlying condition becomes available.

People with FMS often describe numbness or tingling of the hands or lips and a sense of hand or finger swelling. On questioning, however, they will usually acknowledge that the fingers do not really look swollen. This phenomenon sometimes resembles the symptoms of hyperventilation syndrome, but the respiratory component is usually lacking. Not uncommonly, patients with FMS complain of dyspnea. That symptom is often associated with chest discomfort resulting from attempts to take a deep breath. The cause is believed to be chest wall discomfort, but that issue has not been adequately studied.

Irritable bowel-like symptoms are seen in approximately 40% of patients with FMS.[162] Patients may complain of troublesome constipation interspersed with painful cramping and diarrhea. Seldom will the patient have noticed mucus on the surface of the excreted stool. Clinical examination often discloses tenderness to palpation in the left upper quadrant or the whole left side of the abdomen.

The bladder may also be involved, with complaints of urgency, frequency, a sense of incomplete voiding, and sometimes culture-negative dysuria. These symptoms mimic the syndrome of interstitial cystitis, but it is not yet clear whether the tissue of the bladder is involved similarly in both conditions.

Amplification of the tenderness and referred pain caused by MTrPs can be an important comorbidity of FMS. It is especially likely to be a factor in the muscle tension-type headaches so troublesome for FMS patients. This apparent overlap between MPS and FMS seems to be sufficiently common to warrant serious consideration in every FMS patient.

9. Secondary Fibromyalgia

A curious finding has been that FMS may be associated with a number of other medical conditions. In the past, the view of such associations was that the other condition was primary and the FMS was somehow secondary. Of course, the existence of a secondary FMS implies that there is also a primary FMS and that the two are somehow different. The ACR criteria study[153] included subjects with secondary FMS and concluded that there was no difference between the clinical pattern of primary and secondary FMS. Although that may be true clinically, this may be the shining moment for laboratory support of a subset designation for FMS. In a study of nerve growth factor,[48] only persons with primary FMS exhibited elevated levels of the nerve growth factor, in contrast to patients with secondary FMS and inflammatory conditions not exhibiting FMS. Despite this, the distinction is unavoidable because most therapeutic research studies on FMS have specified that the patient population be primary FMS to avoid potential confusion contributed by another associated disorder.

Table 9-5 lists a classification of medical conditions that are suspected of a more-than-chance association with FMS. They are divided into three headings: rheumatic diseases, chronic infectious and/or inflammatory disorders, and endocrine disorders. The current dogma is that none of these conditions has developed from FMS and that FMS is not really caused by the concomitant medical condition. It is beyond the scope of this chapter to provide a detailed description of the relationships between FMS and each of these other conditions. In some cases, there would not be much to say; in others, there is a growing database regarding the overlap.

Nearly one third of all patients with RA will be found to have concomitant FMS. A clinical observation is that the RA patients

Table 9-5   *Clinical Conditions That May Accompany Fibromyalgia and Screening Evaluation for Them*

Illness/Condition	Screening	Appropriate Tests
Rheumatic disease		
Systemic lupus erythematosus	Hx & Px	ANA, ESR
Rheumatoid arthritis	HX & Px	RF, ESR
Sjögren's syndrome	Hx & Px	ANA, ASSA, ASSB
Polymyositis	Hx & Px	CPK, EMG, Bx
Chronic infection/inflammation		
Tuberculosis	Hx & Px	PPD, ESR
Chronic syphilis	Hx & Px	VDRL, FTA
Bacterial endocarditis	Hx & Px	Blood culture, ESR
Lyme disease	Hx & Px	Lyme serology, PCR
Acquired immunodeficiency	Hx & Px	AIDS serology, CD_4
Breast implantation[a]	Hx & Px	Possibly serology
Endocrine disorders		
Hypothyroidism	Hx & Px	T_4, TSH, CPK
Hypopituitary	Hx & Px	Prolactin, others

Adapted from Russell IJ: Fibromyalgia syndrome: approaches to management. *Bull Rheum Dis* 45(3): 1–4, 1996.

Hx & Px, insightful medical history and physical examination; *ANA*, antinuclear antibody; *ESR*, erythrocyte sedimentation rate; *RF*, rheumatoid factor; *ASSA*, antibody to SSA; *ASSB*, antibody to SSB; *CPK*, creatine phosphokinase; *EMG*, electromyography; *Bx*, biopsy of labial minor salivary glands; *PPD*, delayed hypersensitivity skin test for tuberculosis; *VDRL*, serologic test for syphilis; *FTA*, fluorescent treponemal antibody; *PCR*, polymerase chain reaction; *AIDS*, acquired immunodeficiency syndrome; *CD_4*, lymphocytes positive for the CD_4 surface antigen; *T_4*, thyroid hormone; *TSH*, thyroid-stimulating hormone.

[a]Association is probably spurious, but the reason is debatable.

who also have FMS seem to have pain that is out of proportion to the amount of synovitis exhibited. This must be taken into account in treating such a patient because increasing the methotrexate dosage may not be the best solution for the pain amplified by the FMS. In fact, the best results are obtained by treating each of the conditions separately.

The prevalence of FMS in people with systemic lupus erythematosus (SLE) was 22% in one study,[80] while another 23% clinically seemed to have FMS but fell short of meeting full classification criteria for FMS. Shin tenderness was more prevalent in SLE patients with concomitant FMS than in either condition alone.[134] The SLE patients who met the criteria for FMS exhibited more severe symptoms and were more likely to have difficulty performing their daily activities. They were less likely to be employed, more likely to be divorced, and more likely to receive welfare or other medical disability benefits. SLE patients

with and without FMS did not differ, however, with respect to the severity of their SLE activity, as evidenced by laboratory testing or progressive organ injury.

An important observation has been that the FMS symptoms may become more clearly apparent as the SLE symptoms resolve with treatment. The FMS symptoms seem to emerge with too rapid a taper of the corticosteroid dosage. If not recognized as being distinct from the SLE, the FMS symptoms could prompt inappropriate immunosuppressive therapy. To reduce the likelihood of the SLE patient developing emergent FMS symptoms with a steroid taper, it is best to decrease the dosage in graduated steps at approximately 2-week intervals. A suggested tapering protocol is based on the current dosage (from a prednisone-equivalent dosage of 30 to 60 mg/day, each step would reduce the daily dosage by 10 to 20 mg; from 15 to 30 mg/day, it would reduce the daily dosage by 2.5 to 5 mg/day; and from 1 to

15 mg/day, it would reduce the daily dosage by 1 to 2 mg/day).

Similarly, approximately 50% of patients with Sjögren's syndrome meet clinical criteria for FMS.[15] This statement must be qualified, however, because the usual index symptoms of Sjögren's syndrome are dry mouth and/or dry eyes. Those symptoms can also occur in primary FMS patients as side effects from taking tricyclic medicines. In some patients with combined symptoms, it may be necessary to obtain a labial biopsy in order to exclude Sjögren's syndrome.

Any association there may be between FMS and polymyositis, dermatomyositis, or polymyalgia rheumatica is less well defined. Infectious and/or inflammatory conditions that seem to be associated with FMS include tuberculosis, syphilis, and Lyme disease. Of course, the prevalence of overlapping conditions depends on the community prevalence of both conditions. Where these infections are rare, the prevalence of the infection in people with FMS will be low.

There are no formal studies with TB and syphilis, but more consideration has been given to the relationship between Lyme disease and FMS.[36] A university hospital practice in a Lyme-endemic area monitored 287 patients with apparent infection for a mean of 2.5 years (range, 1 to 4 years). Eight percent met classification criteria for FMS, clearly more than would be expected by chance, based on a community prevalence of 2% for FMS. The symptoms of FMS tended to develop within 1 to 4 months after infection, often in association with Lyme arthritis. Most of the Lyme/FMS patients had typical serology, but a subset were seronegative while exhibiting cellular immune responses to borrelial antigens, cerebrospinal fluid (CSF) pleocytosis, or even specific antibody formation in the CSF.

The signs and symptoms of Lyme disease have generally resolved with antibiotic therapy (e.g., intravenous ceftriaxone, 2 g/d for 2 to 4 weeks), but usually the FMS symptoms have persisted. Clinicians who practice in Lyme-endemic areas indicate that they diagnose many more patients with primary FMS than with concomitant Lyme/

FMS. Both the aggressiveness with which an infection should be sought and the decision whether to administer antibiotic therapy to a new FMS patient with a borderline Lyme serology should depend on the regional prevalence of Lyme disease and the clinical judgment of the physician.

An interesting controversy has surrounded the issue of silicone breast implants and FMS. In one large study,[44] soft tissue pain was substantially more common in patients with implants than in persons who had reduction mammoplasty or breast cancer without implantation, but FMS was not specifically identified as the pain condition present. When women with implants are troubled by musculoskeletal pain symptoms, consideration of FMS is warranted.[42]

An association between subacute bacterial endocarditis and FMS has not really been proven by using the current ACR criteria for classification of FMS,[153] but the description of the characteristic musculoskeletal symptoms (arthralgias, myalgias) associated with subacute bacterial endocarditis[30] certainly suggests the possibility of an overlap of the two conditions. Of course, fever, a new heart murmur, and embolic phenomena should never be attributed to FMS. The most serious consequence of misdiagnosis would be a delay in antibiotic therapy of endocarditis.

Mention was made earlier of the hypothalamic-pituitary-adrenal axis abnormalities in FMS. There is evidence for abnormal production of cortisol,[35] growth hormone,[14] hypothyroidism,[26] and prolactin.[21, 64, 112] Presently, the only generalization that can be made from this information is that careful clinical assessment of people with FMS is warranted, with the intent to correct neuroendocrine abnormalities when they are important contributors to the clinical symptoms.

10. Disability

It is easy to believe that a person with a bleeding comminuted fracture is experiencing discomfort. Conversely, there is natural skepticism when an apparently healthy individual with FMS dramatically complains of unbearable pain.

Several sets of circumstances tend to support that measure of doubt. In FMS, routine laboratory test results have usually been normal, failing to implicate inflammation or dysfunction of a major organ system. Affective pathology, such as depression and anxiety, is present in a substantial proportion of FMS patients, raising the specter of psychic distortion of the perceived physical symptoms. Finally, some FMS patients have observed a temporal relationship between a physical injury and the onset of their symptoms. A common legal implication has been that "someone should pay." Naturally, the accused will mount a defense, which often takes the form of a counteroffensive. Disproportionate resources available to such a defender can prove formidable. Legal attempts to discredit both the person and the disorder reverberate widely, whether or not they bear scientific merit.

One problem in such proceedings is that pain is a subjective sensation for which modern medicine still lacks any objective measure to prove the case in favor or against. FMS is one of the disorders in which this shortcoming is critically apparent. Although that issue is troublesome clinically, it is even more difficult when it relates to decisions regarding certification for disability support. In the United States, FMS is not specifically listed as a disabling condition, although RA and osteoarthritis are included. Yet, it is clear that some people with FMS are physically and/or emotionally incapable of full-time, daily physical work. Not only does the constant pain nag at the affected person's attention, but also morning stiffness can interfere with preparation for work, and cognitive difficulties (probably resulting from insomnia and medication effects) can impair concentration. These are most likely problems of degree and probably are not incapacitating in most patients.

The dilemma for any society willing to support its ailing members is to determine who is deserving of the limited compensatory support available and who should be expected to plug along in spite of their symptoms. This decision is made even more difficult when it has appeared from research evidence[76] that people with FMS should be involved in an active exercise program to maintain aerobic fitness and to increase their whole blood (platelet) serotonin levels (Geel, I. J. Russell, *et al.*, 1998, unpublished data).

All would agree that the task of the health care provider in the clinical setting is different from what is called for in the highly charged atmosphere of the courtroom. The objective should be to guide the patient on a path toward better health and function. No matter how obtuse the complaint, illness is evidenced by virtue of presentation. It is therefore incumbent on medicine to find solutions and to make them available to the patient. The search for solutions requires a knowledge base and an open mind on the part of both clinician and patient. Management of the condition must then proceed despite a substantial measure of remaining uncertainty.

Conversely, it must be acknowledged that there is a rapidly growing, critical mass of information about the pathogenesis, natural history, and management of FMS. Objective measures of an FMS diagnosis will likely be available soon, and severity measures may follow. Certainly, the best solution for any physical limitations of FMS would be a cure, but that is not yet available. Short of that, effective symptomatic therapy should be sought for all who exhibit its symptoms. Until more effective options are available to patients with FMS, clinicians in all fields who evaluate patients with pain must use their best judgment in relating to the issue of disability.

Of course, in the United States, the actual decision regarding disability support is not made by physicians anyway. That decision is a legal one made by judges empowered by the Social Security Administration (SSA). Recommendations made by patients' physicians are basically ignored. Independent examiners working directly for the SSA evaluate each candidate and provide an independent clinical database.

D. EPIDEMIOLOGY

Since aches and pains are common to the human condition, it is easy to argue that FMS is merely one end of a discomfort spectrum. Of course, most clinical disorders represent pathologic extremes of a spectrum—consider hypertension, diabetes mellitus, or alcoholism. Like the clinical

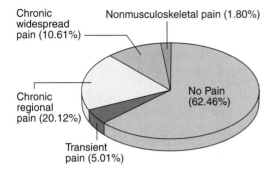

Figure 9-6. Prevalence of pain categories in the general population. About 60% of persons in the general population report having no pain. Of those with pain, the categories represent transient and chronic pain and regional and widespread pain. About 10% of the general population report having chronic widespread pain, but only 2% of the population meet examination criteria for FMS.

or laboratory criteria that define the beginning of a clearly abnormal state, there are criteria by which FMS can be distinguished from the general population.

Besides simply distinguishing FMS from the general population and from other painful disorders, there are three aspects of the epidemiology of FMS that show promising progress. The frequency with which FMS is found in a number of subpopulations permits increasingly sophisticated estimates of the actual prevalence of the disorder. Little information about the incidence of FMS is known, but preliminary data now available are certain to prompt growth in this arena over the next few years. Equally important is an improved understanding of the natural history of FMS.

1. Prevalence

Fibromyalgia occurs in all ages, ethnic groups, and cultures studied to date. Its gender distribution is nearly equal in childhood[22] but is fourfold to sevenfold more common in adult females than adult males (Table 9-2). Most of the FMS epidemiologic studies conducted to determine the prevalence of FMS in the community have been accomplished by administration of a screening questionnaire, followed by confirmatory examination of those individuals who have reported widespread body pain. Surveys of this kind have been conducted

in Canada, Denmark, England, Finland, Germany, Israel, Mexico, Norway, Poland, South Africa, and the United States. In addition, there are less complete reports of cases or case studies from Brazil, China, England, France, India, Japan, Pakistan, and Russia. Fibromyalgia does not seem to be a disorder limited to affluent peoples or to industrialized nations.

Two formal studies conducted in Canada and the United States[148, 155] have produced similar results (Fig. 9-6). These studies showed that approximately 65% of the general population are free of pain, 5% have transient pain, 20% have regional pain, and 10% have widespread pain (the group most likely to include people with FMS). Examination of those with widespread pain has established that approximately 2% of the general population have FMS, which meets ACR criteria.[153] The overall adult population average of 2% was composed of approximately 0.5% males and 1.5% females. Gender distributions varied with age by decade, with the highest prevalence exhibited in women 50 to 60 years of age[155] (Fig. 9-7).

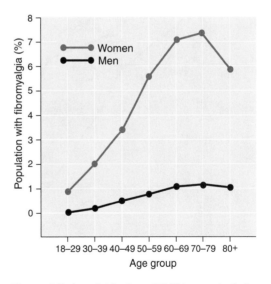

Figure 9-7. Age distribution of FMS by gender in the general population. Although the prevalence of fibromyalgia was consistently higher among females than males, it increased with age in both sexes to approximately age 70 years. The explanation for the decline thereafter is elusive. (Adapted from Wolfe F, Ross K, Anderson J, et al.: The prevalence and characteristics of fibromyalgia in the general population. *Arthritis Rheum* 38:19–28, 1995.)

A partial explanation for the female predominance in FMS is the fact that females exhibit lower pain thresholds to deep palpation than do males (Fig. 9-8).

More relevant to practicing physicians is the finding that 6 to 10% of patients in a typical waiting room[25] and 15% of those evaluated by a rheumatologist have FMS.[4] Patients seen in physiatry and pain clinics would likely exhibit a prevalence of FMS similar to that seen in rheumatology clinics. The implication is that for every 7 to 10 patients examined, at least one will likely have FMS. If the numbers of diagnoses of FMS actually being made are substantially less than that, then patients with this condition are likely being missed.

2. Incidence

Prospective research capable of documenting the incidence of a medical condition that occurs at a 2% prevalence in the general public would be prohibitively costly. For example, if the incidence were 2%, 1500 children or young adults free of symptoms at the time of enrollment would need to be monitored serially for years until each had reached age 80 years in order to identify 30 potential cases.

A group of Israeli investigators has discovered a surprising way to substantially enhance the yield of prospectively monitoring for the development of FMS.[24] The investigators enrolled subjects who had just suffered a whiplash injury to the soft tissues of their necks in a rear-end automobile accident. The recruited control group had just suffered a lower extremity fracture in an industrial accident. By the completion of follow-up, 18 months later, nearly 22% of the whiplash injury subjects had developed FMS, compared with less than 2% of the control group. In most cases, the diagnostic symptoms had developed within 3 months of the whiplash injury. Compared with following the general population from age 20 to 80 years for a 2% incidence, whiplash injury represents a 2400-fold enrichment of case identification and clearly makes prospective monitoring cost-effective.

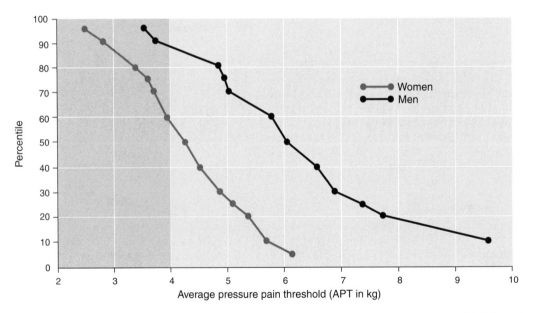

Figure 9-8. Average pressure pain threshold (*APT*) values by gender in the general population. Females exhibit generally lower APT values than males in each percentile. If the cut for an abnormal APT were set below 4 kg, a greater proportion (those within the *shaded area*) of females than males would be identified as having an abnormally low APT. (Adapted from Wolfe F, Ross K, Anderson J, et al.: Aspects of fibromyalgia in the general population: sex, pain threshold, and fibromyalgia symptoms. *J Rheumatol* 22:151–156, 1995.)

From a separate study[98] comes the observation that the dimensions of the cervical canal, as assessed by MRI, are an important risk factor for the development of chronic pain symptoms following a whiplash injury.

Based on these independent observations, there is reason to believe that monitoring whiplash injury subjects, especially those with narrow cervical canals, will prospectively allow the development of FMS to be observed and characterized.

3. Natural History

Extended follow-up (7+ years) studies have shown that FMS is not a disorder in transition to becoming another medical condition.[12, 158] Although FMS commonly accompanies RA, SLE, and Sjögren's syndrome, the associated condition is usually apparent at the time of diagnosis of FMS or shortly thereafter. There is currently no cure for FMS; thus, people who develop FMS will be affected for the rest of their lives. No information available, to date, suggests that FMS contributes to a shortening of life span, but longer follow-up studies will be needed to be certain that mild limitation is not present or even that drug therapy may have some effect on longevity.

4. Economics

There is growing awareness that the impact of FMS on an individual's quality of life and physical function is substantial and may be comparable with that of RA.[28] Although considerable variation exists across the United States,[158] approximately 30% of FMS patients find it necessary to accept shorter work hours or less physically taxing work to maintain employment, and approximately 15% currently receive disability funding because of their symptoms.[29, 157, 158, 159] As a result, the direct cost of FMS to the U.S. economy is in excess of $16 billion annually. This appears to be true proportionately in every country in the world from which data are available. These values certainly justify a moderate research expenditure on the part of governments and health industry companies, which is just beginning to occur.

Another apparent message from the cost assessment data on FMS is that hospitaliza-

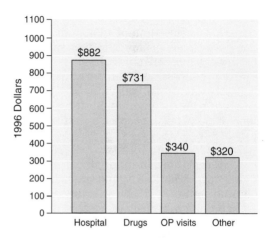

Figure 9-9. Annual direct medical costs of fibromyalgia in the United States. Five hundred thirty-eight representative patients with fibromyalgia were recruited from across the United States. Based on 1996 dollars, the direct medical costs alone for each individual averaged $2,274 annually. If this number is multiplied by 5 million affected persons in the U.S. general population, the result is over $11 billion. That total does not account for loss of work time, work productivity, assisted living, compromised quality of life, personal self-esteem, and effects on other family members. (Adapted from Wolfe F, Anderson J, Harkness D, et al.: A prospective, longitudinal, multicenter study of service utilization and costs in fibromyalgia. *Arthritis Rheum* 40:1560–1570, 1997.)

tion is the single most expensive line item in the cost profile (Fig. 9-9). FMS can usually be managed in the outpatient arena. Clinicians must carefully assess pain complaints that would ordinarily lead to hospitalization but that can also be mimicked by FMS. Doing so may help patients avoid unnecessary diagnostic procedures, surgical risks, and medical costs.

E. PATHOGENESIS

The cause of FMS is still unknown. Theories regarding its cause or causes have undergone a transition historically, from a psychiatric disorder, to a muscle disorder as currently classified in the MEDLINE Index, to a CNS disorder of nociception, as it should most likely now be classified.

1. Psychologic Associations

One of the most prevalent clinical impressions about FMS among health care providers who have not really studied the disorder carefully is that it is merely a somatic manifestation of an affective disorder.[63] Some physicians have perceived it to be a sign of masked depression or merely an aberrant expression of anxiety in psychologically disturbed individuals. That notion is further supported by the fact that there is no widely accepted specific laboratory test for FMS.

In 1982, Payne et al.[96] studied 30 hospitalized inpatient individuals in each of three groups: FMS, RA, and other forms of chronic arthritis. The arthritic patients were included as disease controls because no one then doubted that RA was an objective, painful disorder with inflammatory, destructive synovitis. Twenty years earlier, however, before the roles of rheumatoid factors, inflammatory cells, and lymphokines were recognized as objective factors in the pathogenesis of RA, some physicians viewed RA as an emotively driven disorder.[85, 89] Responses by FMS patients to questions on a Minnesota Multiphasic Personality Inventory (MMPI) resulted in variably higher scores on many of the scales (hypochondriasis, hysteria, psychotic, paranoia, schizophrenia) than were seen from responses by arthritic patients.

These findings were echoed and expanded by another study reported in 1985.[63] Those authors conducted a systematic evaluation of 31 FMS patients and 14 RA patients. They used the National Institute of Mental Health Diagnostic Interview Schedule to identify affective symptoms in both groups. The authors found a higher lifetime rate of major affective disorder among the FMS patients (70% versus 13%). In 64% of the FMS patients with major depression, the affective symptoms anteceded the onset of FMS by at least 1 year. Only approximately 30% were depressed at the time of the study, which raised a question regarding the relevance of the depression to the patient's current somatic symptoms. Perhaps the most interesting observation was a higher prevalence of major affective disorder in the families of the FMS patients. There was a 10% frequency of depression among first-degree relatives of FMS patients, while only approximately 3% of RA patients' first-degree relatives were similarly affected.

The authors concluded that patients with FMS were "psychologically disturbed," but the authors were somewhat ambivalent about the interpretation of their findings. They were not quite willing to conclude that the psychologic disturbances were pathogenic and thus suggested that the psychologic milieu of the involved individuals may have contributed to the development of the somatic manifestations. The researchers implied that the familial association disclosed by this study may pertain to a hereditary or environmental relationship between FMS and major depression.

Several other investigators have concluded that FMS patients are more depressed than RA patients,[5, 152] but many other investigators have found no difference between these two groups with regard to the prevalence of depression.[32, 67, 99, 103] The issue is clouded by the fact that prior to conduction of these studies, there was considerable bias regarding the role of depression in FMS relative to RA. That bias was, in part, responsible for the choice of RA as the control. Conversely, the choice of RA as a disease control was logical. The perceived severity of pain (self-report by VAS), the severity of morning stiffness (self-report by VAS), and the extent of physical function limitation (Baltimore work simulator testing) have been comparable for FMS and RA,[28] while these variables are generally more severe in both RA and FMS than they are in osteoarthrosis.

Many of the psychologic studies comparing FMS with RA involved interview methods in which the investigator was required to make subjective judgments. In most cases, the interviewer was not blinded to the group designation. One study,[2] which made a concerted point of blinding the evaluator to the prestudy diagnosis, found no difference in the prevalence of depression between FMS and RA.

Another potential problem with some of the older studies was that the original MMPI was validated against normal controls. Some of the questions used to identify somatization were not adequately validated against medical conditions in which people would be expected to exhibit symptoms such as pain. Thus, MMPI testing of patients with chronic pain is more likely to reflect the nature of the painful condition than indicate a true psychologic disturbance.[132] This notion is further supported by a study in which patients with RA showed similarly elevated MMPI scores for hypochondriasis, depression, and hysteria.[99]

Generalizations from all sources would now suggest that 30 to 40% of FMS patients are depressed, that this frequency is higher than expected in HNCs (<10%), and higher than expected for persons hospitalized with a variety of medical illnesses (20%).[55, 57] Conversely, this frequency is not consistently greater than is observable with RA patients. Despite their continuing pain and morning stiffness, 40 to 60% of FMS patients fail to meet criteria for a current affective disorder. That fact alone would raise doubt that an affective disorder is the initiating cause or even a perpetuating factor responsible for the painful FMS symptoms.

Another view has been that the pain and fatigue of FMS might be inappropriately amplified by the presence of depression or anxiety. A study described by Ward[145] was designed to evaluate the roles of mood or depression in modifying the perception of painful stimuli administered to RA patients. Objective measures of the arthritis severity, pain, mobility, and affective measures were documented every 2 weeks for 60 weeks. Mood, as measured by a validated self-report questionnaire scale, explained only approximately 2.0% of the variation in longitudinal changes in each of the self-report pain measures, after controlling for the effects of the clinical measures of arthritis activity. Depression, as measured by the Center for Epidemiology Studies Depression (CESD) scale, explained less than 1.0% of the changes in pain and global arthritis status. It was concluded that depression was an unlikely cause for the pain of RA. Considering other factors of similarity discussed above, it seems reasonable to similarly extrapolate that conclusion to most patients with FMS.

It seems likely, though not proven, that the excessive (that which exceeds the level of depression in the general population or in hospitalized persons) depression in both

FMS and RA is likely to represent reactive depression as a natural consequence of experiencing chronic pain, insomnia, physical limitation, compromised quality of life, and demotion from status as an equal competitor in the arena of life to a person with an incurable illness.

The relationship between depression and the somatic manifestations of FMS was explored by correlative analysis with 78 FMS patients at entry into a therapeutic intervention study.[116] When the Hamilton Anxiety Scale administered by an unblinded clinical psychologist was used, the frequency of anxiety was only 5%. Depression was assessed by the Hamilton Depression Scale administered by the same psychologist. He found possible depression at a frequency of 38%, but only 13% exhibited depression at a level that would indicate a probable need for directed therapy.

Those findings were confirmed by the self-administered CESD instrument, which identified 9% of the 78 fibromyalgia patients as being sufficiently depressed to merit treatment. These frequencies of depression are not actually elevated, compared with the prevalence of depression in the general population and in patients with a variety of medical conditions.[55, 57] More than 60% of the 78 fibromyalgia patients were judged free of both anxiety and depression by the specialized assessment instruments.

The same data were used to determine whether the psychiatric and somatic manifestations correlated with each other.[116] Physician-derived assessments of the somatic variables were compared by analysis of variance with the psychologic measures. The degree of interaction is shown in Table 9-6. High intercorrelational relationships were observed between the various somatic clinical measures. Similarly, the psychologic measures exhibited a pattern of internal correlation but failed to cross-correlate with the clinical measures. This observation does not perfectly fit either the "etiologic role" or the "resultant role" hypothesis for depression in FMS but must be explained when either hypothesis is considered. The lack of correlation between the physician-derived, semiobjective clini-

Table 9-6   *Correlational Analysis of Baseline Physical and Psychologic Variables[a]*

	TPI	APT	PHY	HAQ	HDS	HAS	CES
TPI	1.0	−.6	0.7	0.4	NS	NS	NS
APT		1.0	−.5	−.3	NS	−.3	NS
PHY			1.0	0.4	NS	NS	0.3
HAQ				1.0	0.3	0.5	0.4
HDS					1.0	0.3	0.4
HAS						1.0	0.6
CES							1.0

Adapted from Russell IJ, Fletcher EM, Michalek JE, *et al*: Treatment of primary fibrositis/fibromyalgia syndrome with ibuprofen and alprazolam. A double-blind, placebo-controlled study. *Arthritis Rheum* 34:552–560, 1991.

TPI, tender point index; *APT*, dolorimeter tenderness; *PHY*, physician global assessment of disease severity; *HAQ*, Health Assessment Questionnaire; *HDS*, Hamilton Depression Scale; *HAS*, Hamilton Anxiety Scale; *CES*, National Institute of Mental Health Depression Scale.

[a]Values shown are Pearson product moment correlational R values. Correlation coefficients greater than or equal to 3 ($R \geq 3.0$), between two measured values, indicate significant ($P \leq 0.05$) correlations.

cal measures and the psychologic measures in these patients would imply that they are independent of each other (Table 9-6).

Another view of the possible relationship between affective and somatic manifestations of FMS comes from the concept of the "nonpatient." In this case, the nonpatient with FMS is an individual in the community who meets the published criteria for classification of FMS,[153] having widespread pain for at least 3 months and exhibiting tenderness at 11 or more of the anatomically defined TPs, but who had not sought medical attention despite these symptoms. By contrast, a FMS "patient" was defined as an individual who met the criteria and was receiving professional care for the painful symptoms.

In a cohort study[18] comparing FMS patients and nonpatients in Birmingham, the prevalence of affective manifestations in the patients was significantly higher than in the nonpatients. In fact, the investigators reported that depression was the single most important predictor of health care-seeking behavior among individuals meeting criteria for FMS. A community study[154, 155] conducted in Wichita also identified nonpatients, but this study exhibited levels of affective symptoms among the nonpatients that were nearly identical with those of the patients receiving care for FMS at Wichita-area clinics.

A critical appraisal of these two studies does not provide an easy explanation for the observed differences in outcome. The racial admixture, weather climate, and economic backgrounds of the communities were different. There were differences in the methods used to recruit the community subjects. The subjects in the Wichita study were contacted at random by mail or by telephone and asked to answer a series of questions. Their responses, in some cases, disclosed symptoms identifying them as nonpatients. By contrast, the nonpatients in the Birmingham study would have had to first see a newspaper advertisement, make the decision to participate in the study, and then exert the voluntary effort to make a call to the research study center. If the conclusion of Birmingham investigators is correct, that health care seeking is mediated by depression, one might expect the Birmingham nonpatients to be slightly more symptomatic (more depressed) by virtue of the effort required for self-selection, compared with the randomly recruited Wichita nonpatients.

Like the proverbial question of which came first, the chicken or the egg, one could ponder whether people with both FMS and depression were in some way predisposed to develop FMS because of an underlying tendency to depression or whether they developed depression as a reaction to a devastatingly painful illness. It may actually happen both ways, but one should not ignore the relevant point that body pain is not a characteristic manifestation of major depression or anxiety. A number of interesting investigational approaches will likely be devised to better answer this question.

2. Muscle Physiology and Pathology

The perception of many FMS patients is that they experience deep muscle or even bone pain. An important minority of the TPs are located over muscle masses (lateral border of the trapezius, supraspinatus, lateral epicondyle, upper gluteal, and medial knee). Adding these observations to the perception of fatigue and exercise-induced pain in FMS logically led to the concept that there may be some form of anatomic abnormality or at least an energy deficit in the skeletal muscles of people with FMS.[11, 71, 73]

Other authors have disagreed because their controlled studies have failed to identify any histologic or electron microscopic abnormality specific for FMS when contrasted with muscle tissue from normal controls.[163] It has been argued[126] that the abnormal findings in FMS skeletal muscle, disclosed by nuclear magnetic resonance spectroscopy (^{31}P-NMR) and other methods of study, were actually the result of chronic deconditioning, which is prevalent among patients with FMS. This lack of a satisfying muscle-related explanation for the painful symptoms of FMS provided further support to the search for central nociceptive mechanisms.

3. Genetic Predisposition

It is quite common for a patient with FMS to report that a relative, usually a female ancestor or older sibling, has had similar symptoms. Several published studies[23, 97, 104] have documented familial patterns and predicted an autosomal dominant mode of inheritance for FMS. A study by Yunus et al.[164] examined linkage with the histocompatibility locus, by the sibship method, and found supportive evidence. To date, there are no identified abnormal genes, but several candidate genes have been proposed to explain metabolic abnormalities observed in these patients.

4. Gender Selection

The much higher prevalence of FMS among females than among males has led to speculation regarding gender-specific causes. For example, in an epidemiologic study of a midwestern community,[155] the curves representing pain thresholds (sensitivity to a pressure stimulus) in men and women consistently showed lower values for women (Fig. 9-8). Since the examination component of the ACR criteria for FMS[153] involves the response to a fixed pressure stimulus of 4 kg, it is not surprising that the ACR criteria have identified more women than men with FMS.

Understanding of the mechanisms responsible for this gender-related difference in pain thresholds is incomplete. Measurements of female hormones have not been particularly fruitful.[146] A highly probable explanation for gender-related differences in pain perception has come from an unlikely source—positron emission tomography of the brain. A group of Canadian radiologists[91] were studying the CNS synthesis and metabolism of serotonin (5-hydroxytryptamine [5-HT]), one of the key neurotransmitters of the descending antinociceptive system (see Chapter 7). They administered a methylated analog of tryptophan (5-methyl TRP) to healthy adults of both sexes and measured the rate of its conversion through labeled 5-HT to methylated 5-hydroxyindole acetic acid (Me-5-HIAA). The ligand conversion rate was significantly lower (by approximately sevenfold) in women than in men, providing a logical basis for a gender-related differential in antinociceptive activity. In addition, depletion of endogenous, unlabeled TRP by administration of a TRP-depleted amino acid mixture resulted in a 7-fold drop in 5-HT synthesis among men and an even more dramatic 42-fold decrease among women (Fig. 9-10). These findings have not been confirmed by other investigators, nor has the technology been applied to people with FMS, but they do provide a model to explain the observed gender-related differences in pain sensitivity and potentially could explain why females might be at

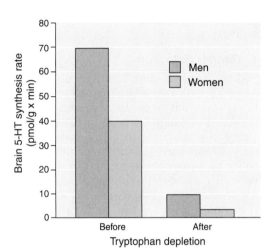

Figure 9-10. The rates of serotonin (5-HT) synthesis in the brains of healthy men and women before and after tryptophan depletion. A radioactive ligand (^{11}C-5-methyl tryptophan) was injected intravenously into healthy subjects before tryptophan depletion (*Women–Before, Men–Before*). The rates of serotonin synthesis and conversion to 5-methylindole acetic acid were monitored by positron emission tomography. The rate of serotonin synthesis in women was lower than in men. Tryptophan was later depleted in the same subjects by feeding them an amino acid mixture lacking tryptophan. Serotonin synthesis under those conditions (*Women–After, Men–After*) was reduced more in women than in men. One could speculate from the data that females in the general population may be more at risk of developing serotonin deficiency, inadequately regulating substance P release, and thus perhaps FMS. (Adapted from Nishizawa S, Benkelfat C, Young SN, et al.: Differences between males and females in rates of serotonin synthesis in human brain. *Proc Natl Acad Sci U S A* 94:5308–5313, 1997.)

greater risk for developing chronic allodynia (read FMS) in response to painful injury.

5. Low Chemical Energy

Two research groups[39, 111] have detected lower-than-normal levels of adenosine triphosphate (ATP) in FMS red blood cells, but the significance of that finding is still uncertain, since it does not correlate with the subject's perception of fatigue.[111] If ATP is also low in FMS platelets, it could explain the low platelet serotonin, because energy is required for serotonin uptake and the serotonin complexes with ATP would help to retain it internally.[151]

6. Neuroendocrine Dysfunction

Many of the symptoms of FMS resemble those observed in patients with hormone deficiencies. That observation has led to several studies examining neuroendocrine function in FMS.[1, 35, 43, 53] From them, a pattern has emerged.

The subsets of those people with FMS exhibit functional abnormalities in the hypothalamic-pituitary-adrenal axis, in the sympathoadrenal system, in the hypothalamic-pituitary-thyroid axis, or in the hypothalamic-pituitary-growth hormone axis. For example, the adrenocorticotropic hormone response to administered corticotropin-releasing factor (Fig. 9-11) to insulin-induced hypoglycemia was abnormal in FMS, but the responsible mechanisms have not yet been clearly delineated. It appears that there may be diurnal rhythm abnormalities in cortisol production and that the epinephrine response to physiologic stress may be blunted. Growth hormone was studied because it was known to be produced during delta-wave sleep which many FMS patients fail to achieve or spend enough sleep time in. Growth hormone is difficult to measure because its release is pulsatile and its plasma half-life is short. An alternative means of monitoring growth hormone production is to measure the plasma levels of insulin-like growth factor-1 (IGF-1), which has a long half-life. An age-adjusted deficiency of IGF-1 has been documented in a large number of FMS patients relative to normal controls[13] (Fig. 9-12).

The reasons why these endocrinopathies would be associated with a chronic pain syndrome are not clear. It may be that CNS abnormalities in the availability of biogenic amines such as norepinephrine or serotonin are responsible for the abnormal regulation of one or more components of the neuroendocrine system.[118] These systems interact and are interdependent, so in susceptible individuals, a partial failure of one system may lead to subtle malfunction of others.

Administration of glucocorticosteroid medications to persons with primary FMS does not seem to improve their symptoms.[33] Conversely, substantial improve-

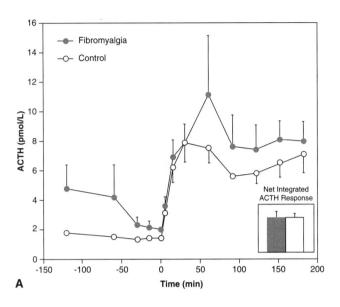

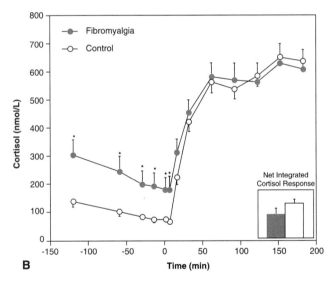

Figure 9-11. Adrenocorticotropic hormone (ACTH) produced in response to corticotropin-releasing hormone in patients with FMS compared with healthy normal controls. Ovine corticotropin-releasing hormone (oCRH, 1 μg/kg) was administered intravenously at time 0. The net integrated ACTH response represents the stimulated area under the curve from 0 to 180 minutes, minus the basal integrated area under the curve. **A.** There was a nonsignificant trend toward increased ACTH production in response to oCRH. **B.** Cortisol production after the administration of oCRH. The total cortisol levels were significantly higher in patients with FMS at all basal time points, but the net integrated cortisol response was significantly lower in FMS patients than in the normal controls. *Asterisk* indicates P < 0.05. (Adapted from Crofford LJ, Pillemer SR, Kalogeras KT, *et al*.: Hypothalamic-pituitary-adrenal axis perturbations in patients with fibromyalgia. *Arthritis Rheum* 37:1583–1592, 1994.)

ment of FMS symptoms may result from otherwise-indicated corticosteroid treatment of patients with FMS concomitant with RA or SLE. Fibromyalgia-like symptoms in such inflammatory disorders may be exacerbated by too rapidly tapering the corticosteroid dosage. Whether that happens only when there is already an underlying FMS is unknown. Some clinicians have observed that administra-

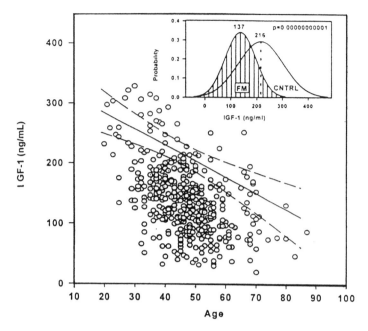

Figure 9-12. Insulin-like growth factor-1 (IGF-1) levels in 500 patients with fibromyalgia and in 152 controls. The *solid line* is the regression for the normal controls, flanked by the 99% confidence limits above and below the mean. The *circles* represent individual values of IGF-1 for individual patients. The *inset* graph shows Gaussian distributions for the FMS and control populations. (Reproduced with permission from Bennett RM, Cook DM, Clark SR, *et al.* Hypothalamic-pituitary-insulin-like growth factor-I axis dysfunction in patients with fibromyalgia. *J Rheumatol* 24:1384–1389, 1997.)

tion of mineralocorticoids can reduce the severity of the neurally mediated hypotension that occurs in some FMS patients.[17]

Parenteral therapy with human growth hormone was effective in reducing the severity of FMS symptoms (Fig. 9-13). But regular injection therapy with this hormone is not universally appealing to FMS patients, and the cost of such therapy is currently prohibitive.[14]

7. Autonomic Nervous System Dysfunction

Orthostatic dizziness and lightheadedness are fairly common complaints among patients with FMS and are particularly noticeable when patients rise from a recumbent or seated position, when they are required to stand still for prolonged periods of time, or when they are unusually tired. While frank syncope is uncommon, many patients report having felt faint at times. Among the various potential explanations, the most probable now seems to be a complex dysfunction in the autonomic nervous system. When subjected to tilt-table testing, a substantial proportion (approximately one third) of FMS and chronic fatigue syndrome patients will exhibit a drop in their blood pressure, some to the point of syncope.[17] Another manifestation of dysfunctional autonomic regulation is the power spectral findings on examination of heart rate with physiologic challenge.[33a, 75a] Finally, a remarkable observation derived with such technology was that the ratios of the slow (sympathetically mediated) spectral bands divided by the faster (parasympathetically mediated) spectral bands of the heart rate exhibit diurnal variations.[75b] Normally, this ratio falls substantially at night and rises again in the morning, but that pattern of change failed to occur or was blunted in FMS (Fig. 9-14). The implication was that sympathetic tone in FMS patients is inappropriately sustained when it should be reduced or that the parasympathetic activity seen in normal controls fails to rise in FMS. The relationship of this finding to insomnia, morning stiffness, and daytime fatigue in FMS must be carefully assessed.

8. Neurosensory Dysfunction

The nociceptive pain model relates to central amplification of pain or reduced antinociception, respectively. It combines information available from animal systems and data already collected from FMS studies in order to predict that central sensitization has resulted in an increase in the

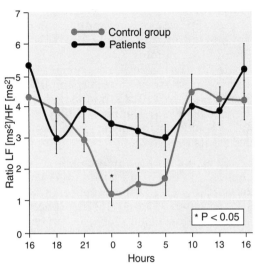

Figure 9-14. Circadian record of heart rate variability in 30 fibromyalgia patients and 30 matched controls. Normal rhythm variability is seen in the control group with enhanced high-frequency (HF) band oscillations during the night. Tracings in the patients were characterized by persistent predominance of the low-frequency (LF) band. Significant differences were found at 0 and 3 hours (asterisks). Values are mean ± SEM. (Reproduced with permission from Martinez-Lavin M, Hermosillo AG, Rosas M, Soto M-E: Circadian studies of autonomic nervous balance in patients with fibromyalgia: a heart rate variability analysis. *Arthritis Rheum* 41:1966–1971, 1998.)

magnitude of afferent stimuli to increase their impact on pain perception. This model also predicts that chronic sensitization to pain might adversely alter the mechanisms involved in signal transmission. There is already sufficient evidence to implicate this model, or at least some aspects of it, in the pathogenesis of FMS. In the following paragraphs are briefly provided some basic terminology, some evidence from animal systems, and finally, some evidence from studies of people with FMS.

Nociception. The term "nociception" refers to the physiologic process of transmitting the electrical signal elicited by a painful stimulus from the periphery to the cerebral cortex, where the body location and the physiologic consequences of the stimulus are consciously interpreted. The process of nociception is accomplished by a series of electrical and chemical neurotransmission and neuromodulation

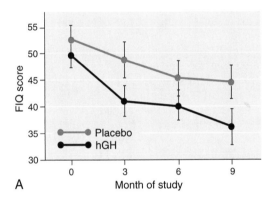

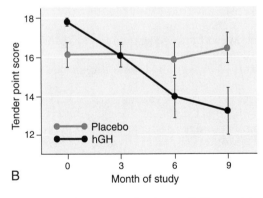

Figure 9-13. Responses of patients with fibromyalgia to parenteral administration of human growth hormone (*hGH*). **A.** Mean scores for the Fibromyalgia Impact Questionnaire (*FIQ*) decreased progressively over the 9 months of the study, reaching significance (P < 0.05) by favoring hGH treatment by month nine. **B.** The tender point score started marginally higher in the hGH-treated group but fell significantly relative to the control by month nine (P < 0.05). (Adapted from Bennett RM, Clark SC, Walczyk J: A Randomized, double-blind, placebo-controlled study of growth hormone in the treatment of fibromyalgia. *Am J Med* 104:227–231, 1998.)

steps involving excitatory amino acids, neuropeptides, prostaglandins, biogenic amines, nitrous oxide, mineral ions, and endogenous opioids (Chapters 1 and 7).[74] Some of those agents are pronociceptive, meaning that they carry or amplify the signal induced by the stimulus; others are antinociceptive, meaning that they inhibit transmission of the nociceptive signal or reduce its amplitude.

Allodynia. The International Association for the Study of Pain has defined the term "allodynia" as the situation in which pain is caused by a stimulus that should not normally cause pain (i.e., an innocuous [non-noxious] stimulus).[16] This contrasts with the definition of hyperalgesia, in which the finding is an increased response to a stimulus that would cause pain in normal individuals (i.e., a noxious stimulus). The low pain threshold in FMS can be viewed as a human model for chronic, widespread deep pressure allodynia in response to deep pressure and may extend to heat-induced cutaneous pain perception in the same individuals with FMS.[47] It is acknowledged, but not relevant to this discussion, that people with FMS may also exhibit hyperalgesia.

Neurochemicals. The roles of neurochemicals as neurotransmitters in the process of nociception and allodynia have been studied extensively in animals,[74] and the findings are now at least theoretically relevant to human FMS.[107] This line of reasoning has led to the measurement of neurotransmitter levels in biologic fluids obtained from FMS patients. Two participants in the nociceptive process that appear to be important to FMS are serotonin (5-HT) and substance P. Both animal and human data are available.

Serotonin. Animal studies have provided some fascinating clues regarding the function of 5-HT in the mammalian CNS. Dietary protein is digested in the gut, and the resulting TRP is absorbed through the intestinal mucosa. It is carried by albumin to the blood-brain barrier, where TRP is taken up by an energy-dependent process for delivery to the brainstem raphe nuclei. One important nucleus in this regard is the nucleus raphe magnus, which forms an essential part of the descending antinociceptive system (see Chapter 7 and Fig. 7-12). The raphe neurons oxidatively decarboxylate TRP to 5-HT and package it for axonal delivery at synapses in brain and spinal cord locations. For example, 5-HT is released by raphe axons into the caudate nucleus[10] and within the dorsal horn region at all levels of the spinal cord.[135] In the spinal cord, 5-HT is known to inhibit the release of substance P by afferent neurons responding to peripheral stimuli.[38, 70, 90, 101] A dysfunction of the descending antinociceptive system as a possible mechanism for the pain of fibromyalgia has been discussed by Henriksson and Mense.[56a]

In this regard, note that raphe neurons also contain substance P,[8] whose concentration in those neurons is inversely related to the 5-HT concentration.[143] The role of 5-HT in the caudate nucleus is less clear, but it most likely is involved in reducing the magnitude of the signal relayed on the cerebral cortex.

A surprising observation, from a murine model, is that increased substance P in the brain increases 5-HT levels in the spinal cord, which in turn decreases release of substance P into the spinal cord.[88, 125, 144] There seems to be an inverse relationship between brain substance P and spinal cord substance P concentrations. If these observations are applicable to human FMS, one would expect low brain tissue levels of both 5-HT and substance P, while spinal cord 5-HT concentrations would be low and spinal cord substance P would be high.

Moldofsky and colleagues[82, 84] were the first to suggest that 5-HT might be involved in the pathogenesis of FMS, in failing both to attenuate its gnawing pain and to overcome its persistent insomnia. Twenty years ago, 5-HT was already believed to regulate pain perception and induce deep, restful sleep. Moldofsky found a clinical correlate between FMS pain and the plasma concentration of the essential amino acid TRP that can be metabolized by oxidative decarboxylation to 5-HT. The serum and CSF of FMS patients were found to exhibit low concentrations of TRP.[115, 119] Early findings of a low serum concentration of 5-HT[117] were supported by other investigators (Fig.

9-15).[62] In addition, a population study[156] disclosed that serum 5-HT correlated with the numbers of TPs only among those individuals who met clinical criteria for FMS. It is now apparent that the low serum 5-HT in FMS patients results from low levels of 5-HT in the peripheral platelets of these patients.[113]

The levels of 5-HT have not yet been reported in FMS CSF, but the levels of its immediate precursor, 5-hydroxy-TRP, and its metabolic product, 5-hydroxyindole acetic acid (5-HIAA), have been. Both were found to exhibit lower-than-normal concentrations in FMS CSF relative to the CSF of HNCs.[118, 119] In addition, 5-HIAA was measured in the 24-hour urine samples of patients with FMS and compared with the results from HNCs.[66] The rate of 5-HIAA excretion was significantly lower in FMS patients than in the HNCs (Fig. 9-16). These findings are only indirect evidence to suggest that something is really amiss bodywide with the production and/or metabolism of 5-HT in FMS. Perhaps the most critical location for such a deficiency would be in the CNS, where 5-HT is needed to regulate nociception.

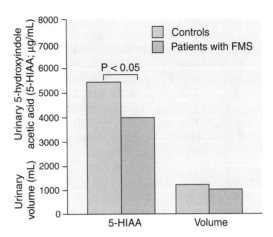

Figure 9-16. Urine volume (mL/24 hours) and 24-hour urinary 5-hydroxyindole acetic acid (5-HIAA) excretion (μg/24 hours) in 19 patients with fibromyalgia syndrome (FMS) and in 19 healthy normal controls. Excretion of 5-HIAA was significantly lower in the patients with FMS than in the normal controls (P < 0.05). (Adapted from Kang Y-K, Russell IJ, Vipraio GA, et al.: Low urinary 5-hydroxyindole acetic acid in fibromyalgia syndrome: evidence in support of a serotonin-deficiency pathogenesis. *Myalgia* 1:14–21, 1998.)

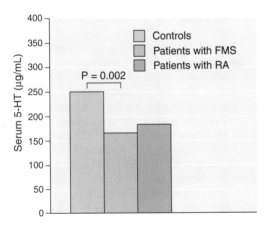

Figure 9-15. Serum serotonin in 38 healthy normal controls, in 38 patients with primary fibromyalgia syndrome (FMS), and in 38 patients with rheumatoid arthritis (RA). The average value (in μg/mL) for fibromyalgia patients is significantly lower than in the normal controls (P = 0.002). The other comparisons are not significantly different. (Adapted from Russell IJ, Vaeroy H, Javors M, et al.: Cerebrospinal fluid biogenic amine metabolites in fibromyalgia/fibrositis syndrome and rheumatoid arthritis. *Arthritis Rheum* 35:550–556, 1992.)

A novel and rather appealing hypothetical explanation for both the low serum TRP and 5-HT in people with FMS was proposed by Klein et al.[68] They reported finding high titers of antibodies (immunoglobulins G and M [IgG, IgM] and anti-5-HT that cross-reacted with TRP) in the serum of FMS patients compared with normal controls and in controls with rheumatic conditions. Their data raised the possibility that an autoimmune process might be responsible for the low levels of 5-HT in FMS sera and platelets.

Two groups in the United States[121, 142] have reexamined this question, using solid-phase radioimmunoassays for both IgG and IgM antibodies to 5-HT. Sera were obtained from individuals in each of three clinical groups (FMS, RA, and HNCs). Each serum sample was tested for IgG and IgM antibodies to 5-HT or to neurophysiologically important gangliosides (monosialo- and asialo-Gm1), which are believed to be involved in the effector receptor for 5-HT.[9] Neither group was able to demonstrate consistently higher titers of anti-5-HT antibodies from either immunoglobulin class in FMS, compared with either of the control groups. Both groups came to the same conclusion: Serum antibodies to 5-HT or to 5-HT receptors are not increased in FMS.

Substance P. Substance P is an 11-amino acid neuropeptide that has several important roles in the process of nociception.[74] Activated, thinly myelinated A-δ and unmyelinated C-fiber afferent neurons release substance P into laminae I, II, and V of the spinal cord dorsal horn. Following release into the synaptic cleft or into the interstitial space from extrasynaptic varicosities, substance P or its C-terminal peptide fragment makes contact with its effector neurokinin-1 (NK-1) receptors. The mechanism of substance P action in the dorsal horn of the spinal cord is not entirely clear, but it apparently facilitates nociception by "arming" or "alerting" spinal cord neurons to incoming nociceptive signals from the periphery. Of course, substance P, released by the afferent nerve fibers into the dorsal horn of the spinal cord, can also diffuse out into the extracellular space and from there to the CSF, where it can be measured as CSF substance P.[61]

As one of several neuropeptides, substance P can be manipulated to induce allodynia in animal models. In the laboratory of one of the authors (SM), the effects of administering substance P intrathecally to rats were examined.[58] In these experiments, substance P induced a dose-dependent increase in the number of peripheral nerves and/or fiber types that were effective in driving the dorsal horn neuron to relay a nociceptive message to the brain. Substance P caused an increase in the size or number of mechanosensitive receptive fields involving nociceptive neurons and induced a lowering of the threshold for postsynaptic potentials. All of these effects were consistent with the model, which views substance P as a facilitator of nociception.

Substance P has been measured in the serum (Ref. 102 and I. J. Russell, unpublished data) and in the urine (I. J. Russell and D. J. Clauw, unpublished data) of people with FMS. In both of these biologic fluids, the levels of substance P were normal.

Working in Norway and Sweden, Vaeroy *et al.*[139] were the first to recognize that the concentration of substance P was elevated (approximately threefold) in the CSF of FMS patients compared with HNC subjects. Their findings have now been reproduced in three other clinical studies.[19, 120, 147] In each case, the average CSF substance P level in FMS was twofold to threefold higher than in the HNCs.

In one of the author's (IJR) original studies of FMS patients,[120] 87.5% exhibited CSF substance P concentrations greater than the highest HNC value (Fig. 9-17). Age and gender had no influence on the measured CSF substance P levels, but minor differences were related to ethnicity. In an attempt to further characterize the nature of the CSF substance P abnormality, a number of lumbar-level CSF samples were collected in three sequential numbered fractions. The CSF substance P concentrations in these samples failed to define a cranial-to-caudal gradient of CSF substance P concentration. Another experiment involved inducing noxious pressure on the lower body TPs to see if it would have any effect on the lumbar-level CSF substance P concentration. There was no significant increase in the levels of CSF substance P, as might have been expected if the substance P were coming primarily from local primary afferent neurons.

The clinical relevance of elevated CSF substance P in FMS has been questioned. In each of the original studies on CSF substance P, the conclusions were based on only a single value for CSF substance P in each subject. It was not possible from such data to know whether the abnormal CSF levels of substance P were stable or were fluctuating with the patients' symptoms. To answer those questions, 30 lumbar level CSF samples were collected from the same medication-free patients an average of 12 months after the first sample had been obtained.[123] As in the prior studies, the FMS patients were asked to discontinue, for 2 weeks, all medications believed to be helpful in treatment of FMS symptoms. There was, on average, a slight increase in the concentration of CSF substance P over time, which correlated directly with a small clinical change in pain/tenderness occurring over the same period of time. These findings imply that CSF substance P may be

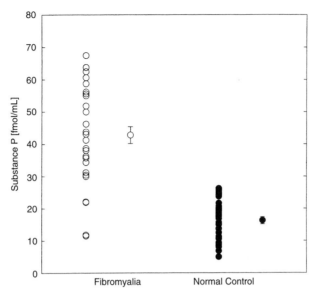

Figure 9-17. Substance P concentrations in CSF samples. FMS patients (*open dots*) exhibited significantly (P < 0.001) higher mean levels (*open dot* with standard error bars) than did healthy normal controls (*closed dots*). Each *dot* represents an individual patient or a normal control. There was little overlap of values between the two groups. Eighty-seven percent of FMS patients exhibited CFS substance P levels higher than the highest normal control value. (Adapted from Russell IJ, Orr MD, Littman B, et al.: Elevated cerebrospinal fluid levels of substance P in patients with fibromyalgia syndrome. *Arthritis Rheum* 37: 1593–1601, 1994.)

integrally related to changes in the severity of the symptomatic pain of FMS.

An important question that eventually must be settled is whether elevated CSF substance P is unique to FMS. An earlier report[130] indicated that substance P was lower than normal in a variety of chronic painful conditions, such as low back pain. In two studies, CSF substance P was lower than normal in idiopathic pain diseases[6] and in chronic neurogenic pain syndromes, including diabetic neuropathy.[138] Finally, both CSF substance P and CSF metenkephalin were normal in chronic pain patients.[54] By contrast, CSF substance P was mildly elevated in patients with severely painful osteoarthritis of the hip and normalized in those same subjects after most of the pain was relieved by total hip arthroplasty.[93]

Two other observations of interest relate substance P to depression. In a small study, mention was made of finding substance P to be increased in the CSF of depressed individuals.[75] In another study, an NK-1 inhibitor was found to be as effective as

paroxetine for the control of depressive symptoms.[40]

The experience with this model in San Antonio now includes analysis of substance P in CSF collected from more than 300 clinical subjects (I. J. Russell, unpublished data). Among them are 156 primary FMS patients whose average CSF substance P was over 33 fmol/mL compared with that of 57 HNCs whose average CSF substance P was only 22 fmol/mL. Disease control groups, including 34 subjects with FMS associated with another painful condition (secondary FMS), exhibited an average CSF substance P similar to that of the primary FMS patients at 30 fmol/mL. A smaller group of 14 subjects with other painful conditions but lacking FMS revealed an average CSF substance P of 32 fmol/mL. Only the HNC CSF substance P values were meaningfully different from those found in the primary FMS patients.

The FMS study group at the University of Alabama at Birmingham[19] shows that the higher CSF substance P levels in FMS correlated with a decrease in regional cerebral blood flow within the caudate nucleus and thalamus of the same FMS patients. The reason for this relationship is not yet clear. It is not likely that the high levels of substance P caused the apparent vasoconstriction because substance P is known to be a potent dilator of cerebral vessels,[78] provided the vascular endothelium of those vessels is intact.

It is possible that the decrease in blood flow could have been caused by neuropeptide Y[35] or dynorphin A,[72, 140] since both are known to be potent vasoconstrictors and both are elevated in FMS. One could speculate, then, that the excess substance P is produced in response to tissue hypoxia as an attempt on the part of the CNS to restore more normal blood flow.[78] That explanation seems unlikely, however, because major brain hypoxic injury, caused in neonatal rats by ligation of an internal carotid artery, resulted in a substantial decrease in brain tissue levels of substance P.[65]

Of course, not being able to immediately explain a biologic finding does not in any way negate it. As with many past observations, this one may need to hibernate for a while until the key to understanding it is disclosed by further research.

Nerve Growth Factor. The anatomic source of the elevated substance P in FMS CSF is still unclear. As mentioned earlier, it is known that painful signals from the periphery normally result in the release of substance P in the dorsal horn of the spinal cord, from which it can find its way, by simple diffusion, to the CSF.[61] It is also clear, from a murine system, that substance P is present in brain tissues[125] and that some of the substance P found in the CSF may have had its origin in the brain or brainstem.

An exciting recent development in the study of CSF substance P in FMS was the finding of elevated levels of nerve growth factor in the CSF of some people with primary FMS, but not in those with an associated painful condition (secondary FMS).[48] This peptide is believed to facilitate the growth of substance P-containing neurons[37, 95] and to be involved in the process of neuroplasticity.[7, 160] For these reasons, nerve growth factor could be critical to the initiation or perpetuation of the painful symptoms of FMS. If so, the next task would be to learn why nerve growth factor would be elevated in the CSF of people with primary FMS.

Calcitonin Gene-Related Peptide (CGRP). This neuropeptide is currently somewhat of a mystery because it colocalizes with substance P in many neurons of afferent neural pathways,[136] but the main function attributed to it is competitive inhibition of the peptidase enzymes that degrade substance P. In patients with diabetic neuropathy,[138] CSF CGRP correlated highly with the concentration of CGRP in the peripheral nerves undergoing ischemic injury. In FMS CSF, CGRP was found to be numerically but not significantly higher than in HNC CSF (I. J. Russell, unpublished data). It was surprising, therefore, that CGRP in FMS CSF correlated inversely with the pain threshold, directly with the number of TPs by dolorimetry, directly with depression, and indirectly with the CSF 5-HIAA concentration. The inverse correlation with 5-HIAA ties the 5-HT pathway to peptide mediators at the spinal cord level CSF. No such clinical correlations were found with CGRP in the normal control CSF. The only prior measurement of CGRP in FMS was obtained by Vaeroy et al.,[138a] but precise comparison with the current data is not possible because the prior authors did not have normal controls with which to compare CGRP levels and did not report contrasts with any clinical variables.

Antinociceptive Activities. The data from one study suggested that there might be a weak negative correlation between CSF substance P levels and pain in FMS.[120] That is the opposite of the strong direct correlative relationship predicted. An intriguing hypothetical explanation for that relationship in FMS related to a proteolytic product of substance P.[120] Intact substance P can be proteolytically cleaved by substance P endopeptidase to produce two main peptide fragments, the C-terminal (substance P5-11) and the N-terminal (substance P1-7).[92] Intact substance P and its C-terminal peptide bind to the NK-1 receptor in order to facilitate nociception. The N-terminal fragment of enzymatically cleaved substance P apparently activates another receptor to effect potent antinociception. As the measured concentration of substance P increases, activation of the N-terminal receptor could progressively counteract the nociceptive effect of the C-terminal portion of substance P on the NK-1 receptor.[61, 131, 161] For example, the N-terminal fragment is known to decrease the numbers of NK-1 receptors on the surfaces of the spinal neurons.[161]

Conversely, the concentration of met-enkephalin-arg-phe, which is supposed to exert an antinociceptive effect in the spinal cord, was found to be significantly decreased among a group of Swedish FMS patients compared with HNCs.[147] This is the expected finding if one were to predict that an enkephalin deficiency would increase the magnitude of nociception. The problem with it is that just the opposite was found by an earlier study using the same laboratory.[140]

Endogenous endorphins represent another group of antinociceptive mediators that have been studied.[140] The title of that publication implied that further pursuit of endorphins in the study of FMS pathogenesis would not be fruitful. The authors reported that neither CSF β-endorphin (acting on the μ-opioid receptor) nor dynorphin A (acting on the κ-opioid receptor) exhibited low levels in FMS CSF. They concluded that the cause of the pain in FMS was not a lack of endogenous opioid. Viewed another way, however, the data clearly indicated that the concentration of dynorphin A in FMS CSF was actually elevated. That finding could indicate an attempt on the part of the endogenous opioid system to balance the increased nociception with increased antinociception. Alternatively, it could have different potential implications, which could not have been predicted with the prevalent understanding of dynorphin A activities in 1991.

Dynorphin A. A combination of recent data from animal systems has led this author (I. J. R.) to develop a hypothesis around CSF dynorphin A in FMS,[109] which must be followed up with a prospective study. When high concentrations of dynorphin A were administered intrathecally to rats, the animals developed a flaccid paraly-

sis.[72] Intermediate concentrations of dynorphin A were less damaging but caused a persistent allodynia.[141] The mechanism responsible for these effects appeared to involve N-methyl-D-aspartate receptors, not the expected κ-opioid receptors. Increased production of dynorphin A has been known to occur in animal experiments in which the spinal cord was constricted or otherwise injured.[41] Under those circumstances, antibodies to dynorphin A reduced the severity of the deficit ultimately resulting from such injury. Conversely, when spinal cord injury resulted from dynorphin A excess, it appeared to be irreversible.

Recall (see Section D1) the study conducted in Israel,[24] which showed that previously healthy people who suffered a whiplash injury in an automobile accident were much more likely (21% versus 2%) to develop symptomatic FMS than were individuals who broke a lower extremity bone in an industrial accident. One could speculate that the reason for the differential effect on development of FMS was that whiplash-induced cervical spine injury led to the production of neurotoxic dynorphin A levels.

Recall also (from above) that dynorphin A was found to be elevated in FMS CSF samples.[140] One puzzle that must be solved is the elevated substance P in the same CSF samples, since dynorphin A can inhibit the release of substance P after an acute noxious stimulus.[165] The theoretical inverse relationship between dynorphin A and substance P may be concentration- or time-dependent in the human exposed to spinal cord injury.

Note that people who develop chronic pain after sustaining a whiplash injury have been found by imaging methodology to have smaller cervical canals. Thus the spinal cords of these people may be at greater risk of compressive myelopathy at the time of sudden impact or even hyperextension trauma during anesthetized surgery or dental procedures.[98]

Obstructive Myelopathy. An additional clinical observation (M. J. Rosner, unpublished personal communication) in support of this hypothesis was that patients with CNS compressive neuropathy (of the brainstem in the area of the posterior fossa, e.g., Arnold-Chiari malformation, or of the cervical spinal cord with cervical spinal stenosis) exhibited symptoms similar to those of FMS. In a recent study of FMS patients with Chiari malformation, as evidenced by magnetic resonance imaging,[3] the levels of CSF substance P were numerically higher than in the CSF of FMS patients who exhibited no such evidence of brainstem compression.

It even appears that syringomyelia may have a similar pathogenesis and similar manifestations. A paper by Milhorat et al.[81] indicated that autopsy specimens from people who have died with this condition have exhibited a high tissue concentration of substance P caudal to the lesion, extremely low levels at the level of the syrinx, and normal levels cranial to it. This finding would be consistent with the proposed model that under circumstances of occluded or distorted spinal axonal flow, caudally directed flow of 5-HT or other inhibitors of substance P release may be inhibited. Of course, there may be several other explanations for this finding. Clearly, this issue must be further explored as a treatable etiology for symptoms like those of FMS.

9. Conclusions Regarding Pathogenesis

In contrast with the situation just a few years ago, when FMS patients were often viewed as healthy complainers without any examination findings, there are now classification criteria to aid in making the diagnosis. Whereas patients were earlier considered to be depressed somatizers, the psychiatric model now appears to be an inadequate explanation. Whereas the pathogenesis was once diligently sought in "painful muscles," the symptoms now appear to better fit a nociceptive model. Although it was said that there were no abnormal test findings in FMS, abnormalities in neurochemical mediators of CNS nociceptive function are clearly abnormal in ways that are consistent with the observed patterns of symptoms (Fig. 9-18).

The recognition of allodynia as a manifestation of abnormal central nociceptive processing has changed the collective view of FMS. It has led research on this condition in a new direction, toward the study of nociceptive neurotransmission in FMS. Some of the abnormalities found in FMS, namely, the low 5-HT and the elevated substance P, are logically consistent with a pain amplification syndrome. The extent to which these mechanisms are unique to FMS will be critical in determining the direction that future research should take. Certainly, a better understanding of the cause of FMS represents an important step toward the development of more effective therapy.

F. MANAGEMENT

No single treatment is completely effective in controlling the symptoms of FMS, and no published management program has achieved universal acceptance. The management approach to be recommended (Table 9-7) was recently reviewed.[108] It begins with an accepting attitude toward the disorder, progresses to a comprehensive clinical evaluation to establish accurate diagnoses, requires concerted education of affected individuals to involve them directly in the care process, and then enters the realm of medicinal interventions whose benefits are maintained by close follow-up.

1. Attitude

If the physician's attitude is that "FMS does not exist," that it is a "diagnosis by exclusion," or that it is a "somatic manifestation of self-induced affective psychopathology," there probably is no value in that clinician's working with patients who have pain. Conversely, for the physician who is willing to approach body pain with an inquisitive mind that is open to understanding the patient's perception of their symptoms, FMS can be gratifying to diagnose and manage.

2. Diagnosis

When a clinician evaluates an individual with a history of body pain, the examination should include a careful assessment both of joints for evidence of arthritis and of the soft tissues around the joints for sites of painful tenderness. In most patients with FMS, nearly all of the TP sites will be symptomatic and painful to palpation at the first clinical presentation. Occasionally, a patient will present with a

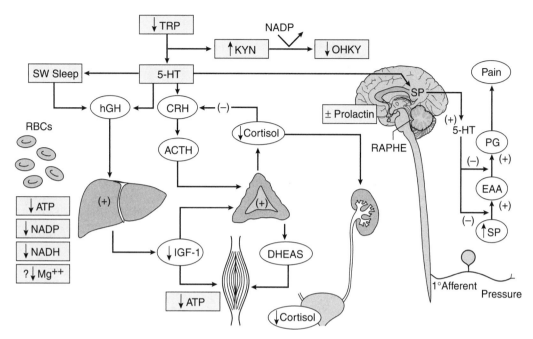

Figure 9-18. Laboratory abnormalities in FMS are reported to include lower-than-normal serum and CSF tryptophan (*TRP*); increased CSF kynurenine (*KYN*); decreased CSF 3-hydroxykynurenine (*OHKY*); lower-than-normal red blood cell (*RBC*) adenine nucleotides, such as adenosine triphosphate (*ATP*), and a functionally abnormal RBC transketolase enzyme, which can be partially corrected by an increased concentration of thiamine pyrophosphate in vitro; decreased production of hypothalamic/pituitary hormones such as human growth hormone (*hGH*), corticotropin-releasing hormone (*CRH*), and adrenocorticotropic hormone (*ACTH*); decreased production of liver insulin-like growth factor-1 (*IGF-1*); decreased production of dehydroepiandrosterone sulfate (*DHEAS*) and cortisol from the adrenal gland; decreased ATP in certain areas of skeletal muscle; and finally, increased levels of CSF substance P (*SP*). (Adapted from Russell IJ: Neurochemical pathogenesis of fibromyalgia syndrome. *J Musculoskeletal Pain* 1(1&2):61–92, 1996.)

single area of symptomatic pain ("chest pain" and "sciatica") but on examination will be found to exhibit tenderness of which they were unaware at most of the other TPs. At times, the generalized pain presentation can so be dramatic that it is referred to as a "flair" or as a "fibromyalgia storm."

When FMS coexists with another condition, both disorders should be managed as separate entities because the FMS in those situations is not different from primary FMS and because there is no evidence that the FMS symptoms will respond to treatment directed only at the associated condition.

3. Tests

Despite the research recognition of reproducible biochemical abnormalities in FMS, none of those measures is yet indi-

Table 9-7   Outline of Multimodal Management for FMS

- Accepting attitude from both physician and patient
- Comprehensive clinical evaluation, accurate diagnosis
- Education for affected individuals, family, society
- Encourage patient to take an active role in self-care
- Psychologic or psychiatric support, biofeedback training
- Physical therapy, physical modalities, exercise program
- Sparing use of medications proven to be effective
- Regular monitoring and follow-up

Adapted from Russell IJ: Fibromyalgia syndrome: approaches to management. *Bull Rheum Dis* 45(3): 1–4, 1996.

cated for routine use in clinical diagnosis. The diagnosis of FMS is adequately made by a typical history and TP examination. The value of laboratory screening (e.g., blood cell counts, sedimentation rate, chemistry panel, creatine kinase, antinuclear antibody, rheumatoid factor, thyroid function tests, skin test for tuberculosis, and perhaps serologic tests for syphilis, the Lyme spirochete, or acquired immunodeficiency syndrome virus in individuals at risk) is to help screen for other clinical disorders that would require separate treatment. There is no diagnostic dependence of FMS on X-rays, electromyography, computed tomography, magnetic resonance imaging, or radioisotope scans. Thus, those tests should only be used if otherwise clinically indicated.

4. Education

Making a confident diagnosis of FMS reduces that patient's utilization of medical resources, such as emergency visits and expensive imaging tests. Benefit results principally from the patient's better understanding of symptoms. Education may not reduce the severity of the pain experienced but can decrease the patient's concern that another condition, such as cancer, has been missed. Women who are being subjected to "wife-battery" will benefit from proper referral. Accurate reading materials (Fibromyalgia Network Newsletter, call USA 602-290-5508), video programs (Fibromyalgia and You, call USA 210-567-4661), and support group interaction resources are increasingly available to assist the health care provider in this area (Table 9-8), but

---

Table 9-8   *Materials Available for Patient Education*

Pamphlet

Fibromyalgia Syndrome. A regularly updated, 11-page primer by one of the authors (I. J. R.). Available as follows: single copies free with a self-addressed, 33¢ stamped, legal-sized envelope—donations accepted; bulk copies to health care professionals at 25¢ per copy; address requests to The University of Texas Health Science Center, c/o I. Jon Russell, MD, PhD, Department of Medicine, 7703 Floyd Curl Drive, San Antonio, TX 78284-7868, USA.

Fibromyalgia Syndrome. An up-to-date summary brochure free to patients, from The Arthritis Foundation (phone USA 800-283-7800) or via any of its branch offices.

Periodical

Fibromyalgia Network. A periodical newsletter for patients with fibromyalgia syndrome. Available from Health Information Network, Inc., P.O. Box 31750, Tucson, AZ 85751-1750, USA.

Regional Newsletters. Publications for patients from local or regional support organizations.

The Journal of Musculoskeletal Pain. A quarterly journal for health care professionals, focusing on soft tissue pain; sixth year of publication; Voice of the International MYOPAIN Society, offers research, clinical reviews, letters, books, news. Available from Haworth Press, Binghamton, NY 13904-1580, USA, phone 800-342-9678, 9-5.

Book

The Fibromyalgia Helpbook. By Jenny Fransen, RN, and I. Jon Russell, MD, PhD. Available from local bookstores or Fibromyalgia Information Resources, P.O. Box 690402, San Antonio, TX 78269, USA.

Fibromyalgia Workbook. By The Arthritis Foundation. Available from The Arthritis Foundation Catalog #835203, phone USA 800-283-7800.

Video

"Fibromyalgia and You." A 90-minute video program, produced by I. Jon Russell; features many of the U.S. experts on fibromyalgia and five patients; a woman TV news anchor moderates. Fibromyalgia Information Resources, P.O. Box 690402, San Antonio, TX 78269, USA.

Fibromyalgia Exercise Videos. Two interactive 30-minute programs produced by exercise expert Sharon Clark, PhD, and Robert Bennett, MD. Available from Oregon Fibromyalgia Foundation, 1221 SW Yamhill, Suite 303, Portland, OR 97205, USA.

---

there is no substitute for some quality physician time. The first few visits should be used to instill confidence in the diagnosis and to directly involve the patient in responsibility for the outcome of the FMS care program. It is important to inform the patient up front that a cure is not available but that teamwork between clinician and patient can usually result in substantial and sustained benefit. In some institutions, psychologists are available to offer biofeedback modalities.

For patients with troublesome fatigue, especially toward the end of the day, an alternating work and rest program for daytime has been helpful. The actual details of the program would be determined by trial and error. The patient would begin by setting a timer in the morning for perhaps 1 hour of work. When the timer rings, the patient would rest for a period of time, perhaps 10 minutes. The timer would then be reset for the next cycle. No matter what is happening at the end of the work period, the patient would stop and rest. At the end of the day, the results should be assessed and adjusted for the next day until a workable program has been found. Many women with FMS who do their work at home have found that a regimen of 20 to 30 minutes of work followed by 10 minutes of rest is effective for them. Adapting this to a workplace setting is obviously more problematic but often can be arranged.

5. Physical Modalities

Research has established that physical exercise is important to the maintenance of physical functions in patients with FMS. The problem is that unaccustomed physical exertion can induce severe body pain for a FMS patient, which will result in near incapacitation for several days thereafter. Gradual adaptation to a routine progressive exercise program, such as alternate-day bicycle ergometry, walking, or water exercise, will usually be well tolerated. Most patients report benefit from heat in the form of a bath or a professional modality, and gradual introduction of massage is similarly appreciated, but neither enjoy the status of proven benefit. The roles of acupuncture and laser therapy are still uncertain.

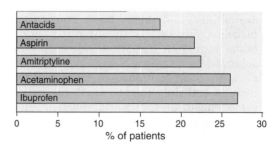

Figure 9-19. Drugs most commonly used by patients with FMS. The most common NSAID in current use is ibuprofen, and the most commonly used sedative hypnotic is amitriptyline. Note that propoxyphene includes various propoxyphene compounds. (Adapted from Wolfe F, Anderson J, Harkness D, *et al.*: A prospective, longitudinal, multicenter study of service utilization and costs in fibromyalgia. *Arthritis Rheum* 40:1560–1570, 1997.)

There is a considerable body of evidence, however, to suggest that both manual therapy techniques and injections can be effective in the treatment of MTrPs (see Chapter 8), with due consideration given to the differences that the additional presence of FMS introduces.

6. Use of Medications

Even though most patients with FMS regularly use one or more oral medications, none in common use can be said to be specific for FMS, and none is dramatically effective. The development of specific therapy will necessitate a better understanding of the underlying biochemical abnormalities. Perhaps future medications will be found to increase platelet serotonin, increase serum IGF-1, or decrease spinal fluid substance P concentration or effect for greater symptomatic benefit. Nevertheless, there is some biochemical logic to the medications that have proven somewhat beneficial in FMS.

The most commonly advocated medication programs involve the use of low-dose, tricyclic, sedative, hypnotic medication and analgesic-level dosage of a nonsteroidal anti-inflammatory drug (NSAID) (Fig. 9-19). There is evidence for benefit from amitriptyline, cyclobenzaprine, and alprazolam, which theoretically increase serotonin availability and have been studied in placebo-controlled trials. Marginal additional reduction in pain severity may be achieved by adding a NSAID if well tolerated. A typical maintenance regimen might include amitriptyline (10 to 35 mg hs) or cyclobenzaprine (2.5 to 10 mg hs) along with ibuprofen (400 to 800 mg bid) or another NSAID.

Several potential adverse effects can limit the usefulness of tricyclic drug therapy. Most patients have some trouble with anticholinergic effects such as dry mouth, which can be managed with sips of water, but tachycardia can be intolerable. An error frequently made is in initiating therapy at too high a dosage. The chronically tired FMS patient may sleep continuously for 2 or more days after a single first dose of 10 to 25 mg amitriptyline or 5 to 10 mg of cyclobenzaprine and then discontinue the drug without an adequate trial. Tachyphylaxis with either amitriptyline or cyclobenzaprine is another problem, which appears to occur after 90 to 120 days of continuous use. Taking a 2- to 4-week holiday from the drug may reestablish more normal nerve cell receptor density and restore effective-

ness (Table 9-9). When the tricyclic drugs are discontinued for a "holiday," all 5-HT reuptake drugs (including fluoxetine, paroxetine, etc.) should also be held, to allow CNS readaptation. During the holiday from the tricyclic drugs or when they are poorly tolerated, alprazolam (0.5 to 1.0 mg hs) is a reasonable substitute. Clonazepam has been advocated especially when the insomnia is caused by nocturnal myoclonus. The beneficial action of carisoprodol (Soma, 350 mg hs) may also relate to sedation.

In a recently completed study,[122] tramadol was used in divided dosages ranging from 50 to 400 mg/day. It was tolerated poorly by approximately 20% of FMS patients, who experienced nausea, somnolence, dizziness, pruritus, constipation, or headache. For those who tolerated at least 50 mg/day, relief from pain was quite uniform and persisted for at least 6 weeks. It is likely that this drug will find considerable utility in the management of FMS. Many questions about its use in FMS remain to be answered. Will it be subject to tachyphylaxis and benefit from periodic "holidays," as is seen with the tricyclic drugs? Will it prove to be synergistic with other analgesic medications? Will concomitant sleep medications still be needed?

Since one of the theoretical goals with the tricyclic drugs was to increase the availability of 5-HT, it seemed likely that the new, highly selective serotonin reuptake inhibitors might also be useful. To date, only the first approved in this class (fluoxetine HCl, Prozac) has been tested, but most have been tried clinically. Fluoxetine reduced the overall severity of depression in the treatment group but did not significantly alter the painful symptoms. One hypothetical explanation may be that the muscarinic, histaminergic, or adrenergic receptors, which are influenced substantially more by the tricyclic drugs than by fluoxetine, may be more important to the mechanism of benefit than previously suspected. When given to patients with FMS, fluoxetine should be given in the morning to avoid worsening the insomnia.

Two enzymes in the glycolytic pathway that depend on thiamine pyrophosphate (from vitamin B_1) as a cofactor appear to require higher-than-normal levels of the

---

Table 9-9   *Drug Holiday Concept*

For Use of Low-Dosage Serotonin Reuptake Inhibitors

Three to four months of serotonin reuptake inhibition:

Four months amitriptyline 10–25 mg (or cyclobenzaprine 5–10 mg) hs:

Possibly fluoxetine 10–20 mg in morning

Possibly ibuprofen 800 mg (or other propionic acid NSAID) bid

Possibly tramadol 50–300 mg in divided dosages

One month of serotonin reuptake inhibitor holiday:

Alprazolam 0.5–1.0 mg hs or clonazepam 1.0 mg hs

Resume serotonin reuptake inhibition for another cycle:

Usually at lowest dosage at first

Adapted from Russell IJ: Fibromyalgia syndrome: approaches to management. *Bull Rheum Dis* 45(3): 1–4, 1996.

vitamin for optimal activity. It is not clear whether administration of large doses of the vitamin will correct the problem, but a trial (thiamine HCl 100 mg/day) might be reasonable, considering its safety profile.

A proprietary combination of malic acid and magnesium (Super Malic, 200/50 mg/ tablet) was tested in FMS and was found useful in fairly high doses (600 to 1200 mg bid). The dosage-limiting factor may be loose stools caused by the magnesium. Caution is also advised when administering magnesium to renal insufficiency patients.

Topical capsaicin cream appears to be beneficial in FMS and can be used on locally painful areas in addition to a regimen of oral agents. The limiting factor may be the cutaneous burning sensation, which may decrease with use and may respond to topical lidocaine or eutectic mixture of local anesthetics (EMLA) cream.

It was earlier mentioned that parenteral administration of human growth hormone was helpful in treating the symptoms of FMS[14] but that the price was prohibitive. As time passes, the cost of this biologic may be reduced, and it may become a more viable alternative for some people with FMS. For the short term, side effects were minimal, but long-term treatment with growth hormone could result in acromegalic changes in body habitus, as occurs with tumors that actively secrete growth hormone.

The biologic effect that 5-hydroxytryptophan has is a committed intermediate in the conversion of TRP to 5-HT. It was theorized that administration of this oral agent would increase 5-HT levels and decrease FMS symptoms if a 5-HT deficiency was a contributor to the pathogenesis. In fact, it was found to be effective at a dosage of 100 mg three times daily.[27] A concern was recently raised that most of the commercial preparations available contain an impurity that may contribute to the development of the eosinophilia myalgia syndrome.[150]

A wide range of other medications used in the treatment of painful neuropathic conditions could be considered, but research supporting their role in FMS is lacking. They include other tricyclic antidepressants not formally tested in FMS (imipramine, doxepin, desipramine, nortriptyline, amoxapine, trazodone), anxiolytics (buspirone); anesthetics (lidocaine, mexiletine); α_2-agonists (clonidine); γ-aminobutyric acid agonists (baclofen); anticonvulsants (clonazepam, carbamazepine); neuroleptics (fluphenazine, chlorpromazine, pimozide); and calcitonin. Opioid analgesics, including codeine admixtures with non-narcotic analgesics, are currently not recommended in the treatment of FMS because of the perceived risk of habituation in patients with chronic pain.

7. Follow-up

It is difficult to extrapolate what may be optimal follow-up in a variety of physician–patient relationships and in other health care delivery settings. It is generally observed that FMS patients appreciate access to the physician at fairly frequent intervals (perhaps every 1 to 2 months for three visits) immediately after diagnosis and then do well with less frequent visits (perhaps every 3 to 4 months) thereafter. Visits can be used to document the severity of the TP pain and to supportively monitor patient progress with the exercise program, the use of medications, the quality of sleep, and efforts toward self-education. The tone of the interaction should not be "I'm not better; what are you going to do about it?" but rather "You are still having quite a bit of trouble; let's see how we can work together more effectively to optimize the growing availability of useful treatment options."

8. Medications

The following descriptions of representative medications were abstracted from standard reference services.[46, 77, 94, 129] They provide useful data about the medications listed above. For ease in finding a given agent, they are listed alphabetically by category and then by generic name. It is the responsibility of the health care provider to appropriately apply this information to a given patient or clinical situation. Most of the listed medications require careful monitoring for continued benefit and adverse effects.

Analgesics

Generic Name: *ibuprofen*
Brand Name: Motrin (over the counter in United States)
Dosage: 200 mg, 400 mg, 600 mg, or 800 mg every 8 to 12 hours with food or fluid.
Action: The analgesic effect is comparable to that of aspirin and occurs by similar mechanisms, except that the antiplatelet effects with ibuprofen are reversible. Its plasma half-life is 2 to 3 hours.
Side Effects: The most frequent adverse effects involve the gastrointestinal tract (gastritis, peptic ulceration, bleeding, perforation, and diarrhea), but the frequency and severity of these effects may be less than with aspirin and more than with acetaminophen. Peptic ulceration can occur *de novo* or can be exacerbated in approximately 1% of patients after 6 months of therapy or in 2 to 4% of patients after 12 months of therapy. Taking ibuprofen with food, or concomitant use of misoprostol at 200 µg qid, can reduce the risk of gastric mucosal injury. CNS effects can include dizziness, headache, confusion, aseptic meningitis, and tinnitus. Inhibition of platelet function is reversible with discontinuance of the drug. Potentially serious gastric, hepatic, renal, hematologic, and cutaneous effects can occur.
Considerations: Coadministration with other analgesic agents should be avoided, but coadministration with amitriptyline has been found useful in some pain states. The relative benefit/risk ratio should be reassessed after 10 days of therapy and periodically thereafter.

Generic Name: *naproxen, naproxen sodium*
Brand Name: Naprosyn, Anaprox, and Aleve (over the counter in United States)
Dosage: 250 mg, 375 mg, or 500 mg every 8 to 12 hours with food or fluid.
Action: The analgesic effect is comparable to that of aspirin and occurs by similar mechanisms, except that the antiplatelet effects with naproxen are reversible. Naproxen may be more effective than aspirin for dysmenorrhea. Its plasma half-life is 10 to 20 hours.
Side Effects: The most frequent adverse effects involve the gastrointestinal tract (gastritis, peptic ulceration, bleeding, perforation, and diarrhea), but the frequency and severity of these effects may be less than with aspirin and more than with acetaminophen. Peptic ulceration can occur *de novo* or can be exacerbated in approximately 1% of patients after 6 months of therapy or in 2 to 4% of patients after 12 months of therapy. Taking naproxen with food, or concomitant use of misoprostol at 200 µg qid, can reduce the risk of gastric mucosal injury. CNS effects can include dizziness, headache, confusion, aseptic meningitis, and tinnitus. Inhibition of platelet function is reversible with discontinuance of the drug.

Potentially serious gastric, hepatic, renal, hematologic, and cutaneous effects can occur.
Considerations: Coadministration with other analgesic agents should be avoided, but coadministration with amitriptyline has been found useful in some pain states. The relative benefit/risk ratio should be reassessed after 10 days of therapy and periodically thereafter.

Generic Name: *tramadol hydrochloride*
Brand Name: Ultram
Dosage: 50 to 400 mg/day in three divided doses.
Action: Tramadol is a synthetic centrally active analgesic. The drug (and its substantially more active M1 metabolite) acts as an opiate agonist, apparently by selective activity at the µ-receptor. In addition, it inhibits reuptake of certain monoamines (serotonin, norepinephrine), which appears to contribute to the drug's analgesic effect, since its analgesic effect is only partially reduced by naloxone. The analgesic effect is comparable with some of the less potent narcotic medications, but its abuse potential appears to be low. There are few or no antiplatelet effects. Its peak analgesic effect is reached 2 to 4 hours after an oral dosage and lasts for 3 to 6 hours.
Side Effects: The most frequent adverse effects are shared by other opiates and include nausea, weight loss, dizziness, somnolence, constipation, dry mouth, diaphoresis, and pruritus. It exhibits minimal cardiovascular risk of hypotension, syncope, and tachycardia. Seizures have occurred during tramadol therapy, so it should be used with caution in people with a recognized risk of seizures and as cotherapy with drugs that lower the seizure threshold.
Considerations: Coadministration with other analgesic agents may provide additional benefit. Coadministration with amitriptyline at night has provided additional desirable sedation for patients with FMS, but because both are inhibitors of biogenic amine uptake, care should be exercised to avoid added toxicity. Initial intolerance can sometimes be avoided by beginning therapy with a half tablet at bedtime and increasing the dosage gradually. The relative benefit/risk ratio should be reassessed after 4 weeks of therapy and periodically thereafter.

Anticonvulsants

Generic Name: *clonazepam*
Brand Name: Klonopin
Dosage: When used for periodic leg movements during sleep, 0.5 to 2.0 mg hs may be effective. Notice that the dosage is lower than is indicated for anxiety or panic. Although parenteral forms are available, oral therapy is the usual route of adminis-

tration for treatment of pain, sleep, and movement disorders.

Action: The mechanism associated with benefit is uncertain, but the anxiolytic or sedating effects may be responsible. There is evidence that benzodiazepines cause skeletal muscle relaxation by facilitating the inhibitory action of γ-aminobutyric acid in the brain or spinal cord. There may also be direct depression of motor nerve and muscle function. The duration of benefit from a single dose may be up to 8 hours.

Indication: The main uses of this drug have been in treatment of petit mal seizures and as concomitant therapy for seizures resistant to other agents alone. It has been used with benefit in patients with akinetic or myoclonic seizures. It has also been somewhat useful with other drugs in the treatment of partial complex seizures. In parenteral form, it has been used to control status epilepticus. Its value as a sedative hypnotic is inadequately evaluated.

Side Effects: The most frequent untoward effects associated with short-term use of clonazepam are similar to those of other benzodiazepine drugs. CNS effects can be sedation, abnormal mentation, nightmares, dysarthria, and extrapyramidal reactions. Chronic usage can contribute to dependency. Acute discontinuation of large dosages can result in breakthrough seizures. Less common are hepatic, hematologic, and cutaneous effects.

Considerations: Administration at night for myoclonic movements offers the potential additional benefit of improved sleep for patients with chronic pain. There may be synergy with other analgesic drugs. The relative benefit/risk ratio should be reassessed after 2 to 3 months of therapy because dependency may occur. When discontinuation of chronic therapy is indicated, the dosage should be tapered down at a rate of approximately 0.5 mg every 3 days.

Sedative Hypnotics

Generic Name: *alprazolam*
Brand Name: Xanax

Dosage: When used for treatment of insomnia and pain in patients with fibromyalgia, the dosage is much lower than is indicated for the treatment of anxiety or panic.[116] Although parenteral forms are available, oral therapy is typically used for the treatment of pain. The dosage is 0.25 to 1.0 mg PO every hour, and in some patients an additional 0.25 to 0.5 mg is given every morning.

Action: The mechanism associated with benefit in fibromyalgia is uncertain, but the drug's anxiolytic or sedating effects may be responsible. There is evidence that benzodiazepines cause skeletal muscle relaxation by facilitating the inhibitory action of γ-aminobutyric acid in the brain or spinal cord. There is also evidence that alprazolam may increase

platelet serotonin by inhibiting platelet turnover induced by platelet-activating factor.[29a] There may also be direct depression of motor nerve and muscle function. The duration of benefit from a single dose may be up to 8 hours.

Side Effects: The most frequent adverse effects associated with short-term use of alprazolam are similar to the benzodiazepine drugs. CNS effects can be sedation, abnormal mentation, nightmares, dysarthria, and extrapyramidal reactions. Chronic usage may contribute to dependency, and acute discontinuation of large dosages can lead to seizures. Less common are hepatic, hematologic, and cutaneous effects.

Considerations: Administration of alprazolam at night offers the benefit of improved sleep for patients with chronic pain. There may be synergy with analgesic drugs. The relative benefit/risk ratio should be reassessed after 2 to 3 months of therapy because dependency may occur. When discontinuation of chronic therapy is indicated, the dosage should be tapered down at a rate of approximately 0.5 mg every 3 days.

Generic Name: *amitriptyline hydrochloride*
Brand Name: Elavil

Dosage: When used for insomnia or pain, the dosage is usually lower than is indicated for major depression. Although parenteral forms are available, oral therapy is typically used for treatment of pain. The dosage is usually 10 to 50 mg PO qhs.

Action: The analgesic effect is apparently independent of its antidepressant effect. The plasma half-life is 10 to 50 hours.

Side Effects: The most frequent adverse effects associated with short-term use relate to the anticholinergic effects, with xerostomia, palpitations, constipation, and urinary retention. CNS effects can include somnolence, dizziness, psychosis, confusion, and even coma. Less common are hepatic, hematologic, and cutaneous effects.

Considerations: Administration at night offers the benefit of improved sleep for patients with chronic pain. There may be synergy with other analgesic drugs. The relative benefit/risk ratio should be reassessed after 2 to 3 months of therapy because tachyphylaxis may occur.

Generic Name: *fluoxetine hydrochloride*
Brand Name: Prozac

Dosage: For major depression and FMS, the usual adult starting dosage is 5 to 10 mg every morning; 20 mg is occasionally used as a maintenance dosage. It should not be administered at night because the stimulatory effect is likely to impair sleep.

Action: There is little or no analgesic effect aside from the antidepressant effect. The plasma half-life is 10 to 50 hours. It is indicated for the treatment of depression and obsessive-compulsive disorder. Although it was not independently effective in the treatment of FMS symptoms other than depression, it was found to be synergistic with amitriptyline in management of FMS.

Side Effects: The list of adverse effects includes anxiety, nervousness, insomnia, drowsiness, fatigue, tremor, diaphoresis, gastrointestinal distress, anorexia, nausea, diarrhea, and dizziness.

Considerations: Administration should be in the morning to avoid insomnia. Substantial weight loss can occur, especially in the elderly. The relative benefit/risk ratio should be reassessed after 2 to 3 months of therapy.

Nutritional/Metabolic

Generic Name: *L-5-hydroxytryptophan*
Brand Name: Not established, but it has orphan drug status with the U.S. Food and Drug Administration (FDA). There are several commercial suppliers.
Dosage: For postanoxic myoclonus, the usual adult starting dosage is 25 mg PO four times daily; the dose may be increased by 100 mg/day every 3 to 5 days as tolerated. A typical dosage for FMS is 100 mg tid.
Action: L-5-Hydroxytryptophan (5-HTP) is a natural aromatic amino acid that is the immediate precursor of the neurotransmitter serotonin. It is metabolically beyond a committed enzyme reaction that begins the conversion of tryptophan to serotonin. 5-HTP is absorbed from the small intestine, with peak plasma concentrations occurring 1 to 2 hours after administration. Approximately 25% of the administered dose is eliminated by first-pass metabolism. The major metabolic pathway is decarboxylation by L-aromatic amino acid decarboxylase to serotonin. The average half-life of the parent compound is 4.3 hours.
Indication: Orphan indication is as treatment of postanoxic intention myoclonus. It has been found in one study[27] to reduce the severity of FMS symptoms, but that application would be considered off label because it is not an officially approved indication.
Side Effects: The most frequently occurring adverse effects include anorexia, diarrhea, nausea, and vomiting. Gradual increases in dose may alleviate some of these effects.
Considerations: 5-HTP is currently an investigational agent intended for use in the treatment protocol of patients with postanoxic myoclonus (cited 12/30/97). There is current concern about subjects taking this agent contaminated with a peak "X" who develop symptoms such as those seen in eosinophilia syndrome. For more information about orphan product designations, contact the Office of Orphan Products Development, available on the World Wide Web at http://www.fda.gov/orphan. The Orphan Drug Sponsor is Circa Pharmaceuticals, Inc., Copiaque, NY; Phone (U.S.A.): (516) 842-8383; Fax (U.S.A.): (516) 842-8630; Designation Date: 11/01/1984.

Generic Name: *malic acid with magnesium*
Brand Name: SuperMalic (200 mg malic acid/50 mg magnesium per tablet), the only one of many over-the-counter preparations that has been studied
Dosage: For FMS, the usual adult starting dosage is 3 tablets twice daily. Gradual increase in dosages (3 to 4 tablets tid) may disclose greater effectiveness.
Action: Malic acid is a naturally occurring intermediate in the Krebs cycle of oxidative metabolism of glucose to produce ATP. Magnesium is a cofactor in the production of ATP. Whether these are responsible for any benefit has not been established.
Indication: Fibromyalgia is not an officially approved indication for use or administration of malic acid or magnesium.
Side Effects: Adverse effects are infrequent even at moderately high dosage. Diarrhea may be related in some persons taking it. In renal insufficiency, caution is advised to avoid hypermagnesemia.
Considerations: In a placebo-controlled study, fibromyalgia patients received 3 tablets of Super-Malic bid but experienced no significant benefit. The basis for use of higher dosages was an open-label follow-up study in which the dosage was escalated to 12 tablets/day in some subjects. In open-label therapy, most subjects reported benefit. They reported less fatigue, greater exercise tolerance, and less pain.

Hypotensive Agents

Generic Name: *clonidine*
Brand Name: Catapres, available in oral and transdermal forms (a parenteral form has been studied)
Dosage: For management of hypertension, clonidine is begun with 0.05 to 0.1 mg bid, and the daily dosage is increased by 0.1 to 0.2 mg every 3 days until the least effective dosage or a maximum of 2.4 mg/day in two to three divided doses is achieved. Transdermal dosage begins with a single patch applied every 7 days, which delivers 0.1 mg/day. Dosage for other applications is extrapolated from the antihypertensive therapy dosage. For sharp, shooting, chronic body pain, a 12-day trial of a patch may be effective in some patients.
Action: Clonidine appears to stimulate α_2-adrenergic receptors in the CNS (mainly in the medulla oblongata), causing inhibition, but not blockade, of sympathetic vasomotor centers. That result is a reduction in peripheral sympathetic nervous system activity and a decrease in the excretion of urinary catecholamines. Clonidine transiently stimulates the release of growth hormone, but chronic administration does not result in a persistent elevation of growth hormone levels. Clonidine reduces heart rate, blood pressure, intestinal motility

in diarrhea states, and intraocular pressure in glaucoma. To the extent that some musculoskeletal pain disorders are sympathetically maintained, clonidine may represent a theoretical solution. It is somewhat sedating, so it may help people with insomnia if it is given only at bedtime. Regarding the antihypertensive effects of clonidine, onset occurs 30 to 60 minutes after oral or intravenous dosing, it reaches its peak within 2 to 4 hours, and it has a duration 6 to 10 hours. Clonidine's oral bioavailability ranges from 65 to 96%, with an elimination half-life of 6 to 23 hours and approximately 20 to 40% bound to plasma proteins. Hepatic metabolism of clonidine to inactive metabolites is accompanied by renal and fecal excretion of unchanged compound (65 and 22%, respectively). Since the drug is excreted by the kidney, the dosage must be decreased in severe renal insufficiency. The tricyclic antidepressant drugs and ibuprofen may reduce the antihypertensive effects of clonidine.

Indication: Currently, the main approved indication for use of clonidine is systemic hypertension. Other uses have included treatment of pheochromocytoma, vasodilation states such as migraine headache, dysmenorrhea, menopausal flushing, opiate withdrawal, and glaucoma. Other potential uses are listed under "Considerations."

Side Effects: The most common adverse effects include sedation (12%), xerostomia, and constipation. Clonidine can cause headache, dizziness, nausea, vomiting, fatigue, weakness, weight gain, gynecomastia, pruritus, and even alopecia. Approximately 20% of patients using the transdermal patch form develop hypersensitivity to clonidine. Impotence or loss of libido has occurred with the oral form in approximately 3% of patients but is rarely problematic with the transdermal form. Muscle pain, muscle spasm, and joint pain have occurred in 3 to 6% of patients.

Considerations: Clonidine can be therapeutic for pain. It has orphan drug status for use in the treatment of cancer pain. Potentially unapproved uses include profound analgesia that can result from injecting the parenteral form epidurally, but it should not be given by this route above the C4 dermatome. Clonidine has been used to treat Tourette's syndrome, in which nearly 50% of patients report beneficial effects of the drug, but when it is taken orally, bothersome side effects reduce compliance. Clonidine has been successful in the treatment of the restless leg syndrome. It is also effective in controlling postoperative shivering. Epidural or subarachnoid or transdermal clonidine can provide symptomatic pain relief from a variety of chronic pain states in which the onset of relief begins within 20 minutes and lasts up to 6 hours. Clonidine is probably helpful as adjunctive therapy in baclofen-refractory cases of spinal cord injury spasticity. Quadriplegics may be more responsive than paraplegics. There is some

evidence for improved mortality in tetanus when clonidine is used to control autonomic dysfunction The tricyclic antidepressant drugs and ibuprofen may reduce the antihypertensive effects of clonidine. A potentially important use in patients with FMS is reduction of symptoms associated with withdrawal from narcotic abuse.

N-Methyl-D-aspartate Antagonist
Generic Name: *ketamine*
Brand Name: Ketalar solution for injection (10, 50, and 100 mg/mL)

Dosage: For induction of dissociative anesthesia, recommended dosages of ketamine are 1 to 4.5 mg/kg IV or 5 to 10 mg/kg IM; maintenance of anesthesia is achieved with an intravenous infusion of 0.1 to 0.5 mg/min or one-half to full induction dose intravenously or intramuscularly, repeated as required. For sedation and analgesia, intramuscular doses of 2 to 4 mg/kg or intravenous doses of 0.2 to 0.75 mg/kg have been employed; ketamine has also been given orally, rectally, and epidurally.

Action: Ketamine is a nonbarbiturate anesthetic/analgesic agent that should be viewed as another CNS depressant. Peak serum levels of ketamine occur 5 to 30 minutes after intramuscular injection and 30 minutes following oral doses; anesthesia is usually induced within 30 seconds and 4 minutes following intravenous and intramuscular induction doses, respectively. Similar to thiopental, ketamine is rapidly distributed to highly perfused tissues (e.g., brain, heart, lungs) following parenteral doses and then redistributed to muscle, peripheral tissues, and fat.

Ketamine is metabolized in the liver, and hepatic clearance is required for termination of clinical effects. A prolonged duration of action may occur in patients with cirrhosis or other types of liver impairment; thus, dose reductions should be considered in these patients. Norketamine is an active metabolite of ketamine; most of a dose of ketamine is excreted in the urine as hydroxylated and conjugated metabolites. Less than 4% appears in urine as unchanged drug or norketamine; the elimination half-life of ketamine is 2 to 3 hours. Its duration of action is not prolonged in the presence of decreased renal function, so dose adjustments do not appear warranted in renal insufficiency.

Unlike inhalational agents and narcotics, which suppress the reticular activating system, ketamine induces a dissociative anesthesia, described as a functional and electrophysiologic dissociation between the thalamoneocortical and limbic systems; this prevents the higher centers from perceiving auditory, visual, or painful stimuli. With adequate anesthetic doses, a trance-like, cataleptic state with amnesia is produced with no impairment of laryngeal and pharyngeal reflexes or depression of respiration. The eyes remain open with a "disconnected" stare, and nystagmus is usually observed; the patient may appear to be awake but is dissociated from the environment, immobile, and unresponsive to pain.

Indication: Ketamine is useful as an anesthetic and analgesic/sedative in a variety of specialized procedures and clinical settings, particularly in children and asthmatics for relief of severe bronchospasm. Ketamine may be used in conjunction with anesthetic agents for the purpose of inducing and maintaining anesthesia, postoperative pain control, chronic pain control, radiologic and diagnostic procedures, and conscious sedation. Epidural ketamine has been useful in treating various types of pain, but it does not appear to offer much advantage over epidural morphine. It may prove particularly useful in severe FMS exacerbations.

Side Effects: Adverse effects associated with ketamine include emergence phenomena (vivid dreams, hallucinations, delirium), cardiovascular stimulation (tachycardia, hypertension), hypersalivation, elevation of intracranial and intraocular pressures, nausea, vomiting, skeletal muscle hyperactivity, nystagmus, and skin rash; respiratory depression is usually not observed. Benzodiazepines or clonidine have been useful in attenuating cardiovascular effects and preventing emergence phenomena. Low-dose ketamine is safe for administration to obstetric patients. Ketamine is contraindicated in cases of hypersensitivity to the drug and when a significant elevation of blood pressure is hazardous (e.g., patients with poorly controlled hypertension, aneurysms, acute right- or left-sided heart failure, angina, cerebral trauma, recent myocardial infarction). Special caution must be exercised when administering ketamine to patients with hypertension, chronic congestive heart failure, tachyarrhythmias, or myocardial ischemia. The same applies when administering ketamine to patients with neurotic traits or psychiatric illness, alcohol intoxication or alcohol abuse, acute intermittent porphyria, seizure disorders, glaucoma, or hyperthyroidism, to patients receiving thyroid replacement (increased risk of hypertension, tachycardia, pulmonary or upper respiratory infection—ketamine sensitizes the gag reflex, potentially causing laryngospasm), or to patients with intracranial mass lesions, the presence of head injury, globe injuries, or hydrocephalus.

Considerations: Unapproved potential uses of ketamine include phantom limb pain, priapism, acute pain resulting from musculoskeletal trauma, and FMS.

REFERENCES

1. Adler JE, Kinsley BT, Hurwetz S, et al.: Reduced hypothalamic-pituitary and sympathoadrenal responses to hypoglycemia in women with fibromyalgia syndrome. *Arthritis Rheum* 39(Suppl. 9): S276, 1996.

2. Ahles TA, Khan SA, Yunus MB, et al.: Psychiatric status of patients with primary fibromyalgia, patients with rheumatoid arthritis, and subjects without pain: a blind comparison of DSM-III diagnoses. *Am J Psychiatry* 148:1721–1726, 1991.

3. Alarcon GS, Bradley LA, Hadley MN, et al.: Does Chiari formation contribute to fibromyalgia (FM) symptoms? *Arthritis Rheum* 40(Suppl. 9):S 190, 1997.

4. Alarcon-Segovia D, Ramos-Niembro F, Gonzalez-Amaro RF, et al.: One thousand private rheumatology patients in Mexico City. [Letter]. *Arthritis Rheum* 26:688–689, 1983.

5. Alfici S, Sigal M, Landau M, et al.: Primary fibromyalgia syndrome—a variant of depressive disorder? *Psychother Psychosom* 51:156–161, 1989.

6. Almay BG, Johansson F, von Knorring L, et al.: Substance P in CSF of patients with chronic pain syndromes. *Pain* 33:3–9, 1988.

7. Andreev NY, Dimitrieva AN, Koltzenburg M, et al.: Peripheral administration of nerve growth factor in the adult rat produces a thermal hyperalgesia that requires the presence of sympathetic postganglionic neurones. *Pain* 63:109–116, 1995.

8. Arvidsson U, Cullheim S, Ulfhake B, et al.: Quantitative and qualitative aspects on the distribution of 5-HT and its coexistence with substance P and TRH in cat ventral medullary neurons (published erratum appears in *J Chem Neuroanat* Oct;7(4):285–287, 1994.) *J Chem Neuroanat* Jul;7(1–2):3–12, 1994.

9. Baba H, Kaune GC, Ilyas AA, et al.: AntiGm1 ganglioside antibodies with differing fine specificities in patients with multifocal motor neuropathy. *J Neuroimmunol* 25:143–150, 1989.

10. Becquet D, Faudon M, Hery F, et al.: The role of serotonin release and autoreceptors in the dorsalis raphe nucleus in the control of serotonin release in the cat caudate nucleus. *Neuroscience* 39:639–647, 1990.

11. Bengtsson A, Henriksson KG, Larsson J, et al.: Reduced high energy phosphate levels in the painful muscles of patients with primary fibromyalgia. *Arthritis Rheum* 29:817–821, 1986.

12. Bengtsson A, Backman E, Lindblom B, et al.: Long-term follow-up of fibromyalgia patients: clinical symptoms, muscular function, laboratory tests—an eight year comparison study. *J Musculoskeletal Pain* 2(2):67–80, 1994.

13. Bennett RM, Clark SR, Burckhardt CS: IGF-1 assays and other GH tests in 500 fibromyalgia patients. *J Musculoskeletal Pain* 3(Suppl. 1):109, 1995.

13a. Bennett RM, Cook DM, Clark SR, et al. Hypothalamic-pituitary-insulin-like growth factor-I axis dysfunction in patients with fibromyalgia. *J Rheumatol* 24:1384–1389, 1997.

14. Bennett RM, Clark SC, Walczyk J: A Randomized, double-blind, placebo-controlled study of growth hormone in the treatment of fibromyalgia. *Am J Med* 104:227–231, 1998.

15. Bonafede RP, Downey DC, Bennett RM: An association of fibromyalgia with primary Sjögren's syndrome: a prospective study of 72 patients. *J Rheumatol* 22:133–136, 1995.

16. Bonica JJ: Definitions and taxonomy of pain. *The Management of Pain, Volume I.* Ed. 2. Edited by Bonica JJ, Loeser JD, Chapman CR, Fordyce WE. Lea & Febiger, Philadelphia, 1990 (pp 18–27).

17. Bou-Holaigah I, Calkins H, Flynn JA, *et al.*: Provocation of hypotension and pain during upright tilt table testing in adults with fibromyalgia. *Clin Exp Rheumatol* 15:239–246, 1997.

18. Bradley LA, Alarcon GS, Triana M, *et al.*: Health care seeking behavior in fibromyalgia: associations with pain thresholds, symptom severity, and psychiatric morbidity. *J Musculoskeletal Pain* 2(3): 79–87, 1994.

19. Bradley LA, Alberts KR, Alarcon GS, *et al.*: Abnormal brain regional cerebral blood flow (rCBF) and cerebrospinal fluid (CSF) levels of substance P (SP) in patients and non-patients with fibromyalgia (FM). *Arthritis Rheum* 39(Suppl.): S212, 1996.

20. Buskila D: Fibromyalgia in children—lessons from assessing nonarticular tenderness. [Editorial]. *J Rheumatol* 23:2017–2019, 1996.

21. Buskila D, Fefer P, Harman-Boehm I, *et al.*: Assessment of nonarticular tenderness and prevalence of fibromyalgia in hyperprolactinemic women. *J Rheumatol* 20:2112–2115, 1993.

22. Buskila D, Neumann L, Press J, *et al.*: Assessment of nonarticular tenderness of children in different ethnic groups. *J Musculoskeletal Pain* 3(1):83–90, 1995.

23. Buskila D, Neumann L, Hazanov I, *et al.*: Familial aggregation in the fibromyalgia syndrome. *Semin Arthritis Rheum* 26:605–611, 1996.

24. Buskila D, Neumann L, Vaisberg G, *et al.*: Increased rates of fibromyalgia following cervical spine injury: a controlled study of 161 cases of traumatic injury. *Arthritis Rheum* 40:446–452, 1997.

25. Campbell SM, Clark S, Tindall EA, *et al.*: Clinical characteristics of fibrositis. I. A "blinded" controlled study of symptoms and tender points. *Arthritis Rheum* 26:817–824, 1983.

26. Carette S, Lefrancois L: Fibrositis and primary hypothyroidism. *J Rheumatol* 15:1418–1421, 1988.

27. Caruso I, Sarzi Puttini P, Cazzola M, *et al.*: Double-blind study of 5-hydroxytryptophan versus placebo in the treatment of primary fibromyalgia syndrome. *J Intern Med Res* 18:201–209, 1990.

28. Cathey MA, Wolfe F, Kleinheksel SM: Functional ability and work status in patients with fibromyalgia. *Arthritis Care Res* 1:85–98, 1988.

29. Cathey MA, Wolfe F, Roberts FK, *et al.*: Demographic, work disability, service utilization and treatment characteristics of 620 fibromyalgia patients in rheumatologic practice. *Arthritis Rheum* 33:S10, 1990.

29a. Chesney CM, Pifer DD, Cagen LM: Triazolobenzodiazepines competitively inhibit the binding of platelet activating factor (PAF) to human platelets. *Biochem Biophys Res Commun* 144(1):359–366, 1987.

30. Churchill MAJ, Geraci JE, Hunder GG: Musculoskeletal manifestations of bacterial endocarditis. *Ann Intern Med* 87:754–759, 1977.

31. Clark GT, Rugh JD, Handelman SL: Nocturnal masseter muscle activity and urinary catecholamine levels in bruxers. *J Dent Res* 59:1571–1576, 1980.

32. Clark S, Campbell SM, Forehand ME, *et al.*: Clinical characteristics of fibrositis II. A "blinded" controlled study using standard psychological tests. *Arthritis Rheum* 28:132–547, 1985.

33. Clark S, Tindall E, Bennett RM: A double-blind crossover trial of prednisone versus placebo in the treatment of fibrositis. *J Rheumatol* 12:980–983, 1985.

33a. Clauw DJ, Radulovic D, Heshmat Y, Barbey JT: Heart rate variability as a measure of autonomic function in patients with fibromyalgia (FM) and chronic fatigue syndrome (CFS). *J Musculoskeletal Pain* 3(Suppl. 1):78, 1995.

34. Cohen MM Jr: Syndromology: an updated conceptual overview. *Int J Oral Maxillofac Surg* 18:216–222, 1989.

35. Crofford LJ, Pillemer SR, Kalogeras KT, *et al.*: Hypothalamic-pituitary-adrenal axis perturbations in patients with fibromyalgia. *Arthritis Rheum* 37:1583–1592, 1994.

36. Dinerman H, Steere AC: Lyme disease associated with fibromyalgia. *Ann Intern Med* 117:281–285, 1992.

37. Donnerer J, Schuligoi R, Stein C: Increased content and transport of substance P and calcitonin gene-related peptide in sensory nerves innervating inflamed tissue: evidence for a regulatory function of nerve growth factor in vivo. *Neuroscience* 49:693–698, 1992.

38. Eide PK, Hole K: Interactions between serotonin and substance P in the spinal regulation of nociception. *Brain Res* 550:225–230, 1991.

39. Eisinger J, Plantamura A, Ayavou T: Glycolysis abnormalities in fibromyalgia. *J Am Coll Nutr* 13:144–148, 1994.

40. Elwood W: Treatment of depression with MK-869, an NK1 receptor inhibitor. *Inpharma Weekly* 1154:9–10, 1998.

41. Faden AI: Opioid and nonopioid mechanisms may contribute to dynorphin's pathophysiological actions in spinal cord injury. *Ann Neurol* 27:67–74, 1990.

42. Fenske TK, Davis P, Aaron SL: Human adjuvant disease revisited: a review of eleven post-augmentation mammoplasty patients. *Clin Exp Rheumatol* 12:477–481, 1994.

43. Ferraccioli G, Cavalieri F, Salaffi F, *et al.*: Neuroendocrinologic findings in primary fibromyalgia and in other chronic rheumatic conditions. *J Rheumatol* 17:869–873, 1990.

44. Friis S, Mellemkjaer L, McLaughlin JK, *et al.*: Connective tissue disease and other rheumatic conditions following breast implants in Denmark (see comments). *Ann Plastic Surg* 39:1–8, 1997.

45. Fukuda K, Straus SE, Hickie I, *et al.*: The chronic fatigue syndrome: a comprehensive approach to its definition and study. *Ann Intern Med* 121:953–959, 1994.

46. Gelman CR, Rumack BH, Hess AJ (Eds.): *DRUGDEX System.* MICROMEDEX Inc., Englewood, CO, revised June 1997.

47. Gibson SJ, Littlejohn GO, Gorman MM, *et al.*: Altered heat pain thresholds and cerebral event-related potentials following painful CO_2 laser stimulation in subjects with fibromyalgia syndrome. *Pain* 58:185–193, 1994.

48. Giovengo SL, Russell IJ, Larson AA: Increased concentrations of nerve growth factor in cerebrospinal fluid of patients with fibromyalgia. *J Rheumatol* 26:1564–1569, 1999.

49. Goldenberg DL, Simms RW, Geiger A, *et al.*: High frequency of fibromyalgia in patients with chronic fatigue seen in a primary care practice. *Arthritis Rheum* 33:381–387, 1990.

50. Gowers WR: Lumbago: its lessons and analogues. *Br Med J* 1:117–121, 1904.

51. Granges G, Littlejohn G: Prevalence of myofascial pain syndrome in fibromyalgia syndrome and regional pain syndrome: a comparative study. *J Musculoskeletal Pain* 1(2):19–36, 1993.

52. Greenfield S, Fitzcharles MA, Esdaile JM: Reactive fibromyalgia syndrome. *Arthritis Rheum* 35:678–681, 1992.

53. Griep EN, Boersma JW, deKloet ER: Evidence for neuroendocrine disturbance following physical exercise in primary fibromyalgia syndrome. *J Musculoskeletal Pain* 1(3, 4):217–222, 1993.

54. Guieu R, Tardy-Gervet MF, Giraud P, *et al.*: Met-enkephalin and substance P. Comparison of CSF levels in patients with chronic pain based on a sampling procedure. (French). *Rev Neurol* 149:398–401, 1993.

55. Hader N, Rimon D, Kinarty A, *et al.*: Altered interleukin-2 secretion in patients with primary fibromyalgia syndrome. *Arthritis Rheum* 34:866–872, 1991.

56. Hawley DJ, Wolfe F, Cathey MA: Pain, functional disability, and psychological status: a 12-month study of severity in fibromyalgia. *J Rheumatol* 15:1551–1556, 1988.

56a. Henriksson KG, Mense S: Pain and nociception in fibromyalgia: clinical and neurobiological considerations on aetiology and pathogenesis. *Pain Rev* 1:245–260, 1994.

57. Hernanz W, Valenzuela A, Quijada J, *et al.*: Lymphocyte subpopulations in patients with primary fibromyalgia. *J Rheumatol* 21:2122–2124, 1994.

58. Hoheisel U, Mense S, Ratkai M: Effects of spinal cord superfusion with substance P on the excitability of rat dorsal horn neurons processing input from deep tissues. *J Musculoskeletal Pain* 3(3):23–43, 1995.

59. Holmes GP, Kaplan JE, Gantz NM, *et al.*: Chronic fatigue syndrome: a working case definition. *Ann Intern Med* 108:387–389, 1988.

60. Hong C-Z, Hsueh T-C, Simons DG: Difference in pain relief after trigger point injections in myofascial pain patients with and without fibromyalgia. *J Musculoskeletal Pain* 3(Suppl. 1):60, 1995.

61. Hornfeldt CS, Sun X, Larson AA: The NH2-terminus of substance P modulates NMDA-induced activity in the mouse spinal cord. *J Neurosci* 14:3364–3369, 1994.

62. Hrycaj P, Stratz T, Müller W: Platelet 3H-imipramine uptake receptor density and serum serotonin in patients with fibromyalgia/fibrositis syndrome [Letter]. *J Rheumatol* 20:1986–1987, 1993.

63. Hudson JI, Hudson MS, Pliner LF, *et al.*: Fibromyalgia and major affective disorder: a controlled phenomenology and family history study. *Am J Psychiatr* 142:441–446, 1985.

64. Jara LJ, Gomez-Sanchez C, Espinoza LR: Prolactin in primary fibromyalgia and rheumatoid arthritis. *J Rheumatol* 18:480–481, 1991.

65. Johnson M, Hanson GR, Gibb JW, *et al.*: Effect of neonatal hypoxia-ischemia on nigro-striatal dopamine receptors and on striatal neuropeptide Y, dynorphin A and substance P concentrations in rats. *Brain Res Dev Brain Res* 83:109–118, 1994.

66. Kang Y-K, Russell IJ, Vipraio GA, *et al.*: Low urinary 5-hydroxyindole acetic acid in fibromyalgia syndrome: evidence in support of a serotonin-deficiency pathogenesis. *Myalgia* 1:14–21, 1998.

67. Kirmayer LJ, Robbins JM, Kapusta MA: Somatization and depression in fibromyalgia syndrome. *Am J Psychiatry* 145:950–954, 1988.

68. Klein R, Bansch M, Berg PA: Clinical relevance of antibodies against serotonin and gangliosides in patients with primary fibromyalgia syndrome. *Psychoneuroendocrinology* 17:593–598, 1992.

69. Kosek E, Ekholm J, Hansson P: Increased pressure pain sensibility in fibromyalgia patients is located deep to the skin but not restricted to muscle tissue. *Pain* 63:335–339, 1995.

70. Larson AA, Igwe OJ, Seybold VS: Effects of lysergic acid diethylamide (LSD) and adjuvant-induced inflammation on desensitization to and metabolism of substance P in the mouse spinal cord. *Pain* 37:365–373, 1989.

71. Lindman R, Hagberg M, Bengtsson A, *et al.*: Capillary structure and mitochondrial volume density in the trapezius muscle of chronic trapezius myalgia, fibromyalgia and healthy subjects. *J Musculoskeletal Pain* 3(3):5–22, 1995.

72. Long JB, Rigamonti DD, Oleshansky MA, *et al.*: Dynorphin A-induced rat spinal cord injury: evidence for excitatory amino acid involvement in a pharmacological model of ischemic spinal cord injury. *J Pharmacol Exp Therapeut* 269:358–366, 1994.

73. Lund N, Bengtsson A, Thorborg P: Muscle tissue oxygen pressure in primary fibromyalgia. *Scand J Rheumatol* 15:165–173, 1986.

74. Malmberg AB, Yaksh TL: Hyperalgesia mediated by spinal glutamate or substance P receptor blocked by spinal cyclooxygenase inhibition. *Science* 257:1276–1279, 1992.

75. Martensson B, Nyberg S, Toresson G, *et al.*: Fluoxetine treatment of depression. Clinical effects, drug concentrations and monoamine metabolites and N-terminally extended substance P in cerebrospinal fluid. *Acta Psychiatr Scand* 79:586–596, 1989.

75a. Martinez-Lavin M, Hermosillo AG, Mendoza C, *et al.*: Orthostatic sympathetic derangement in subjects with fibromyalgia [see comments]. *J Rheumatol* 24:714–718, 1997.

75b. Martinez-Lavin M, Hermosillo AG, Rosas M, Soto M-E: Circadian studies of autonomic nervous balance in patients with fibromyalgia: a heart rate variability analysis. *Arthritis Rheum* 41:1966–1971, 1998.

76. McCain GA: Nonmedicinal treatments in primary fibromyalgia. *Rheum Dis Clin North Am* 15:73–90, 1989.

77. McEvoy GK (Ed.): *AHFS Drug Information*. American Society of Health-Systems Pharmacists, Bethesda, MD, 1996.

78. Mejia JA, Pernow J, von Holst H, *et al.*: Effects of neuropeptide Y, calcitonin gene-related peptide,

substance P, and capsaicin on cerebral arteries in man and animals. *J Neurosurg* 69:913–918, 1988.

79. Melzack R,: The short-form McGill Pain Questionnaire. *Pain* 30:191–197, 1987.

80. Middleton GD, McFarlin JE, Lipsky PE: The prevalence and clinical impact of fibromyalgia in systemic lupus erythematosus. *Arthritis Rheum* 37:1181–1188, 1994.

81. Milhorat TH, Mu HT, LaMotte CC, et al.: Distribution of substance P in the spinal cord of patients with syringomyelia. *J Neurosurg* 84:992–998, 1996.

82. Moldofsky H: Rheumatic pain modulation syndrome: the interrelationships between sleep, central nervous system, serotonin and pain. *Adv Neurol* 33:51–57, 1982.

83. Moldofsky H: Sleep and fibrositis syndrome. *Rheum Dis Clin North Am* 15:91–103, 1989.

84. Moldofsky H, Warsh JJ: Plasma tryptophan and musculoskeletal pain in nonarticular rheumatism ("fibrositis syndrome"). *Pain* 5:65–71, 1978.

85. Moos RH, Solomon GF: Minnesota multiphasic personality inventory response patterns in patients with rheumatoid arthritis. *J Psychosom Res* 8:17–28, 1964.

86. Mountz JM, Bradley LA, Modell JG, et al.: Fibromyalgia in women: abnormalities of regional cerebral blood flow in the thalamus and the caudate nucleus are associated with low pain threshold levels. *Arthritis Rheum* 38:926–938, 1995.

87. Muizelaar JP, Kleyer M, Hertogs IA, et al.: Complex regional pain syndrome (reflex sympathetic dystrophy and causalgia): management with the calcium channel blocker nifedipine and/or the alpha-sympathetic blocker phenoxybenzamine in 59 patients. *Clin Neurol Neurosurg* 99:26–30, 1997.

88. Murphy RM, Zemlan FP: Differential effects of substance P on serotonin-modulated spinal nociceptive reflexes. *Psychopharmacology (Berlin)* 93:118–121, 1987.

89. Nalven FB, O'Brien JF: Personality patterns of rheumatoid arthritic patients. *Arthritis Rheum* 7:18–28, 1964.

90. Naranjo JR, Arnedo A, Molinero MT, et al.: Involvement of spinal monoaminergic pathways in antinociception produced by substance P and neurotensin in rodents. *Neuropharmacology* 28:291–298, 1989.

91. Nishizawa S, Benkelfat C, Young SN, et al.: Differences between males and females in rates of serotonin synthesis in human brain. *Proc Natl Acad Sci U S A* 94:5308–5313, 1997.

92. Nyberg F, LeGreves P, Sundqvist C, et al.: Characterization of substance P (1–7) and (1–8) generating enzyme in human cerebrospinal fluid. *Biochem Biophys Res Commun* 125:244–250, 1984.

93. Nyberg F, Liu Z, Lind C, et al.: Enhanced CSF levels of substance P in patients with painful arthrosis but not in patients with pain from herniated lumbar discs. *J Musculoskeletal Pain* 3(Suppl. 1):2, 1995.

94. Olin BR, Editor in Chief: *Facts and Comparisons.* Facts and Comparisons, St. Louis, MO, 1992.

95. Otten U, Goedert M, Mayer M, et al.: Requirement of nerve growth factor for the development of substance P containing neurones. *Nature* 287:158–159, 1980.

96. Payne TC, Leavitt F, Garron DC, et al.: Fibrositis and psychologic disturbance. *Arthritis Rheum* 25:213–217, 1982.

97. Pellegrino MJ, Waylonis GW, Sommer A: Familial occurrence of primary fibromyalgia—Department of Physical Medicine, Ohio State University, Columbus. *Arch Phys Med Rehabil* 70:61–63, 1989.

98. Pettersson K, Karrholm J, Toolanen G, et al.: Decreased width of the spinal canal in patients with chronic symptoms after whiplash injury. *Spine* 20:1664–1667, 1995.

99. Pincus T, Callahan LF, Bradley LA, et al.: Elevated MMPI scores for hypochondriasis, depression, and hysteria in patients with rheumatoid arthritis reflect disease rather than psychological status. *Arthritis Rheum* 29:1456–1466, 1986.

100. Quimby LG, Block SR, Gratwick GM: Fibromyalgia: generalized pain intolerance and manifold symptom reporting. *J Rheumatol* 15:1264–1270, 1988.

101. Raffa RB, Friderichs E, Reimann W, et al.: Opioid and nonopioid components independently contribute to the mechanism of action of tramadol, an 'atypical' opioid analgesic. *J Pharmacol Exp Therapeut* 260:275–285, 1992.

102. Reynolds WJ, Chiu B, Inman RD: Plasma substance P levels in fibrositis. *J Rheumatol* 15:1802–1803, 1988.

103. Robbins JM, Kirmayer LJ, Kapusta MA: Illness worry and disability in fibromyalgia syndrome. *Int J Psychiatry Med* 20:49–63, 1990.

104. Rosenblatt RM, Reich J, Dehring D: Tricyclic antidepressants in treatment of depression and chronic pain. *Anesth Analg* 63(11):1025–1032, 1984.

105. Russell IJ: Fibrositis/fibromyalgia syndrome. *The Clinical and Scientific Basis of Myalgic Encephalomyelitis Chronic Fatigue Syndrome.* Ed. 1. Edited by Hyde BM II, Goldstein JA, Levine PH. The Nightingale Research Foundation, Ottawa, 1992 (pp. S663–S690).

106. Russell IJ: Thank you reviewers! *J Musculoskeletal Pain* 3(4):1–2, 1995.

107. Russell IJ: Neurochemical pathogenesis of fibromyalgia syndrome. *J Musculoskeletal Pain* 1(1&2):61–92, 1996.

108. Russell IJ: Fibromyalgia syndrome: approaches to management. *Bull Rheum Dis* 45(3):1–4, 1996.

109. Russell IJ: Advances in fibromyalgia: possible role for central neurochemicals. *Am J Med Sci* 315:377–384, 1998.

110. Russell IJ, Michalek JE: Comparative reliability of digital palpation and algometry-based pain measures in patients with fibromyalgia syndrome. *J Rheumatol* [Submitted for publication].

111. Russell IJ, Vipraio GA: Red cell nucleotide abnormalities in fibromyalgia syndrome. *Arthritis Rheum* 36(9):S223, 1993.

112. Russell IJ, Vipraio GA: Serum prolactin in fibromyalgia syndrome, rheumatoid arthritis, osteoarthritis, and healthy controls. *Arthritis Rheum* 36(Suppl. 9):S222, 1993.

113. Russell IJ, Vipraio GA: Serotonin (5-HT) in serum and platelets (PLT) from fibromyalgia patients (FS) and normal controls (NC). *Arthritis Rheum* 37(Suppl.):S214, 1994.

114. Russell IJ, Vipraio GA, Morgan WW, *et al.*: Is there a metabolic basis for the fibrositis syndrome? *Am J Med* 81:50–56, 1986.

115. Russell IJ, Michalek JE, Vipraio GA, *et al.*: Serum amino acids in fibrositis/fibromyalgia syndrome. *J Rheumatol* 19(Suppl.):158–163, 1989.

116. Russell IJ, Fletcher EM, Michalek JE, *et al.*: Treatment of primary fibrositis/fibromyalgia syndrome with ibuprofen and alprazolam. A double-blind, placebo-controlled study. *Arthritis Rheum* 34:552–560, 1991.

117. Russell IJ, Michalek JE, Vipraio GA, *et al.*: Platelet 3H-imipramine uptake receptor density and serum serotonin levels in patients with fibromyalgia/fibrositis syndrome. *J Rheumatol* 19:104–109, 1992.

118. Russell IJ, Vaeroy H, Javors M, *et al.*: Cerebrospinal fluid biogenic amine metabolites in fibromyalgia/fibrositis syndrome and rheumatoid arthritis. *Arthritis Rheum* 35:550–556, 1992.

119. Russell IJ, Vipraio GA, Acworth I: Abnormalities in the central nervous system (CNS) metabolism of tryptophan (TRY) to 3-hydroxy kynurenine (OHKY) in fibromyalgia syndrome (FS). *Arthritis Rheum* 36(9):S222, 1993.

120. Russell IJ, Orr MD, Littman B, *et al.*: Elevated cerebrospinal fluid levels of substance P in patients with fibromyalgia syndrome. *Arthritis Rheum* 37:1593–1601, 1994.

121. Russell IJ, Vodjani A, Michalek JE, *et al.*: Circulating antibodies to serotonin in fibromyalgia syndrome, rheumatoid arthritis, osteoarthrosis, and healthy normal controls. *J Musculoskeletal Pain* 3(Suppl. 1):143, 1995.

122. Russell IJ, Bennett RM, Katz WA, *et al.*: Efficacy of Ultram (tramadol HCl) treatment of fibromyalgia syndrome: preliminary analysis of a multi-center, randomized, placebo-controlled study. *Arthritis Rheum* 40(9):S117, 1997.

123. Russell IJ, Fletcher EM, Vipraio GA, *et al.*: Cerebrospinal fluid (CSF) substance P (SP) in fibromyalgia: changes in CSF SP over time parallel changes in clinical activity. *J Musculoskeletal Pain* 6(Suppl. 2):77, 1998.

124. Salit IE, The Vancouver Chronic Fatigue Syndrome Consensus Group. The chronic fatigue syndrome: a position paper. *J Rheumatol* 23(3):540–544, 1996.

125. Sharma HS, Nyberg F, Olsson Y, *et al.*: Alteration of substance P after trauma to the spinal cord: an experimental study in the rat. *Neuroscience* 38:205–212, 1990.

126. Simms RW: Is there muscle pathology in fibromyalgia syndrome? *Rheum Dis Clin North Am* 22:245–266, 1996.

127. Simms RW, Goldenberg DL, Felson DT, *et al.*: Tenderness in 75 anatomic sites. Distinguishing fibromyalgia patients from controls. *Arthritis Rheum* 31:182–187, 1988.

128. Simons DG: Clinical and etiological update of myofascial pain from trigger points. *J Musculoskeletal Pain* 4(1&2):93–121, 1996.

129. Siston DW, Special Projects Editor: *Physicians' Desk Reference.* Medical Economics, Montvale, NJ, 1997.

130. Sjostrom S, Tamsen A, Hartvig P, *et al.*: Cerebrospinal fluid concentrations of substance P and (met)enkephalin-Arg6-Phe7 during surgery and patient-controlled analgesia. *Anesth Analg* 67:976–981, 1988.

131. Skilling SR, Smullin DH, Larson AA: Differential effects of C- and N-terminal substance P metabolites on the release of amino acid neurotransmitters from the spinal cord: potential role in nociception. *J Neuroscience* 10:1309–1318, 1990.

132. Smythe HA: Problems with the MMPI. [Editorial]. *J Rheumatol* 11:417–418, 1984.

133. Smythe HA, Moldofsky H: Two contributions to understanding the "fibrositis syndrome." *Bull Rheum Dis* 28:928–931, 1977.

134. Smythe HA, Lee D, Rush P, *et al.*: Tender shins and steroid therapy. *J Rheumatol* 18:1568–1572, 1991.

135. Sorkin LS, McAdoo DJ, Willis WD: Raphe magnus stimulation-induced antinociception in the cat is associated with release of amino acids as well as serotonin in the lumbar dorsal horn. *Brain Res* 618:95–108, 1993.

136. Tamatani M, Senba E, Tohyama M: Calcitonin gene-related peptide and substance P-containing primary afferent fibers in the dorsal column of the rat. *Brain Res* 495:122–130, 1989.

137. Travell JG, Simons DG: *Myofascial Pain and Dysfunction: The Trigger Point Manual, Volume 2.* Williams & Wilkins, Baltimore, 1992.

138. Tsigos C, Diemel LT, Tomlinson DR, *et al.*: Cerebrospinal fluid levels of substance P and calcitonin-gene-related peptide: correlation with sural nerve levels and neuropathic signs in sensory diabetic polyneuropathy. *Clin Sci* 84:305–311, 1993.

138a. Vaeroy H: Modulation of pain in fibromyalgia (fibrositis syndrome): cerebrospinal fluid (CSF) investigation of pain-related neuropeptides with special reference to calcitonin gene-related peptide (CGRP). *J Rheumatol* 16(Suppl. 19):94–97, 1989.

139. Vaeroy H, Helle R, Forre O, *et al.*: Elevated CSF levels of substance P and high incidence of Raynaud's phenomenon in patients with fibromyalgia: new features for diagnosis. *Pain* 32:21–26, 1988.

140. Vaeroy H, Nyberg F, Terenius L: No evidence for endorphin deficiency in fibromyalgia following investigation of cerebrospinal fluid (CSF) dynorphin A and Met-enkephalin-Arg6-Phe7. *Pain* 46:139–143, 1991.

141. Vanderah TW, Laughlin T, Lashbrook JM, *et al.*: Single intrathecal injections of dynorphin A or des-tyr-dynorphins produce long-lasting allodynia in rats: blockade by MK-801 but not naloxone. *Pain* 68:275–281, 1996.

142. Vedder CI, Bennett RM: An analysis of antibodies to serotonin receptors in fibromyalgia. *J Musculoskeletal Pain* 3(Suppl. 1):73, 1995.

143. Walker PD, Schotland S, Hart RP, *et al.*: Tryptophan hydroxylase inhibition increases preprotachykinin mRNA in developing and adult medullary raphe nuclei. *Brain Res* 8:113–119, 1990.

144. Walker PD, Riley LA, Hart RP, *et al.*: Serotonin regulation of tachykinin biosynthesis in the rat neostriatum. *Brain Res* 546:33–39, 1991.

145. Ward MM: Are patient self-report measures of arthritis activity confounded by mood? A longitudinal study of patients with rheumatoid arthritis. *J Rheumatol* 21:1046–1050, 1994.

146. Waxman J, Zatzkis SM,: Fibromyalgia and menopause. Examination of the relationship. *Postgrad Med* 80:165–167, 1986.

147. Welin M, Bragee B, Nyberg F, *et al.*: Elevated substance P levels are contrasted by a decrease in metenkephalin-arg-phe levels in csf from fibromyalgia patients. *J Musculoskeletal Pain* 3(Suppl. 1):4, 1995.

148. White K, Speechley M, Harth M, *et al.*: The London Fibromyalgia Epidemiology Study: the prevalence of fibromyalgia in London, Ontario. *Arthritis Rheum* 39(Suppl.):S212, 1996.

149. Wigers SH, Skrondal A, Finset A, *et al.*: Measuring change in fibromyalgic pain: the relevance of pain distribution. *J Musculoskeletal Pain* 5(2):29–41, 1997.

150. Williamson BL, Klarskov K, Tomlinson AJ, *et al.*: Problems with over-the-counter 5-hydroxy-L-tryptophan. *Nat Med* 4(9):983, 1998.

151. Wojenski CM, Schick PK: Development of storage granules during megakaryocyte maturation: accumulation of adenine nucleotides and the capacity for serotonin sequestration. *J Lab Clin Med* 121:479–485, 1993.

152. Wolfe F, Cathey MA, Kleinheksel SM, *et al.*: Psychological status in primary fibrositis and fibrositis associated with rheumatoid arthritis. *J Rheumatol* 11:500–506, 1984.

153. Wolfe F, Smythe HA, Yunus MB, *et al.*: The American College of Rheumatology 1990 criteria for the classification of fibromyalgia. *Arthritis Rheum* 33:160–172, 1990.

154. Wolfe F, Ross K, Anderson J, *et al.*: Aspects of fibromyalgia in the general population: sex, pain threshold, and fibromyalgia symptoms. *J Rheumatol* 22:151–156, 1995.

155. Wolfe F, Ross K, Anderson J, *et al.*: The prevalence and characteristics of fibromyalgia in the general population. *Arthritis Rheum* 38:19–28, 1995.

156. Wolfe F, Russell IJ, Vipraio GA, *et al.*: Serotonin levels, pain threshold, and FM. *J Rheumatol* 24:555–559, 1997.

157. Wolfe F, Anderson J, Harkness D, *et al.*: Work and disability status of persons with fibromyalgia. *J Rheumatol* 24:1171–1178, 1997.

158. Wolfe F, Anderson J, Harkness D, *et al.*: A prospective, longitudinal, multicenter study of service utilization and costs in fibromyalgia. *Arthritis Rheum* 40:1560–1570, 1997.

159. Wolfe F, Anderson J, Harkness D, *et al.*: Health status and disease severity in fibromyalgia: results of a six center longitudinal study. *Arthritis Rheum* 40:1571–1579, 1997.

160. Woolf CJ, Shortland P, Coggeshall RE: Peripheral nerve injury triggers central sprouting of myelinated afferents. *Nature* 355:75–78, 1992.

161. Yukhananov RYU, Larson AA: An N-terminal fragment of substance P, substance P (1–7) downregulates neurokinin-1 binding in the mouse spinal cord. *Neurosci Lett* 178:163–166, 1994.

162. Yunus M, Masi AT, Calabro JJ, *et al.*: Primary fibromyalgia (fibrositis): clinical study of 50 patients with matched normal controls. *Semin Arthritis Rheum* 11:151–171, 1981.

163. Yunus MB, Kalyan-Raman UP, Masi AT, *et al.*: Electron microscopic studies of muscle biopsy in primary fibromyalgia syndrome: a controlled and blinded study. *J Rheumatol* 16:97–101, 1989.

164. Yunus MB, Rawlings KK, Khan MA, *et al.*: Genetic studies of multicase families with fibromyalgia syndrome with HLA typing. *Arthritis Rheum* 38(Suppl.):S247, 1995.

165. Zachariou V, Goldstein BD: Dynorphin-(1–8) inhibits the release of substance P-like immunoreactivity in the spinal cord of rats following a noxious mechanical stimulus. *Eur J Pharmacol* 323:159–165, 1997.

Glossary

These definitions apply to their use in this book; some have additional meanings when used in another context.

A band: dark (anisotropic) band that can be seen running across muscle fibers in the light microscope. It is formed by the aligned myosin filaments of many myofibrils and causes the visible striations of skeletal muscle fibers.

Abscess: a circumscribed collection of pus appearing in acute or chronic localized infection and associated with tissue destruction and, frequently, with swelling (Sted).

Acetylcholine (ACh): neurotransmitter of the neuromuscular endplate (junction between a motor fiber and a muscle cell) and of many synapses in the peripheral and central nervous system.

Acetylsalicylic acid (ASA): aspirin is one of the nonsteroidal anti-inflammatory drugs.

Action potential: propagated change of the membrane potential of a nerve or muscle cell. If the membrane is depolarized (its inside made more positive) to threshold, a sudden influx of sodium ions occurs that makes the membrane potential transiently positive. It becomes negative again by an outflux of potassium ions.

Activation: stimulation of a receptor or

neuron so that it starts firing action potentials or increases its discharge frequency.

Active TrPs: trigger points (TrPs) that cause a clinical pain complaint or other abnormal sensory symptoms. Latent TrPs may show all the other characteristics of active TrPs but usually to a lesser degree; often they are pain-free. Both active and latent TrPs can cause significant motor dysfunction. It appears that the same factors responsible for the development of an active TrP can, to a lesser degree, cause a latent TrP.

Acute pain: pain caused by a short-lasting noxious stimulus acting on normal nociceptive structures. Acute pain does not lead to long-lasting changes in the nervous system; i.e., after the end of the acute pain, the nociceptive system returns to its normal state.

Adenitis: inflammation of a lymph node or gland (Sted).

Adenosine triphosphatase (ATPase): an enzyme that splits adenosine triphosphate (ATP) into adenosine diphosphate (ADP) and phosphate (P) plus energy.

Adenosine triphosphate (ATP): a molecule that provides energy for energy-dependent cell processes by splitting into adenosine diphosphate (ADP) and energy. ATP is also assumed to be a cotransmitter in sympathetic efferent neurons and analgesic substance.

Adhesions: inflammatory bands that bind surfaces together that are covered by mucous membranes.

The Glossary contains the terms and definitions as used in the book. Definitions adopted from *Stedman's Concise Medical Dictionary* (Ed. 2., Edited by McDonough JT. Williams & Wilkins, Baltimore, 1994) are marked with "(Sted)"; definitions adopted from the *Classification of Chronic Pain* (Ed. 2., Edited by Merskey H, Bogduk N. IASP Press, Seattle, 1994) with "(IASP)."

Adventitia: connective tissue surrounding blood vessels and some inner organs.

A-δ fiber: a thin myelinated nerve fiber that conducts action potentials at a velocity of approximately 2.5 to 30 m/s in humans.

Affective-motivational component of pain: pain component that mediates the suffering associated with pain.

Afferent fiber or nerve cell: a neuron or its fiber that conducts action potentials from the periphery to the central nervous system (primary afferent fiber) or to higher centers within the central nervous system (secondary or higher order afferent neurons). Often, sensory is used as a synonym for afferent.

Afferent unit: an afferent (sensory) fiber together with its receptive ending and cell body.

Afterdischarge: a discharge of neurons outlasting the duration of the stimulus. Afterdischarges in nociceptors are likely to be the cause of painful aftersensations following strong painful stimuli.

Algesic: pain-producing.

Algesic substance: one of the substances that cause pain and/or increase the sensitivity of nociceptors (e.g., bradykinin, serotonin, high concentrations of potassium ions, protons).

Algogenic: pain-producing.

Algometer: an instrument for measuring the degree of sensitivity to a painful stimulus; syn: algesiometer (Sted).

Algometry (measurement of pain): in practice, measurement of tenderness in response to a force applied perpendicularly to the skin.

Allodynia: pain caused by a stimulus that does not normally provoke pain (decreased pain threshold: the stimulus and response are of different sensory modalities [categories], e.g., tactile stimuli evoke pain).

Amino acid transmitters: neurotransmitters that consist of amino acids such as glutamate and aspartate.

γ-Aminobutyric acid (GABA): an inhibitory neurotransmitter in the central nervous system.

Amyloidosis: a disease of unknown cause characterized by the extracellular accumulation of amyloid (protein fibrils) in various organs and tissues of the body (Sted).

Analgesia: absence of pain in response to a stimulus that would normally be painful.

Anaphylaxis: immediate transient kind of immunologic (allergic) reaction characterized by contraction of smooth muscle and dilation of capillaries, resulting from the release of pharmacologically active substances such as histamine, bradykinin, and serotonin (Sted).

Angina pectoris: severe constricting pain in the chest, often radiating from the precordium to the left shoulder and down the arm as a result of ischemia of the heart muscle; it is usually caused by coronary disease; syn: stenocardia (Sted).

Anorexia: diminished appetite, aversion to food (Sted).

Antidromic: an impulse propagation against the normal direction; mainly used for action potentials in sensory fibers when they propagate toward the body periphery.

Aponeurosis: a fibrous sheet or expanded tendon giving attachment to muscular fibers and serving as the means of origin or insertion of a flat muscle (Sted).

Arterioles: small arterial vessels of a size between arteries and capillaries. In contrast to capillaries, the wall of arterioles contains a thin layer of smooth muscle cells.

Arteritis: inflammation involving an artery (Sted).

Asepsis: a condition in which living pathogenic organisms are absent (Sted).

Association cortex: those parts of the cortex that are not specialized as target areas of the special sense organs (e.g., eye and ear). In the association cortex, information processing at a high level takes place, and for this purpose, information from many different cortical areas as well as from previous experiences is used.

Atrophy (of a muscle): a wasting of tissue (e.g., from disuse).

Autoimmune disease: a disease arising from and directed against the individual's own tissues (Sted).

Autonomic nervous system: those efferent parts of the nervous system that are not under voluntary control. It consists of two main parts: the sympathetic and the parasympathetic nervous system. Some authors distinguish a third part, the enteric system.

Average pain threshold (APT): sum of dolorimeter readings at the 18 designated tender point sites (usually kg/cm^2) divided by 18. This value correlates well with, but is inversely proportional to, the tender point index.

Axial muscles: head and trunk muscles that are situated in the central part of the body.

Axodendritic synapse: a contact between the axon of one neuron and the dendrite of another nerve cell.

Axon: a process of a neuron that conducts action potentials away from the cell body. The axon is the output portion of a neuron.

Axon reflex: in sensory nerve fibers, the invasion of nonexcited branches of a receptive ending by antidromic action potentials arising in other excited branches of the ending or in the axon. The invasion is followed by the release of neuropeptides and other substances from the ending.

Axotomy: transection of nerve fibers or a nerve.

Basal ganglia: originally, all of the large masses of gray matter at the base of the cerebral hemisphere; currently, the corpus striatum (caudate and lentiform nucleus) and cell groups associated with the corpus striatum (Sted).

Benign: denoting the mild character of an illness or the nonmalignant character of a neoplasm (Sted).

Biofeedback: a training technique that enables an individual to gain some element of voluntary control over autonomic (or other involuntary) body functions (Sted). In electromyographic feedback training, the patient sees or hears the electromyogram of the affected muscle and thus receives information (feedback) about the contractile state of the muscle he or she is trying to relax or activate.

Biogenic amines: substances formed by decarboxylation of amino acids. Examples are serotonin, norepinephrine, epinephrine, dopamine, and histamine.

α-Blocking drug: synonymous with α-adrenergic blocking agent. A compound that selectively blocks or inhibits responses to sympathetic adrenergic nerve activity mediated by α-adrenoceptors (Sted).

Botulinum A toxin: one of a series of toxins from the bacterium *Clostridium botulinum*, which may be present in improperly preserved food and acts by permanently inactivating acetylcholine release and destroying the neuromuscular junction. The toxin is used in the therapy of spasticity.

Bradykinin (BK): a molecule composed of nine amino acids (a nonapeptide). One of the so-called vasoneuroactive substances; it dilates blood vessels and sensitizes or excites nociceptors. BK is cleaved from a precursor protein (kallidin) in the blood plasma.

Brainstem (syn: hindbrain): mesencephalon plus rhombencephalon (other definitions also exist). The rhombencephalon includes the pons, cerebellum, and medulla oblongata (Sted).

Brawny edema: a thickening and dusky edema (Sted).

Brodmann area: a region of the cortex characterized by a particular cytoarchitecture, i.e., size, arrangement, and density of nerve cells.

Bruxism: a clenching of the teeth, resulting in rubbing, gritting, or grinding together of the teeth, usually during sleep (Sted).

Bundle of muscle fibers: a muscle fascicle. A group of muscle fibers surrounded by perimysium.

Calcitonin gene-related peptide (CGRP): a neuropeptide composed of 37 amino acids. CGRP has a strong vasodilating action.

Calcium pump: energy-dependent transport mechanism that transports Ca^{++} across a membrane. For instance, it returns Ca^{++} ions into the sarcoplasmic reticulum to terminate muscle contraction following their release to activate the contraction.

Calculosis: tendency to form calculi or stones (Sted); also used to describe the presence of stones in the urinary or biliary tract.

Calculus: a stone-like concretion formed in the passages of the biliary and urinary tracts; it is usually composed of salts of inorganic or organic acids or of other material, such as cholesterol (Sted).

cAMP: *see* Cyclic AMP.

Capillary: the smallest blood vessel. Here, the exchange processes between blood and tissue take place. Capillaries consist of an inner layer of endothelial cells and a basal lamina. They lack a muscle layer.

Capsaicin: the active ingredient of the chili pepper that causes the burning sensations after ingestion. It is a powerful stimulating agent for afferent C fibers. Its stimulating action is often followed by reduced sensitivity of C nociceptors (i.e., by desensitization).

Carrageenan: a sulfated polysaccharide derived from Irish moss; it is used in animal experiments to induce a sterile inflammation.

Catalepsy: a morbid state in which there is a waxy rigidity of the limbs, which may be placed in various positions that can be maintained for a time; there is unresponsiveness to stimuli, pulse and respiration are slow, and the skin is pale (Sted).

Catecholamines: pyrocatechols with an alkylamine side chain; e.g., epinephrine, norepinephrine, dopamine (Sted).

Caudal: related to or in the direction of the tail end of an organism.

Causalgia: a syndrome of sustained burning pain, allodynia, and hyperpathia after a traumatic nerve lesion, often combined with vasomotor and sudomotor dysfunction and later trophic changes.

Cellulitis: inflammation of cellular or connective tissue (Sted).

Central nervous system (CNS):   the brain and the spinal cord.

Central pain: pain initiated or caused by a primary lesion or dysfunction in the central nervous system (IASP); it may result, for example, from spinal cord injury, central nervous system ablative surgery, or a stroke lesion in the thalamus.

Central sensitization: increase in excitability of central nervous system neurons; this excitability can last for long periods of time following an acute painful stimulus.

Cerebral ventricles: normal cavities in the brain that are interconnected and filled with cerebrospinal fluid. The third ventricle is located in the midline diencephalon; its lateral walls are partly formed by the thalamus and hypothalamus.

C fiber: an unmyelinated nerve fiber that conducts action potentials at a velocity of less than 2.5 m/s in humans.

c-fos: cellular (c) oncogene that controls the growth of osteosarcoma (os). It is one of the immediate-early genes that are expressed in neurons within a few hours following stimulation of sensory endings or fibers.

c-FOS: the transcription factor (protein) synthesized by the c-fos gene.

c-jun: a cellular oncogene that—similarly to c-fos—is expressed in neurons in response to input from the body periphery.

c-JUN: the protein synthesized by the oncogene c-jun.

Cholecystitis: inflammation of the gallbladder (Sted).

Chorea: irregular, spasmodic, involuntary movements of the limbs or facial muscles (Sted).

Chronic pain: pain that persists past the normal time of healing; in clinical practice, a period of 3 months is recognized as a convenient dividing line between acute and chronic pain (IASP).

Cingulate cortex or gyrus: a gyrus on the medial aspect of a hemisphere located directly above and running parallel to the corpus callosum.

Clearance: removal of a substance from the blood (Sted).

Colic: spasmodic pain in the abdomen (Sted).

Collateral: a side branch of an axon.

Complex regional pain syndrome (CRPS): forms of pain (e.g., causalgia, Sudeck syndrome) that are associated with signs of sympathetic disturbances and therefore suggest an involvement of the sympathetic system; formerly called reflex sympathetic dystrophy.

Compliance: the compressibility, for example, of a muscle that can be assessed clinically by pressing a finger into it or by squeezing it between the fingers to determine how easily it is indented and how "springy" it is.

Compound action potential: summed action potentials of many fibers in a nerve that are excited simultaneously, for example, by an electrical stimulus.

Concentric (shortening) contraction: a reduction of muscle length produced by generation of muscle force.

Contractile activity: forms of activation of the contractile apparatus of a muscle: 1. electrogenic contraction or stiffness (muscle tension coming from voluntary muscle contraction, accompanied by observable electromyographic activity and seen in normals who are not completely relaxed. The term "electrogenic" refers to propagated action potentials originating in the α-motor neurons and transmitted by the neuromuscular junctions). 2. electrogenic spasm that specifically identifies pathologic involuntary electrogenic contraction. 3. contracture in the physiologic (dynamic) sense, arising endogenously within the muscle fibers, independent of electromyographic activity.

Contraction-sensitive receptor: a muscle receptor that responds strongly to physiologic contractions. The receptors are probably identical with the "ergoreceptors" that mediate circulatory and respiratory adjustments during muscle work.

Contracture: 1. in the clinical (static) sense: shortening of muscle caused by remodeling of connective tissue that may include joint capsules and ligaments and reduction in the number of sarcomeres. These changes occur when the muscle remains in a shortened position for a prolonged period of time. Like the contracture in the physiologic sense, this condition lacks electromyographic activity, but for a different reason. 2. in the physiologic (dynamic) sense or rigor: an activation of the contractile mechanism of a muscle (sliding of actin and myosin filaments), unaccompanied by electrical activity of the muscle cell, i.e., in the absence of electromyographic activity.

Convergence: a neuroanatomic connection implying that inputs from many sources make synaptic contacts with a single neuron in the central nervous system.

Convergence-facilitation theory: a theory put forward by McKenzie that assumes that a continuous impulse traffic from one peripheral source can enhance the responses of a central nervous system neuron to the input from a second source.

Convergence-projection theory: a theory put forward by Ruch for the explanation of referred pain. It states that a dorsal horn neuron receives synaptic connections from two separate body areas (convergent input) and that the neuron elicits subjective pain in only one (and always the same) area, regardless from which area it is excited.

Coronary infarction: a sudden insufficiency of the blood supply in the coronary arteries (arteries that supply the heart muscle) as a result of emboli, thrombi, or external pressure (Sted).

Coryza: syn: acute rhinitis; mucous discharge from the nostrils, running at the nose (Sted).

Cramp: a painful muscle spasm associated with electromyographic activity, such as nocturnal leg cramp. Sometimes, without electromyographic activity, contracture (as observed in McArdle's disease) is also called cramp, but it is actually a dynamic contracture in the physiologic sense.

Cranial: relating to the head end of an organism.

Cranial nerve: a large peripheral nerve whose fibers originate and terminate in supraspinal portions of the central nervous system (brainstem and diencephalon). The cranial nerves are numbered with the Latin numerals I to XII. For instance, cranial nerve X is the vagus nerve.

Cross excitation: transmission of action potentials between neighboring nerve fibers; impulses in one fiber elicit action potentials in the other fiber. Under normal circumstances, cross excitation is prevented by Schwann cells around the axons, which provide electrical insulation. In contrast to cross talk, cross excitation does not show a close coupling between transmitted action potentials; i.e., there is no one-to-one transmission.

Curare: a plant extract that produces paralysis of skeletal muscle by blocking the receptor molecule for acetylcholine in the postsynaptic portion of the neuromuscular endplate.

Cyclic AMP (cAMP): cyclic adenosine monophosphate, an intracellular second messenger that is part of the cascade of events that transforms the action of neurotransmitters or other substances into metabolic changes in the affected cell.

Cyclo-oxygenase (COX): an enzyme that synthesizes prostaglandins from arachidonic acid.

Deafferentation: abolition of the influence of afferent fibers (or afferent activity) from central nervous system neurons. Dorsal root avulsion is an example of traumatic deafferentation.

Decarboxylation: a chemical reaction involving the removal of a molecule of carbon dioxide from a carboxylic (—COOH) group (Sted).

Decerebration: the removal of the brain above the lower border of the corpora quadrigemina of the mesencephalon or a complete section of the brain at about this level (Sted). The respiratory and circulatory centers in the medulla oblongata are still functioning after decerebration; i.e., respiration and circulation are maintained spontaneously; sensory awareness is eliminated.

Deep somatic tissues: subcutaneous tissues such as muscle, tendon, joint capsule, and ligaments. The term excludes viscera.

Demyelination: destruction of the myelin sheath of thick nerve fibers, caused by degenerative and metabolic diseases (e.g., diabetes).

Dendrite: a process of a neuron where most of the synaptic contacts with axons of other neurons are located. A dendrite is the main input region of a neuron.

Depolarizing muscle relaxants (e.g., succinylcholine): agents that block neuromuscular transmission by binding to the acetylcholine receptors of the muscle membrane and depolarizing the membrane for a prolonged period of time. The depolarized membrane is not excitable. Nondepolarizing agents (e.g., tubocurarine chloride, gallamine triethiodide, vecuronium bromide) bind to the acetylcholine receptor without causing ion fluxes. They compete with acetylcholine for the binding sites and, in proper dosage, reduce the amplitude of the endplate potential to a subthreshold level.

Dermatome: area of skin supplied by cutaneous branches from a single spinal nerve (Sted).

Descending antinociceptive system: a pain-suppressing network of neurons that originate in the mesencephalon and medulla and inhibit the activity of spinal nociceptive neurons via descending axons.

Descending facilitation: pain-enhancing activity of a network of spinal nociceptive neurons that originate in the mesencephalon and medulla and influence spinal neurons via descending axons. These pain-facilitating neurons are intermingled with the pain-inhibiting neurons of the antinociceptive system.

Descending inhibition: a network of neurons that originate in the mesencephalon and medulla oblongata and inhibit spinal nociceptive neurons; syn: descending antinociceptive system.

Desensitization: a reduction in sensitivity of a neuron to a stimulus, caused by the same or another stimulant. An example is the desensitization of receptors caused by capsaicin after initial excitation.

Desmin: an intracellular protein filament of intermediate size (between microfilaments and microtubules). It forms bundles that enhance the mechanical stability of cells.

Diaphoresis: perspiration (Sted).

Diastolic (blood pressure): blood pressure during the period of relaxation of the heart ventricles. It is the minimum blood pressure that occurs between two contractions of the heart musculature.

Discectomy: excision, in part or whole, of an intervertebral disc (Sted).

Disinhibition: the abolition of an existing inhibition of a neuron. In terms of discharge frequency of a spontaneously active neuron, disinhibition is equivalent to activation.

Distal: situated away from the center of the body, or from the point of origin; applied to the extremity or distant part of a limb or organ (Sted).

Divergence: a neuroanatomic connection implying that a single afferent fiber has synaptic contacts with more than one central nervous system neuron.

Dolorimeter: an instrument for measuring the intensity of a painful stimulus.

Dorsal horn: dorsal (posterior) portion of the gray matter in the spinal cord. Sensory neurons are located here.

Dorsal root: nerve fiber bundles that enter the spinal cord at the dorsolateral circumference of the spinal cord. It contains primary afferent fibers that originate in cell bodies of the dorsal root ganglion.

Dorsal root ganglion: an accumulation of sensory nerve cell bodies forming part of a dorsal root. The cell bodies in the ganglion have a central process that terminates in the spinal cord and a peripheral process that forms one or several receptive nerve endings. The dorsal root ganglia of spinal nerves are located in the intervertebral foramen.

Dysarthria: disturbance of articulation as a result of emotional stress or paralysis, incoordination, or spasticity of the muscles (Sted).

Dysesthesia: is an unpleasant abnormal sensation, whether spontaneous or evoked (IASP).

Dysphagia: is difficulty in swallowing (Sted).

Dystonia: an abnormal tonicity in any of the tissues (Sted).

Dysuria: difficulty or pain in urination (Sted).

Eccentric (lengthening) contraction: an increase in muscle length, with muscle force resisting the lengthening of the muscle by external forces.

Ecchymosis: a purplish patch caused by extravasation of blood into the skin (Sted).

Ectopic: out of place (Sted). With regard to neuronal activity, the term means that the discharges originate at an abnormal location, i.e., not at the receptive ending (in the case of an afferent fiber), or in the soma of a motor neuron or postganglionic autonomic cell.

Edema: an accumulation of an excessive amount of watery fluid in cells, tissues, or serous cavities (Sted).

Effusion: escape of fluid from the blood vessels or lymphatics into the tissues or a cavity (Sted).

Elastic stiffness: elastic part of the viscoelastic component of resistance to movement. It is clinically tested by performing slow movements (where the viscosity does not influence the measurement).

Electrogenic contraction: a contraction elicited by electrical activity of the motor nerve and muscle cell (in contrast to a contracture, which occurs without electrical activity in both structures).

Elevation: lifting a part of the body.

Emotional-affective component of pain: pain component identified with suffering.

Endogenous: originating   or   produced within the organism (Sted).

Endomysium: loose   connective   tissue around a single muscle cell (a muscle fiber).

Endorphin: an endogenous opioid with morphine-like actions. It is an inhibitory transmitter and leads to activation of the descending antinociceptive system.

Endplate potential (EPP):   short-lasting positive change of the normally negative membrane potential of a muscle cell. The EPP is caused by acetylcholine; it is normally suprathreshold; i.e., it reaches threshold and makes the muscle cell fire an action potential (to be distinguished from a miniature endplate potential).

Endplate zone: that part of a skeletal muscle where the endplates are located; now also called the motor point.

Enkephalin: an endogenous opioid derived from endorphin by splitting. Like endorphin, it is used by central nervous system neurons to activate the descending antinociceptive system. Neurons that use enkephalin as a transmitter are called enkephalinergic.

Enthesitis: painful inflammation of the insertion region of a muscle provoked by muscle stress (Sted).

Enthesopathy: a disease process occurring at the site of insertions of muscle tendons and ligaments into bones or joint capsules (Sted).

Ephapse: synapse-like close apposition between neighboring fibers in a damaged nerve or neuroma, which may provide direct electrical coupling, leading to cross talk between the fibers.

Epigastric (region): topographic area of the abdomen located between the costal margins and the subcostal plane (Sted), which is the level of the bottom of the rib cage.

Epimysium: connective tissue that encloses a whole muscle. In most muscles a separate fascia surrounding the epimysium is also present.

Ergonomics: a scientific discipline dedicated to providing a work situation that provides optimal trunk and limb support and placement of work materials. A goal of ergonomics is to eliminate strained posture and unnecessary motor activity, especially repetitive and sustained muscle contraction.

Ergoreceptor: a non-nociceptive group III or IV muscle receptor that is activated during physiologic contractions. It is presumed to mediate respiratory and circulatory adjustments during physical work.

Evoked potential: a change in voltage usually recorded from the somatosensory cortex surface following stimulation of a peripheral nerve or another sensory input. The potential consists of several waves that are named according to their polarity (N for negative, P for positive) and their latency (time between onset of the stimulus and occurrence of the potential) in milliseconds (ms).

Exacerbation: an increase in the severity of a disease or in any of its signs or symptoms (Sted).

Excitatory postsynaptic potential (EPSP): a short-lasting depolarization of the membrane of the postsynaptic neuron, caused by a small amount of excitatory neurotransmitter (e.g., glutamate). The normal excitatory postsynaptic potential is subthreshold; i.e., it is too small to initiate an action potential.

Extrapyramidal reactions: motor reactions that are caused by activation of the extrapyramidal motor pathways (pathways outside the pyramidal tract). Disturbances of these pathways express themselves not in paralysis but in the way movements are performed.

Facet joints: small joints connecting the vertebrae.

Fascia: a sheet of fibrous tissue that envelops the body beneath the skin; it also encloses muscles and muscle groups and separates structural components of a muscle (Sted).

Fascicle: a bundle of nerve or muscle fibers that are enclosed in perineurium or perimysium, respectively.

Fasciculations: involuntary contractions or twitchings of individual motor units, a coarser form of spontaneous muscular contractions than the fibrillation of individual muscle fibers.

Fibrillation: involuntary contraction of individual muscle fibers.

Fibromyalgia (FM) or fibromyalgia syndrome (FMS): a chronic condition of increased pain sensitivity, characterized by widespread pain and *tender* points at 18 designated locations (in contrast to central myofascial *trigger* points that can be located in the endplate zone of any muscle). Fibromyalgia can be thought of as a set of core features and two types of ancillary features. The core features are generalized pain and tenderness at 11 of 18 prescribed anatomic sites. Frequent ancillary features are fatigue, impaired concentration, difficulty recalling names, nonrestorative sleep, and morning stiffness. Less common findings include irritable bowel syndrome, Raynaud's phenomenon, headache, subjective swelling, nondermatomal paresthesia, psychologic stress, and marked functional disability.

Fibrosis: formation of fibrous tissue as a reparative or reactive process (Sted).

Fibrositis: an historical and outdated term describing muscle pain radiating from a small tender spot within the muscle. The term is largely synonymous with nonarticular rheumatism. In patients diagnosed with fibrositis, the pain was probably not caused by inflammation but was caused by either myofascial trigger points or fibromyalgia, which were not identified as such at that time.

Filament: 1. one of the contractile proteins of the muscle (actin and myosin). The filaments consist of a chain of amino acids. The myosin filament has so-called "heads" that attach to the actin filaments during contraction and make repeated flexing movements to cause movement between the filaments. 2. in neurophysiologic animal experiments, a filament is a thin bundle of nerve fibers dissected from a nerve for recording the impulse activity in single fibers.

Flare: a redness of the skin extending beyond the local reaction to the application of an irritant or a noxious stimulus; it is assumed to be the result of vasodilation caused by the release of histamine from mast cells and of neuropeptides (calcitonin gene-related peptide and substance P) from sensory nerve endings.

Flexion (or flexor) reflex: a reflex leading to the contraction of a flexor muscle. Usually, the reflex occurs in response to a painful stimulus to the skin. The effect of the reflex is to move the limb away from the source of pain.

Flexor reflex afferents (FRA): afferent fibers that can elicit the flexion reflex. The fibers comprise not only nociceptive afferents but also non-nociceptive ones belonging to groups II, III, and IV.

Free nerve ending: main type of receptive ending of small-diameter afferent fibers (A-δ and C fibers). The name is derived from the fact that in the light microscope, the endings lack identifiable structural specialization. Functionally, they are nociceptors, thermoreceptors, and mechanoreceptors.

Funiculus: synonymous with a column. The largest subdivision of the white matter in the spinal cord (e.g., dorsal funiculus between the two dorsal horns).

GABA: *see* γ-Aminobutyric acid.

Galactorrhea: a continued discharge of milk from the breasts between intervals of nursing or after weaning (Sted).

Gate-control theory: a spinal mechanism for the modulation of pain, which assumes that impulse activity in small-diameter (nociceptive) fibers elicits pain (opens the gate), whereas activity in large-diameter (non-nociceptive) fibers inhibits the pain (closes the gate).

Glaucoma: an increase in the inner pressure of the eye. One possible mechanism is closure of the angle between iris and cornea. The closure inhibits the efflux of the fluid from the anterior eye chamber into the veins of the eyeball.

Glycolysis: anaerobic conversion of glucose to lactic acid, which yields much less energy per molecule of glucose than does oxidative metabolism.

Gray matter: tissue component of the central nervous system that contains the cell bodies of the neurons together with other structures. The processing of impulse activity takes place in the gray matter.

Group Ia fiber: an afferent (sensory) fiber with origin in a primary ending of a muscle spindle. Ia fibers have monosynaptic excitatory connections with the α-motor neurons of the homonymous muscle.

Group Ib fiber: an afferent (sensory) fiber originating in a Golgi (tendon) organ. Ib fibers have disynaptic inhibitory connections with the α-motor neurons of the homonymous muscle.

Group III fiber: a thin myelinated muscle afferent (sensory) fiber that conducts action potentials at a velocity of 2.5 to 30 m/s. The term is used only for afferents in muscle nerves; the same fibers in other nerves are called A-δ fibers.

Group IV fiber: an unmyelinated muscle afferent (sensory) fiber that conducts action potentials at a velocity of less than 2.5 m/s. The term is synonymous with a C fiber in other than muscle nerves.

Gynecomastia: excessive development of the male mammary glands (Sted).

Gyrus: one of the prominent, folded elevations that form the cerebral hemispheres. Each gyrus is separated from the next by a sulcus (Sted).

H (Hensen) band: a pale inner zone of the A band of the striation pattern of a skeletal muscle. It marks that region of the A band where only myosin (and no actin) filaments are present.

Half-life (or half-time):   time for half of a substance to be converted or disappear from the tissue.

Hamstring muscles: semimembranosus, semitendinosus, and biceps femoris muscles. The tendons of these muscles attach to the ischial tuberosity.

Hematoma: a localized mass of usually clotted blood outside blood vessels, confined within an organ, tissue, or space (Sted).

Hemiparesis: a slight paralysis affecting one side of the body (Sted).

Hemiplegia: paralysis of one side of the body (Sted).

Hemolysis: alteration, dissolution, or destruction of red blood cells in such a manner that hemoglobin is liberated (Sted).

Herniated disc: a protrusion of the soft center of a vertebral disc into the vertebral canal. The protrusion can compress the spinal cord or nerve roots and cause pain and other symptoms.

Hertz: a measure of frequency in cycles per second.

Heterosynaptic facilitation: increase in responsiveness of a central nervous system neuron by an input that does not excite the cell, meaning that the input excites another neuron, which in turn facilitates the cell under study.

High-threshold mechanosensitive (HTM) receptor: a mechanoreceptor with a high stimulation threshold in the noxious range. The term is often used to describe nociceptors that have not been tested with chemical or thermal stimuli. High-threshold mechanosensitive receptors in a muscle probably mediate the pain caused by mechanical traumas.

Hippocampus: convoluted structure that forms the caudal medial margin of the cerebral hemisphere. The hippocampus is a part of the limbic system.

Histamine: a biologic amine derived from histidine by decarboxylation. It stimulates gastric secretion, constricts bronchial smooth muscle, and dilates blood vessels. It is stored in mast cells and can be released from these cells under pathophysiologic circumstances (Sted.), e.g., by substance P liberated from nociceptive nerve endings.

Hoarseness: a rough, harsh quality of voice (Sted).

Homonymous: having the same name (Sted). When used with regard to muscle reflexes, it means that the receptor eliciting the reflex and the contracting motor units are located in the same muscle.

5-Hydroxytryptamine (5-HT):   *see* Serotonin.

Hyperalgesia: an increased pain response to a stimulus that is normally painful (stimulus and response are in the same mode).

Hyperesthesia: an increased sensitivity to stimulation, excluding the special senses (the increased sensation is in the same category as the applied stimulus).

Hyperexcitability: an abnormal increase in responsiveness of a central nervous system neuron to synaptic input. Hyperexcitability is assumed to be the cause of various forms of pain, such as phantom pain and hyperalgesia.

Hyperpathia: a painful syndrome characterized by abnormally painful reaction to a stimulus, especially a repetitive stimulus, as well as an increased threshold (increased threshold and increased response: stimulus and response are in the same mode).

Hypertonia: an increased muscle tone for any reason. It includes a variety of conditions, such as spasticity, rigidity, dystonia, and muscular contracture.

Hypertonic saline: a salt solution that has a higher osmotic pressure than serum. In pain research, it is used as a painful chemical stimulus.

Hypoalgesia: diminished pain sensation in response to a normally painful stimulus (increased threshold and decreased response: stimulus and response are in the same mode).

Hypochondriasis: a false belief that one is suffering from some disease.

Hypoesthesia: a decreased sensitivity to stimulation, excluding the special senses (IASP).

Hypothalamus: ventral region of the diencephalon forming the walls of the ventral half of the third ventricle. It controls the autonomic nervous system and, through its vascular connections with the anterior lobe of the hypophysis, is involved in endocrine mechanisms.

Hypothenar: fleshy mass at the medial ulnar side of the palm (Sted).

Hypotonia: a loss of normal elastic stiffness that may relate to thixotropy. It is characteristic of so-called "floppy infants."

Hypoxia: a reduction in the level of oxygen pressure in body tissues.

Hysteria: diagnostic term referable to a wide variety of psychogenic symptoms involving disorders of function that may be mental, sensory, motor, or visceral (Sted).

I band: isotropic area of the striation pattern of a muscle. The band is located outside the region of the myosin filaments adjacent to the Z band. The I band contains actin filaments only; it looks pale in the light microscope.

Idiosyncrasy: an unusual individual mental, behavioral, or physical characteristic.

Immediate-early gene (IEG): a gene that is expressed in neurons within a few hours following stimulation by peripheral input. An immediate-early gene can produce a transcription factor (a protein) that moves to another area of the chromosome and induces the synthesis of other molecules such as neuropeptides.

Immunoreactive: a tissue component (antigen) that is stained histologically with labeled antibodies.

Immunoreactivity: staining produced in histologic sections by labeled antibodies in order to visualize antigens in the tissue.

Inhibitory postsynaptic potential (IPSP): a short-lasting hyperpolarization of the membrane of the postsynaptic neuron, caused by a small amount of inhibitory neurotransmitter (e.g., glycine). The IPSP shifts the membrane potential away from threshold, which reduces the excitability of the cell.

Innocuous stimulus: a weak stimulus that is not normally painful. In skeletal muscle, small deformation of the tissue or contractions under physiologic conditions are innocuous.

Insula: an oval region of the cerebral cortex; it is buried in the depth of the sylvian (lateral) fissure (Sted).

Integration of neuronal activity: processing of simultaneous excitatory and inhibitory synaptic potentials in a neuron. As a result of the integration, the neuron may become more or less active (or stay the same).

Interleukin-1 (IL-1): a polypeptide hormone that is synthesized by monocytes and acts on the hypothalamus to induce fever and on the muscle to promote protein degradation (Sted). IL-1 is an important signal for cell-to-cell communication in pathophysiologically altered tissue.

Interneuron: a nerve cell that is interposed between two others and has no long axons in ascending or descending tracts; for instance, the activity from group II muscle spindle afferents is transmitted to α-motor neurons by interneurons with short axons.

Intracerebroventricular (injection): an injection into one of the cerebral ventricles.

Intrafusal muscle fiber: a muscle fiber inside a muscle spindle. Intrafusal muscle fibers contract in response to activity in efferent γ-motor fibers and change the sensitivity of the spindle to stretch.

Intrathecal: into the subarachnoid space; usually refers to administration of a drug into the space around the spinal cord, which contains the cerebrospinal fluid.

Intrinsic: inherent. Applied to neuronal activity, it refers to discharges that occur in neurons in the absence of a recognizable external stimulus.

In vitro: from Latin "in the glass." An experimental setup (organ bath) for studying isolated organs or cells that are immersed in or superfused with artificial extracellular fluid and kept alive by gassing the fluid with a mixture of oxygen and carbon dioxide.

Ion channel: a large channel protein present in the membrane of nerve cells. The protein consists of several subunits that, in the open state, form a pore-like opening through which ions can flow. The channel protein can be opened either by a change in the membrane potential or by binding to a neurotransmitter molecule.

Irritable bowel syndrome: troublesome constipation interspersed with painful cramping and diarrhea, often accompanied by tenderness to palpation in the left upper quadrant or the whole left side of the abdomen. The syndrome is seen in approximately 40% of patients with fibromyalgia.

Ischemia: a reduction in blood flow in an organ or a part of an organ.

Isometric contraction: an increase in muscle force without length change.

Isotonic contraction: a reduction in muscle length without change in the force exerted.

Kinesiology: the science or study of movement and of the active and passive structures involved (Sted).

Kyphosis: dorsal flexion (forward bending) of the spine. A small degree of kyphosis in the thoracic spine is normal. Opposite to lordosis.

Lamina: Latin for "layer." In this book, the term is used for the layers of the dorsal horn of the gray matter of the spinal cord (see Fig. 7-2).

Latent (silent) connections: ineffective synaptic connections in the central nervous system that may become effective under pathologic conditions.

Latent TrPs: trigger points (TrPs) that often cause motor dysfunction (stiffness and restricted range of motion) *without causing pain,* in contrast to the pain-producing *active* TrPs.

Leukotrienes (LTs): substances released from damaged tissue by activation of the enzyme lipoxygenase. Some LTs promote inflammatory processes and lead to hyperalgesia (e.g., LT B_4); others (e.g., LT D_4) have been shown to depress the activity in muscle nociceptors.

Local muscle pain: pain caused by excitation of muscle nociceptors (in contrast to other forms of muscle pain that are caused, for example, by lesions of the muscle nerve or by alterations of central neurons mediating muscle pain).

Local twitch response (LTR): a twitch response of the taut band fibers evoked by snapping palpation or needle penetration of the trigger point. Twitch responses can be elicited from both active and latent trigger points. The spinal reflex twitch response is also present in anesthetized animals and, therefore, can be used to identify trigger points in animal experiments.

Lockjaw: an example of trismus, which may be caused for example by tetanus infection.

Locomotor muscle: a skeletal muscle that is mainly used for body movement. In contrast, postural muscles are mainly used for maintaining body posture.

Long-term potentiation (LTP): in the hippocampus, LTP represents a neuroplastic change that is characterized by a long-lasting increase in neuronal excitability following a short-lasting high-frequency input. LTP is considered an important component of learning processes in the hippocampus and of hyperalgesia in the spinal cord.

Lordosis: curvature of the spine with the convexity looking anteriorly. A small degree of lordosis in the lumbar region is normal.

Low-threshold mechanosensitive (LTM) receptors: mechanoreceptors with a low stimulation threshold in the innocuous range. LTM receptors in muscle probably mediate subjective sensations of pressure or tension.

Lumbago: pain in the mid and lower back (a descriptive term not specifying cause) (Sted).

Luxation: complete dislocation of a joint.

Malignant: (in reference to a neoplasm) having the property of locally invasive and destructive growth and metastasis (Sted).

Mast cells: free tissue cells that are frequently located in the connective tissue around blood vessels. They contain and release (among other substances) histamine and serotonin. Substance P depletes the substances stored in mast cells.

Masticatory muscles: muscles involved in chewing (temporal m., masseter m., medial and lateral pterygoid m., and digastric m.)

Medulla oblongata: caudalmost part of the brainstem, just rostral to the spinal cord.

Membrane depolarization: a change of the membrane potential of a neuron or muscle cell that makes the normally negative potential on the inside more positive. A strong depolarization can reach the electrical threshold of the cell and initiate action potentials (spikes). Longer-lasting and severe depolarizations of a neuron are likely to block the spike-generating mechanism; i.e., the cell is no longer excitable.

Membrane potential: difference in electric charge between the two sides of a cell membrane. The resting membrane potential of most muscle and nerve cells is around -90 mV (inside negative).

Meningitis: inflammation of the membranes of the brain or spinal cord.

Mesencephalon: syn: midbrain; characterized by the lamina tecti dorsally and the crus cerebri ventrally. Important cell groups include the red nucleus, the substantia nigra, and the periaqueductal gray matter. The mesencephalon is located between the hypothalamus (rostrally) and the pons (caudally).

Mesothelium: a single layer of flattened cells forming an epithelium that lines serous cavities (Sted).

Metabotropic receptor: a receptor molecule for neurotransmitters that is located in the postsynaptic membrane and, after binding to the transmitter, activates G proteins and other membrane-bound molecules. These processes lead to metabolic changes in the cell; in neurons, they can cause an increase or decrease in excitability.

Metenkephalin: an endogenous opioid that is used as an inhibitory neurotransmitter by neurons of the descending antinociceptive system. Its action results in decreased pain sensitivity.

Micromolar (μM): a measure of concentration of a substance in a solution. A micromolar solution contains 1/1,000,000 of the molecular weight of the substance in grams per liter.

Microneurography: a technique of recording impulse activity from single nerve fibers in humans by inserting thin needle electrodes through the skin into a peripheral nerve.

Microsome: one of the small spherical vesicles derived from the endoplasmic reticulum after disruption of cells by centrifugation (Sted).

Miniature endplate potential (MEPP): small, spontaneous synaptic potentials (depolarizations) of the muscle cell membrane in the endplate region in the absence of electrical activity of the α-motor neuron. MEPPs are always subthreshold for the muscle cell; they are caused by random release of single packets of acetylcholine from the presynaptic nerve terminal. (*See also* Endplate potential.)

Mitochondrion: a cell organelle (structure within the cytoplasm) that supplies the cell with energy; it contains the enzymes of the citric acid cycle.

Moderate pressure: a weak mechanical stimulus used in animal experiments to stimulate low-threshold mechanosensitive receptors. It leads to a small local deformation of the muscle.

Monosynaptic: a neuronal connection that includes only one synapse.

Morning stiffness: stiffness felt by patients with, for example, rheumatoid arthritis. It is not accounted for primarily by changes in measurable stiffness and relates more to subjective discomfort associated with movement than to a change in soft tissue viscoelastic properties. The common stiffness of old age, following periods of a fixed position (when traveling), may well be another example of such a subjective stiffness and reduced pain-free range of motion.

α-Motor fiber: a thick myelinated nerve fiber of a somatomotor neuron that supplies striated muscle.

γ-Motor fiber: a thin myelinated motor nerve fiber that supplies the muscle fibers within a muscle spindle (the intrafusal muscles). Excitation of the γ-motor fibers leads to contraction of the intrafusal muscle fibers and thus changes the sensitivity of the spindle.

Motor (neuromuscular) endplate: structure that links a terminal nerve fiber of the α-motor neuron to a muscle fiber. It contains the synapse where the electrical signal of the nerve fiber is converted to a chemical messenger (acetylcholine), which in turn initiates another electrical signal (the action potential) in the cell membrane of the muscle fiber.

Motor point: that part of a skeletal muscle where the endplates are located. Now used as synonymous with the endplate zone. Previously defined as the region where the motor nerve entered the muscle.

Motor unit: all muscle fibers supplied by the same α-motor neuron.

Mucosa: (short for tunica mucosa) mucous membrane lining the inner wall of the gastrointestinal tract and other inner organs.

Multireceptive neurons: nerve cells with convergent input from various receptor classes, such as mechanoreceptive and nociceptive. Some authors call these cells wide dynamic range neurons.

Muscle fatigue: a progressive reduction in force of maximum voluntary contraction of a muscle, accompanied by a progressive reduction in median frequency of the electromyogram, an increasing electromyographic amplitude, and associated with an increasing sense of muscle tiredness.

Muscle fiber: synonymous with muscle cell. A muscle fiber contains many nuclei and can extend over the whole length of a muscle.

Muscle spasm: *spasm* is a persistent contraction of striated muscle that cannot be released voluntarily. If the contraction is painful, is of sudden onset, and involves only part of the muscle, it is called a *cramp*. Spasm and cramp in the sense of this definition are associated with electromyographic activity. If involuntary shortening of a muscle occurs without electromyographic activity, the term *contracture* is more appropriate.

Muscle spindle: a muscle receptor that measures the length of a muscle and is excited by muscle stretch. The spindle is arranged parallel to the skeletal muscle fibers. It contains (intrafusal) muscle fibers that, when contracted, increase the sensitivity of the spindle.

Muscle stiffness: a term commonly used to describe discomfort with movement of a joint. It is also used in the engineering sense: With increased stiffness, greater force is required to produce the same movement, or the same force produces smaller movement. In this sense, spastic muscles have increased stiffness.

Muscle tension: an increase in resistance to passive joint movement commonly described as muscle tone or muscle spasm.

It depends on two factors: (1) the basic viscoelastic properties of the soft tissues and/or (2) the degree of the activation of the contractile apparatus of the muscle.

Muscle tone: resting tension of a muscle, clinically determined as resistance to passive movement or to deformation. Muscle tone has two components: (1) the viscoelastic component, which is independent of nervous activity and reflects the passive physical properties of muscle tissue (tension of elastic fibers, osmotic pressure of cells); and (2) the contractile component, whose presence can be detected in the electromyogram.

Muscle twitch: a single (or short-lasting) activation of the contractile apparatus of a muscle, e.g., by a short electrical stimulus or during a monosynaptic reflex. Twitches cannot be performed voluntarily; voluntary contractions consist of repeated sliding movements of the contractile apparatus and are controlled by higher motor centers.

Myalgia: pain in a muscle or muscle group.

Myasthenia gravis: a chronic progressive muscular weakness, beginning usually in the face and throat, unaccompanied by atrophy; it is caused by a defect in myoneural conduction; syn: Goldflam disease (Sted).

Myelinated nerve fiber: a process of a neuron that is surrounded by a myelin sheath. Myelin consists of multiple layers of the membrane of Schwann cells (in peripheral nerves) or of glial cells (in the central nervous system).

Myoclonus: twitching of a muscle or group of muscles (Sted).

Myoedema: a mounding of the muscle without electromyographic activity following percussion. Myoedema is caused by nonpropagated local contracture of the muscle. It is seen in some individuals with normal muscle relaxation and is a common postmortem phenomenon.

Myofascial pain syndrome (MPS): a term used for two different concepts: (1) in a *general sense* that applies to a regional muscle pain syndrome of any soft tissue origin; or (2) in the *specific sense* of that syndrome, which is caused by trigger points within a muscle belly (not scar, ligamentous, or periosteal trigger points). In this book, the term is used according to concept 2.

Myofibril: contractile element of a muscle cell. Each myofibril consists of a chain of sarcomeres, which are the basic contractile units and contain the actin and myosin filaments.

Myogelosis: a term derived from the older German literature, describing a localized hardening in muscle caused by a hypothetical increase in muscle colloid (literally translated as "muscle gellings"). To date, the tender nodule of myogelosis is thought to be a myofascial trigger point.

Myotome: muscles supplied by muscular branches from a single spinal nerve.

Nausea: sick at the stomach; an inclination to vomit (Sted).

Necrosis: death of tissue cells as a result of pathologic changes.

Neoplasia: pathologic process that results in the formation and growth of a neoplasm.

Neoplasm: an abnormal tissue that grows more rapidly than normal, shows lack of structural organization, and usually forms a distinct mass of tissue that may be either benign or malignant (Sted).

Nerve fiber: an axonal process of a neuron together with its sheath. The sheath consists of glial cells in the central nervous system and of Schwann cells in the peripheral nervous system. Notice also that unmyelinated nerve fibers have a sheath of glial or Schwann cells.

Neuraxis: axial unpaired part of the central nervous system: the spinal cord, rhombencephalon, mesencephalon, and diencephalon (Sted).

Neurite: synonymous with axon; at the neurite, the action potentials leave the neuron.

Neurobiology: a term including neuroanatomy, neurophysiology, and neuropharmacology.

Neurogenic inflammation: a sterile inflammation caused by antidromic neuronal activity in a spinal nerve or parts of it. The antidromic activity releases endogenous substances with vascular and cellular actions (e.g., substance P, calcitonin gene-related peptide). "Antidromic" means that in afferent (sensory) fibers, the propagation of the action potentials occurs in the efferent direction, i.e., toward the body periphery.

Neurokinin A (NKA), neurokinin B (NKB): peptides that together with substance P form the tachykinin group.

Neurokinin-1 receptor (NK-1): a receptor molecule in the membrane of nerve cells that binds substance P and mediates its intracellular effects.

Neuroma: (traumatic) the proliferative mass of Schwann cells and axons that develops at the proximal end of a severed or injured nerve (Sted). Besides Schwann cells and sprouting axons, a neuroma also contains fibroblasts and fibrocytes.

Neuromuscular endplate: junction between a motor nerve fiber and a muscle cell.

Neuron: a nerve cell.

Neuropathy: a disturbance of function or pathologic change in a nerve: in one nerve, mononeuropathy; in several nerves, neuropathy multiplex; if diffuse or bilateral, polyneuropathy (IASP).

Neuropeptide: a molecule consisting of a chain of amino acids that is found in the cytoplasm of neurons and other cells. A prominent example of a neuropeptide is substance P (SP), which consists of 11 amino acids. Neuropeptides are considered to be neuromodulators (substances that *modulate* the neuronal activity produced by neurotransmitters) and are not themselves neurotransmitters (substances that elicit and transmit neuronal activity). Most neuropeptides do not open ion channels (as neurotransmitters do) but influence the intracellular metabolism by acting on G proteins. G proteins are membrane-associated proteins that influence cell metabolism, for example, by the synthesis of second messengers.

Neuroplasticity: capability of the central nervous system to react to a (short-lasting) input with a long-lasting deviation from normal synaptic function. Nociceptive input from muscle is known to be particularly effective for inducing neuroplastic changes in the central nervous system.

Neurosis: a psychologic or behavioral disorder in which anxiety is the primary characteristic; in contrast to the psychoses, the neuroses do not involve gross distortion or disorganization of personality (Sted).

Nitric oxide (NO): a gaseous neuromodulator that is synthesized by the enzyme NO-synthase in neurons. It can also be produced by endothelial and microglial cells. It has a strong dilatory action on blood vessels.

NMDA receptor: *N*-methyl-D-aspartate receptor, one of the receptors of glutamate. Activation of the NMDA receptor is assumed to be involved in the transition from acute to chronic pain.

Nociception: events in the peripheral and central nervous system that are associated with the processing of electrical signals elicited by tissue-threatening stimuli. Most of these events also occur under anesthesia and can be studied in experiments on anesthetized animals.

Nociceptive neuron: a nerve cell that signals the presence of tissue-threatening stimuli. Excitation of nociceptive cells elicits pain if the frequency of the induced activity is high enough and the pain-inhibiting mechanisms are not activated.

Nociceptor: a free nerve ending that is specifically activated by noxious (tissue-threatening, subjectively painful) stimuli. A nociceptor is capable, by its response behavior, of distinguishing between innocuous and noxious stimuli and signaling the intensity of a noxious stimulus.

Nonarticular rheumatism: a commonly used, but not clearly defined, general term for soft tissue pain syndromes that are not associated with a specific joint dysfunction or disease; generally considered synonymous with soft tissue rheumatism. This term was commonly used to describe a range of conditions that also include myofascial pain caused by trigger points. Currently, the term "nonarticular rheumatism" is used to identify pain syndromes of deep somatic tissue that are *not* fibromyalgia and are *not* attributed to myofascial trigger points. They include conditions such as adhesive capsulitis, periarticular arthritis, bursitis, epicondylitis, insertion tendinosis, and tennis elbow, which are frequently myofascial trigger points masquerading as another diagnosis.

Nonsteroidal anti-inflammatory drug (NSAID): a nonsteroidal drug (e.g., aspirin) that inhibits inflammatory processes. Aspirin blocks the enzyme cyclooxygenase, which synthesizes proinflammatory prostaglandins.

Noxious stimulus: a tissue-threatening, subjectively painful stimulus. Nociceptors respond in a specific way to noxious stimuli.

Nucleus: an aggregation of neuronal cell bodies within the central nervous system, typically belonging to the same sensory or motor system.

Nucleus raphe magnus (NRM): an aggregation of neuronal cell bodies in the midline region of the ventral medulla oblongata. The NRM is an important nucleus of the descending antinociceptive system.

Occupational myalgia: muscle pain induced by muscular activity at work that is at or near the muscle's tolerance (because of intensity of work or frequent repetition). Often the muscle activity has activated myofascial trigger points. Other terms used to describe this condition are repetitive strain injury and cumulative trauma.

Opiate: any derivative or preparation from opium (Sted).

μ-Opiate agonist: an agonist that acts on the μ-receptor molecule for opiates.

Opioid: any (synthetic) narcotic that resembles opiates in action but is not derived from opium (Sted).

Oxidative metabolism: energy-yielding degradation of metabolites (glucose, fat, protein) that requires consumption of oxygen.

p: pond; 1 p is the force a mass of 1 g exerts under the influence of earth's gravity.

Pain: an unpleasant sensory and emotional experience associated with actual or potential tissue damage or described in terms of such damage (IASP).

Pain-facilitating system: a system of neurons in the reticular formation of the upper medulla, which, by their activity, enhance the discharges of spinal nociceptive neurons.

Pain memory: a hypothetical mechanism implying that a peripheral lesion induces a memory trace in the central nervous system (cerebrum or spinal cord), which reproduces or maintains the pain even after (surgical) removal of the pain source. An example is the phantom pain in amputees that often is felt in those areas of the amputated limb that were painful before amputation.

Pain-producing substances: in this book, the term is used only for *endogenous* substances that can excite nociceptors. Among these substances are bradykinin, serotonin, and high concentrations of potassium ions.

Palpitation: perceptible pulsation of the heart, often with an increase in frequency or force.

Pancytopenia: pronounced reduction in the number of erythrocytes, all types of white blood cells, and the blood platelets in the circulating blood (Sted).

Paralysis: loss of power of voluntary movement in a muscle through injury or through disease of its nerve supply (Sted).

Paranoid: relating to paranoia, a mental disorder characterized by the presence of delusions, often of a persecutory character, in an otherwise intact personality (Sted).

Paraplegia: paralysis of both lower extremities and of the lower trunk in general.

Paraspinal muscles: muscles that attach to or near vertebrae.

Parenteral: by some other means than through the gastrointestinal tract or lung; introduction of substances by intravenous, subcutaneous, or intramuscular injection (Sted).

Paresthesia: an abnormal sensation, whether spontaneous or evoked. In contrast to dysesthesia, the term is used to describe an abnormal sensation that is not unpleasant (IASP).

Parietal peritoneum: serous sac consisting of mesothelium and a thin layer of irregular connective tissue that lines the abdominal cavity (Sted).

Peptic ulcer: a lesion characterized by loss of tissue of the mucous surface of the stomach or duodenum, where the mucous membrane is exposed to acid gastric secretion (Sted).

Peptide: a molecule composed of two or more amino acids connected by peptide bonds.

Periaqueductal gray matter (PAG): an aggregation of neuronal cell bodies around the cerebral aqueduct (a tube-like structure in the mesencephalon that connects the third with the fourth cerebral ventricle).

Perimysium: connective tissue around a muscle fascicle (a bundle of muscle fibers).

Periosteum: thick layer of connective tissue that covers the surface of a bone except for its articular cartilage.

Peritendineum: connective tissue around a tendon.

Periumbilical: around the umbilicus.

Petechia: minute hemorrhagic spot in the skin (Sted).

Phantom pain: pain referred to (felt in) a surgically removed limb or part thereof (IASP).

Phlebitis: inflammation of a vein.

Phosphorylation: addition of phosphate to an organic compound, such as glucose or a protein, through the action of a phosphorylase or kinase (Sted). The phosphorylation of ion channel proteins in neuronal membranes is an effective means of increasing the excitability of neurons.

Pia mater: a thin membrane of connective tissue that firmly adheres to the surface of the brain and spinal cord. The pia mater is one of the membranes of the central nervous system.

Pitting edema: an edema that retains for a time the indentation produced by pressure (Sted).

Polymodal nociceptors: nociceptors that can be excited by a variety of noxious stimuli, such as mechanical, chemical, and thermal.

Postexercise muscle soreness: the pain caused by excessive or unaccustomed eccentric (lengthening) contractions (e.g., following unaccustomed descent from a mountain climb or other vigorous activity). Soreness, tenderness, and stiffness appear between 8 and 24 hours after the activity.

Postganglionic fibers: fibers of the sympathetic and parasympathetic nervous system between the autonomic ganglion and the innervated tissue. In both systems, the efferent pathway consists of two cells: (1) a preganglionic neuron whose cell body is located in the central nervous system and which conducts its activity via a preganglionic fiber to the ganglion, and (2) a postganglionic neuron whose cell body is located in the ganglion and which terminates with its postganglionic fiber in the innervated organ or tissue. In the ganglion, the neuronal activity is synaptically transmitted from the preganglionic to the postganglionic neuron.

Postsynaptic inhibition: an inhibition of a postsynaptic cell effected by a hyperpolarization (an inhibitory postsynaptic potential [IPSP]) of the membrane of the postsynaptic neuron.

Postural muscle: a skeletal muscle that is (mainly) used for maintaining body posture.

Potentiation: an influence between stimuli that leads to an enhancement of the effect of one stimulus by the other in a more than additive way.

Poupart's ligament: inguinal ligament.

Prefrontal cortex: a large portion of the frontal lobe, including all areas ventral to the motor cortex on the lateral and medial aspects of the hemispheres.

Presynaptic bouton: a widening of the axon that forms the presynaptic portion of a synapse. The bouton (French for button) contains the neurotransmitter.

Presynaptic inhibition: an inhibition of a postsynaptic cell effected by a reduction of the amount of neurotransmitter released by the presynaptic bouton; i.e., the inhibitory transmitter does not influence the postsynaptic neuron directly (in contrast to postsynaptic inhibition, there is no inhibitory postsynaptic potential in the postsynaptic membrane).

Prevalence: number of existing cases of a disease in a given population at a specific time (Sted).

Preventive (preemptive) analgesia: local anesthesia applied immediately before and while a painful therapy or operation is being performed under general anesthesia. The concept behind preventive analgesia is that operations excite nociceptors, whose activity is likely to cause sensitization of central nervous system neurons. By preventing the nociceptive impulses from reaching the spinal cord or brainstem, central sensitization and other neuroplastic changes in central nervous system neurons do not occur. Therefore, postoperative pain and the danger of a transition to chronic pain should be reduced.

Priapism: abnormally persistent erection of the penis (Sted).

Primary afferent fiber: sensory nerve fiber in a peripheral nerve. It extends from a receptive ending in the body periphery to its terminals in the spinal cord or brainstem. In primary afferent fibers, action potentials propagate toward the central nervous system.

Primary ending of muscle spindle: a receptive nerve ending that wraps around the central portion of an intrafusal muscle fiber in a spiral course. The afferent fiber of the primary ending is a group Ia (thick myelinated) fiber that has monosynaptic connections with α-motor neurons.

Primary hyperalgesia: increased pain in the region of a peripheral lesion (see also secondary hyperplasia). It can be explained by increased excitability (sensitization) of nociceptors and/or dorsal horn neurons supplying the traumatized region.

Processing of nociceptive information: all neuronal events associated with the transmission of nociceptive impulses in the central nervous system. The processing consists of many synaptic events, such as excitation, inhibition, sensitization, desensitization, and facilitation.

Projected pain: pain caused by a lesion of nerve fibers along their course in a peripheral nerve or dorsal root. At the site of the lesion, action potentials are generated that reach the central nervous system neurons via the same afferent fibers that normally signal the presence of a stimulus at the receptive ending. The central nervous system neurons cannot recognize the origin of the action potentials and interpret any activity in a nerve fiber as coming from the receptive ending. Therefore, projected pain is felt in the innervation territory of the damaged (overactive) nerve fibers.

Proprioceptive cells: neurons that are dominated by input from muscle spindles and tendon organs. These cells mediate the sensation of joint angle and body posture and are involved in locomotor control.

Prostaglandins (PGs): biologically active substances that were first found in genital fluids and accessory glands (Sted). Some belong to the vasoneuroactive substances (particularly those of the E type) that dilate blood vessels and sensitize or excite nociceptors. PGs are synthesized from arachidonic acid by cyclo-oxygenases in endothelial and other tissue cells.

Protraction: drawing a part of the body forward.

Proximal: nearest the trunk or the point of origin (Sted).

Pruritus: itching.

Psychosis: a mental disorder causing gross distortion or disorganization of a person's mental capacity, emotional response, and capacity to recognize reality, communicate, and relate to others (Sted).

Pyogenic: related to pus formation (Sted).

Quadriplegia: syn: tetraplegia; paralysis of all four limbs.

Radiation of pain: subjective spreading of pain from a lesion to neighboring areas. The term is mainly used to describe spreading that is continuous with the site of the original pain, compared with referred pain, which appears separately in another location. Whether the mechanisms underlying radiation or spreading are different from those underlying referral is unknown.

Radiculopathy: pain caused by compression or another lesion of a dorsal root. The pain of radiculopathy is similar to that caused by a lesion of a spinal or cranial nerve (peripheral neuropathy).

Ramus: (dorsal or ventral) the main divisions of a spinal nerve. A muscle system supplied by the dorsal ramus is the erector spinae muscle; the ventral rami supply the ventral body wall and form nerve plexuses for the innervation of the limbs.

Rash: a cutaneous eruption (Sted).

Receptor potential: a local change in the membrane potential of a receptive nerve ending, caused by a stimulus. If the receptor potential is large enough, action potentials are elicited in the afferent fiber.

Receptive field (RF): body region from which a neuron can be excited or inhibited.

Receptor: 1. a receptive nerve ending, i.e., all peripheral branches of a sensory nerve fiber that are located in a small volume of tissue and possess specialized membrane areas for the transduction of a stimulus into an electrical signal (the receptor potential). 2. a large molecule (often glycoprotein) built in the cell membrane. Specific agonist molecules (e.g., neurotransmitters, hormones) can bind to a receptor molecule and thus induce reactions in the cell.

Reciprocal inhibition: a spinal mechanism by which an antagonist muscle is inhibited whenever the agonist muscle is activated.

Red muscle fibers: muscle cells that contain quantities of myoglobin and oxidative enzymes but are poor in phosphorylases. The red fibers are slow-twitch fibers and are also called type I fibers.

Referral of pain: a central nervous system mechanism by which pain is not felt at the site of a lesion but remote from it. Referral is prominent in pain from muscle and viscera, but not in pain from the skin. The cause of referral is probably the unmasking of formerly ineffective (silent) connections in the central nervous system. The unmasking is the reason nociceptive input from a lesion excites central nervous system neurons that are not normally driven by that input.

Referred hyperalgesia: a hyperalgesia in one tissue induced by a painful lesion in another tissue or organ. An example of referred hyperalgesia in muscle is the hyperalgesia of the obliquus externus muscle in patients with calculi (stones) in the upper renal tract.

Referred inhibition: an inhibition of one muscle caused by abnormal input from another site.

Referred pain: referred pain is felt not at the site of its origin but remote from it. Pain referral is probably caused by unmasking of ineffective synapses in the spinal cord (see Referral of pain). Typically, the area of referred pain is discontinuous with the site of the lesion.

Referred spasm: a spasm caused in a muscle by a painful disorder in another muscle or other body structure.

Reflex: an involuntary reaction to a stimulus. The reflex consists of an afferent arc that conducts the information about the stimulus to the spinal cord or brain, one or more central nervous synapses, and an efferent arc that activates the effectors of the reflex (e.g., skeletal muscle).

Reflex sympathetic dystrophy: is now called complex regional pain syndrome (CRPS); characterized by forms of pain (e.g., causalgia, Sudeck syndrome) that are associated with signs of sympathetic disturbances and therefore suggest an involvement of the sympathetic system.

Refractory period: that period of time directly following an action potential, during which a muscle or nerve cell is not excitable (absolute refractory period) or requires a stronger than normal stimulus for excitation (relative refractory period).

Repetitive strain injury: muscle pain induced by muscular activity at work, which is at or beyond the muscle's tolerance. Other terms used to describe this condition are occupational myalgia and cumulative trauma.

Resonant frequency: frequency of minimum resistance to movement of a mechanical system that has a certain weight and elasticity. At resonant frequency, resistance to motion comes from viscosity and not from elasticity.

Resting (background) discharge: impulse activity of neurons in the absence of external stimulation. Sometimes, the term "spontaneous" discharge is also used. The latter term must be used with caution, however, because in most situations, the presence of a stimulus cannot be excluded with certainty.

Rigidity: stiffness and inflexibility of muscles, caused by muscle spasm (involuntary contraction), such as in Parkinson's disease. In contrast to spasticity, rigidity is caused by imbalance between the direct and indirect pathways of the basal ganglia and is characterized by cocontraction of antagonist muscles.

Rigor mortis: irreversible contracture (in the physiologic sense) of all muscle fibers after death. Normally, the binding of myosin to actin is terminated by the consumption of energy, which is provided by adenosine triphosphate (ATP). After death, the intracellular ATP is used up after a while and not restored. Without ATP, the myosin heads cannot separate from the actin.

Rippling muscle syndrome: a dysfunction of skeletal muscle characterized by a rolling wave of contraction that spreads laterally across the muscle in both directions following percussion of the muscle.

Rostral: relating to the snout end of an organism (Sted).

Rupture (of muscle): tearing of a muscle or its tendon.

Sarcomere: smallest functional unit of a muscle cell. A sarcomere has three main constituents: actin filaments, myosin filaments, and the Z band or disc. The actin filaments are attached to the Z band and interdigitate with the myosin filaments. The filaments slide against each other during shortening of a muscle. A sarcomere extends from one Z band to the next.

Sarcoplasmic reticulum: the reticulum (network) within the sarcoplasm (cytoplasm of a muscle cell). The reticulum consists of branching and anastomosing tubules that form a reservoir for calcium. The reticulum occupies the space between the myofibrils within a muscle cell.

Satellite cells: 1. cells that are present underneath the basement membrane of normal muscle cells. Satellite cells are thought to be myoblasts, i.e., cells that develop into muscle cells during development. The satellite cells also can probably repair small muscle lesions. 2. cells that are found around dorsal root ganglion cells and are derived from Schwann cells.

Satellite TrPs: trigger points (TrPs) that develop from a key TrP in another muscle. They are prone to develop in muscles that lie within the pain reference zone of key myofascial TrPs.

Schwann cells: non-neuronal cells that form a sheath around axons in the peripheral nervous system.

Sciatica: pain in the lower back and hip radiating down the back of the thigh into the leg; it is usually attributed to a herniated lumbar disc but may come from muscles.

Sclerosing agent: an injectable irritant that causes tissue induration and scarring by eliciting a sterile inflammation.

Secondary ending of muscle spindle: receptive nerve ending that wraps around the intrafusal muscle fiber on both sides of the central region. The afferent fiber of the secondary ending is a group II fiber that contacts α-motor neurons via an interneuron.

Second messenger: intracellular signal molecules that activate enzymes in response to an external stimulus and change the metabolism of cells. In neurons, second messengers can change the excitability of the cells following activation of receptor molecules in the cell membrane. Examples of second messengers are Ca^{++}, cyclic adenosine monophosphate (cAMP), and protein kinases. In this context, neurotransmitters are the first messengers.

Secondary hyperalgesia: increased pain and allodynia in body regions surrounding a lesion (where the tissue and receptors are completely intact). Secondary hyperalgesia can be explained by assuming that *nociceptive* central nervous system neurons have become hyperexcitable. Because of this, they can be driven by input from regions they do not normally supply, and they can respond to innocuous input.

Secondary muscle spindle afferents: myelinated (group II) fibers from muscle spindles that, in contrast to the primary muscle spindle afferents, do not arise from the receptive endings in the center of the intrafusal muscle fibers but on both sides of the central region.

Segment: applied to the spinal cord: a section where one spinal nerve originates with its dorsal and ventral roots.

Segmental (afferent) inhibition: inhibition of local pain caused by input via thick myelinated (non-nociceptive) afferent fibers from the same region. An example of segmental inhibition is the reduction of the pain following a blow to the shin, brought about by rubbing the skin of the knee region.

Sensitization of a nociceptor: an increase in the nociceptor's sensitivity to stimulation. The sensitization leads to a lowering of the excitation threshold; a sensitized nociceptor can be excited by nonpainful stimuli and elicits pain in response to an innocuous stimulus. The sensitization of nociceptors is assumed to be the main peripheral mechanism for the tenderness of damaged tissue.

Sensory-discriminative component of pain: pain component that mediates the identification of the modality (mechanical, chemical, thermal), the site, intensity, and time-course of a painful stimulus. This component is probably the result of activity in the postcentral gyrus of the cortex.

Sensory modalities: all sensations originating in special sense organs (e.g., vision, hearing, touch, pain).

Serotonin (5-hydroxytryptamine [5-HT]): one of the vasoneuroactive substances; it constricts blood vessels, sensitizes or excites nociceptors, and is released from blood platelets. Serotonin is also important as one of the main neurotransmitters in the descending pain-inhibiting tracts. A serotonin deficiency is thought to be a causal factor for the development of the fibromyalgia syndrome.

Silent nociceptors: nociceptors that cannot be activated by mechanical stimuli under normal circumstances but respond readily to these stimuli in inflamed tissue. Whether such receptors are present in skeletal muscle is unexplored.

Sinusitis: an inflammation of the lining membrane of any sinus, especially one of the paranasal sinuses (Sted).

Slowly conducting fiber: a nerve fiber that has a conduction velocity of below 30 m/s. Morphologically, the fiber is either thin myelinated or unmyelinated.

Soft tissue pain disorders: a term including more than 100 different painful conditions of muscle, fascia, tendon, ligament, joint capsule, bursae, periosteum, and subcutaneous tissue. This term has replaced the outdated designation "nonarticular rheumatism." Fibromyalgia is an example of a soft tissue pain disorder.

Somatic reference zone: that region of the body (skin or deep somatic tissues) to which pain from a trigger point is referred.

Somatization: a process characterized by the development of physical signs and symptoms, including pain, in response to psychic stress.

Somatomotor cortex: that cortical region where motor information to skeletal muscle groups originates. The primary motor cortex comprises large portions of the precentral gyrus, the secondary motor cortex, and a small, medially adjacent region on the medial surface of the brain.

Somatosensory: relating to sensory information from receptors of the body, excluding those of such special sensory organs as eye and ear.

Somatosensory cortex: that cortical region where the information from mechanoreceptors, thermoreceptors, and possibly also nociceptors is processed. Anatomically, the primary somatosensory cortex comprises the central sulcus and the postcentral gyrus. The secondary somatosensory cortex includes a small region at the lower end of the postcentral gyrus.

Somatostatin (SOM): one of the neuropeptides. SOM has mainly inhibitory influences on nerve cells. It is also present in other tissues (e.g., pancreatic islets).

Somatotopy: topographic association of positional relationships of receptors in the body via respective nerve fibers to their terminal distribution in specific functional areas of the cerebral cortex (Sted) and other areas of the central nervous system. The somatotopy reflects itself in a projection of a (distorted) image of the body onto neuron populations.

Somnolence: drowsiness; sleepiness; an inclination to sleep (Sted).

Soreness: *see* Postexercise muscle soreness.

Spasm: Longer-lasting contraction of a muscle that is not under voluntary control and is not dependent on posture. A muscle in spasm exhibits electromyographic activity. Spasm may or may not be painful.

Spasticity: muscle spasm observed in conditions such as hemiplegia, brain injury, or spinal cord injury. It is associated with hyperactivity of stretch reflexes and tendon jerks, which is probably caused by a loss of supraspinal inhibitory influence on the α-motor neurons.

Spatial summation: the mechanism by which subthreshold inputs to a neuron add up (and may become suprathreshold) if inputs from many body regions act on the same neuron simultaneously.

Spinal nerve: a large peripheral nerve whose fibers originate or terminate in one segment of the spinal cord. For instance, the human lumbar spinal cord has five segments (and vertebrae) and hence five spinal nerves.

Spinal stenosis: a narrowing of the vertebral canal that encroaches on the spinal cord.

Spread of pain: term used for describing the expansion of a region in which pain is felt. In contrast to referral of pain, the expansion is continuous with the origin of the site of pain.

Static contraction: maintained contraction without phases of relaxation.

Stellate blockade: a block of the stellate ganglion by injection of a local anesthetic. The block interrupts any conduction in sympathetic efferent fibers to the head-neck region.

Striatal-frontal circuits: neuronal connections between the striate body (a complex formed by the caudate nucleus and the putamen, two nuclei belonging to the basal ganglia) and the cortex of the frontal lobe.

Striatum (or corpus striatum): striate body, a complex formed by the caudate and putamen, two nuclei in the cerebrum.

Subluxation: an incomplete dislocation of a joint.

Substance P (SP): a neuropeptide. It consists of a chain of 11 peptides, has strong vasodilatory actions, and is a neuromodulator for nociceptive processes in the central nervous system.

Substantia gelatinosa: second lamina (layer) of the dorsal horn in the spinal cord.

Sudomotor fibers: sympathetic efferent fibers that activate sweat glands.

Superfusion: a method of administering active agents to tissues: a constant stream of fluid containing the agent is applied to the surface of the tissue so that it is always covered with a thin film of the solution.

Supine: the body lying face upward.

Supplementary motor area: a part of the motor cortex that is located on the medial surface of the hemispheres, ventral to the precentral gyrus.

Sympathectomy: excision of a segment of a sympathetic nerve or of one or more sympathetic ganglia (Sted).

Synapse: a connection between two neurons in the central nervous system. It consists of a presynaptic terminal or bouton that contains the neurotransmitter and a specialized portion of the membrane of the postsynaptic neuron. Between these two structures is the synaptic cleft, which is several nanometers wide. When an action potential arrives in the presynaptic bouton, it releases neurotransmitters into the synaptic cleft. The transmitter molecules diffuse across the synaptic cleft and bind to molecular receptors in the postsynaptic membrane. This leads to the opening of ion channels in the membrane. The ion flux causes membrane changes, the postsynaptic potentials, which increase or decrease the excitability of the postsynaptic neuron.

Syncope: a fainting or swooning; a sudden fall of blood pressure or failure of the cardiac systole, resulting in cerebral ischemia and subsequent loss of consciousness (Sted).

Syringomyelia: presence in the spinal cord of fluid-filled longitudinal cavities; it is marked clinically by pain and paresthesia followed by muscular atrophy of the hands (Sted).

Systemic lupus erythematosus (SLE): an inflammatory connective tissue disease with variable features, frequently including fever, weakness, and fatigability, joint pain or arthritis resembling rheumatoid arthritis, diffuse erythematous skin lesions on the face, neck, or upper extremities, with liquefaction degeneration of the basal layer and epidermal atrophy, lymphadenopathy, pleurisy or pericarditis, glomerular lesions, anemia, hyperglobulinemia, a positive lupus erythematosus test, and other evidence of an autoimmune phenomenon (syn: disseminated lupus erythematosus) (Sted).

Systremma: another term for calf cramps or nocturnal leg cramps.

Tachyphylaxis: rapid appearance of progressive decrease in response following repetitive administration of a pharmacologically or physiologically active substance (Sted).

Tardive dystonia: a late, tardy form of dystonia.

Taut band: a palpable rope-like hardening of a muscle harboring a myofascial trigger point. Taut bands are a group of tense muscle fibers that may be passively stretched by the contracture of contraction knots in a trigger point in the center of the fibers.

Temporal summation: a mechanism by which subthreshold inputs to a neuron sum up (may become suprathreshold and elicit action potentials) if a given input from the same source acts on a neuron at a high frequency.

Tender point: one of eighteen designated soft tissue body sites that, when tender to palpation, help to identify fibromyalgia.

Tender point index: the sum of tenderness ratings (on a scale of 0 to 4) for each of the 18 designated tender point sites (see Table 9-4).

Tenderness: pain elicited by weak (pressure) stimuli that are not normally painful. The reason for tenderness is sensitization of nociceptors or of central nervous system neurons.

Tendomyopathy: a painful condition of the insertion zone of a muscle. The term usually includes a distinction between generalized tendomyopathy (largely identical with fibromyalgia) and localized tendomyopathy (pain in one or a few insertion regions) that corresponds to attachment trigger point characteristics.

Tendon (Golgi) organ: a mechanoreceptor in the tendon that measures the tension of the muscle. It is arranged in series with the muscle. Activation of tendon organs inhibits the homonymous muscle.

Teratogenicity: property or capability of producing fetal malformation (Sted).

Tetanic muscle contraction: repeated muscle contractions at such a high frequency that the single contractions merge. In recordings of the muscle mechanics, the muscle force is a straight line under these circumstances.

Tetrodotoxin (TTX): a powerful neurotoxin found in the ovaries of the Japanese pufferfish (Sted) that blocks impulse conduction in nerve fibers.

Thixotropy: change (reduction) in the viscosity of a fluid following movements. The viscoelastic tone of skeletal muscles exhibits marked thixotropy.

Threshold: 1. electrical. The minimum change in membrane potential that leads to the generation of action potentials in an excitable cell (nerve or muscle cell). Normally, the electrical threshold is approximately 30 mV more positive than the resting membrane potential. 2. mechanical, thermal, chemical. When using these less well-defined stimuli, the lowest intensity of a stimulus that leads to a just-recognizable response of a neuron or individual is taken as its threshold.

Tinel sign: pain, dysesthesia, or paresthesia on percussion of a neuroma or nerve lesion. The peripheral basis of the Tinel sign is the mechanosensitivity of sprouting nerve fibers in the neuroma or in the nerve lesion.

Tinnitus: sensation of noises in one or both ears (Sted).

Topography: description of any part of the body, especially in relation to a definite and limited area of the surface (Sted).

Tract: a bundle of nerve fibers that connect two centers (nuclei) within the central nervous system. An exemption from this rule is primary afferent fibers in the dorsal columns that run from mechanoreceptors in the body periphery to the dorsal column nuclei (gracile and cuneate nuclei).

Transcription factor: the intermediate gene product (e.g., of immediate-early genes) that is involved in the transcription of a DNA (deoxyribonucleic acid) sequence into an mRNA (messenger ribonucleic acid) sequence.

Transcutaneous electrical nerve stimulation (TENS): therapeutic method that is used to inhibit nociceptive neurons in the central nervous system by stimulating myelinated afferents in a peripheral nerve through the intact skin.

Tremor: an involuntary trembling movement (Sted).

Triad: electron microscopic structure of a muscle cell, formed by two cisternae (terminal expansions of the sarcoplasmic reticulum) and a tubular invagination (transverse tubule) of the cell membrane. The triad is an essential structure for electrogenic activation of muscle contraction.

Trigger point (TrP):   1. central TrP: a tender localized hardening in a skeletal muscle. *Clinical characteristics* include circumscribed spot tenderness in a nodule that is part of a palpably tense band of muscle fibers, patient recognition of the pain evoked by pressure on the tender spot as being familiar, pain referred in the pattern characteristic of TrPs in that muscle, a local twitch response, painful limitation of stretch range of motion, and some weakness of that muscle. *Diagnostic criteria* of an active TrP are circumscribed spot tenderness in a nodule of a palpable taut band and patient recognition of the pain, evoked by pressure on the tender spot, as being familiar. Latent TrPs cause no clinical pain complaint. 2. attachment TrP: tenderness in the region of muscle attachment caused by enthesitis or enthesopathy induced by the persistent tension of the taut band muscle fibers.

Trismus: a firm closing of the jaw as a result of tonic spasm of the muscles of mastication. In practice, the term is commonly applied to restricted opening of the mouth, not only because of muscle spasm but also because of fibrotic contractures and/or adhesions.

Tropomyosin: a protein molecule associated with the actin filament, which (together with troponin) masks the binding site for myosin in a resting muscle.

Troponin: a protein molecule associated with the actin filament, which (together with tropomyosin) masks the binding site for myosin in a resting muscle.

Twitch: a momentary contraction of a muscle fiber (Sted) or of a group of muscle fibers.

Unmyelinated fiber: a nerve fiber that lacks a myelin sheath. Notice that these fibers still have a thin sheath formed by Schwann or glial cells.

Varicosities: expanded portions of nerve endings and preterminal fibers that contain neuropeptides and other substances stored in vesicles. When the receptive ending is excited, the stored substances are released from the fiber.

Vasomotor fibers: sympathetic efferent fibers that innervate smooth muscle of blood vessels.

Vasoneuroactive substances: substances that dilate or constrict blood vessels and increase the sensitivity of nociceptors or excite them. Examples are bradykinin (BK), serotonin (5-HT), and prostaglandins (PGs, particularly PGE_2). The substances are ubiquitously present in the organism and are released by tissue lesions.

Ventral root: fiber bundles leaving the spinal cord at the ventrolateral circumference of the spinal cord. They contain efferent somatomotor and preganglionic autonomic fibers.

Ventricle: in this book, the term is used for cerebral ventricles. The ventricles are interconnected cavities in the brain filled with cerebrospinal fluid.

Ventrobasal complex (VB):   the combination of two nuclei of the thalamus: nucleus ventralis posterolateralis (which receives somatosensory input from the body except the head) and nucleus ventralis posteromedialis (which receives somatosensory input from the head region).

Verbal rating scale (VRS):   verbal estimate of pain severity by the patient, on the same scale of 0 to 10 that is used for the visual analog scale values.

Vesicle: in neurons: a microscopic sac inside the presynaptic portion of a nerve cell and also within receptive nerve endings. Vesicles are formed by membrane material and contain neurotransmitters and other substances.

Vicious cycle: a positive feedback mechanism that is self-sustaining. In such a system, the result of a chain of events is fed back to the starting point of the chain, maintaining the process.

Viscoelastic tone: combined viscous and elastic tension of a resting muscle, caused by the physical properties of the soft tissues. One causal factor seems to be that in a resting muscle, a certain proportion of the actin filaments stick to the myosin filaments. Viscoelastic tone occurs without electromyographic activity.

Visual analog scale (VAS): a tool for measuring the severity of a patient's pain. The patient is asked to mark on a line, usually 10 cm long, that has 0 designated at one end and 10 at the other end. Zero represents no pain, and 10 represents the most severe pain that the patient can imagine. In clinical practice, a simplified version, the corresponding verbal rating scale (VRS), is easier to administer and shows a high correlation with the VAS.

von Frey hairs: synthetic or natural hairs used for quantitative mechanical stimulation of skin receptors. They are mounted on a short handle so that they can be placed vertically (with their long axis perpendicular to the surface) on the skin. Hairs of different thickness can be calibrated by placing the tips on an analytic scale with slight pressure until the hair bends. The force exerted by the hair can be read off the scale.

Warfarin: an anticoagulant derived from coumarin, it is also used as a rat poison.

Wheal: a circumscribed evanescent area of edema of the skin, appearing as a urticarial lesion, slightly reddened, and accompanied by itching (Sted). The wheal around a lesion is probably the result of an increase in the permeability of blood vessels, caused by the release of substance P.

Whiplash injury: a hyperextension-hyperflexion injury of the neck (Sted). Often, this injury occurs in a car accident when one car (which may be stopped) is hit from behind by another (moving) car.

White matter: a tissue component of the central nervous system that contains many fiber tracts and only a few neuronal cell bodies. In the white matter, the conduction of impulse activity between central nervous system centers occurs, but no information processing takes place.

White muscle fibers: muscle cells that have a pale appearance because they contain less myoglobin than do red fibers. The white fibers are also called type II fibers; they have predominantly glycolytic metabolism and are fast twitch.

Wind-up: increase in the magnitude of response in dorsal horn neurons to repeated C-fiber input. The increase occurs if the identical input is repeated at short intervals (less than 2 seconds).

Winging (of the scapula): an abnormal scapular posture characterized by lifting of the medial margin of the scapula from the thorax wall as a result of muscle weakness.

Xerostomia: dryness of the mouth, resulting from diminished or arrested salivary secretion (Sted).

Z band: the borderline region between two sarcomeres. Actin filaments are fixed to the Z bands.

Zygapophyseal joints: small joints connecting the vertebrae.

Index

Page numbers in *italics* denote figures; those followed by a "t" denote tables.